Psychosomatic Medicine and Liaison Psychiatry

Selected Papers

Psychosomatic Medicine and Liaison Psychiatry

Selected Papers

Z. J. LIPOWSKI
Clarke Institute of Psychiatry
Toronto, Canada

PLENUM MEDICAL BOOK COMPANY
New York and London

Library of Congress Cataloging in Publication Data

Lipowski, Z. J. (Zbigniew Jerzy)
  Psychosomatic medicine and liaison psychiatry.

  Includes bibliographies and index.
  1. Medicine, Psychosomatic. 2. Psychiatric consultation. I. Title. [DNLM: 1. Psy-
chiatry—collected works. 2. Psychosomatic Medicine—collected works. 3. Referral and
Consultation—collected works. WM 90 L764p]
RC49.L524   1985   616.08   85-12474
ISBN-13: 978-1-4612-9517-4   e-ISBN-13: 978-1-4613-2509-3
DOI: 10.1007/978-1-4613-2509-3

©1985 Plenum Publishing Corporation
Softcover reprint of the hardcover 1st edition 1985
233 Spring Street, New York, N.Y. 10013

Plenum Medical Book Company is an imprint of Plenum Publishing Corporation

For Anne and Christopher

Foreword

Men born to distinction do not always develop it in their homeland. Sometimes transplantation taps routes to hidden sources of concern for the embracing of novel concepts or the clarification of man's behavior, illuminating this understanding in the language of their adopted tongue. Such a one was Joseph Conrad, the Polish sailor whose new vision graced our literature long after his death in 1924. Such a one also is the author this book, who was born in that same year to carry on his country's vigor and resourcefulness in our time. He is numbered among those distinguished emigrés whose contributions to our culture and progress emanated from the trials and tribulations of the political upheavals, persecutions, and wars of Europe. Like many others, he has brought sound traditions and learning from his native land to enhance the new and less developed of what was only recently a frontier land.

Watersheds in world events impose themselves willy-nilly on our lives. One such time was 1946, when the author of this book left his native land and set out for the West. He spent six months in London learning English and then moved to Ireland, where he trained in medicine and also absorbed novel ways and a new culture, including the writings of Swift and Joyce. This young medical graduate's potential was soon recognized by his teacher in neurology at Belfast, who with foresight predicted great accomplishment. As a trainee at McGill his exceptional competence emerged first as a student, and later after appointment to staff. This lasted for the next twelve years, during which period I was privileged to watch his development and appreciate his distinction in thought and action. Subsequently, by reading his papers and attending meetings over the following fifteen years, I have retained contact with his learning and maintained his friendship.

It is not my function to itemize in detail the many contributions made by Zbigniew Lipowski in his career since his gazetting as a psychiatrist in 1959. However it is necessary to point out the critical part he played as a constructive participant in the dual novel programs of psychosomatic medicine and liaison psychiatry at a time when they were in a midcentury doldrums. His efforts count high among those whose efforts, thoughts, teaching, and writing propelled these approaches back into the mainstream of progress. One most significant aspect of his considerations over the years has been a return to emphasis upon the neurological basis of patients' illnesses as a frequent cause of mental symptoms. This is particularly true of the topic of "delirium," to which he has addressed himself in considerable detail, bringing this rather common phenomenon out of the clouded medical scene to be included in the orbit of the psychiatrist's concern.

My main objective in this foreword is not to signify those important chapters and critical contributions in the following pages, since they speak for themselves. I would

like not to stress the professional academic work but to emphasize the holistic knowledge and wisdom of the author. In a brilliant paper entitled ''The Conflict of Buridan's
Ass,'' he offers a commentary on the disturbing affluence of our time. More recently
he has written of Benjamin Franklin as a psychotherapist with insight and relevance.
He is a modern man with genuine roots in the fertile past. It is not fortuitous that he
has recently rejoiced in his most significant recognition, an honorary degree from Helsinki, accompanied by all the panoply of medieval pomp and circumstance. Dr.
Lipowski is a man for the present season on our troubled planet because his efforts
help to point the direction and to initiate therapeutic measures for the sick in body and
soul. Still, he is not beyond engaging in lively discussion with pundits on the nefari-
ous influence of Descartes' dualism on medical thought while clarifying his own
philosophical eclecticism.

Cataclysmic events cast up men to grapple with the problems of their times. History commonly cites national leaders' names more often than those original perceptive minds which grace the history of our discipline. These, by their sensitivity, intelligence, imagination, originality, and literary gifts permit them to foresee and
influence trends beyond their times. Such men were Hippocrates, Vesalius, and Coper-
nicus, the Polish divine whose revolutionary heliocentric theories led, along with the
anatomist's innovation, to the destruction of medieval theories in their respective subjects. So also were greats such as Pinel, Kraepelin, and Freud. Now, although we have
advanced with chemistry to a level of therapeutic effectiveness hardly foreseen thirty
years ago, we are still left with psychosocial problems which demand relief in another
way. These still subtle approaches will not be neglected but promoted if we pay due
attention to the holistic concepts expounded in the following pages.

R.A. Cleghorn, M.D., D.Sc., F.R.C.P.(C),
F.R.C.P.sych.

Past Chairman, Department of Psychiatry, McGill
University, Montreal
Past President, American Psychosomatic Society
Emeritus Professor of Psychiatry, Department of Psy-
chiatry, McGill University, Montreal

Preface

The purpose of this book is to present a broad overview of psychosomatic medicine in its historical, theoretical, investigative, and clinical aspects. The papers selected for inclusion span 17 years of a sustained effort to develop a comprehensive conceptual framework for this whole field and to fill it with currently available information. As the volume and complexity of the relevant information continue to grow, it is necessary to try to organize it in a coherent manner.

The decision to publish a selection of my papers has been prompted by indications that many of them are used for teaching and continue to be quoted. Bringing them out together should facilitate access to them for their potential readership and thus enhance whatever value they may possess as teaching material and as an introduction to psychosomatic medicine and liaison psychiatry. The included articles cover a wide range of topics and, I hope, offer a broad enough conceptual framework to accommodate new research findings, theoretical formulations, and therapeutic advances.

A measure of unavoidable overlap and repetition exists among the selected papers and reflects, in part, a consistency in my approach to the subject over the years. It is a deliberately eclectic approach, which as a clinician and chronicler I have found to be the most cogent and satisfying. I have never been satisfied with any single and narrow theoretical stance from which to interpret the complex mind–body–environment transactions in health and disease. Such a reductionistic viewpoint would be, in my opinion, incompatible with the traditional conception of psychosomatic medicine as a unifying and integrating scientific and clinical discipline. An eclectic approach is, I believe, the only one able to do justice to that conception and consonant with it.

In selecting papers for this book, I have tried not only to offer a conceptual framework and a body of information, but also to convey some of my personal fascination with the subject. I hope that at least some of the younger readers of this book will find my fascination contagious and feel challenged to contribute to the field.

The development of my thinking about psychosomatic medicine has been strongly influenced by the writings of Dr. George L. Engel, who also offered me generous encouragement and helpful criticism in the early years of my writing career. I wish to acknowledge my debt of gratitude for his inspiration and help.

Psychosomatic medicine, as I see it, represents continuation in modern and scientific dress of a long tradition in Western thought and medicine. Its origins go back to the writings of Hippocrates and the Greek philosophers of antiquity. That tradition is based on a view of the human being as a mind–body complex in ceaseless interaction with its environment, both social and physical. It is a predualistic, Aristotelian conception, one that asserts indivisible unity of mind and body. Applied to issues of health and disease, and to medical practice, this conception calls for a unified approach, one combining a biological and a psychosocial perspective in research and in clinical work with patients. I hope that this collection of papers will in a small way contribute toward the continuation of this line of thought and approach in the future.

I acknowledge with gratitude the receipt of a grant-in-aid from the Commonwealth Fund, which has enabled me to prepare this book.

Z.J. Lipowski

Introduction

Psychosomatic medicine and consultation–liaison psychiatry are two fields inextricably tied together. The former has, by definition, a much broader scope, one encompassing a body of research and theory as well as a set of guidelines for medical practice. Liaison psychiatry embodies clinical application of the psychosomatic approach to problems at the interface of psychiatry and medicine. Both these fields emerged, more or less simultaneously, half a century ago and have shared changing fortunes. After a period of initial popularity, both of them experienced a rather dormant phase in the 1950s and 1960s, only to develop rapidly in the past 15 years or so. The articles I have selected for this book trace the historical antecedents as well as the recent growth of the two fields in all their major aspects. In order to round out my overview I have supplemented the already published articles with seven previously unpublished papers. The selection of topics for the book reflects my own conception of the fields under discussion and calls for comment and clarification.

The contents of this book are divided into four parts, each of which deals with a different topic and consists of related papers presented, in most cases, in the order in which they were written. Part I includes articles concerned with the field of psychosomatic medicine as a whole in its theoretical and historical aspects. This part may be viewed as an introduction to the entire volume and presents a conceptual framework into which the remaining parts fit. It also advocates the value of a holistic approach to both medicine and psychiatry, even though the latter subject has been traditionally, if not entirely logically, regarded as falling outside the purview of psychosomatic medicine proper.

Part II deals with the modes and the determinants of psychological and social reactions to physical illness regardless of its postulated etiology. This area has been relatively neglected by psychosomatic writers, who have put more emphasis on the proposed etiological role of psychosocial factors in the development of various bodily diseases. Yet the matter of how people respond to physical illness and injury, and what determines the common types of such a response, clearly falls within the scope of psychosomatic inquiry and is crucially important for the practice of medicine as well as liaison psychiatry.

Part III is concerned with another neglected aspect of psychosomatic medicine which, in my opinion, should be viewed as its integral part. The complex relationship between physical, including cerebral, disorders and psychiatric morbidity represents but one more facet of the psychosomatic relationships. It is an area straddling the boundaries of medicine and psychiatry, that is, two fields whose separation strikes me as artificial and conventional rather than logically and scientifically sound. Its importance to all health professionals hardly needs to be argued.

Finally, part IV consists of a set of articles dealing with consultation–liaison psychiatry, which may be viewed as a clinical offshoot of psychosomatic medicine. It includes a two-part review which, when originally published, offered the first comprehensive survey of this field. The subsequent papers trace the development of consultation–liaison psychiatry over the past decade, when the field experienced rapid growth. Taken together, these articles offer the reader a rather comprehensive overview and bibliography of the subject.

Biographical Note

Zbigniew J. Lipowski was born in Warsaw, Poland, in 1924. He completed his secondary education in Nazi-occupied Warsaw, after attending clandestine high school courses, in 1943. Having survived the Warsaw Uprising in 1944, he began to study medicine at the Jagiellonian University of Cracow in 1945. In 1947 he enrolled in medicine at University College, Dublin, Ireland, and graduated in 1953. After general internship in Dublin and work at a neurological hospital in Belfast, he began postgraduate training at the Allan Memorial Institute of Psychiatry in Montreal in 1955. In 1957–1958 he worked as a Research Fellow in Psychophysiology under Charles Shagass and completed a thesis on the effect of methedrine on critical flicker fusion and its relation to personality and affect. In 1958–1959 he worked as a Fellow on the Psychiatric Consultation Service at the Massachusetts General Hospital in Boston and held a Teaching Fellowship in Psychiatry at Harvard. In 1959 he received his Postgraduate Diploma in Psychiatry (with distinction) from McGill University.

From 1959 to 1971, Lipowski directed the Psychiatric Consultation Service to the Royal Victoria Hospital in Montreal and the Montreal Neurological Institute. He organized the first such service in Canada. Concurrently, he held staff positions at the Allan Memorial Institute and academic positions in the Department of Psychiatry at McGill. Throughout his years there he was actively engaged in teaching psychosomatic medicine (as a successor to Eric D. Wittkower), liaison psychiatry, and general psychopathology, at both the undergraduate and postgraduate levels. While at McGill, he published (in 1967–1968) his tripartite "Review of Consultation Psychiatry and Psychosomatic Medicine," which met with considerable acclaim and is still widely used for teaching liaison psychiatry in North America and beyond. He also edited a volume on *Psychosocial Aspects of Physical Illness* (Basel, Karger, 1972).

In the years 1971–1983, Lipowski was director of the Psychiatric Consultation Service at the Dartmouth–Hitchcock Medical Center in Hanover, New Hampshire, and a Professor of Psychiatry at the Dartmouth Medical School. During those years he lectured widely in the United States, Canada, Europe, Australia, and New Zealand. While at Dartmouth, he published extensively on psychosomatic medicine, liaison psychiatry, information overload, and organic psychiatry and contributed chapters to the *American Handbook of Psychiatry* and the *Comprehensive Textbook of Psychiatry*, among others. In 1974–1975 he edited a special issue of the journal *Psychiatry in Medicine*, which was subsequently published, in 1977, as *Psychosomatic Medicine: Current Trends and Clinical Applications* (New York, Oxford University Press). In 1980 he wrote a monograph, *Delirium: Acute Brain Failure in Man* (Springfield, Illinois, Charles C Thomas).

Lipowski's professional activities have included membership in the American Psychiatric Association's Task Force on DSM-III, where he was mainly concerned with revising the classification of organic mental disorders. He has repeatedly served as a consultant to the World Health Organization on matters of psychiatric classification and the health-related psychosocial factors. He is a member of the editorial boards of *General Hospital Psychiatry,* the *Journal of Psychosomatic Research,* and the *International Journal of Psychosomatics.* He is a Fellow of the American Psychiatric Association and a Founding Fellow of the International College of Psychosomatic Medicine, and a member of many other professional organizations.

Among his special honors are a Doctor of Medicine *honoris causa* from the University of Helsinki (1981) and a Master of Arts *honoris causa* from Dartmouth College (1981).

In 1983, Lipowski returned to Canada and became Psychiatrist-in-Chief of the Psychosomatic Medicine Unit at the Clarke Institute of Psychiatry, Coordinator of Liaison Psychiatry in the Department of Psychiatry, and a Professor of Psychiatry at the University of Toronto. He is currently coediting a forthcoming volume on *Viruses, Immunity, and Mental Disorders,* to be published by Plenum Press.

Contents

IV. Consultation–Liaison Psychiatry

Psychosomatic Medicine

Theoretical Concepts

I

The articles in this section deal with three related topics: psychosomatic medicine, the holistic approach to medicine and psychiatry, and the impact of certain environmental factors on health and behavior. The main focus is on such issues as the development of psychosomatic conceptions from a historical perspective, the definition of the relevant terms, and the current scope of psychosomatic medicine. This section may be viewed as a general introduction to the psychosomatic field in all its major aspects.

Review of Consultation Psychiatry and Psychosomatic Medicine

1

III. Theoretical Issues

In the first two parts of this review[75,76] an attempt was made to define the scope and functions of psychiatric consultative activity in the nonpsychiatric divisions of general hospitals. Part I dealt primarily with the various aspects of psychiatric consultations in this type of setting. Part II included a critical survey of the studies of psychiatric morbidity among medical and surgical patients as well as an overview of psychological problems encountered by the consultants. One of the main purposes of Parts I and II was to emphasize (1) the wealth and diversity of the clinical material accessible to psychiatric study and (2) the expanding scope of the consultants' work. Both of these factors have an important bearing on the development of psychosomatic medicine. The latter has now entered a new phase, characterized both by increased clinical application of its principles as well as by a siginificant broadening of its theoretical perspectives. The preceding phase was marked by the predominant interest in the groups of so-called psychosomatic disorders; a great deal of research, theorizing, and therapeutic endeavor was devoted to them. There have been gains in factual knowledge and a considerable yield of explanatory hypotheses which; however, largely failed to achieve satisfactory validation. The efficacy of psychotherapeutic intervention based on the theoretical assumptions about the role of psychological etiological factors has been unimpressive.[19] The overall result has been a spreading sense of disenchantment with the whole concept of psychosomatic medicine. But is it really the *whole* concept that has reached an impasse or just one particular methodological approach? This writer believes that it is the latter, and will try to support his view in this section of the review.

Many writers have attempted to define the meaning and goals of psychosomatic medicine.[1,8,20,38,43,49,66,80,86,91,103] These writings, and the often divergent views they contain, are scattered in the literature, and it seems worthwhile to try and present a comprehensive statement of the scope and conceptions of psychosomatic medicine as seen by a clinician. There is increasing demand at present for the training of psychiatric residents in consultative skills.[84] The continuing trend to develop psychiatric units in the general hospitals and to offer consultations to other physicians, in and out

---

Reprinted from *Psychosomatic Medicine* 30(4):394–422, 1968. Copyright © 1968 by The American Psychosomatic Society, Inc. Reprinted by permission of Elsevier Science Publishing Co., Inc.

of hospital, makes this demand imperative. Yet, the teaching of techniques of consultation is not enough. Talking about techniques is meaningless unless one specifies what types of questions the consultant may be expected to answer, who asks them, who is to benefit from the answers and how, and in what setting the whole process takes place. Furthermore, teaching of techniques is not likely to inspire a postgraduate student unless he is given a broad view of the field in which he is to work and the theoretical issues relevant it it. Only then is he likely to approach his work as an exciting intellectual challenge, as well as a service to the community. Hence the need to teach psychosomatic medicine as a distinct discipline, one practical application of which is psychiatric consultation with other physicians. Yet the very conception of psychosomatic medicine is at present vague, its semantic and epistemological aspects confusing. To attempt clarification may appear quixotic and may provoke the ire of colleagues who hold different views and may be better qualified to speak about the subject than this reviewer. Yet the demands for better teaching are so pressing that the challenge must be met. The following attempt may at least have the merit of stimulating discussion about the basic assumptions of our discipline.

THE MEANING AND SCOPE OF PSYCHOSOMATIC MEDICINE

The writer will not attempt to trace the historical development of the psychosomatic conception, since this task has been adequately accomplished by others.[2,3,62] The word "psychosomatic" has been used in a variety of contexts: psychosomatic medicine, movement, approach, research, disorders, sysmptoms, etc. Some rather futile discussions have raged about its alleged metaphysical connotation, that is, whether it affirmed the unity or duality of mind and body. The term, however, means no more than we agree that it should mean, and we delimit its boundaries by defining it. Such a definition should aim at expressing the actual scope of interests and activities of individuals who believe themselves to be working in the field of psychosomatic medicine; additionally, it should be sufficiently comprehensive, clear, and useful.

No matter which noun it qualifies, "psychosomatic" connotes an assumption that there exist two classes of phenomena, i.e., psychic (mental) and somatic, which require separate methods of observation and distinct languages for their description. If dualism is implied here, it is a deliberately imposed, methodological and semantic dualism,[45] One reflecting current scientific strategy and relaity but neutral with regard to metaphysical questions concerning the nature of the mental and the physical. A viewpoint which this reviewer considers as particularly cogent for this discussion is that put forth by Woodger:[138]

> The view I shall take is simply this: that the notions of body and mind are both reached by abstraction from something more concrete. For these more concrete objects we have the convenient and familiar word persons...But even the notion of person is abstract in the sense that every person is a member of some community of persons, upon which the kind of person he is, and even his continued existence, as a person, depends.

The task of psychosomatic medicine is to attempt to integrate the three modes of abstraction, viz., biological, psychological, and social.

''Psychosomatic'' does not imply a value judgment that psychic events are more important than somatic or vice versa. Nor does it connote the assumption of specific causal relationships, i.e., psychic events causing somatic ones and somatic causing psychic. The use of terms ''psychosomatic'' and ''somatopsychic'' does give the impression of implied causal sequences, but this is only a problem of semantics and not of causality. Both the psychic and somatic phenomena are aspects (or modes of abstraction) of persons. Their separation is artifical but heuristically useful. A person is and responds as a unity, but the limitations of man as an investigator necessitate the breakdown of the unity for the purpose of observation, description, and the study of relationships among selected variables. Whatever the merits of the holistic conception as a theoretical construct, the study of the person-as-a-whole is wishful fiction.

This brief general discussion may help clarify some basic assumptions underlying psychosomatic medicine. The latter had its modern origin as a movement directed against what Whitehead[133] might have called an ''intolerant use of abstractions'' practiced by medical investigators and practitioners. Thus the psychosocial aspects of persons called patients were abstracted from and regarded as irrelevant. The psychosomatic movement has displayed two basic attitudes: The reformist and the scientific. The former was an expression of discontent with the state of medicine and resulted in postulates, exhortations, and practical suggestions about how medical practice should be changed to give substance to the fact that patients are persons, with all that this implies. The scientific attitude evolved into a systematic search for the role of psychosocial variables as etiological factors in human diseases. These two attitudes are still with us and any definition of psychosomatic medicine must give justice to both of them but also reflect broader contemporary concerns.

It follows from the preceding discussion that a composite definition of psychosomatic medicine is most likely to encompass the scope of its meaning. Many writers have insisted that, as Alexander put it,[1] the term ''psychosomatic'' should be ''used only to indicate a method of approach.'' Grinker[49] asserts that ''psychosomatic'' means ''a conceptual approach to relationships, not new physiological or psychological theories or new therapeutic approaches to illness.'' Mirsky[91] suggests that psychosomatic medicine is not a distinct body of knowledge nor even a distinct division of the general field of medicine.'' These views are debatable. It seems to this reviewer that confining the psychosomatic conception to that of an approach is too vague and one-sided. It expresses no more than the reformist attitude. But as Walker[129] rightly points out, we must distinguish factual statements and general laws from the practical precepts that can be based on them; he calls these precepts ''techniques.'' Psychosomatic medicine is more than a set of techniques, more than an approach; it is also a science. There is at present no other discipline whose avowed purposes are to study, and to formulate explanatory hypotheses about, the relationships between biological, psychological, and social phenomena as they pertain to persons.

The word ''medicine'' in this context, fixed by traditional usage, is unfortunate. It connotes a primary concern with diseases and is thus unduly restricting. The term ''psychosomatics'' is more neutral in this regard and therefore preferable. In any case, these two terms will be used synonymously here. The following definitions express both the scientific and applied aspects of psychosomatic medicine:

A *science*; one which studies the relationships between psychological and biological phenomena in humans, as they occur in and are influenced by the human and nonhuman enviroment, in both health and disease.

An *approach* to the practice of medicine; one formulated in various postulates and norms as guidelines for action. The hallmark of the psychosomatic approach is the insistence that psychosocial as well as biological factors be considered in the diagnosis, treatment, and prevention of all diseases.

Consulting activities (and related techniques) of psychiatrists with other physicians.

The three aspects of psychosomatics will now be reviewed.

I. PSYCHOSOMATICS AS A SCIENCE

The subject matter of psychosomatics as a science are the psychosomatosocial relationships. There are no specific psychosomatic methods of study. What distinguishes psychosomatics as a science is its mode of abstraction, that is, what it concentrates on and what it leaves out.[139] Grinker[49] states that it is "the development and functioning of patterns of relationships among somatic and psychological systems that properly defines the psychosomatic study that is evolving in our time." Our proper concern then is observing, describing, and formulating explatory hypotheses about the relationships between psychological and biological dispositions, states, processes and events occurring in persons. The methods used, as well as the descriptive languages, are those of biology and psychology, respectively. The relevant explanatory hypotheses may be expected to be formulated, at least at their highest level of abstraction, in what von Bertalanffy[128] calls neutral models superordinated to the conceptual systems of both psychology and biology. This may be regarded as the ultimate goal of psychosomatic as a science. At a lower level of abstraction, there are possible crossconnection laws, which state an observable connection at the same time between a psychological and a physiological event.[13]

TRENDS IN PSYCHOSOMATIC RESEARCH

A survey of trends and methods in contempory psychosomatic research would be beyond the scope of this review. Several recent publications deal with these issues.[14,27,49,72,91,103,131,136] The following areas of research are seen as directly relevant to the subject matter of psychosomatics.

Psychophysiological Research[4,11,121]

Psychophysiology has been defined as "the study of the interrelationships between the physiological and psychological aspects of behavior. It typically employs human subjects, whose physiological responses are usually recorded on a polygraph while stimuli are designed to influence mental, emotional, or motor behavior."[121] Psychophysiological research involves manipulation of psychological variables, often conceptualized as contrived analogues of naturally occurring psychological stress, and simultaneous recording of one or more physiological variables regarded as measurable indicators of the evoked psychological change. The application of computers to this type of research is a promising development.[140] Psychophysiological laws are an example of the cross-connection laws mentioned earlier.

Psychosomatic Clinical Research

This type of research focuses on the interplay of psychological, biological, and social factors which predispose to, precipitate, maintain, and counteract those states of the human organism which we call diseases. Since experimental production of disease in humans is generally regarded as unethical, clinical research is largely confined to the observation of the "experiments of nature" in the form of pathological processes. However, current experimental methods for the study of psychopathology, such as drug-induced "model psychoses," manipulation of sensory input and sleep, and hypnosis-induced pathological states, provide experimental methods of value for investigation of psychosomatic relationships in abnormal states.

Significant areas of clinical study include such problems as the doctor–patient relationship and the psychological reactions of patients to illness, hospitalization, medical and surgical procedures, disability, etc. There is no sharp boundary between clinical psychosomatic research and that falling within the province of social and preventive medicine.

It must be clear that psychosomatic research has gone far beyond the early preoccupation with the so-called psychosomatic disorders. Engel's[27] plea for such an expansion has been vindicated, as exemplified by a recent symposium on the psychophysiological aspects of cancer.[102] There is no logical reason for excluding any disease for the purpose of psychosomatic research. Furthermore, too sharp a distinction has often been drawn between the concepts of etiological and reactive psychological factors in the study of disease. As Grinker[51] points out, "crude linearity has to be abandoned, since in nature most tranactions are curvilinear." Thus the distinction between psychosomatic and somatopsychic disorders, which implies linear causal chains, seems to be an arbitrary dichotomy of limited methodological usefulness. Psychosomatic research has gone beyond the frantic search for psychogenicity of somatic disorders. Engel[129] has recently emphasized that the main current task for psychosomatic investigators is the study of simultaneity or sequence, i.e., of temporal relationships, of psychic and somatic phenomena. This new trend may at last direct psychosomatic research to the largely neglected field of the so-called somatopsychic reactions[39]—such as delirium,[74] in which psychic and organic factors interact in close temporal proximity—so that no tenuous retrospective reconstruction of alleged causal sequences is needed. The problems of psychogenicity and causality will be further discussed in subsequent sections of this review.

Study of Mediating Mechanisms

This research is concerned with the elucidation of neurophysiological and neuroendocrine processes which enable transactions between the highest neural activity necessary for symbolic activity and the rest of the body. Langer[70] has recently suggested that a crucial question is "how the phase of being felt is attained, and how the process may pass into unfelt phases again, and furthermore how an organic process in psychical phase may induce others which are unfelt." Much of the relevant work has been lately reviewed.[11,18,31,37,40,80,81,95,109,113,131,136]

Epidemiological and Ecological Research

Methodological problems of epidemiological research in psychosomatic medicine have recently been discussed.[21,67] The ecological approach is stressed by Hinkle,[56,57] who predicts that the processes whereby man adapts to his external environment and tries to maintain his relationship to it will be a primary concern of future medicine. He formulates the key questions, which human ecologists attempt to answer, as follows:

1. What determines how a man evaluates his external environment and reacts to it?
2. How does the neural apparatus accomplish integration, evaluation, and organization of reaction patterns?
3. How do neurally integrated, adaptive reaction patterns affect the structure and function of organs so as to cause disease?
4. How can the understanding of these phenomena be utilized by physicians in the prevention and treatment of illness?[57]

A relation between psychosomatic processes and the patterns of dynamic interaction within the family is attracting increasing attention.[44,83,132] The role of disruption of important interpersonal relationships and the ensuing difficulties in replacing the loss of the relationship as antecedents of any illness—somatic or psychiatric—has been postulated.[28,30,94,100,112,126]

Study of the Psychophysiology of Human Development from Conception to Senility

Grinker[49] asserts that the crucial problem for psychosomatic research is the study of the period of differentiation from "total hereditary to individual learned patterns and their integration into a new personal system." Other relevant topics studied involve the influences of prenatal environment,[33,118] individual differences at birth,[48] mother–child relationships,[132] functions of the autonomic nervous system in infancy,[77] psychobiology of aging,[10] etc.

The above classification of research directly relevant to psychosomatic medicine is not complete. It is actually desirable to avoid premature closure of the boundaries of relevance in this area. The reviewer believes, however, that stressing the broad scope of investigative activities necessary for the formulation of psychosomatic hypotheses has heuristic value. All above classes of research supplement one another and their integration should be the task of psychosomatic theoreticians. The reviewer expects to be criticized for what may seem to be a quixotic attempt to advocate a "superscience" of psychosomatics. What matters, however, is the potential usefulness of the conception of psychosomatics presented here, for the purpose of teaching and theory development. As factual knowledge progresses by leaps and bounds, attempts at integration, however crude they may be, are necessary for further progress and for development of practical applications of value for the practice of medicine.

THEORETICAL CONCEPTS AND EXPLANATORY HYPOTHESES

It has been proposed that the task of empirical science is the acquisition and systematization of knowledge about observed things and phenomena. Systematization includes formulation of explanatory hypotheses which go beyond observation in that they introduce unobservable explanatory or theoretical concepts.[139] Psychosomatic theory is still in an early stage of development. There is a current fashion to talk about theoretical "models" in psychosomatic medicine.[85] It is preferable to discuss this area in terms of hyotheses and concepts. One may distinguish for the purpose of this discussion between psychophysiology and psychopathophysiology. What methodological and theoretical advances have been made by the former are reviewed by Sternbach[121] and Ax.[4] Psychosomatic theory concerned with *morbid* conditions consists largely of hypotheses about the role of specific psychological factors—personality traits, intrapsychic conflicts, dysphoric affects, defensive or adaptive patterns, etc.—in bringing about physiological dysfunction and somatic disease. Galdstron[38] criticizes this trend and complains that psychosomatic medicine "specializes in the psychogenesis of organic disease" and is concerned with the psyche as a "morbific agent." In his view, such concern compounds two fallacies of organicist medicine: the conceptions of specificity and of time—sequential causality.

The prevalent conceptual tendencies in psychosomatic medicine have been reviewed by a number of writers.[8,20,43,49,51,64,85,86,91,103,136] Historical roots of these trends are traced to medical and psychoanalytic viewpoints on etiology[43] and to the fact that the psychosomatic movement was spearheaded by psychoanalysts. A priori assumptions, no less than empirical observations, have influenced the choice of clinical material for psychosomatic study, the explanatory hypotheses about data of observation, and the language of descriptive and theoretical statements. The reformist zeal in the search for psychological causality of somatic disorders has predominated despite solemn declarations about multicausality, holism, and the like. Such an attitude could hardly result in a balanced appraisal of observed facts but it had a salutary effect in stimulating research.

The Concept of Psychogenesis (Psychogenicity)

Gitelson[43] asserts that the term "psychosomatic" implies that somatic symptoms are "caused" by psychic contents or by affects. He adds that this implication is a carryover from psychoanalytic ideas about conversion and anxiety hysteria, and asks: "What are the common factors which are at once physiological and psychological; which do not 'cause' each other yet are reflected in each other, are contingent and affect each other, and taken together, produce disease?" This question expresses, with admirable clarity, one of the main contemporary concerns of psychosomatic medicine. It does away with the concept of psychogenesis but the latter still survives and invites examination.

A lengthy discussion of psychogenicity in a recent book[66] illustrates the confusion surrounding this concept. It is stated there that "psychogenic" should refer to the psychic aspect of function, i.e., that which is "mediated through the mind." Psychogenesis is defined as having origin within the mind or psyche.[58] For some writers, psychogenesis connotes "a causal chain of psychic phenomena only."[41] Others have extended the meaning of the term to include the effect of those aspects of cerebral activity—which are subjectively experienced and described in psychological terms—on bodily functions expressed in the language of physiology. A typical example of a general statement expressing psychogenetic proposition is this:

> All such processes, in which the first links in a chain of events are perceived *subjectively* as emotions and the subsequent links are objectively observed as changes in body functions, are called psychosomatic phenomena.[3]

Note that the first links in this formulation are emotions, the subsequent ones are somatic changes. This statement typifies the confused thinking found in many psychosomatic writings. It implies a causal chain beginning at an arbitrary point, without specifying what is meant by emotions and what time spans between the "links" are considered significant. Furthermore, as Engel[127] points out, such statements tend to encourage equation of "psychosomatic" with "psychogenic" and thus result in single-factor concepts, which psychosomatic medicine has strived to eliminate. Bahnson[102] remarks that it is naive to think that the level on which a phenomenon is first observed is the casual level and that phenomena on other levels (psychological, physiological, biochemical, molecular) must be regarded as results. He further suggests that it is a meaningless question whether a psychological process is causing a physiological state or vice versa, since both are arbitrary descriptions, in abitrary terms, of a global process.

Should the concept of psychogenesis be abandoned? The reviewer does not believe so, but is of the opinion that its meaning should be redefined to suit current needs. It is assumed that the unique feature of humans is the creation of a universe of symbols in thought and language.[127] Von Bertalanffy[127] defines symbols as signs that are freely created, represent some content, and are transmitted by tradition. The fact of symbolic activity, conscious and unconscious, adds a set of variables to the repertoire of the human organism. Perceptions of the external and internal environments provide information whose significance or meaning for the given person determines his affective and motor responses. The process of appraisal of sensory input and the meaning resulting from the appraisal are aspects of cerebral activity. These aspects, as well as the concomitant (or subsequent) response, are partly described in psychological terms and explained by psychological hypotheses. At another level of abstraction, the same processes and events may be described in terms of physiology, biochemistry, etc. The concept of psychogenesis pertains to those aspects (or "phase" in Langer's[70] terminology) of neural activity which are felt, and their effects on physiological processes, which are not felt. Of course, these effects may *become* felt—e.g., as pain or some other sensation—and exert a feedback effect on the psychic phase. The crucial concept for our view of psychogenesis is that of *meaning*, whether conscious or unconscious. Miller[87] defines it as the significance of information to a system which processes it. The meaning of an event is, of course, influenced by the person's past experience in the broadest sense, and reflects the influence of his transactions with his environment. Since meaning is the result of cognitive processes, the latter require more attention from psychosomatic investigators than has often been the case. It has been observed[129] that the psychic causes to which somatic symptoms are attributed are almost always emotions, which of all psychic phenomena appear the least psychic and the most somatic. It is proposed that the emphasis in psychogenetic statements should shift towards cognition and perception as the crucial psychological variables.

The search for psychogenic factors in illness is not the only concern of psychosomatic medicine. On the contrary, it is one of the basic psychosomatic hypotheses that there can be no psychogenesis, sociogenesis, or somatogenesis alone.[51] What concerns us is the establishment of the relative relevance of psychogenic factors in the genesis, course, and outcome of any illness in the given individual.

The Concept of Psychosomatic Disorder

The concept of a psychosomatic disorder has been one of the dominant themes in psychosomatic medicine. It has both a classificatory and an explanatory connotation. It implies the existence of a class of diseases which have some common characteristic which differentiates them from other diseases. Furthermore, this distinguishing characteristic is purported to have explanatory value, in that in its absence the disease in question could not have come about; it is thus a necessary condition for its occurrence. This general line of reasoning seems to underlie the concept of a psychosomatic disorder. It is a controversial concept, whose acceptance is far from general. To examine it critically one should attempt to answer the following questions:

1. What is the meaning of the term "psychosomatic disorder"?
2. To what extent does its definition correspond to observable facts?
3. What is the value of including certain disorders under the rubric "psychosomatic," for the purposes of research and medical practice?
4. Is it methodologically sound and practically useful to distinguish psychosomatic from nonpsychosomatic disorders?

Szasz[123] maintains that the problem of definition of a "psychosomatic disorder" is a pseudoproblem. However, one cannot afford to dismiss without discussion and argument a problem which has occupied many investigators in our field for some three decades. Psychosomatic or psychophysiological disorders are included in official classifications, discussed in psychiatric textbooks, and have papers and books written about them—a widespread pseudoproblem!

Halliday's[53] definition of a psychosomatic disorder (affection) seems to be the one most commonly accepted: "A bodily disorder in which the application of the psychological approach provides information of high aetiological relevance." Walker[129] tries to make this definition more "operational" by modifying it thusly: "Somatic symptoms that can be successfully treated by methods effective in treating psychic symptoms." Walker's definition has been criticized by Szasz[123] as a caricature of operationalism. Wisdom[135] contends that whole-person medicine necessitates the reality of psychosomatic disorder and expresses the fundamental hypothesis of psychosomatic medicine, that "a mental factor pays a direct part in the pathology of a disorder with a somatic syndrome, and plays the same sort of part as, say, hypersecretion of a gland." Wisdom refutes the opinion held by some writers, such as Alexander,[1] that *all* disease is psychosomatic, as an attempt to bring every type of disease under mental dominance. Obviously this statement is misleading and a reductio ad absurdum of the psychosomatic approach. Furthermore, Wisdom seems to imply that the "true" psychosomatic disorders are "under mental dominance," a viewpoint which is directly contrary to the widespread psychosomatic assumption that all disease is multicausal and that this applies to the traditional psychosomatic disorders. The hypothesis of "mental dominance" can neither be proved nor disproved and is really a value judgment and thus scientifically irrelevant. Engel's[28] conclusions from his study of patients with ulcerative colitis may be regarded as representative of current psychosomatic thinking. He says:

> No assumption is made that such factors (i.e., psychological) have primary etiologic significance. We are only attempting to establish the existence and nature of conditions which may contribute to or even be necessary for the development of the process in the colon now known as ulcerative colitis, but which may not be sufficient in themselves for this development. We do not concern ourselves here with the problem of psychogenesis in the sense of psychologic processes *causing* ulcerative colitis.

Recent reviews of the role of psychological factors in the development and course of the "classical" psychosomatic disorders as well as of the effectiveness of psychotherapy in them are characterized by cautious statements. A typical conclusion, drawn from appraisal of the role of psychological variables in allergic disease, reads:

> From this appraisal of recent research comes the conclusion that the catalogue of methodological shortcomings is lengthy and the number of well-established findings small.[32]

Critical reviews of such conditions as ulcerative colitis,[28,82] duodenal ulcer,[89] hypertension,[115] thyrotoxicosis,[42] rheumatoid arthritis,[92] and skin disorders[104] tend to stress multiple etiology, reject dominance of psychogenesis, call for refinement of methodology, and largely cast doubt on the existence of disease-specific personality or psychodynamic constellations. Engel and Schmale[30] sum up the contemporary position clearly:

> ...diseases differ in respect to the degree to which some are associated with specific psychological features and others not ...with such entities as ulcerative colitis or hyperthyroidism, patients with the same disease appear to resemble each other psychologically to an appreciable extent.

The authors conclude that there is at present insufficient knowledge to ascertain whether these differences are spurious or real.

The related problem of the postulated alternation of somatic and psychic symptoms in psychosomatic disorders has not been substantiated, although such substitution does occasionally occur.[98] Psychosis may coexist with a psychosomatic disorder, such as ulcerative colitis, and influences overall prognosis adversely.[97]

What then is the present state of the concept of a psychosomatic disorder? Its critics are many, and a few utterances by leaders in the field may illustrate dissatisfaction with the whole idea:

> Multicausality and the varying distribution of psychological and nonpsychological factors from case to case invalidates the concept of a "psychosomatic disease" as a specific diagnostic group.[1]
>
> There has been a tendency to limit the illness labelled as psychosomatic to certain syndromes such as ulcerative colitis, asthma, peptic ulcer, etc. This is a misapprehension of a basic concept.[65]
>
> The term "psychosomatic disorder" (or disease) is misleading since it implies a special class of disorders of psychogenic etiology and by inference, therefore, the absence of a psychosomatic interface in other diseases. ...Strictly speaking, there can be no "psychosomatic diseases," just as there can be no "biochemical diseases" or "physiological diseases."[29]

This controversial issue is discussed at some length, and without agreement, in a recent publication by the World Health Organization.[103]

It is appropriate to return now to the four questions posed at the beginning of this discussion. The meaning of the term "psychosomatic disorder" remains unclear and no generally agreed upon definition of it exists. Since no such definition can be regarded as a standard one, the question of its correspondence to current factual knowledge cannot be answered meaningfully. The value of distinguishing a separate category of psychosomatic disorders is doubtful. It has tended to prejudice the selection of material for psychosomatic research and has led to an undesirable impasse.[26,27,29,72] It has focused clinical research and psychotherapeutic endeavor on a limited group of conditions and eventually impeded progress of psychosomatic investigation and theory building. It has had the undersirable effect of diverting attention from a great many problems, practical and theoretical, discussed in Part II of this review,[76] problems which fall logically into the orbit of psychosomatic medicine. It has tended to alienate other physicians from the psychosomatic approach by virtue of what is often felt to be a "territorial invasion" by psychiatry into the field of medicine. Such as impression could do little to facilitate the spread of the practically valuable psychosomatic approach to all phases of medical practice. In conclusion, the concept of a psychosomatic disorder is methodologically and practically unsound. It has created a false dichotomy of diseases and encouraged futile speculation about psychological characteristics of "psychosomatic patients" as if they constituted a homogenous population about whom generalizations could be made. This concept has had some merit in stimulating research but has outlived its usefulness and should be abandoned.

Should one accept the proposition that *all* disease is psychosomatic? This is an ambiguous statement unless its meaning is specified. If we assume that diseases are states which invariably affect the whole person, then all diseases are in this sense psychosomatic. If we assume that "psychosomatic" equals "psychogenic," then the above statement is unwarranted or even nonsensical. Talking of etiology, we can state that aspects of cerebral activity which are expressed in psychological terms may be looked upon as a class of etiological factors. These are relevant to all disease, although this relevance varies in its weight from disease to disease, from person to person, and from one episode of the same disease in the same person to another episode. To draw a boundary between more or less psychogenic diseases seems to be an arbitrary and futile exercise. What matters is to determine in each individual patient how the interplay of psychological and other etiological factors influences the onset, course, and outcome of his illness, by what psychophysiological mechanisms these processes are brought about, and what practical conclusions for prevention and management of illness can be drawn from this knowledge. As observations accrue, some general statements may become possible about the relative role of psychological factors in each particular disease.

The Concept of Specificity

This concept is logically related to the concepts of psychogenesis and psychosomatic disorder. If one accepts the hypothesis that cerebral processes which are conveniently described in psychological terms form a class of etiological factors, then one may postulate that specific psychological states, processes, or events can have specific effects on the function of tissues and organs. Such effects may result in specific dysfunctions or diseases. As formulated by Alexander,[1] specificity theory postulates that "physiological responses to emotional stimuli, both normal and morbid, vary according to the nature of the precipitating emotional state." Furthermore, Alexander hypothesized that every emotional state has its own physiological syndrome.

For the past three decades or so a variety of hypotheses have been put forth about alleged specific psychological factors playing an etiological role in a variety of disorders, mostly those belonging to the so-called psychosomatic group. Personality profiles, nuclear intrapsychic conflicts, attitudes, have been described and their specificity for the given disease has been posulated. The questions that one may ask in this regard are:

1. Does specificity necessarily imply etiological relevance or causality?
2. If so, is the postulated specific factor regarded as a *necessary* condition for the occurrence of the disease in question or not?
3. Are diseases themselves sufficiently "specific" phenomena invariably brought about by the same set of causal, including psychological, factors?
4. Does validation of a given specificity hypothesis allow practical guidelines for the prevention and treatment of a given diesase?

A great deal of research has been stimulated by the specificity hypotheses and therein lies their methodological merit. All too often, however, hypotheses have been accepted as statements of facts, with the resulting devaluation of psychosomatic medicine as a scientific discipline. The present state of the various specificity hypotheses is characterized by more cautious formulations and more rigorous attempts at their validation, and by widespread skepticism about the methodological value of specificity as an explanatory concept in general. Gitelson[43] expressed it most succinctly: "There is no doubt that 'specificity' as it has until now been understood has been discarded." Many other writers[8,14,17,24,43,49,63,69,85,103] have reached similar conclusions. What answers may be tentatively offered to the questions asked above?

First, even if the observation that a certain cluster of personality traits, dispositions, or events antedates a given disorder and achieves statistical validation, it does not logically follow that a causal relationship between the two has been established. In fact, it is difficult to see how even an adequate degree of probability of such a causal relationship can be achieved until the mediating physiological mechanisms are known. Second, it follows that specificity does not imply etiologic necessity. It has been stated[24] that there is no conclusive evidence as yet that a specific psychodynamic pattern is either a sufficient or a necessary condition in the pathogenesis of any psychosomatic disorder. This is not surprising in view of the increasing recognition that in biology and psychology the same antecedent may have different effects, and different antecedents may lead to the same end-effect. Third, the specificity hypotheses have generally been applied to diseases of unkown etiology, with inadequately known pathophysiology and possibly not "specific" disease entities at all. Fourth, whether appropriate preventive and/or remedial measures can be based on the finding of a concomitance or antecedence of a specific set of psychological variables for a given disorder is of particular practical importance. It has been asserted that identification of a specific psychological conflict for some somatic disorders has had practical usefulness for treatment.[63] It is an open question, however, whether any of the specificity hypotheses proposed to date have led to therapeutic advances.[63] In an article dealing with the management of psychosomatic disorders, Rosenbaum and Reiser[108] discuss the variables which they believe should be considered in planning treatment of "psychosomatic" patients, but make no reference to specificity hypotheses and state: "In many chronic diseases, specificity both of etiology and treatment may be lacking." Sperling[119] in a recent paper discusses psychoanalytic treatment of patients suffering from a "psychosomatic disorder proper." She proposes that the most fundamental dynamic hypothesis about psychosomatic illness is that patients suffering from it had a specific mother–child relationship, characterized by rewarding the child for being sick and rejecting him for being healthy. Her analytic techniques aim at helping the patients unlearn the pathological results of the above interaction. There is no mention of any disease-specific psychodynamic patterns in Sperling's paper.

In conclusion, there is no evidence that the proposed specificity hypotheses have offered useful clues to the treatment of patients. One exception may be Sperling's hypothesis of a specific mother–child relationship which, however, seems to apply to a number of syndromes, not only the psychosomatic ones. In the reviewer's opinion, crucial concepts in the treament of any disorder are those of reversibility, modifiability, and compensability of the patient's personality dynamics, physiological dysfunction, or structural damage, as well as of his social situation. All three of these concepts are relative in that they may obtain to varying degrees in different patients and change with time in the same patient. Any treatment plan implies predictions about the feasibility of change according to the above three parameters in the given patient. It appears that no concept of specificity available today has significant relevance for such predictions.

There is evidence that the search for specific psychological variables antedating or concomitant with various somatic syndromes continues. Current interest in the so-called coronary personality[93] is an example of this. Grinker[102] complains about the tendency to search for psychological specificity in the development and location of cancer and says:

> One is struck with the tenuousness of the theoretical concepts and the weakness of evidence for specificity—the same continually reiterate unscientific statements of correlation between disease or the organ involved with an interminable time-span and a spatial discrepancy which is insoluble by our present methods.

Bahnson,[102] in his discussion of Grinker's above remarks, points out that while trait description of people has proved unreliable for prediction, the study of psychodynamic mechanisms may yield evidence of specificity which discriminates between coronary heart disease and cancer, for example.

Clearly, the issue of specificity is far from being closed but there seems to be no doubt that its meaning has changed. Grinker[52] asserts that psychosomatic diseases do not have a specific emotional etiology but are characterized by *response specificity*. There is less tendency to assign to a given psychological variable, or set of variables, the weight of a necessary or sufficient condition for the development of a disease or the "choice" of an organ.

It is increasingly realized that any illness is a final state which may be reached by the interaction among a number of diverse variables and processes. The ultimate goal of etiological research is to determine the pathways to the end-point of illness.[51] Furthermore, illness is not a static but a dynamic state, one in which the interaction among the biological, psychological, and social factors continues unabated and determines the course, modes of coping with, and thus the outcome of the illness. The viewpoint implies that there is no sharp boundary between etiological and reactive factors but a continuity of processes which we artifically classify as causative or reactive. Such distinction, however, is of value for the practice of medicine, which needs the concept of cause for the planning of remedial and preventive measures.[129] It is this consideration which makes the concept of specificity of psychological variables a useful one. If we can identify those of them which contribute to or facilitate the development of any illness, then preventive psychological intervention may become possible. This does not, of course, imply that faultless psychological functioning would ensure eternal life!

The Concept of Psychological Stress

This concept has recently attained prominence in psychosomatic literature and is likely to stay with us for some time. A recent book by Lazarus[71] is an attempt at systematic presentation of the research on, as well as theoretical aspects of, psychological stress. Lazarus points out that for a stimulus to evoke a stress reaction by psychological means it must have a meaning or significance of harm and be *communicated symbolically*. The individual must regard the stimulus as dangerous to his psychological well-being. Lazarus introduces the intervening variable of *threat*, i.e., "a state in which the individual anticipates a confrontation with a harmful condition of some sort." Stimuli are evaluated as threatening by the cognitive process of *ap-*

praisal. The latter depends upon two types of antecedents: factors in the stimulus configuration and factors within the psychological structure of the individual. When a stimulus has been appraised as threatening, there follow processes aimed at reduction or elimination of the anticipated harm and these are called *coping processes*. The end results observed in behavior (such as affective experiences, motor manifestations, alterations of adaptive functioning, and physiological reactions) are understood in terms of the coping processes. The latter depend on cognitive activity termed secondary appraisal. Psychological stress in this theoretical approach includes the stimulus, intervening variables, and response as aspects or components of the total concept.

This thumbnail presentation of Lazarus' conception of psychological stress does not give justice to the rich contents of his book and the value of the conception as an attempt to organize a great mass of data. His proposed theoretical framework integrates many concepts and approaches which are usually considered separately, such as conflict, emotions, defenses, ecology, physiological reactions to symbolic stimuli, etc. As central issues in psychological stress he regards:

1. The conditions and processes which determine when stress reactions will be produced.
2. The consequence of the reaction to a stimulus as a stressful one.
3. The patterns of reaction that define the presence of stress.

Lazarus discusses these three issues in considerable detail.

A different formulation of psychological stress is offered by Engel.[25] According to him, such stress designates

> ...all processes, whether originating in the external environment or within the person which impose a demand or requirement upon the organism, the resolution of which necessitates work or activity of the mental apparatus before any other system is involved or activated.

One feels that Engel's definition includes an unnecessary temporal stricture implied by the adverb "before." As he himself states, a somatic disorder can also be a psychological stress and in this case other systems will be involved before the mental apparatus. Engel distinguishes three broad and overlapping categories of psychological stress: (1) loss or threat of loss of psychic objects; (2) actual or threatened injury to the body; and (3) frustration of drives.

The following criteria seem to define the theoretical concept of psychological stress:

1. The stimuli qualifying as psychologically stressful, whether they originate within or without the person, must be perceived.
2. Such stimuli have to be evaluated by the perceiving individual as dangerous or threatening to him; the results of such evaluation, as well as the process itself, may be partly or totally outside the person's awareness.
3. The response to a psychologically stressful stimulus includes one or more dysphoric affect as well as coping processes and activities.

4. All these processes are experienced, communicated, and described in psychological terms, i.e., in person-language.[139]

Thus conceived, psychological stress is thought to be an important variable in
human health and disease. Physiological concomitants of affects, such as anxiety,
depression, anger, etc., have widespread organismic effects which may facilitate the
onset of, maintain, or exacerbate those states which we call diseases. In general, one
may depict psychological stress and its effects as a series of linked and interacting
loops. Thus, affective arousal in response to appraisal of threat may influence cognitive processes in the direction of magnification of threat, with resulting increase in
affective arousal. Perception of peripheral physiological concomitants of affect may
have a positive feedback effect on the latter and on the evaluative processes, etc.
Much current research is concerned with identification of relevant variables and
processes and their interaction. Such research has direct bearing on our understanding of disease and on medical practice. Several representative examples of such current research may be mentioned.

The work of the Rochester group has focused on the settings in which illness occurs.[30,112] The onset situation has been proposed as the period in which to study the
nature of the psychological stress involved in the development of illness. As one nonspecific onset situation, they have described the giving up–given up complex, involving affects of helplessness and hopelessness. It is proposed that this complex is neither necessary nor sufficient for, but only contributory to, the emergence or
exacerbation of both somatic and psychiatric illness. The most common situations
provoking the complex involve real, threatened, or symbolic psychic object losses.
The crucial question—what are the mediating biological mechanisms whereby the
proposed psychological state may have pathogenic influence—remains unanswered.
Perhaps the immunological and endocrinological approaches will offer new insights
here.[31,37,50,52,90,102,109,117]

A different approach to the study of illness onset has focused on social changes
which threaten the security of the person and lead to attempts at adaptive behavior.[56,94,100,105,106,126] Changes in social status, conceptualized as a "life crisis,"
are said to antedate illness or a clustering of illnesses of many kinds. It is postulated
that psychosocial stress may result in the lowering of bodily resistance to disease and
thus, by constituting a necessary, but not sufficient, cause of diesase, may help determine the timing of its onset.[105,106] It is pertinent at this point to quote Schilder's[111]
warning:

> We often wonder why organic diseases occur at times when the life situation of the in-
> dividual has come to a crisis, and why they do occur where the individual seems to need
> them out of his innermost strivings. Even then we have to be careful. How many normal in-
> dividuals do we meet who are not at a given time more or less in serious stress?

Other approaches to the study of psychological stress have attempted to identify
personality variables which may determine a person's evaluation of a given stimulus
or set or stimuli. Graham[46] asserts that patients with different diseases describe
differently the situations which provoke attacks of their disease. This characteristic
mode of description is called "attitude." It is hypothesized that those events which

induce in the patient the appropriate specific attitude are relevant to the production or exacerbation of a particular disease process.

An interesting approach to personality characteristics relevant to psychological stress is that concerned with *perceptual reactance*. According to Petrie,[101] individuals differ with regard to their tendency to reduce, augment, or leave unchanged what is being perceived. Thus, tolerance for pain as well as for sensory over- or underload varies according to the person's characteristic perceptual modulation, i.e., reduction or augmentation. It is suggested that physiological concomitants of emotions may give rise to sensations which are reduced by some persons and augmented by others, and thus influence the intensity of the emotional experience and the person's reaction to it.

Other investigators have been concerned with affect as a "bridging concept between the psychological and somatic spheres."[103] Anxiety, anger, and depression have attracted particular attention in this regard since they have measurable somatic concomitants and behavioral manifestations.[50] Anxiety has been singled out by some as both an indicator or response to stress and a precursor of further stress responses.[52,63] The concept of anxiety presents a considerable epistemological and semantic muddle, well brought out by a recent monograph.[120] Rarely is distinction made between anxiety as a theoretical and a descriptive term. Defined as an affect, anxiety is characterized by anticipation of an imminent but intangible danger. One of the most perceptive descriptions of this experiential characteristic of anxiety can be found in Chekhov's "A Dreary Story."[125] The main character in this short story experiences a nocturnal anxiety attack which he sums up thusly: "I was possessed by unaccountable animal terror, and I cannot understand why I was so frightened." The neuroendocrine substrate of the anxiety experience, as outlined by Mirsky,[90] suggests possible mechanisms by virtue of which this affect may exert influence on the function of many organs. Its pathogenic significance in somatic disease has been postulated[63] but, as Grinker[50] points out, there is as yet no proved relationship between emotional processes and a specific disease. The effects of anxiety on an already present somatic disease are often profound, as is clearly exemplified by cardiac disease.[107] One may expect that further clarification of the physiological processes concomitant with the various affects will result in specification of the mediating mechanisms whereby psychological stress may influence the onset and course of many diseases.

Some investigators emphasize the importance of the role of defenses and of their breakdown in determining the consequences of psychological stress.[99] It is increasingly recognized that the classical ego mechanisms of defense do not fully account for a person's modes of coping with psychologically stressful stimuli and the resulting affective arousal. Hamburg and Adams[54] have studied the importance of the seeking and utilization of information as a way of coping with stressful experience. This is surely an area of study which has practical implications for preventive and remedial measures in medicine and public health. How do people cope with the stress of somatic disease, for example, and how can the efficacy of such coping be increased by psychological means? Can the maintenance of adequate coping techniques have benefical effect on progressive disease, such as cancer? Grinker[102] suggests that "growth and development leading to pride, productivity, and creativity are significant antidotes to disease." There is a good deal of "anecdotal" evidence that this may be true, but how it works and how it can be deliberately induced are problems for the future psychosomatic research.

An interesting commentary on the relativity of the concept of psychological stress is the observation that among concentration camp inmates psychosomatic disease were "extremely rare."[68] It was suggested that in extreme situations such diseases, as well as psychoneuroses, tend to be ameliorated. Equally rare were common colds. Does it mean that under extreme stress all these conditions become, as it were, a biological luxury?

In summary, the theoretical concept of psychological stress is in the foreground of psychosomatic theory today. It is a useful construct whose defining empirical properties are in the process of elaboration by experimental and clinical research. This concept unifies a wide range of interactions between man and his enviroment and highlights the role of the uniquely human capacity for symbolic activity as a crucial variable among the factors determining health and disease. The varied conceptual and research approaches to psychological stress have been illustrated here. They indicate the multifaceted character of the concept and the interplay of many variables determining which inner or outer stimuli are psychologically stressful to the given individual at any particular time, and how he responds psychologically, behaviorally, and physiologically. All these approaches are complementary rather than mutually exclusive, and each expresses the position of the observer and his theoretical bias. Taken together, they bring out the complexity of this whole area and put in proper perspective the reductionist trends of the earlier phase of psychosomatic medicine. We are no longer satified with the relatively simple notions of specificity, psychogenesis, and linear causality as formulated by some pioneers in our field. The present trend is more truly holisic and open to new theoretical formulations less exclusively inspired by the psychoanalytic theory.

The Concept of Body Image

This concept is seldom adequately discussed in psychosomatic literature. Its importance as a bridging construct between the psychological, biological, and social modes of abstraction should be brought into prominence. Its relevance to psychosomatic theory is obvious, as are its practical implications for medical practice.[88] Several recent reviews deal with various aspects of the body image and its abnormalities.[35,78,130]

As defined by Schilder,[111] body image or schema designates the tridimensional mental picture of our own body. In Schilder's conception, the body image has the following main features:

1. It is dynamic, in the sense that it is in a continual process of contruction and reconstruction.
2. It is developmental, i.e., it is a process going on throughout the whole life with the gradual increase in the knowledge about our body.
3. It has a physiological basis.

4. It is dependent on our emotional life and conflicts, and changes with the emotional attitude towards the body.
5. There is a continual interchange between our own own body image and the body images of others; body image is a social phenomenon.
6. It is an expression of the total personality.
7. It is part of every experience and all life experiences influence it.

It is impossible to do justice to Schilder's work in a few lines but they may encourage others to read his book. His concept has considerable explanatory value and practical relevance for all diseases which give rise to somâtic symptoms. He stresses that organic disease provokes abnormal sensations, and that these at once become part of the individual's general attitude and experience and change his body image. The latter is also helpful in explaining the choice of somatic symptoms in hysteria and hypochondriasis as well as certain symptoms in schizophrenia.

More recent studies which have utilized the concept of the body image include many disorders. Some representative examples follow. Bruch[15] emphasizes that a disturbance in the body image of delusional proportions is the cardinal feature of true anorexia nervosa. She points out that without correction of the patient's body image, improvement is likely to be only temporary. The same author found disturbances of the body image in obesity.[16] Phantom phenomena following amputation,[116] mastectomy,[61] facial disfiguration,[59] and orchidectomy[55] have been explained by invoking the body image concept. Hollender[60] stresses that the intensity of the reaction to the loss of a body part depends on the representation it has in the body image. The latter has been particularly stressed in relation to plastic surgery. It is suggested that patients with an unimpaired body image tend to benefit from plastic surgery, while those whose image is distorted tend to continue having emotional difficulties after surgery.[124]

An experimental approach to the study of the body image of particular interest to psychosomatic medicine has been elaborated on by Fisher and Cleveland.[34-36] They postulate that a fundamental aspect of the body image is the manner in which a person perceives his body boundaries. Individuals are said to vary in the degree of definiteness or clarity of the perception of their body boundaries. To study this variability, Fisher and Cleveland developed a method which involves scoring the properties of the boundary regions of percepts elicited in the blot stimuli (e.g., Rorschach or Holtzman blots). Boundary definiteness was related to the degree to which definite structure, substance, and surface qualities were assigned to the periphery of ink-blot images. Two basic boundary indices were formulated: "barrier responses" indicating perception of definite boundaries, and "penetration responses" characterized by perceived penetrability of persons and objects. Applying these concepts and method of research to clinical problems the investigators observed that patients with rheumatiod arthritis, neurodermatitis, and conversion symptomss involving the musculature were characterized by higher barrier and lower penetration scores than patients with gastric ulcer or spastic colitis. A hypothesis was then put forth that the choice of psychosomatic symptoms developed in response to stress was partly determined by the degree of definiteness of perceived body boundaries. Thus persons with definite boundaries tend to develop symptoms in the exterior body layers (skin and muscle); persons with indefinite boundaries are more likely to show symptoms in the internal organs. This approach was extended to the study of reactions to body disablement, as in poliomyelitis or after amputation, and the finding made was that adjustment to such disability was better in individuals with definite boundaries, as indicated by higher barrier scores.

Williams and Krasnoff[134] have cross-validated Fisher and Cleveland's findings regarding differentiation of patients with peptic ulcer and rheumatoid arthritis on the basis of body image scores. Furthermore, they attempted to determine if patients with symptoms involving the body exterior had different physiological responses from individuals with symptoms involving the body interior. They confirmed their prediction that peptic ulcer patients had higher heart rates than the arthritic patients under all experimental conditions. They concluded that some support was found for a relationship between a person's attitude towards his body and his physiological responses. Nichols and Tursky[96] report that persons with definite body boundaries, as measured by the barrier score, tolerate pain better than those with indefinite boundaries.

In summary, the concepts of the body image and its boundaries appear to be of value for the study of various aspects of psychosomatic relationships. They reflect both cognitive and affective attributes and processes of persons, and seem to show some correlation with physiological reactivity. They may help predict what type of somatic symptom and physiological dysfunction a person will develop in response to psychological stress. Here is one more cluster of psychological variables to be considered in the study of and theoretical formulations about the effects of such stress. As de Ajuriaguerra[130] observes:

> The concepts of the body as it is perceived, represented, and experienced, have different meanings at different moments of the development; they depend partly on maturation, and partly on experience. Each of these concepts needs to be made more precise, and to be more thoroughly studied through longitudinal and multidimensional approaches.

THE CONCEPT OF SOMATIZATION

The term "somatization" is often used in psychiatric discussions but its meaning is obscure. It has been stated that Stekel introduced this term to mean "a type of bodily disorder arising from a deep-seated neurotic cause"; "somatization" was thus said to be identical with "conversion."[58] This alleged identity of meaning does not seem to be generally accepted in the literature. A group of psychoanalysts has recently formulated the meaning of somatization in these somewhat cryptic passages:

> The regressed libidinization of an organ or organ system or fantasy of function of an organ system which becomes manifest in symptoms or signs is somatization.... Somatization would be the actual changes within the organ or organ system which may come into the field of awareness.[66]

Elsewhere[110] the process of somatization is defined as the "psychological mechanisms through which the various personality elements—the idealization and rejection of attitudes and self-aspects, body-image distortions, functioning in restitutive direction—are translated in somatic symptoms.'' In an often quoted paper, Schur[114] discusses the metapsychology of somatization without, however, defining the term. He states in a footnote that while his paper is concerned with dermotoses, his concepts apply to all ''psychosomatic'' disorders. His main hypothesis asserts that ego regression, characterized by prevalence of primary process thinking, may result in the ego's incapacity to neutralize aggression and this in turn leads to resomatization of responses. Schur notes the similarity between symptom formation (in some dermatoses) and hysterical conversion, but states that this similarity is limited to the structure of the symptom ''eruption.'' The patients with dermatoses show a tendency to regressive types of anxiety and an inability to neutralize their aggression. They thus possess ego defects analogous to those of schizophrenics but differ from the latter by their ability to restore secondary processes and control of anxiety. Inability to neutralize aggression is seen by Schur as sommon to both schizophrenia and psychosomatic disorders; in the former, regression results in impairment of thought processes and defusion of instinctual drives, while in the latter it results in a resomatization of various responses. Schur points out that the main purpose of his paper was to show how the ''pure analytic approach'' can contribute to the understanding of certain physiological mechanisms.

Gitelson[43] suggests that Schur's work represents ''a most explicit application'' of contemporary psychoanalytic theory to the problems of neurotic organ disease. However this may be, his hypotheses invite a critical examination. First, to what observable phenomena and to what patient populations do Schur's hypotheses apply? He affirms their importance for the ''entire area of psychosomatic manifestations,'' but seems to base them on the study of unspecified numbers of cases of several skin disorders. What are ''psychosomatic manifestations''? Are they defined by Schur's generalizations or by some independent criteria? Second, what is meant by ''resomatization of various responses''? This concept seems to imply partial replacement of cognitive and motor activity by increased autonomic nervous system activity in response to danger, internal or external. This concept is related to the hypothesis of physiological regression, whose methodological sterility has been pointed out.[85] Third, it is not clear how the analytic approach, ''pure'' or otherwise, can help explain physiological mechanisms. This seems to be an example of mixing of categories. Psychological hypotheses may help explain why certain physiological mechanisms occurred in a certain person at a certain time, but cannot add anything to the understanding of the mechanisms as such. Fourth, there seems to be little value in formulating highly abstract hypotheses to explain diverse phenomena put in a single class with undefined characteristics. It is as if the proposed hypotheses were both the explanations and the only criteria for grouping together what is being explained. The current tendency in psychosomatic medicine seems to be to emphasize meticulous psychological description and the formulation of low-level explanatory hypotheses capable of empirical validation, rather than to indulge in sweeping generalizations about ill-defined and poorly understood psychophysiological relationships.

The concept of somatization as reviewed is an example of the semantic muddle in our field. Unless further defined, it remains ambiguous and thus useless. Yet there is a need for a generic term designating the *tendency to experience, conceptualize, and/or communicate psychological states or contents as bodily sensations, functional changes, or somatic metaphors.* Somatization may be adopted as such a generic term. It encompasses a variety of phenomena which need to be classified on a descriptive basis until psychological and physiological mechanisms can be worked out for them. A proposed classification for somatization phenomena follows:

1. Subjectively perceived physiological concomitants of affects which may be regarded as integral components (or equivalents) of the affect and are devoid of primary symbolic meaning.
2. Somatic changes symbolically expressing ideational content, i.e., conversion phenomena.
3. Secondary symbolic elaborations of perceived bodily changes regardless of their origin.
4. Excessive preoccupation with bodily sensations and functions, normal or abnormal, i.e., hypochondriacal syndrome.
5. Nosophobia.
6. Somatic delusions.
7. Communication of psychological distress in bodily metaphors.

There is obviously no sharp demarcation of the above classes, nor are they mutually exclusive. One may postulate a continuum of somatization reactions ranging from objectively observable somatic change, through purely subjective but reportable somatic sensations, to *ideas* about the body and their use as a mode of experiencing and communicating psychic conflict, distress, etc. One may postulate that each of the above types of somatization involves different psychological and physiological processes and determinants. The latter are likely to include, to a varying extent, genic factors, prenatal influences, early learning experiences, past and current vicissitudes in object relations, effects of biological and psychological stress, cultural influences,[22] etc. From the physiological viewpoint, each somatization reaction can be seen as predominantly of either central or peripheral origin and involving, in varying combinations, both the central and the autonomic nervous systems. There is thus no postulated sharp difference between conversion symptoms and "vegetative neurosis" as suggested by Alexander.[1] A detailed discussion of the above classes would be beyond the scope of this review. They will be considered in detail in a future article. Their study is seen as one of the main tasks of clinical psychosomatic research.

II. Psychosomatic Medicine as a Method of Approach

It has been proposed earlier that the psychosomatic approach is expressed in a body of postulates and norms conceived as guidelines for medical practice. It is this aspect of psychosomatic medicine which can be expected to be incorporated in medical teaching and practice and thus lose its rationale as a separate designation. This time has not arrived yet. The present trend in medical education with its stress on the behavioral sciences should speed up the process of assimilation. For the time being it may still be useful to spell out some of the key postulates formulating the psychosomatic approach to medicine.

1. Human health and disease are viewed as states without a sharp dividing line between them. They are determined by multiple factors: biological, psychological, and social.
2. Any event at any level of organization of the human organism—from the symbolic to the molecular—may have repercussions at all the other levels.
3. Medical diagnosis should focus not only on identification of a particular disease but consider the total situation of the patient and the relative contribution of all determinants to the presenting clinical picture.
4. Psychosocial factors must be considered in planning preventive and therapeutic measures.
5. The relationship between the patient and those taking care of him influences the course of illness and efficacy of treatment.
6. Psychotherapy may be of value whenever psychological factors are recognized as significantly contributing to the precipitation, maintenance, or exacerbation of any illness in a given person.

These principles characterize the psychosomatic approach. Their application has practical value and does not have to await definitive results of the study of psychophysiological relationships. Such study, however, may be expected to give increasing precision to remedial action. The need for the latter is particularly pressing in the area of somatization reactions. As defined and classified here, these reactions include the bulk of the so-called functional or "psychosomatic" symptoms frequently encountered in medical practice.[5,9,22,79,122] They may occur in the presence or absence of demonstrable organic disease, and represent the *preferred mode of experiencing, expressing, and/or reporting of psychological distress, i.e., the somatic mode.* This is not to say, of course, that such "preference" is the result of conscious or deliberate choice. Increased efficiency in identifying these reactions as well as their psychophysiological determinants and mechanisms poses a pressing challenge to clinical psychosomatic research. The problems of prevention and management of these reactions involve such measures as individual and group psychotherapy, behavior therapy, family therapy, and the use of psychotropic drugs, as well as environmental manipulation. None of these techniques should be rejected on a priori grounds, but the indications for each must be evaluated in each individual case. While the emphasis is usually, and rightly, on psychodynamic evaluation and psychotherapy, these are not the only contributions a psychiatrist can make and teach, in regard to somatization reactions. There is surely a place for the discerning use of psychotropic drugs whether as adjuncts to psychotherapy or as the main treatment. There is need for long-term studies to find out whether, for instance, the proper use of these drugs may prevent chronic and/or intense anxiety or depression from exacerbating or precipitating serious organic disease. Furthermore, it is possible that effective suppression of physiological concomitants of affects by pharmacological means, such as beta adrenergic blocking agents,[47] may prevent the positive feedback from the periphery and thus facilitate integrative ego mechanisms and related coping devices. In the area of psychotherapy of somatization reactions the work of Balint and his co-workers[6,7] at the Tavistock Clinic in London is particularly promising although a great deal more research is clearly needed to develop precise practical guidelines for the kind of psychotherapy to be chosen for the individual case.

In summary, the psychosomatic approach to medicine has not been so satisfactorily assimilated into practice that it can be said to have lost its pertinence and thus be ready for dissolution. In advocates general propositions about the increasingly precise guidelines for comprehensive diagnosis as well as preventive and therapeutic action in all areas of medicine. It is based on the recognition that patients are persons and that psychosocial variables are relevant, albeit to a varying extent, in all illnesses.

III. CONSULTING ACTIVITIES (CONSULTATION PSYCHIATRY)

This aspect of psychosomatic medicine has been dealt with in the first two parts of this review.[75,76] The activities of psychiatric consultants in general hospitals can be regarded as clinical application and teaching of the psychosomatic approach. The clinical material to which consultants have access is diverse. This fact is reflected in the broadening of research interests within the whole area of psychosomatic medicine. Furthermore, demonstration of the practical usefulness of the psychosomatic approach and psychiatric conceptions and techniques to a wide variety of diagnostic and management problems encountered on the medical wards provides a most promising teaching opportunity. The consultant's daily work can bring home to medical students and the nonpsychiatric physician the truth that the psychosomatic approach is not just a set of abstract generalizations but a means of improving the efficacy of medical care. No amount of theoretical teaching and proselytizing preaching can replace this.

A matter of concern is the apparent cleavage between the laboratory researcher in psychosomatics and the consultant–clinician. This is reflected in the relative dearth of clinical reports in this journal as well as in the programs of the Society's meetings. Such lack of communication is deplorable. Research, theory development, and clinical activity are integral components of psychosomatic medicine. Free flow of communication among those engaged in each of these areas is necessary for the further development of the field as a whole. Clinicians, even if they are not engaged in research, may make observations which are not to be dismissed as "anecdotal" material. Even a single observation may provide a seminal idea to be formulated as a testable hypothesis. It is often a casual observation from which a fruitful hypothesis is born. On their part, clinicians need to know what developments are taking place in the areas of research and theory building. It is ultimately their task to put experimental findings and theoretical statements to the test of practical applicability and to communicate the results to other physicians.

An insufficiently recognized problem is that of training of consultants. A good deal is written about whom they should teach and how,[23] but little attention is paid to the teaching of teachers. A recent survey of training in consultation techniques offered by psychiatric centers in the United States highlights this problem: "Generally there is a great lack of training personnel who are skilled and experienced in doing consultation."[84] It was concluded from the survey that relevant training was insufficient and that knowledge about consultation process and technique should be sought and taught formally. This reviewer is of the opinion that future consultants and teachers should spend at least one year, after completion of their psychiatric training, in supervised consulting work in all nonpsychiatric areas of a general hospital. In addition, they should receive formal training in all aspects of psychosomatic medicine as outlined in this review. Only such comprehensive clinical and theoretical training can qualify a psychiatrist as a competent consultant and teacher of others. This work should not be entrusted to well-meaning amateurs, no matter how well trained in general psychiatry and psychodynamics. Thus the case is made here for regarding psychosomatic medicine and consultation psychiatry as an "area of special interest" (not a subspecialty) within the field of psychiatry.

Summary and Conclusions

An attempt has been made in this tripartite review to present some major current issues in the field of psychosomatic medicine. What was initially intended only as an outline of the work of psychiatric consultants in general hospitals has expanded into a more ambitious project—a survey of the psychosomatic field as a whole. The reviewer felt that such a task, despite its inevitable shortcomings of omission and commission, could have some didactic value. He has often encountered questions from colleagues as well as students about the meaning and scope of psychosomatic medicine. He has read statements purporting that the term "psychosomatic" reflects merely "a rather muddled phase of specialized ignorance."[73] As a consultant and teacher, he has felt the need to clarify for himself the meaning of some terms and conceptions relevant to his work. Without such clarification one feels like a blind man trying to lead the blind—a rather stressful role.

The field of psychosomatic medicine abounds in semantic and conceptual confusion. There is no general agreement regarding the meaning of basic terms, not enough distinction between what are data of observation and theoretical concepts and explanatory hypotheses, and little consensus about the scope of our discipline and its position within the larger fields of medicine, psychiatry, and human biology. A great deal of accumulated relevant observation remains unintegrated or is at times interpreted from a narrow theoretical position. Unless attempts at integration are made, the gap between the mass of accruing data and our ability to evaluate and relate them to one another will grow steadily. We need individuals prepared to scan the field and attempt unification, while being aware that premature closure is neither possible nor desirable.

What are the hallmarks of psychosomatic medicine of the sixties? One may offer a tentative list of them:

1. A trend away from the search for psychogenesis of a limited number of somatic disorders labelled "psychosomatic."

2. A focus on the relationship between specific psychological variables—such as affects—and specific physiological functions and processes rather than disease entities.

3. Elaboration of the multifaceted concept of psychological stress and its aspects, including stimulus, intermediate mechanisms, and behavioral and physiological response.

4. Study of neuroendocrine processes as mediating mechanisms between symbolic activity and the function of organs and tissues. In this area the contribution of so-called corticovisceral medicine is of increasing importance.[18,137]

5. Stress on meticulous psychological description rather than premature interpretation.

6. Awareness of the crucial importance of prenatal and early postnatal influences for the developments of specific and interacting psychological and physiological reaction patterns and vulnerabilities. Stress on longitudinal studies beginning with the embryonic phase of organization.

7. Emphasis on the effects of environmental influences, mediated through symbolic activity, on the maintenance of health and development of illness.

8. Concern with the psychosocial conditions determining the timing of onset of many diseases and their course.

9. The expanding clinical application and teaching of the psychosomatic approach stimulated by the development of general hospital psychiatric units and their liaison with other departments.

10. Growing awareness of the vast complexity of the factors and processes that maintain health and precipitate and determine the course of all diseases. Less enthusiasm for catchy, sweeping, one-factor explanations of somatic disorders by psychological mechanisms, conscious or unconscious. More emphasis on carefully designed clinical and experimental studies.

The writer expects to be criticized for suggesting that psychosomatics be in part designated a science. It is a controversial viewpoint, but it may have the heuristic value of unifying diverse lines of research for the purpose of theory building and teaching. It is not an attempt to achieve respectability for our field by claiming for it the status of a science—a futile quibble over words. What is the value of psychosomatic medicine? In Brecht's play *The Life of Galileo*, the physicist says: "I maintain that the only purpose of science is to ease the hardship of human existence."[12] The reviewer contends that psychosomatics can contribute to this purpose in three ways: by offering means to alleviate some suffering; by expanding the knowledge of man—a cognitive and esthetic value in its own right; and by giving the sense of a meaningful task to the workers in all aspects of our field. Is this not sufficient justification to continue?

REFERENCES

1. Alexander F: *Psychosomatic Medicine.* New York, Norton, 1950.
2. Alexander F: The development of psychosomatic medicine. *Psychosomatic Med* 24:13, 1962.

3. Alexander FG, Selesnick, ST: *The History of Psychiatry*. New York, Harper, 1966, p 389.
4. Ax AF: Goals and methods of psychophysiology. *Psychophysiology* 1:8, 1964.
5. Bain ST, Spaulding WB: The importance of coding presenting symptoms. *Canad Med Assoc J* 97:953, 1967.
6. Balint M: *The Doctor, His Patient and the Illness*. London, Pitman, 1957.
7. Balint M, Balint E: *Psychotherapeutic Techniques in Medicine*. London, Tavistock, 1961.
8. Bandler B: Some conceptual tendencies in the psychosomatic movement. *Am J Psychiatry* 115:36, 1958.
9. Berblinger KW: The functional symptom in psychiatric perspective. *Psychosomatics* 7:205, 1966.
10. Birren JE (ed): *Handbook of Aging and the Individual*, Chicago, University of Chicago Press, 1959.
11. Brady JV: Psychophysiology of emotional behavior in Experimental Foundations of Clinical Psychology, Bachrach AJ (ed). New York, Basic, 1962.
12. Brecht, B: The life of Galileo, in Plays, vol 1. London, Methuen, 1960.
13. Brodbeck M: Models, meaning and theories, in Gross L (ed). *Symposium on Sociological Theory*, New York, Harper, 1959.
14. Brown F: A clinical psychologist's perspective on research in psychosomatic medicine. *Psychosom Med* 20:174, 1958.
15. Bruch H: Anorexia nervosa and its differential diagnosis. *J Nerv Ment Dis* 141:555, 1966.
16. Bruch H: *The Importance of Overweight*. New York, Norton, 1957.
17. Buck C, Hobbs GE: The problem of specificity in psychosomatic illness. *J Psychosom Res* 3:227, 1959.
18. Bykov KM, Gantt HW: *The Cerebral Cortex and the Internal Organs*. New York, Chemical Pub., 1957.
19. Chalke FCR: Effect of psychotherapy for psychosomatic disorders. *Psychosomatics* 6:125, 1965.
20. Cleghorn RA: Message and method. *Psychosom Med* 28:272, 1966.
21. Cooper B: The epidemiological approach to psychosomatic medicine. *J Psychosom Res* 8:9, 1964.
22. Crandell DL, Dohrenwend BP.: Some relations among psychiatric symptoms, organic illness, and social class. *Am J Psychiatry* 123: 1527, 1967.
23. Deutsch F, (ed): *Training in Psychosomatic Medicine*, New York, Hafner, 1964.
24. Editorial: The specificity hypotheses of psychosomatic medicine. *Am J Med* 24:323, 1958.
25. Engel GL: A unified concept of health and disease, *Perspect Biol Med* 3:459, 1960.
26. Engel GL: Psychological factors and ulcerative colitis. *Br Med J* 4:56, 1967.
27. Engel GL: Selection of clinical material in psychosomatic medicine. *Psychosom Med* 16:368, 1954.
28. Engel GL: Studies of ulcerative colitis: V. Psychological aspects and their implications for treatment. *Am J Dig Dis* 3:315, 1958.
29. Engel GL: The concept of psychosomatic disorder. *J Psychosom Res* 11:3, 1967.
30. Engel GL, Schmale AH Jr: Psychoanalytic theory of somatic disorder: Conversion, specificity, and the disease onset situation. *J Am Psychoanal Assoc* 15:344, 1967.
31. Fawcett JA, Bunney W.E. Jr: Pituitary adrenal function and depression. *Arch Gen Psychiatry* 16: 517, 1967.
32. Feingold BF, Singer MT, Freeman EH, Deskins A: Psychological variables in allergic disease: A critical appraisal of methodology. *J Allerg* 38:143, 1966.
33. Ferreira AJ: Emotional factors in prenatal environment. *J Nerv Ment Dis* 141:108, 1965.
34. Fisher S: A further appraisal of the body boundary concept. *J Consult Psychol* 27:62, 1963.
35. Fisher S, Cleveland SE: *Body Image and Personality*. New York, Van Nostrand, 1958.
36. Fisher S., Cleveland SE: The role of body image in psychosomatic symptom choice. *Psych Monogr* 69:1, 1955.
37. Friedman SB, Glasgow LA: Psychologic factors and resistance to infectious disease. *Pediatr Clin North Am* 13:315, 1966.
38. Galdston I: Psychosomatic medicine. *Arch Neurol (Chicago)* 74:441, 1955.
39. Garner HH: Somatopsychic concepts. *Psychosomatics* 7:329, 1966.
40. Gellhorn E: The tuning of the nervous system: Physiological foundations and implications for behavior. *Perspect Biol Med* 10:559, 1967.
41. Gerö G: The idea of psychogenesis in modern psychiatry and in psychoanalysis. *Psychoanal Rev* 30:187, 1943.
42. Gibson JG: Emotions and the thyroid gland: A critical appraisal. *J Psychosom Res* 6:93, 1962.
43. Gitelson M:A critique of current concepts in psychosomatic medicine. *Bull Menninger Clin* 23:165, 1959.

44. Goldberg EM: *Family Influences and Psychosomatic Illness.* London, Tavistock, 1958.
45. Graham DT: Health, disease, and the mind-body problem: Linguistic parallelism. *Psychosom Med* 29:52, 1967.
46. Graham DT, Stevenson I: Disease as response to life stress: 1. The nature of the evidence, in Lief HI, Lief VF, Lief NR (eds).: *The Psychological Basis of Medical Practice,* New York, Harper, 1963.
47. Granville-Grossman KL Turner P: The effect of propranolol on anxiety. *Lancet* 1:788, 1966.
48. Greenberg NH: Studies in psychosomatic differentiation during infancy. *Arch Gen Psychiatry (Chicago)* 7:389, 1962.
49. Grinker, RR: *Psychosomatic Research.* Norton, New York, 1953.
50. Grinker, RR: The physiology of emotions, in Simon A (ed): *The Physiology of Emotions,* Springfield, Ill, Charles Thomas, 1961.
51. Grinker RR Sr: "Open-system" psychiatry. *Am J Psychoanal* 26:115, 1966.
52. Grinker, RR Sr: The psychosomatic aspects of anxiety, in *Anxiety and Behavior,* Spielberger, CD (ed): New York, Academic Press, 1966.
53. Halliday JL: *Psychosocial Medicine.* New York, Norton, 1948.
54. Hamburg DA, Adams JE: A perspective on coping behavior. *Arch Gen Psychiatry (Chicago)* 17:277, 1967.
55. Heusner PA: Phantom genitalia. *Trans Amer Neurol Assoc* 75:128, 1950.
56. Hinkle LE Jr. Ecological observations of the relation of physical illness, mental illness, and the social environment. *Psychosom Med* 23:289, 1961.
57. Hinkle LE Jr; Human ecology, "psychosomatic medicine" and the medical curriculum. *Adv Psychosom Med* 4:23, 1964.
58. Hinsie LE, Campbell RJ: *Psychiatric Dictionary,* ed 3. New York, Oxford, 1960.
59. Hoffman J: Facial phantom phenomenon. *J Nerv Ment Dis* 122:143, 1954.
60. Hollender MH: *The Psychology of Medical Practice.* Philadelphia, Saunders, 1958.
61. Jarvis JH: Post-mastectomy breast phantoms. *J Nerv Ment Dis* 144:266, 1967.
62. Kaplan HI, Kaplan HS: an historical survey of psychosomatic medicine. *J Nerv Ment Dis* 124:546, 1956.
63. Kaplan HI, Kaplan HS: A psychosomatic concept. *Am J Psychother* 11:16, 1957.
64. Kaplan HI, Kaplan HS: Current theoretical concepts in psychosomatic medicine. *Am J Psychiatry* 115:1091, 1959.
65. Kaufman RM: Introduction, in Early recognition and management of psychiatric disorders in general practice. *J Mount Sinai Hosp NY* 25:137, 1958.
66. Kaufman RM, Heiman, M (eds): *Evolution of Psychosomatic Concepts. Anorexia Nervosa: A Paradigm.* New York, International Universities Press, 1964.
67. Kessel N., Munro A: Epidemiological studies in psychosomatic medicine. *J Psychosom Res* 8:67, 1964.
68. Kral VA: Psychiatric observations under severe chronic stress. *Am J Psychiatry* 108:185, 1951.
69. Kubie LS: The problem of specificity in the psychosomatic process, in Deutsch F (ed): *The Psychosomatic Concept in Psychoanalysis* , New York, International Universities Press, 1953.
70. Langer SK: *Mind: An Essay on Human Feeling.* Baltimore, Johns Hopkins Press, 1967, vol 1.
71. Lazarus RS: *Psychological Stress and the Coping Process.* New York, McGrawHill, 1966.
72. Lewin KK: Psychosomatic research: Problems in methodology. *Ann Intern Med* 50:122, 1959.
73. Lewis A: *Inquiries in Psychiatry.* London, Routledge, 1967.
74. Lipowski ZJ: Delirium, clouding of consciousness and confusion. *J Nerv Ment Dis* 145:227, 1967.
75. Lipowski ZJ: Review of consultation psychiatry and psychosomatic medicine. I. General principles. *Psychosom Med* 29:153, 1967.
76. Lipowski ZJ: Review of consultation psychiatry and psychosomatic medicine. II. Clinical aspects. *Psychosom Med* 29:201, 1967.
77. Lipton EL, Steinschneider A. Richmond JB: The autonomic nervous system in early life. *N Engl J Med* 273:147, 1965.
78. Lukianowicz N: "Body image" disturbances in psychiatric disorders. *Br J Psychiatry* 113:31, 1967.
79. Maclay I: The "functional" medical outpatient. *Br J Psychiatry* 111:34, 1965.
80. MacLean PD: Psychosomatics, in Field J (ed): *Handbook of Physiology.* Washington, DC, American Physiology Society, 1960, section 1, vol 3.

81. McCleary AR, Moore RY: *Subcortical Mechanisms of Behavior.* New York, Basic, 1965.
82. McDermott JF Jr., Finch, SM: Ulcerative colitis in children: Reassessment of a dilemma. *J Am Acad Child Psychiatry* 6:512, 1967.
83. Meissner WW: Family dynamics and psychosomatic processes. *Fam Process* 5:142, 1966.
84. Mendel WM: Psychiatric consultation education—1966. *Am J Psychiatry* 123:150, 1966.
85. Mendelson M, Hitsch S, Webber MA. A critical examination of some recent theoretical models in psychosomatic medicine. *Psychosom Med* 18:363, 1956.
86. Meyer E: The psychosomatic concept, use and abuse. *J Chron Dis* 9:298, 1959.
87. Miller JG: Living systems: Basic concepts. *Behav Sci* 10:193, 1965.
88. Miller MH, Greenfield NS: Body image: The value of a psychiatric construct in medical practice. *AP-DT* 10:447, 1959.
89. Mirsky AI: Physiologic, psychologic, and social determinants in the etiology of duodenal ulcer. *Am J Dig Dis* 3:285, 1958.
90. Mirsky AI: Psycho-physiological basis of anxiety. *Psychosomatics* 1:1, 1960.
91. Mirsky AI: The psychosomatic approach to the etiology of clinical disorders. *Psychosom Med* 19:424, 1957.
92. Moos RH: Personality factors associated with rheumatoid arthritis: A review. *J Chron Dis* 17:41, 1964.
93. Mordkoff AM, Parsons OA: The coronary personality: A critique. *Psychosom Med* 29:1, 1967.
94. Mutter AZ, Schleifer MJ: The role of psychological and social factors in the onset of somatic illness in children. *Psychosom Med* 28:333, 1966.
95. Neurophysiology and psychosomatic research. *J Psychosom Res* 9:5, 1965.
96. Nichols DC, Tursky B: Body image, anxiety, and tolerance for experimental pain. *Psychosom Med* 29:103, 1967.
97. O'Connor JF, Daniels G., Karush A, Flood C, Stern, LO: Prognostic implications of psychiatric diagnosis in ulcerative colitis. *Psychosom Med* 28:375, 1966.
98. O'Connor JF, Stern LO: Symptom alternation. *Arch Gen Psychiatry (Chicago)* 16:432, 1967.
99. Oken D: The role of defense in psychological stress. in Roessler R, Greenfield NS (eds). *Physiological Correlates of Psychological Disorder*, Madison, University of Wisconsin Press, 1962.
100. Parens H, McConville BJ, Kaplan SM: The prediction of frequency of illness from the response to separation: A preliminary study and replication attempt. *Psychosom Med* 28:162, 1966.
101. Petrie A: *Individuality in Pain and Suffering.* Chicago, University of Chicago Press, 1967.
102. Psychosphysiological aspects of cancer. *Ann NY Acad Sci* 125:773, 1966.
103. *Psychosomatic Disorders.* WHO Techn. Rep. Ser., 275, 1964.
104. Purchard PR: Some psychiatric aspects of dermatology. *Psychiat Quart* 41:280, 1967.
105. Rahe, RH, McKean JD, Arthur RJ: A longitudinal study of life-change and illness patterns. *J Psychosom Res* 10:355, 1967.
106. Rahe RH, Meyer M, Smith M, Kjaer G, Holmes TH: Social stress and illness onset. *J Psychosom Res* 8:35, 1964.
107. Reiser MF, Bakst H: Psychology of cardiovascular disorders, in *American Handbook of Psychiatry* Arieti, S (ed). New York, Basic, 1959, vol 1.
108. Rosenbaum, M, Reiser, MF: Principles of management of psychosomatic disorders. *Med Clin North Am* 42:769, 1958.
109. Rubin RT, Mandell AJ: Adrenal cortical activity in pathological emotional states: A review. *Am J Psychiatry* 123:387, 1966.
110. Rubins JL: Psychodynamics and psychosomatic symptoms, in *The Collected Award Papers*, New York, Gralnick Foundation, 1966.
111. Schilder, P: *The Image and Appearance of the Human Body*, New York, International Universities Press, 1950.
112. Schmale AH Jr, Engel GL: The giving up-given up complex illustrated on film. *Arch Gen Psychiatry (Chicago)* 17:135, 1967.
113. Schmitt FO: Molecular biology among the neurosciences. *Arch Neurol* 17:561, 1967.
114. Schur M: Comments on the metapsychology of somatization, in *The Psychoanalytic Study of the Child.* New York, International Universities Press, 1955, vol 10.

115. Shapiro AP: Psychophysiologic mechanisms in hypertensive vascular disease. *Ann Intern Med* 53:64, 1960.

116. Simmel ML: On phantom limbs. *Arch Neurol Psychiatry* 75:637, 1956.

117. Solomon GF, Moos RH: Emotions, immunity, and disease. *Arch Gen Psychiatry* (Chicago) 11:657, 1964.

118. Sontag LW: Somatopsychics of personality and body funtion. *Vita Hum* 6:1, 1963.

119. Sperling M: Transference neurosis in patients with psychsomatic disorders. *Psychoanal Quart* 36:342, 1967.

120. Spielberger CD (ed).: *Anxiety and Behavior.* New York, Academic Press, 1966.

121. Sternbach RA: *Prinicples of Psychophysiology.* New York, Academic Press, 1966.

122. Stoeckle JD, Zola IK, Davidson GE: The quantity and significance of psychological distress in medical patients. *J Chronic Dis* 17:959, 1964.

123. Szasz TS: Comments on "the definition of psychosomatic disorder." *Br J Philos Sci* 7:231, 1956.

124. Taylor BW, Litin EM, Litzow TJ: Psychiatric considerations in cosmetic surgery. *Mayo Clin Proc* 41:608, 1966.

125. Tchehov AP: A dreary story, in *Select Tales of Tchehov.* London, Chatto & Windus, 1954.

126. Thurlow JH: General susceptibility to illness: A selective review. *Can Med Assoc J* 97:1397, 1967.

127. Von Bertalanffy L: A biologist looks at human nature. *Sci Monthly* 82:33, 1956.

128. Von Bertalanffy L: The mind-body problem: A new view. *Psychosom Med* 26:29, 1964.

129. Walker N: The definition of psychosomatic disorder. *Br J Philos Sci* 6:265, 1956.

130. Wapner S, Werner H (eds): *The Body Percept.* New York, Random, 1965.

131. Weiner H: Training in psychosomatic research. *Adv Psychosom Med* 5:64, 1967.

132. Wenar C, Handlon MW, Garner AM (eds).: *Origins of Psychosomatic and Emotional Disturbances. A Study of Mother-Child Relationships.* New York, Hoeber, 1962.

133. Whitehead AN, quoted in Woodger JH: *Biological Principles,* New York, Humanities, 1967, p 157.

134. Williams RL, Krasnoff AG: Body image and physiological patterns in patients with peptic ulcer and rheumatoid arthritis. *Psychosom Med* 26:701, 1964.

135. Wisdom JO: Whole-person medicine: Psychosomatic approach or psychosomatic disorder? *Acta Psychother* 12:241, 1964.

136. Wittkower ED, Lipowski ZJ: Recent developments in psychosomatic medicine. *Psychosom Med* 28:722, 1966.

137. Wittkower ED, Solyom L: Models of mind-body interaction. *Int J Psychiatry* 4:225, 1967.

138. Woodger JH: *Biology and Language.* London, Cambridge, 1952.

139. Woodger JH: *Physics, Psychology and Medicine.* London, Cambridge, 1956.

140. Zimmer H (ed): Computers in Psychophysiology. Springfield Ill, Charles C Thomas, 1966.

Psychosomatic Medicine in a Changing Society

2

Some Current Trends in Theory and Research

The scope of psychosomatic medicine has broadened to a point where people begin to wonder what the limits of its boundaries are. A puzzled observer asks: "Has psychosomatic medicine any limits? If so, what and why? If not, has the term outlived its usefulness, being neither definable nor even describable?" These are valid questions. There is justification in talking about the *second phase* of development of our discipline,[2] one whose growing diversity makes attempts at integration difficult but necessary if we are to maintain its identity and sense of direction. This writer has formulated a comprehensive definition of psychosomatic medicine reflecting both its scientific and clinical aspects.[2] It expresses a conception of our field as one whose main goal is twofold: to strive for a unified theory of mind–body–environment interrelations; and to apply what knowledge we gain to improve the care of the sick, to help prevent some illness, and ultimately to enhance the quality of human existence. We do not need to be too concerned with sharp delimitation of the boundaries of our field. To do so might lead to premature closure on many promising lines of unorthodox thought. It would mean missing an opportunity and the intellectual challenge of constructing a unified theory from elements supplied by disparate methods of observation and explanatory systems. To meet this challenge, however, an *ecological perspective* must be added to the traditional focus of our discipline.

As Dubos[3] expressed it, "Psychosomatic medicine, concerned primarily with the causation of organic disease by mental disturbances, was an outgrowth of the enlargement of thought brought about by the Freudian revolution." He goes on to say that the observation that what happens in the mind affects the body and vice versa makes it "misleading to single out certain diseases as having psychosomatic origin.... The understanding and control of disease requires that the body–mind complex be studied in its relations to external environment." This is also the thesis of the present article. It does not call for rejection of what was achieved in the first phase of psychosomatic medicine, but stresses a broadening of the whole conception of the latter, to include environmental variables into our theoretical framework and research projects to a much greater extent than before.[4]

Reprinted from *Comprehensive Psychiatry* 14 (3):203–215, 1973. Copyright © 1973 by Grune & Stratton, Inc.

PSYCHOSOMATIC MEDICINE AND THE SOCIAL ENVIRONMENT

It is often asserted that factors inherent in the social environment are no less relevant to the well-being of individuals, to issues of health and disease, than the biological and physicochemical characteristics of the physical environment. The validity of
this assumption is being tested by research relating specific social factors to psychophysiological processes of individuals and morbidity of various social groups. This calls
for both individual-oriented and epidemiological studies. Psychosomatic medicine has
often ignored social variables. In many psychosomatic studies the main emphasis has
been on psychodynamic explanatory concepts, such as intrapsychic conflicts of the
approach–avoidance type and the related emotions; attitudes; ego defenses; and attempts
at regressive, nonverbal communication utilizing autonomic nervous pathways instead
of language and gesture. These psychological concepts have then been casually related
to particular modes of physiological dysfunction and disease. When the social environment was considered by psychosomatic investigators, it was often in a general sense
as a source of deprivation, temptation, loss, or danger, which elicits specific emotional
responses and their physiological concomitants. Further, psychosomatic research seldom ventured beyond the family environment.

Relevant explanatory hypotheses have revolved around inhibited expression of dependent needs and consequent intensification of intrapsychic conflicts over impulses
to express disavowed desires and emotions, especially aggression. This methodological approach has yielded important observations but it needs to be supplemented by
inclusion into our inquiry and theoretical formulations of the influence of a whole range
of social variables on psychophysiological processes.

We cannot view currently prevalent psychodynamic conceptions as immutable laws
of human behavior. Intrapsychic conflicts, for example, which played such a prominent role in psychosomatic hypotheses of Alexander and his followers, may well undergo significant changes under the influence of changing values and their impact on
psychological development of children. Certain impulses, sexual, dependent, or aggressive, may be losing their pejorative connotation and the consequent need for their
repression and other defenses against their intrusion into consciousness, if not their
outward expression. Thus the most often postulated unconscious approach–avoidance
conflicts may gradually cease being unconscious, and the expression of relevant impulses may lead to conscious, interpersonal conflicts, or even no conflicts at all. And
yet physiological dysfunctions and specific diseases purportedly dependent on the existence of such unresolved conflicts continue to develop with no perceptible change
in their incidence. Further, other psychosocial variables, such as approach–approach,
choice and decision conflicts,[5] value conflicts, status incongruity,[6,7] increased rate of
social change, dissonance between expectations and gratification, and a host of other
currently prevailing factors may well supersede the previously mentioned psychodynamic variables as potential sources of psychic distress, physiological dysfunction, and disease. Their influence may be expressed by nonspecific general susceptibility to any physio- and psychopathological processes. It is psychosomatic research
in all its aspects—experimental and clinical, human and animal, epidemiological as well
as that focused on unique subjective responses of individuals—which should throw light

on these questions. The foundations for this broad approach were laid in the milestones of psychosomatic literature.[8-12]

THE ECOLOGICAL DIMENSION OF PSYCHOSOMATICS

Human ecology has been defined as the study of the relations between man and his environment, both as it affects him and as he affects it.[13] To be methodologically useful, however, the ecological dimension of psychosomatics needs to be defined in more specific terms. Both physical and social environment is relevant to psychosomatic relationships in four overlapping ways: (1) as a source of stimulus and information input; (2) as an instigator of goal-directed thought and action; (3) as a source of stimuli which give rise to somatic perceptions; (4) as a source of factors which alter cerebral function and structure and thus impair adaptive capacities of the individual. Each of these four aspects may influence psychophysiological functioning of man and lead to behaviors which in turn modify the environment. There is thus a dynamic interplay in the man–environment system whose detailed study is the aim of psychosomatic research. Each of these aspects of the environment needs further elaboration for the sake of clarity.

First, environment concerns us as a source of information input in a broad sense. As Hinkle[4] states: "A meaningful hypothesis about the relation of a man to his social and interpersonal environment, and the effect of this upon his health, must take into account the *information* that he receives from this environment, and the way that he *evaluates* it" (italics mine). Thus, the key intervening variable here is a cognitive one, namely subjective *meaning*. This writer has proposed that we may distinguish four major categories of subjective meaning of perceived events, situations, and objects. They are *threat, loss, gain* (or its promise), and *insignificance*.[14] These categories are not necessarily mutually exclusive. The evaluation and meaning are both conscious and unconscious, and the two may be at variance with each other. It is especially in uncovering the unconscious meaning of information for the individual that psychoanalytic method and theory continues to play an indispensable role in psychosomatics. Threat, loss, and gain are classes of meaning of key importance for psychosomatic research and theory. They are so by virtue of their power to evoke emotional, behavioral, and physiological responses. They are also central to the concept of psychological stress and its consequences, whether desirable or pathogenic. Gain is linked conceptually with appetitive drives, hopeful anticipation, striving, pleasure, and satiety.

There are other features of information input relevant to psychosomatics. They include quantity, novelty, clarity, consistency, and attractiveness of information as experienced by its recipients. These characteristics have attracted increasing scientific interest only recently. What concerns a psychosomatic investigator is the psychophysiological effects of these variables. We are especially interested in such effects when there is personally experienced information underload or overload, when information is novel, discrepant, or ambiguous, or when it elicits appetitive drives beyond the individual's capacity for consummation. All these situations are potential sources of information-derived stress with its varied psychological and somatic components.

Second, social environment instigates activity at both cognitive and motor levels. This is the domain of interpersonal relationships, of prevalent values and norms of behavior, of competitive striving and its goals, of feedback in the form of rewards and punishments. There is a growing number of studies attempting to relate these social variables to psychophysiological responses.[15-17]

Third, environment is a source of somatic perceptions. The latter constitute an internal, somatic information input which may be endowed with personal meaning. From then on the four categories of meaning mentioned earlier come into play.

Fourth and last, environmental factors may cause changes in the biological substrate of psychic processes and thereby alter a person's habitual modes of perceiving, thinking, and feeling. This is a class of environmental factors which may influence psychosomatic relationships *without* the interposition of symbolic stimuli.

Application of this schema to a concrete example of an important contemporary problem may help to clarify it further. Let us consider pollution of the physical environment. It may affect individuals and be relevant to psychosomatics in the following ways: First, it gives rise to social communications which alert individuals to the noxious aspects of pollution and may make them view the environment as personally threatening. The alerted subject may then notice and interpret certain sensory cues, such as color of the water or smell of the air, as subjectively meaningful danger signals. These in turn may make him view his physical environment as alien and potentially lethal. It should be feasible to design research to determine how this type of information affects individuals psychologically and physiologically. Second, information about pollution leads to the formulation of values, norms, and problem-solving actions related to the quality of the environment as well as to relevant social interactions, cooperative or hostile. Third, noxious biological, chemical, or physical pollutants may cause tissue changes. These in turn may give rise to somatic perceptions, e.g., of impaired breathing or diarrhea, which become endowed with symbolic meaning in terms of the categories described above. Such a meaning may be both conscious and unconscious and evoke emotional responses with their physiological concomitants, thus giving rise to more somatic perceptions which in turn may be interpreted as threatening. This is an example of positive feedback which magnifies the emotional response to the original somatic perception. Fourth, some pollutants may bring about changes in the physicochemical milieu of the brain and alter its function.

It is clear that each of these aspects of pollution may affect a person's psychophysiological functioning and the study of the effects of pollution on humans would be incomplete if any of these aspects was ignored. This may serve as a paradigm of the psychosomatic approach to certain aspects of the physical environment, or of the ecological dimension of psychosomatics.

SOME RELEVANT SOCIAL VARIABLES

INFORMATION INPUTS

It is difficult to demarcate sharply the social and nonhuman environment since the latter is increasingly modified and shaped by human activity. As the above example of environmental pollution illustrates, man-made influence on the environment results in symbolic and physical stimuli both of which, though by means of different pathways, may result in psychological and physiological changes. Our primary concern in this section is with the *symbolic stimuli*, or *information inputs*, emanating from the social environment.

One aspect of information relevant to psychosomatics is *quantity* of information or stimulus input. Of more particular interest are conditions of information underload and overload because of their potentially detrimental psychophysiological effects. A great deal has been learned about such effects of information underload, usually referred to as sensory deprivation. Knowledge about its effects has been admirably summarized in a volume edited by Zubek.[18] One of the major theoretical formulations attempting to account for the phenomena of sensory underload and overload is Zuckerman's theory of *optimal level of stimulation*.[19] The key postulate of this theory asserts that every individual has characteristic optimal levels of stimulation and arousal for cognitive and motor activity and positive affective tone. It follows that deviations from the optimal level for the given individual at the given point in his life cycle are likely to result in subjectively unpleasant experience and some pattern of psychophysiological derangement. These experiential, behavioral, and physiological responses may be subsumed under the term *stress*.

For some reason studies of *information overload* have lagged behind those of sensory deprivation, despite their obvious relevance to the contemporary environment in technological societies. Miller,[20] a pioneer in this field, describes mechanisms of adjustment to information input overload and suggests that it may have psychopathological consequences. He postulates, for example, that certain conditions, such as infection or trauma, may exacerbate schizophrenic symptoms as a result of lowering of channel capacity for the inflow of information, a capacity perhaps abnormally low in schizophrenics to start with. Spitz[21] proposed that surfeit of emotional stimuli in infancy might have psychopathogenic effects in later life. Ludwig[22,23] reports preliminary results of the first major research project on the effects of sensory overload on human subjects. He describes altered state of consciousness ("psychedelic" effects) in 40% or normal volunteers subjected to two and one-half hours of overload with two types of sensory input: light and sound. These findings seem to support Lindsey's earlier assumption of common factors in sensory deprivation, distortion, and overload.[24] What is still missing is the study of selected physiological variables, along with the behavioral and experiential ones, in states of sensory overload. Experiments in which rats were exposed to intense sound, light, and motion stimuli ("stressors") consistently produced significant increases in systolic blood pressure, hypertrophy of the left ventricle, and evidence of hyperfunction of the adrenal cortex.[25] Relevance of these findings for humans is unknown.

A most recent contribution to this field is a study of Gottschalk et al.[26] It differs in details of design and psychological indices used from Ludwig's study, but it also purports to investigate the effects of visual and auditory stimulus overload on humans. The significant findings include increase in social alienation—personal disorganization scores and cognitive impairment after exposure to overstimulation. The cognitive impairment correlated with preexposure field dependence scores suggesting greater susceptibility of field-dependent subjects to cognitive disorganization under sensory overload.

Both Ludwig and Gottschalk et al., refer to their respective experiments as involving "sensory overload." This term raises the question of the difference, if any, between concepts of stimulus and information overload, respectively. The former concept implies quantity, the latter, meaning. It is questionable, however, if any type, intensity, or patterning of sensory stimuli is anything but variation of information input. Even apparently "meaningless" stimuli, such as white noise or colored lights, may and apparently do evoke associative thoughts and images in the subject and are, in this sense, personally meaningful information, however idiosyncratic the latter may be. This view made the writer include this experimental work under the heading "information overload." The terms "information" and "stimulation" have been used interchangeably here.

The potential importance of this budding shield of inquiry lies in its relevance to environmental psychology, especially problems of urban environment. The latter has been stated to constitute "a continuous set of encounters with overload, and of resultant adaptations."[27] There are other situations where at least some individuals will experience overload. They include overcrowding,[28] driving conditions,[28] certain occupations,[28] exposure to various communication media, etc. Experimental animal research on the effects of crowding led Welch[29] to propose a theoretical principle related conceptually to that derived from work on sensory deprivation: that every environment exerts its own characteristic *mean level of stimulation* which is largely determined by social interaction and emotional involvement. The mean level is reflected in reticular activation and endocrine secretions, and influences the animal's resistance to disease.[29]

Cassel,[30] reviewing epidemiological studies of human populations, suggests that increased population density enhances the importance of the social environment as a source of stimuli which evoke physiological responses influencing general susceptibility to disease. Quality of social interactions and position within the group seem to be important, in addition to the sheer quantity and novelty of stimuli.

We thus have converging lines of evidence which may be tentatively summed up in the following hypotheses:

1. Each individual is characterized by an *optimum level* of stimulus or information input which he can tolerate and process. This level may fluctuate over time and a person's life-cycle.

2. Each individual has a for him characteristic and enduring stimulus or information *need*. This need acts as motivational factor in seeking or avoiding (or oscillation between both) a stimulus level which is consonant with pleasure. There is some evidence that this need is greater in extroverts than introverts.[31]

3. Each social environment is characterized by the *mean level* of stimulation which will affect different individuals according to their individual stimulus tolerance and need.

4. Extreme deviations of stimulus input result in excessive autonomic and cortical arousal leading to cognitive disorganization, unpleasant feelings, and objective

decrement in cognitive and/or motor performance. This state is a form of *psychological stress*, one elicited by excess or deficiency of symbolic stimuli.

5. Contemporary technological society provides numerous opportunities for arousal of stimulus need, its satisfaction, as well as for information overload.

6. Such repeated or sustained arousal may lead to physiological changes as well as behaviors enhancing the subject's general *susceptibility to illness*. The specific form and severity of the latter will be codetermined by intraindividual specific somatic vulnerability as well as current environmental noxae.

These hypotheses await testing through multidisciplinary research. The question of their validation has obvious social and clinical relevance. One notes, however, that investigators often cultivate their respective gardens while ignoring what goes on outside their territorial fence. There is a host of studies pertaining to the tolerance of and need for stimulation from early infancy to old age which await meaningful conceptual integration.

Korner[32] summarizes observations on neonates which reveal individual differences in the responsiveness to and synthesis of sensory stimuli. Thus some infants readily become overwhelmed by overstimulation unless a mothering person provides a "stimulus barrier." Others, by contrast, display high sensory thresholds to all sensory stimuli and need a great deal of stimulation for optimal development. Korner postulates that the most enduring characteristics of an individual derive from his capacity to cope with sensory stimuli and his individual stimulus needs. She proposes that there are two basic regulatory strategies for dealing with overstimulation: one aimed at diminishing the sensory input; the other employing motor or affective discharge and experiencing strong excitation as ego-syntonic. These two basic coping strategies are linked to specific ego defenses and cognitive styles which may be regarded as their enduring characterological derivatives. These basic stimulus needs and coping styles may be reflected in later life in behavioral dispositions referred to as stimulus-seeking,[33] reducing or augmenting sensory inputs,[33] impulsiveness or reflectiveness, field dependence or independence, as well as optimal level of stimulation. These individual differences may also codetermine the modes in which different subjects *cope* with stimulus or information overloads.[34,35] What remains to be investigated is the physiological responses which accompany these different modes of coping with overstimulation and their relevance, if any, to general or specific disease susceptibility. This may well emerge as a major task of psychosomatic research in the coming years.

It may be argued that the concept of quantity of information is more cogent for engineering than psychology. When applied to humans, quantity of information can hardly be teased away from its other attributes, especially the *meaning* of information for the recipient as well as its novelty, consistency, etc. Thus when we talk of informational underload and overload we must consider the effects of these latter characteristics in addition to sheer quantity. They will be discussed briefly.

Novel stimuli induce the orienting reaction. According to Sokolov[36] this reaction includes numerous autonomic arousal responses, such as dilated pupils, increased blood supply to the head, respiratory irregularity, etc. One may postulate that there is an optimal level for such arousal and that its excess is stressful. Inconsistency or ambiguity of information may reflect social change or, more specifically, the spread of discrepant values and guidelines for choice and action. There is some experimental evidence that inconsistent or conflicting information may have a high physiologically arousing potential.[16] Prevalent values influence people's expectations, goals, and striving. They influence the quality of interpersonal relationships and have a decisive effect on which social events and situations will mean threat, loss, or gain, achievement or failure, for the individual, and thus partly determine the psychophysiologic response to information received or action undertaken. Toffler[37] gives an outspoken account of the current value crisis in technological societies and the related choice and decision conflicts. The latter are closely related to this writer's theory of *attractive stimulus overload*.[5] The concept of "attractiveness" in this context refers to the capacity of information to arouse an appetitive state and approach tendencies in the recipient. It is postulated that attractive information overload is a hallmark of affluent societies with pervasive social, psychological, and, one may predict, physiological consequences. On the one hand there is an overabundance of information and stimuli arousing desire for consummation, at both material and symbolic levels. The surfeit coupled with a wide range of available options for choice as well as discrepant value systems results in approach–approach and decision conflicts. Several behavioral coping strategies with this predicament have been described.[34] They are aimed at avoidance or reduction of stimulation, or are ceaseless, repeated attempts at approach and consummation. The poor exposed to this form of overload are aroused and expectant but unable to approach the proffered attractive goals for economic reasons and are frustrated. Those endowed with the economic means are often hampered by psychological and temporal limitations for approach behavior and consummation. For them, the decision and choice conflicts are a potential source of frustration and discontent. These hypothetical formulations await experimental validation through psychosomatic research. The only relevant study to date is Masserman's experiment.[38] He subjected normal monkeys to increasingly difficult choices between nearly equally desirable food. After 10 days in the difficult-choice situation, the animals developed neurotic disturbances, such as tics, agitation, distractibility, and destructiveness. These effects were similar to those induced by aversive conflicts.

SOCIAL CHANGE AND HEALTH

Dubos[3] asserts that social change may be a cause of disease and that prevalent chronic neoplastic and degenerative diseases are "diseases of civilization," in some way related to affluence. This is a vague generalization whose validity may only be tested by identifying and studying those social factors which can be related to social change in specific areas of living and linked causally to affluence. Hypotheses presented above are an attempt at just such identification of some relevant social variables. Three major research approaches attempting to relate social factors to morbidity have employed *epidemiological*, *psychodynamic* (individual), and *experimental animal* approaches, respectively. These approaches are complementary rather than mutually exclusive.

Representative examples of these studies are provided by the work of Hinkle, Holmes, Rahe, and others on the relation between life change and general susceptibility to disease;[39,40] the work by Engel, Schmale, and their collaborators on the giving-up–given-up complex as a common setting for the onset of any illness[41]; and the studies by Henry et al., of effects of social stimulation on hormonal and cardiovascular functions in mice.[42] One may argue that the former two types of study reflect the impact of the social environment on the individual's value system and his consequent evaluation of life events which are, in part at least, an expression of his interaction with, subjective evaluation of, and his coping with his social environment. The informational feedback from the social environment has a crucial influence on man's setting of his goals, definition of his social role and status, his actual behavior, and his evaluation of himself and his actions. These factors are closely related to subjective meaning of social events, to what constitutes social stress,[43] to status integration,[6] and other social variables whose causal relationship to affective response, physiological dysfunction, and disease has been postulated. Reviews of the role of these factors in two prevalent causes of morbidity and mortality, i.e., essential hypertension[44] and coronary heart disease,[7] illustrate this. One may postulate, for example, that particular personality dispositions leading to a behavior pattern characterized by upward social mobility and ceaseless striving in a competitive environment offering an overabundance of options and incentives for striving may represent a constellation of psychosocial factors conducive to the development of coronary artery disease.

THE ROLE OF MEDIATING PHYSIOLOGICAL MECHANISMS

How do social stimuli and the psychological responses to them disturb homeostatic mechanisms of the human organism? What are the physiological pathways which intervene between symbolic stimuli and changes in body cells, tissues, and organs? In other words, by what mechanisms does the information input from the environment bring about somatic changes which may contribute to the development of disease?

These questions are the subject of research cutting across many biological disciplines. Until the above questions are answered, psychosomatic hypotheses will remain only plausible guesses. Yet progress is evident in this difficult area, one which has come to occupy the center of the stage in current psychosomatic research. It would be beyond the scope of this article to summarize the vast number of relevant studies. Only the most prominent and promising lines of investigation will be referred to.

The most intensive research activity has centered on neuroendocrine mechanisms, especially the role of the hypothalamus, reticular activating system, the limbic system, and the pituitary–adrenal axis. The reader is referred to relevant comprehensive reviews.[45-54] Solomon has pursued promising research on the influence of psychological stress on immune reactions.[52] A relationship between social class and achievement and striving for it on the one hand and serum urate levels on the other, has been proposed.[53]

The majority of the studies in question have focussed on physiological correlates of stress and emotion, Both these constructs are not free of ambiguity, although Lazarus must be credited with bringing some order into semantic chaos surrounding them.[54] Of particular interest to our thesis that symbolic stimuli may affect physiological functions is the finding that those stimuli which are subjectively stressful can be discriminated on the basis of EEG tracings.[55]

AN ATTEMPT AT INTEGRATION

An appropriately sceptical and cautious viewpoint widely held among psychosomatic researchers is that to attempt integration of psychosomatic relationships at this stage is both premature and doomed to failure. There is yet a cogent argument that such attempts, however inadequate and tentative they may be, are of value as they point to meaningful relationships not noticed before and pinpoint gaps in our knowledge which stimulate further research. Without theorizing, our field could hardly advance and would likely disintegrate into a mass of unrelated observations and hypotheses. Thus, its potential for developing a unified theory of human behavior as well as its clinical applicability would be impeded. The following attempt at an integrative summary of the preceding discussion may serve as a conceptual framework, tentative and incomplete, bringing together the psychosomatic and ecological dimensions of human psychobiology.

Man's social environment is a source of symbolic stimuli, that is, events and situations which impinge on individuals as information. The latter is processed at the psychological level of organization and endowed with subjective meaning, conscious and unconscious. The nature of the meaning is determined by the person's individual characteristics, innate and learned, enduring and current. Depending on the way in which information is evaluated by the subject, it sets off affective and psychomotor responses as well as physiological changes which provide feedback modifying the cognitive processes whereby information is evaluated. These activities are studied by psychological observation methods and expressed in statements, descriptive and theoretical, couched in the language of psychology, the person language. All these processes are subserved by the activity of the central nervous system. External stimuli undergo screening at the level of the reticular activating system which serves an arousing function for cerebral cortex and prepares it for reception of specific stimulus input and its processing. Some of the incoming stimuli may set off impulses transmitted from the cell assemblies in the reticular activating system to the limbic system and the hypothalamus, and by activating these structures bring about emotional and autonomic arousal. The latter results in affective tone as well as neuroendocrine activities which lead to a homeostatic change whose pattern is partly determined by individual and partly by stimulus-bound response specificity. Affective and autonomic arousal appears to be achieved by both cortical and subcortical activity which function as an intergrated whole. A symbolic stimulus may thus lead to affective and physiological changes both through evaluative, cognitive processes of the cerebral cortex, and by the direct outflow of impulses from the reticular activating system to neural structures controlling all bodily processes. The pattern of physiological changes induced by the central nervous system's integrative activity may give rise to somesthetic perceptions, that is feedback which in turn augments or inhibits the activity of cortical and subcortical neural structures. The result at the psychological level of abstraction involves modification of the information processing, planning of action, and readiness for and direction of the manifest behavior. The somesthetic perceptions elicited by the motor and secretory activity provide somatic information input which may be endowed with any of the subjective meanings mentioned before. Both external and somatic information inputs are evaluated in the light of individual's accrued learning, his values, goals, and motives. These contribute the third information input in the form of memories, imagery, fantasies, and directed throughts. The outcome of the processing of these information inputs, their respective subjective meanings, and related affective concomitants is a pattern of physiological arousal mediated by neuroendocrine regulating mechanisms. If such an arousal exceeds, by virtue of its intensity and/or duration, the person's adaptive capacity, then a state of general susceptibility to illness may ensue. This state may be viewed as the final common path for psychological stress. Whether an illness follows and what form it takes will then depend on additional factors, inherent in the person and his environment. These factors include specific individual predisposition, innate or acquired, to respond with dysfunction of a given organ or tissue as well as on the presence of physical, chemical, or biological noxae within the organism or impinging on it from outside. An additional set of determinants includes the effectiveness of the subject's psychobiological defense mechanisms and the degree of support he receives from his social milieu. If biological, psychological, and social defenses and supports fail, or the individual engages in behavior increasing his illness susceptibility, an organismic state called disease follows. The latter implies failure of adaptive capacity at some level of organization from the molecular to the symbolic. Once disease develops, a new set of psychosocial and physiological processes is set into motion which influence the course and outcome of every disease. It is at this point that a comprehensive diagnosis and management which take cognizance of the patient's psychological, social, and biological liabilities, strains, and strengths may be applied in the service of optimal recovery and rehabilitation.

The task of psychosomatic medicine is threefold: First, to break down the enormous complexity of the above processes into conceptually tractable and researchable interrelationships among selected social, psychological, and biological variables. This is an analytic approach. Second, to integrate the diverse elements of empirical knowledge to formulate higher-order generalizations about environment–mind–body transactions. This is a synthetic approach. And third, to translate the knowledge so gained into guidelines for clinical action: preventive, therapeutic, and rehabilitative. This is the applied, practical approach of direct relevance to medicine. Neither of these three approaches can be dispensed with if psychosomatic medicine is to remain a viable and practically useful field of knowledge.

CONCLUSIONS

This article continues the series of papers in which the writer has attempted to delineate salient issues in contemporary psychosomatic medicine: investigative, clinical, and theoretical.[2,14,56-58] The focus of the present paper is on a relatively neglected aspect of the field, one which may be called its *ecological dimension*. More specifically, a set of postulates is put forth to underscore the various aspects of information or stimulus overload as a class of variables linking conceptually man's social environment with his psychophysiological functioning. Information is seen as a heuristically useful concept for psychosomatic formulations and research on the impact of social events and change on psychological and physiological processes codetermining health and illness. It is a tentative attempt to add a new perspective to psychosomatic theory and integrate it into the main body of its hypotheses relating the psychological and biological factors whose interplay determines human behavior and functions at all levels of organization, from the molecular to the symbolic. No claim is made that information is the only relevant variable. The author does assert, however, that it helps to identify specific aspects of our social environment and lends itself to formulation of testable hypotheses. Their ultimate result is hoped to lead to guidelines for practical action aimed at prevention of some potentially pathogenic aspects of a technological society which exert their effects on the individuals through the medium of symbolic, man-made stimuli.

SUMMARY

This article formulates the ecological dimension of psychosomatic medicine and stresses its indispensability for a comprehensive conception and further development of the latter. Special emphasis is laid on various aspects of information input overload as a paradigm of current social change relevant to psychophysiological functioning of individuals in technological societies and to issues of health and disease. An attempt is also made to outline a comprehensive theoretical framework integrating growing diversity of trends in research, experimental and clinical, pertinent to the central concern of psychosomatics: the interrelationships of psychological, biological, and social variables as they influence health and disease. It is argued that this integrationist approach enhances the dual social role of psychosomatics: to strive for a unified theory of man in a changing social environment, and to work out practical guidelines for preventive and remedial action applicable to medical practice.

REFERENCES

1. Spaulding WB: Psychosocial aspects of physical illness, in Lipowski ZJ (ed): *Advances in Psychosomatic Medicine*. Basel, Karger, 1972, vol VIII.
2. Lipowski ZJ: New perspectives in psychosomatic medicine. *Can Psychiat Assoc J* 15:515, 1970.
3. Dubos R: *Man, Medicine, and Environment*. New York, Praeger, 1968.
4. Hinkle LE: Ecological observations of the relation of physical illness, mental illness, and the social environment. *Psychosom Med* 23:298, 1961.
5. Lipowski ZJ: The conflict of Buridan's ass or some dilemmas of affluence: The theory of attractive stimulus overload. *Am J Psychiatry* 127:273, 1970.
6. Dodge DL, Martin WT: *Social Stress and Chronic Illness*. Notre Dame, Indiana, University of Notre Dame Press, 1970.

7. Jenkins DC: Psychologic and social precursors of coronary disease. *N Engl J Med* 284:244, 1971.
8. Alexander F: *Psychosomatic Medicine.* New York, Norton, 1950.
9. Grinker RR: *Psychosomatic Research.* New York, Norton, 1953.
10. Wolff HG: *Stress and Disease.* Springfield, Ill, Charles C Thomas, 1953.
11. Engel GL: Selection of clinical material in psychosomatic medicine. *Psychosom Med* 16:368, 1954.
12. Mirsky, AI: The psychosomatic approach to the etiology of clinical disorders. *Psychosom Med* 19:424, 1957.
13. Rogers ES: *Human Ecology and Health.* New York, Macmillan, 1960.
14. Lipowski ZJ: Psychosocial aspects of disease. *Ann Intern Med* 71:1197, 1969.
15. Leiderman HP, Shapiro D (eds): *Psychobiological Approaches to Social Behavior.* Stanford, Calif, Stanford University Press, 1964.
16. Shapiro D, Crider A: Psychophysiological approaches in social psychology, in Lindzey G, Aronson E: *The Handbook of Social Psychology,* ed 2. Reading, Mass., Addison-Wesley, 1969.
17. Shapiro D, Schwartz GE: Psychophysiological contributions to social psychology. *Ann Rev Psychol* 21:87, 1970.
18. Zubek JP, (ed): *Sensory Deprivation.* New York, Appleton-Century-Crofts, 1969.
19. Zuckerman M: Theoretical formulations, in Zubek JP (ed): *Sensory Deprivation.* New York, Appleton-Century-Crofts, 1969, pp 407–432.
20. Miller JG: Information input overload and psychopathology. *Am J Psychiatry* 116:695, 1960.
21. Spitz RA: The derailment of dialogue: Stimulus overload, action cycles, and the completion gradient. *J Am Psychoanal Assoc* 12:752, 1964.
22. Ludwig AM: "Psychedelic" effects produced by sensory overload. Read at the 124th annual meeting of the American Psychiatric Association, Washington, DC, 1971.
23. Ludwig AM: Self-regulation of the sensory environment. *Arch Gen Psychiatry* 25:413, 1971.
24. Lindsey DB: Common factors in sensory deprivation, sensory distortion and sensory overload, in Solomon P et al (eds): *Sensory Deprivation.* Cambridge, Mass, Harvard University Press, 1965.
25. Smookler HH, Buckley JP: Effect of drugs on animals exposed to chronic environmental stress. *Fed Proc* 29:1980, 1970.
26. Gottschalk LA, Haer JL, Bates DE: Changes in social alientation, personal disorganizaton and cognitive-intellectual impairment produced by sensory overload. *Arch Gen Psychiatry* 27:451, 1972.
27. Milgram S: The experience of living in cities. *Science* 167:1461, 1970.
28. Carson DH, Driver BL: An environmental approach to human stress and well-being: With implications for planning. Mental Health Research Institute, The University of Michigan, July, 1970.
29. Welch BL: Psychophysiological response to the mean level of environmental stimulation: A theory of environmental integration. Symposium on Medical Aspects of Stress in the Military Climate. Washington, DC, Walter Reed Army Institute of Research, 1964.
30. Cassel J: Health consequences of population density and crowding, in National Academy of Sciences: *Rapid Population Growth.* Baltimore, Johns Hopkins Press, 1971, pp. 462–478.
31. Elliott CD: Noise tolerance and extraversion in children. *Br J Psychol* 62:375, 1971.
32. Korner AF: Individual differences at birth: Implications for early experience and later development. *Am J Orthopsychiatry* 41:608, 1971.
33. Sales SM: Need for stimulation as a factor in social behavior. *J Personal Soc Psychol* 19:124, 1971.
34. Lipowski ZJ: Surfeit of attractive information inputs: A hallmark of our environment. *Behav Sci* 16:467, 1971.
35. Miller JG: Psychological aspects of communication overloads, in Waggoner RM, Carek DJ (eds): *International Psychiatry Clinics: Communication in Clinical Practice.* Boston, Little, Brown, 1964.
36. Sokolov YN: *Perception and the Conditioned Reflex.* New York, Macmillan, 1963.
37. Toffler A: *Future Shock.* New York, Random House, 1970.
38. Masserman J: The effect of positive-choice conflicts on normal and neurotic monkeys. *Am J Psychiatry* 115:481, 1963.
39. Rahe RH: Subjects' recent life changes and their near-future illness susceptibility, in Lipowski ZJ (ed): *Psychosocial Aspects of Physical Illness, Advances in Psychosomatic Medicine,* Basel, Karger, vol VIII, 1972.
40. Wyler AR, Masuda M, Holmes TH: Magnitude of life events and seriousness of illness. *Psychosom Med* 33:115, 1971.

41. Schmale AH: Giving up as a final common pathway to changes in health, in Lipowski ZJ (ed): *Psychosocial Aspects of Physical Illness, Advances in Psychosomatic Medicine*. Basel, Karger, vol VIII, 1972.

42. Henry JP, Meehan JP, Stephens PM: The use of psychosocial stimuli to induce prolonged systolic hypertension in mice. *Psychosom Med* 29:408, 1967.

43. Levine S, Scotch NA (eds): *Social Stress*. Chicago, Aldine, 1970.

44. Henry JP, Cassel JC: Psychosocial factors in essential hypertension. *Am J Epidemiol* 90:171, 1969.

45. Black P (ed): *Physiological Correlates of Emotion*, New York, Academic Press, 1970.

46. Levi L (ed): *Society, Stress and Disease*. London, Oxford University Press, 1971.

47. Mason JW: A review of psychoendocrine research on the pituitary-adrenal cortical system. *Psychosom Med* 30:576, 1968.

48. Mason JW: A review of psychoendocrine research on the sympathetic-adrenal medullary system. *Psychosom Med* 30:631, 1968.

49. Mason JW: "Over-all" hormonal balance as a key to endocrine organization. *Psychosom Med* 30:791, 1968.

50. Teichner WH: Interaction of behavioral and physiological stress reactions. *Psychol Rev* 75:271, 1968.

51. Wolf S: Emotions and the autonomic nervous system. *Arch Intern Med* 126:1024, 1970.

52. Solomon GF, Moos RH: Emotions, immunity and disease: a speculative theoretical integration. *Arch Gen Psychiatry* 11:657, 1964.

53. Mueller EF, *et al*: Psychosocial correlates of serum urate levels. *Psychol Bull* 73:238, 1970.

54. Lazarus RS: *Psychological Stress and the Coping Process*. New York, McGraw-Hill, 1966.

55. Berkhout J, Walter DO, Adey RW: Alterations of the human electroencephalogram induced by stressful verbal activity. *Electroenceph Clin Neurophysiol* 27:457, 1969.

56. Lipowski ZJ: Review of consultaiton psiciatry and psychosomatic medicine, I. General principles. *Psychosom Med* 29:153, 1967.

57. Lipowski ZJ: Review of consultation psychiatry and psychosomatic medicine, II. Clinical aspects. *Psychosom Med* 29:201, 1967.

58. Lipowski ZJ: Review of consultation psychiatry and psychosomatic medicine, III. Theoretical issues. *Psychosom Med* 30:395, 1968.

Sensory and Information Overload 3
Behavioral Effects

One of the most pervasive and novel characteristics of life in technologically advanced societies is the growing prevalence of conditions of sensory and informational overloads. Even though this assertion seems self-evident, or perhaps because of it, little systematic effort has been made to examine its empirical basis and to attempt theoretical integration of the diverse lines of research and hypotheses that apply the explanatory concepts of sensory and information overload. Yet these concepts reflect profound changes in the environment in which we live and their impact on the quality of life, on subjective experience, on individual and social behavior, and on human health and disease. Urbanization, crowding, noise, mass media of communication, revolution in information technology, explosive growth of printed data, conditions of work—these are the major factors that are transforming man's sensory environment. Some of the sensory input that bombards him consists of symbolic stimuli intended as messages and meaningful communication. Some represents physical stimuli, such as noise, which are by-products of technological development and are devoid of informational content. For the purpose of this discussion I shall follow the distinction between *information inputs*, connoting symbolic stimuli on the one hand, and *sensory inputs*, which refer to physical stimuli that do not consist of messages, on the other. Overstimulation, or overload, may result from the excess and other attributes of both symbolic and physical stimuli.

Paradoxically, the much less commonly encountered and practically less important opposite conditions, those of perceptual and sensory deprivation, have given rise to a massive research effort and theorizing. Ingenious experiments carried out by Hebb and his co-workers at McGill University between 1951 and 1954 proved to be methodologically fertile.[1] Reduced and/or monotonous environmental stimulation has evoked in some experimental subjects a set of symptoms including illusions and hallucinations, mostly in the visual sphere; impairment of attention and directed thinking; emotional disturbances, notably anxiety; feelings of unreality; delusions of persecution; increased suggestibility, etc. Numerous explanatory hypotheses have been put forth to accout for these phenomena.[1] Lindsley[2] proposed in 1958 that the behavioral and experiential changes encountered in states of sensory deprivation shared a common neurophysiological mechanism with those provoked by sensory distortion and overload. In each

Reprinted from *Comprehensive Psychiatry* 16(3):199–221, 1975. Copyright © 1975 by Grune & Stratton, Inc. Reprinted by permission.

of these states there would be disturbed balance of the reticular activating system of the brain stem and resulting disturbances of perception, attention, and cognitive performance. Lindsley included sensory overload in his hypothesis even though empirical support was lacking at the time. His formulation implied that psychological functioning was optimal with average levels of environmental stimulation and consequent optimal degree of central-nervous-system activation and cerebral cortical, emotional, and autonomic arousal. Research on sensory deprivation has provided some support for this theory.[1] Experimental work on sensory overload has been, unaccountably, too sparse to allow conclusions. A number of other areas of research, however, have used the concept of overload without referring to it as sensory. Despite their diversity, many unrelated studies have focused on conditions of excessive sensory stimulation and information input. These investigations and theoretical statements related to them share certain common assumptions and concepts. It is my purpose to bring together those disparate lines of inquiry and attempt their integration. As science becomes increasingly fragmented and overspecialized in response to the onslaught of data, efforts at integration become increasingly difficult but necessary. The topics to be discussed have direct relevance to conditions of modern life and should concern behavioral scientists, physicians, and literate people in general.

PROBLEMS OF DEFINITION

Every new area of behavioral research is plagued by semantic ambiguities. Rossi[3] lists 25 terms, used more or less synonymously, that refer to sensory deprivation. Similar problems face a reviewer of the literature on sensory and information overload. Information has been variously defined. Neisser[4] asserts that information is "essentially *choice*, the narrowing down of alternatives." MacKay[5] defines it as that which adds something to our model of the external world, either by introducing new features or increasing confidence in the old. He points out that a person's total state of readiness for adaptive or goal-directed activity and his expectations change when information is gained. MacKay emphasizes that the concept of meaning is inseparable from that of information. Meaning connotes subjective significance of perceived stimuli and represents a relationship between message and receipient. For Jones,[6] information implies the degree of unpredictability or randomness of a series of stimuli from the point of view of the subject. Thus information is a subjective- rather than an objective-stimulus variable. Jones distinguishes meaningful from nonmeaningful stimuli, the latter being usually presented in the form of flashes of light, simple geometric figures, brief tones, etc., which are not built of formal linguistic units or easily identifiable visual images. Mucchielli[7] proposes that the concept *information* connotes every physical influence exerted on a recipient able to retain its significance.

The human organism may be viewed as an information-processing system. The processing capacity is limited, and when it is exceeded by the stimulus input, a state of *information overload* ensues.[8] A person cannot manage within a fixed period of time to cope with more than a finite number of signals. Broadbent[9] hypothesized that the limited capacity of the nervous system to transmit and process information is protected by a selective filter. Defective functioning of this hypothetical filter has been proposed as the core psychobiological impairment in schizophrenia and will be discussed later. Man does not passively transmit incoming information, but actively selects it, adds to it, and interprets and transforms it in complex ways.[4] These cognitive activities show interindividual differences and intrapersonal variation over time. They codetermine, along with various attributes of the information or sensory input, when the state of overload is reached. The latter is not simply a function of the quantity and intensity of stimuli impinging on the person.

The term *sensory overload* connotes for some writers a state occurring in response to "intense multisensory experiences," or one in which two or more sensory modalities are stimulated at higher than normal intensity and this combination of stimuli is introduced suddenly.[2] I shall follow this narrow definition in regard to what I have referred to earlier as physical or nonmeaningful stimuli. It is clear, however, that the concepts of information and sensory overload, respectively, are not sharply delimited and do overlap.

METHODOLOGICAL APPROACHES

I shall include in this discussion several very different methodological approaches whose main common feature is the study of high or excessive levels of environmental stimulation on behavior and on certain psychophysiological variables. Such a treatment may at first appear overinclusive, but it allows integration of conceptually related investigations pursued with little or no regard for theoretically important links among them.

One may distinguish several areas of research using the concept of overload. They include both naturalistic field studies and controlled experimental situations, human and animal, which attempt to replicate various forms and aspects of naturally occurring situations in the laboratory. The following studies are considered relevant: (1) field studies of urban life, (2) studies on the effects of population density and crowding, (3) research on behavioral effects of noise, (4) studies of work and information load, (5) laboratory research on sensory overload, (6) experimental evocation of attractive-stimulus overload and related theoretical formulations, (7) studies of psychopathological conditions.

Only representative examples of the above studies will be discussed as a basis for an attempt at their theoretical integration. Relevance of this research for human behavior and health will be emphasized.

FIELD STUDIES OF URBAN LIFE

Milgram[10] has reviewed several studies of the experience of and adaptation to city life and put forth a set of hypotheses. He postulates that the concept of overload links the objective aspects of an urban social environment, such as large numbers of people and high population density and heterogeneity, with people's subjective experiences related to these demographic factors. Overload, he asserts, influences the daily life of city dwellers at the following levels: role performance, evolution of social norms, cognitive functioning, and the use of facilities. Overload induces a number of adaptive responses in the urbanites. First, they show a tendency to select and allow less time for each information input that is reflected in their dealings with other people in a perfunctory manner. Second, they evolve norms of behavior that facilitate distance, impersonality, and aloofness in social contacts. Third, city dwellers tend to develop cognitive coping strategies aimed at screening out and ignoring a large proportion of the information and sensory inputs impinging on them. Fourth, they compete ruthlessly for the limited facilities in the city, especially the usually insufficient means of transportation and the scarce space for driving, parking, etc. In sum, Milgram characterizes conditions of city life as a "continuous set of encounters with overload" of sensory and information inputs. His paper is already a classic in the growing literature on environmental psychology.

STUDIES ON THE EFFECTS OF POPULATION DENSITY AND CROWDING

This research is relevant to conditions of city life. The literature on this subject is long on speculation but short on empirical data, especially those regarding human crowding. It is important to distinguish the meaning of the terms population density and crowding, respectively. Density refers to a physical condition involving the limitation of space, while crowding connotes subjective perception of restricted space by the people confined to it. Density is a necessary, but not a sufficient, condition for the experience of crowding.[11] The latter results from an interaction of spatial, social, and personal factors and their relative intensity and modifiability. Desor[12] proposes that the experience of being crowded is equivalent to the reception of excessive social stimulation and not to a lack of space. Further, there are marked individual differences in tolerance for and response to crowding. Thus, Desor conceptualizes crowding as a form of perceptual overload, one implying a person's awareness of spatial restriction that is determined by the presence of other people.

Four major methodological approaches to the effects of crowding on behavior may be identified in the literature: animal studies, correlational surveys using census-tract data, experiments on the use of space by man, and laboratory studies of the effects of crowding on human behavior and selected physiological variables.

Calhoun's[13] elegant studies of the effects of increased population density on the behavior of rats have achieved wide publicity. Overcrowded rats showed a gamut of pathological behaviors, such as marked aggressivity, cannibalism, sexual deviation, frantic overactivity or extreme withdrawal, neglect of the young by their mothers, etc. The relevance, if any, of these studies to human behavior is dubious. Available data suggest that high human population density per se is not necessarily associated with social and behavioral pathology. More provocative are the ingenious experiments of Henry and his co-workers.[14] They demonstrated that placing mice in a population cage designed to maximize social interaction among them has resulted in pathophysiological changes. The presumably socially overstimulated mice have developed sustained hypertension, arteriosclerotic degeneration of the intramural coronary blood vessels and aorta, myocardial fibrosis, etc. The degree and persistence of blood-pressure elevation were related to the frequency and duration of the social stimuli. The overstimulated mice showed increased production of the adrenal catecholamine-synthesizing enzymes. Henry et al. have interpreted their findings as suggesting that increased and prolonged social stimulation is accompanied by emotional arousal and concomitant activation of the sympathetic–adrenal medullary as well as the pituitary–adrenal cortical neuroendocrine response patterns. Such sustained activation appears to be responsible for the observed cardiovascular pathology.

Henry and Cassel[15] propose that social stimuli that elicit repeated activation of the defense alarm response patterns may play an etiological role in human essential hypertension. According to Welch,[16] animal studies indicate that with increasing population density there is an increase in the mean level of environmental stimulation, which may reach sensory overloading. The latter results from enhanced social interaction and is accompanied by increased activity of the brainstem reticular formation leading to heightened cerebral cortical and hypothalamic activation, and subsequent increased secretion of ACTH, adrenocortical hormones, and catecholamines. These neurophysiological and neuroendocrine changes in turn influence the individual's subjective experience, observable behavior, and resistance to disease. J.C. Cassel (unpublished findings) concludes from human epidemiological studies that increased population density enhances the importance of the social environment as a source of stimuli that elicit physiological responses and increase general susceptibility to disease. Novelty, unpredictability, and subjectively perceived threatening nature of the social stimuli are important in increasing physiological arousal.

Correlational studies have focused on relationships between various actuarial measures of population density and statistical indicators of deviant behavior and disease rates.[17] Galle et al.[18] distinguish four components of density: the number of of persons per room, the number of rooms per housing unit, the number of housing units per structure, and the number of residential structures per acre. These investigators have developed the concept of interpersonal press as the type of overcrowding composed of two distinct factors: the number of persons per room and the number of rooms per housing unit. These two factors, especially the first one, are believed to influence decisively the degree of perceived social stimulation, privacy, and subjective experience of crowding. Correlational studies using the four factors of population density and several indicators of social pathology, such as juvenile delinquency, have been done in Chicago. The results indicate that the effect of population density on pathology is primarily a consequence of interpersonal press. The data further suggest that, for mortality, fertility, public assistance, and juvenile delinquency, the most important component of density is the number of persons per room.[19] Galle et al. conclude that this type of overcrowding may have a serious effect on human behavior and health, but they caution that specific knowledge about causal links, if there are any, is still lacking.

Experimental studies of the effects of crowding on human behavior are few.[17] One type of study is exemplified by the work of Desor[12] and Cozby.[19] These investigators have used scaled-down model rooms and miniature figures representing people. Experimental subjects were asked to place as many figures in the rooms as possible without overcrowding them. This method was assumed to provide a criterion of "crowded" for each subject and each type of room. Desor[12] hypothesized that varying architectural features, such as partitions, number of doors, and disparity of linear dimensions of the experimental rooms so as to reduce the overall level of social stimulation or interpersonal perception, would influence the subjects to judge a room as less crowded. The results showed that while judgments of crowding varied with space, they were also influenced by partitions, linear dimensions, and number of doors. Subjects allocated less space per person when partitions were added, when the number of doors was less, or when area was rectangular rather than square. The investigators interpreted these results as confirming their hypothesis that judgments of being crowded are controlled by the level of perceived social stimulation. Other relevant variables appeared to include the type of activity in which people are engaged in a given space and the individual differences in tolerance for crowding. Cozby,[19] using a technique modeled after Desor's, investigated the effects of these last two variables. He found that preference for a low- or high-density setting was influenced by the type of ongoing activity. High density was liked or not depending on the person's current goals and the facilitation or inhibition of their attainment by the presence of other people in the physical setting. Thus, attending a party and studying elicited opposite preferences for room density, i.e., high and low, respectively. Cozby found that the experience of being crowded was influenced by personality factors. The individual difference variable studied was "personal space," defined as the distance that subjects place between themselves and others. Close-personal-space subjects preferred a high- to a low-density setting.

In summary, human crowding is defined as an experiential state resulting from interaction of several classes of variables: (1) physical–structural, especially large numbers of people per unit of space (high density) and relative lack of physical barriers to social perceptions and interactions; (2) social, such as types of social interactions and degree of interference with ongoing activities occurring in a given unit of space; (3) psychological, notably individual differences in personal space; (4) temporal, i.e, frequency and duration of exposure to conditions of crowding.[11,17] Sensory and information overload is one way in which crowding may be conceptualized.[10,12,17] Their psychophysiological and social effects have been insufficiently studied. The available data suggest that crowding may result in subjective discomfort, social disorganization, and sustained or repeated physiological and emotional arousal that may contribute to human morbidity, especially to the prevalence of chronic cardiovascular diseases.

BEHAVIORAL EFFECTS OF NOISE

Noise, defined as any sound that is unwanted and produces unwanted effects,[20] is one of the main contributors to the sensory overload characterizing urban environments. It is estimated that the intensity of city noise in the United States doubles every 3 years.[20] Studies of nonauditory effects of environmental roise have focused on its influence on human task performance, subjective comfort, and physiological functioning.[20-22] Glass and Singer[21] have carried out a series of laboratory studies on the direct effects and aftereffects of high-intensity broad-band noise. They hypothesized that one of the necessary conditions for noise-induced performance impairment was overloading the subject—that is, providing task inputs so numerous as to inhibit adequate information processing. Further, they postulated that unpredictable noise would have more deleterious effects on performance than predictable (periodic) noise. In one experiment subjects were given a primary task as well as a subsidiary one. Noise stimuli consisted of white-noise bursts of 80 dbA transmitted to the right ear of each subject over a headphone. The predictable noise condition consisted of 9-sec bursts of noise followed by 3 sec of silence. The unpredictable noise condition consisted of noise bursts of random duration varying in ten 1-sec steps between 1 and 9 sec. Intervals of silence were also random. The results showed significantly more errors on the subsidiary task in the unpredictable noise condition. Glass and Singer[21] draw the following conclusions from their experiments: acute noise for brief periods of time does not affect man's ability to do mental and psychomotor tasks. Noise will, however, produce performance impairments when the individual works on two tasks simultaneously or must maintain vigilance. The deleterious effect is most likely to occur if the noise is experienced as unpredictable and/or uncontrollable. Thus the effects of noise on task performance appear to be related to the extent to which it interferes with some ongoing activity or when it produces disruptive cognitive overload. Tolerance for frustration, quality of proofreading performance, and ability to resolve cognitive conflict were all impaired *after* exposure to unpredictable high-intensity noise. The adverse aftereffects of unpredictable noise were reduced when subjects believed that they could terminate it and thus had control over it. The postnoise impairments may occur in spite of adaptation to noise rather than because of it. These degradations in performance may be due to an overloading of the person's information-processing capacity brought about by accumulated effects of unpredictable noise interfering with task performance. Practical implications of these experiments are suggestive: noise produced by jets, traffic, machinery, etc., is often unpredictable and uncontrollable and provides a potential source of impaired performance, discomfort, and irritability with undesirable psychosocial consequences. Significantly, Glass and Singer report their experiments in a book entitled *Urban Stress*.

The question whether frequent exposure to intense noise has harmful effects on behavior remains unresolved. Kryter[22] states that, with the exception of hearing, the psychological and physiological (arousal) responses to noise are transient and subject to adaptation and do not constitute a health hazard. Yet longitudinal behavioral studies of human subjects exposed to various levels of environmental noise are conspicuously lacking. Glass and Singer[21] propose that there is a psychic cost involved in exposure to noise despite ready adaptation to it. Many investigators have drawn attention to annoyance and increased irritability reported by people questioned about their subjective reactions to noise.[20] Sounds of high frequency are generally more annoying than those of low frequency, and so are sounds emitted randomly or at varying levels rather than unchanging ones. Studies of traffic noise indicate that a complaints of annoyance associated with exposure to it increase there are more reported symptoms, such as headache, insomnia, and nervousness.[20] Interviews with a random sample of 2130 Detroit and 496 Los Angles families indicate that machine, aircraft, and traffic sounds are usually considered noise and are a source of annoyance to about 25% of women and 30% of men.23 Reports of annoyance increase linearly with increasing noise levels above 50 db on the A scale based on a 24-hr average.[20] An earlier study showing that admission rates to a psychiatric hospital in a London borough were higher from the high-noise area close to Heathrow Airport could not be confirmed in a more recent investigation.[24] There are individual differences in noise tolerance. Extroverts have been shown to have higher levels of noise tolerance than introverts.[25]

In summary, noise is one of the main sources of sensory overload for city dwellers and for a substantial proportion of industrial workers. Behavioral effects of noise depend not only on its physical attributes, such as frequency, intensity, and intermittency, but also on the cognitive and soical aspects of the situation in which exposure to it occurs.[21] There is some evidence that feelings of annoyance and irritability are common effects of noise and a potential cause of subjective discomfort and interpersonal conflicts. These effects are likely to vary in severity in relation to individual differences in tolerance to this form of sensory overload. Long-term studies of psychophysiological effects of noise are sorely needed. Noise pollution of our environment deserves as much research and preventive action as does air and water pollution.

WORK LOAD AND OVERLOAD

Modern work methods expose many workers to information overloads. Research in this area of occupational psychology and psychophysiology has included both naturalistic field studies and laboratory experiments. Different investigators have used different terms for what seem to be overlapping, or even coterminous, variables and concepts. Widely used terms, such as work load, mental load, information load, and role overload, contribute to the semantic muddle and impede integration of this practically important area of research.

Important studies on the effects of the work environment and conditions on psychological and physiological variables have been conducted by the Institute for Social Research at the University of Michigan and are summarized by French and Caplan.[26] They use the concept of role overload as one of the key variables contributing to job stress and its undesirable effects on health. They distinguish between objective and subjective as well as quantitative and qualitative overload, respectively. Objective overload refers to the actual volume of information input that the individual is expected to process per unit time. There are two broad methods of determining the presence of objective overload: to calculate the load on the person from a logical analysis of the job, and to use the technique of the secondary task, i.e., to impose an extra task over and above his obligatory one on the subject and to assess the impairment of his performance on the extra task. The number of telephone calls to be answered, office visits to receive, or number of patients to examine in the course of a working day are the type of quantifiable indicators of objective overload. Subjective overload connotes a person's feeling and belief that he has too much work to do. Quantitative overload implies that the person has more work than he can do in a given time period. Qualitative work overload implies that the given job requires skills and knowledge exceeding those of the worker. The former type of overload appears to involve excess of information;

the latter type refers to situations in which the information input is too complex and/or novel for the person. In a national sample survey, 44% of male white-collar employees reported some degree of overload, highlighting its prevalence. A study of university professors showed that many of them suffer from a quantitative work overload that is mostly self-induced and related to achievement orientation.

Both quantitative and qualitative overload correlate with several psychological and physiological indices of stress. Overloaded subjects show increased heart rate and serum cholesterol levels; they smoke more and have more job dissatisfaction and tension as well as lower self-esteem. French and Caplan[28] point out that job dissatisfaction, elevated cholesterol and heart rate, and smoking are considered to be risk factors for development of coronary heart disease. Sales[29] has tried to replicate experimentally the state of role overload, defined as a condition in which the person is faced with a set of obligations which, taken as a set, require him to do more than he is able to in the available time. The actual experiment involved a force-pace task exceeding the subjects' processing capacity. A control group were given the same type of task but were required to carry it out at a rate well below the subjects' ability to do so. The overloaded subjects had a mean increase in blood cholesterol values during the experimental hour, but individuals who enjoyed working on the experiment, regardless of whether they were objectively overloaded or underloaded, showed a mean decrease in serum cholesterol. This work suggests that job satisfaction is a significant variable that co-determines the psychophysiological effects of a given work load.

In order to study the psychological effects of information overload per se, it is necessary to set up an analogue of the work situation in the laboratory and introduce information load as an independent variable. A number of such studies have been reported. Danev et al.[30] attempted to assess the effects of two levels of information load on psychophysiological functioning. Their experiment involved a two-choice and an eight-choice reaction task. They found that behavioral parameters rather than the physiological ones distinguished more reliably between the two levels of information load. Thus reaction time, misses, mistakes, and performance on a secondary task all reflected impaired information processing in the condition of higher information load. Ettema and Zielhuis[31] defined mental load as the amount of information handled per unit time. Their subjects were given a simple binary-choice task. High and low tones were transmitted through earphones in random order. The high tone had to be responded to by pressing a pedal with the right foot, the low tone by pressing a pedal with the left foot. Thus every signal called for a decision between two choices – a binary-choice task. As the number of signals per unit time, and hence the mental or information load, was increased, the subjects showed an increase in heart and respiratory rates and in systolic and diastolic blood pressures as well as a suppression of sinus arrhythmia. Zwaga[32] has recently criticized the mental-load model and proposed that the novelty of the experimental situation increases the subject's general level of arousal, which is then reflected in physiological indices and in impaired performance. As the experimental task is repeated, habituation occurs with decrease in the indicators of arousal. Wilkinson et al.[33] assert that many factors other than arousal level co-determine the level of performance in most situations. Incentive, novelty, and difficulty of the task as well as information load affect performance. Frankenhaeuser et al.[34] compared psychophysiological responses to understimulation and overstimulation. The latter was induced by a complex sensorimotor test requiring simultaneous capacity and involving two consecutive 90-min work periods. Overstimulated (overloaded) subjects reported irritability and unplesant feeling and showed a pronounced increase in heart rate and in the secretion of both adrenaline and noradrenaline, indicative of hightened arousal.

Miller,[8,34] a pioneer in the work on information-input overload, has developed an apparatus for the study of psychological responses to such overload and for measuring human channel capacity. The apparatus, called information overload testing aid, has been used to study performance of subjects exposed to increasing information loads. Miller described several mechanisms of adjustment to the stress of information overload. They include omission of some information under overload conditions; error, i.e., processing information incorrectly and allowing the mistake to stand; queuing, i.e., delaying responses during heavy-lead periods and catching up during lull periods; filtering or systematic omission of some items of information; approximation or giving an imprecise response; multiple channels; decentralization; and escape, either leaving the experiment or cutting off the input of information. Miller suggested that some persons, such as schizophrenics, might have a lowered channel capacity and suffer cognitive and behavioral disorganization when exposed to information-input overload of a degree with which normal people could cope by using one or more of the above adjustment mechanisms. This hypothesis has been tested by other investigators and will be discussed later.

In summary, both field and experimental studies of information-input overload suggest that it elicits autonomic arousal, impairs performance on complex tasks, and produces unpleasant subjective-feeling states. It appears that increasing the information input beyond the person's processing capacity is one of the major factors contributing to the subjectively perceived job pressure and dissatisfaction. Information overload should be a matter of serious concern for occupational health. These are reasons to believe that objective and/or subjective information-input overload has potentially deleterious consequences for job performance, for subjective sense of well-being, and for health. Laboratory studies on the effects of information load involve relatively brief exposures to overload conditions. There is evidence that such exposure results in autonomic and behavioral arousal, which with repeated exposures tends to decrease. This observation, however, tells us nothing about the long-term effects on behavior and physiological functioning of work involving information inputs that are frequently novel, complex, and excessive in amount when a person is exposed to them over months or years. It is reasonable to conjecture that repeated exposure to information-input overload, with its concomitant physiological arousal, is a potential health hazard and a suspected risk factor for the development, course, and outcome of chronic cardiovascular diseases, which are highly prevalent in technological societies.

Overcommitment

There is another interesting aspect of work overload. Some of the studies quoted earlier (those pertaining to professional workers such as the university professors) indicate that the condition of overload is by no means always imposed by factors external to the person. On the contrary, it appears that many of those who responded to relevant questionnaires with complaints about overload indicated that the latter was self-induced. French and Caplan[26] ask: "Then what induces some professors and administrators to overload themselves, to work sixty or even seventy hours per week?" They hypothesize that "achievement orientation," a tendency to engage in multiple activities and strive for success, has something to do with it. Indeed, achievement orientation correlated 0.42 with the number of hours worked per week and 0.25 with the factor score on quantitative overload. Achievement orientation is one of the cardinal features of the so-called Type-A behavior pattern, which has shown significant predictive power for the development of coronary heart disease and its complications, and for death from the latter.[35] This suggests that achievement-oriented professional workers tend to engage in self-generated activities that lead to a quantitative information overload and to related sustained periods of autonomic arousal, thus increasing the risk of developing coronary heart disease.[27,28]

One often hears complaints of "overcommitment" voiced by members of the academic community. This interesting neologism seems to reflect a novel social phenomenon that deserves systematic study. To this writer it connotes a state of role and information overload due in part to unwillingness or inability to set limits to one's pursuit of activities rewarded by approval, success, promotion, money, and other inducements that bolster self-esteem. Overcommitment seems to be brought about by interaction of personality and social factors. The social environment provides abundant opportunities and rewards for ceaseless striving. Persons who display willingness to assume more tasks and ability to cope with them may be pushed to the limits of their capacity by those who derive power and other benefits from their achievements, such as academic administrators. An individual's needs, superego demands, and values may interfere with his ability to limit his involvement. The overload is contributed to by the exponential growth of scientific information and its dissemination by information-transmitting industries. Further, the overcommitted individuals are often those who actively contribute to the glut of printed words. The subjective state of overcommitment is characterized by a feeling that one is subjected to demands that are close to, or actually exceed, one's limits of endurance and are experienced as overwhelming and exhausting. This seems to be a malaise affecting many professional workers today.

STUDIES ON SENSORY OVERLOAD

Only a handful of published studies fall into this class. Several investigators refer to their research explicitly as being concerned with sensory overload. Workers at the Tohoku University in Japan started in 1970 to publish reports on sensory-overload experiments.[36-49] In their first report they comment on the difficulties in defining sensory overload and point out that in contrast to experiments with sensory deprivation many attributes of the stimulus situation need to be taken into account in devising methods of producing the overload. These attributes include the quality, intensity, and duration of the stimuli as well as the amount of information, and the degree of change, meaning, novelty, and complexity of the stimulus input. The Tohoku workers exposed their experimental subjects to intense auditory and visual stimuli presented randomly in a condition of confinement ranging in duration from 3 to 5 hr. The subjects showed heightened and sustained arousal, found sensory overload more aversive than deprivation, and had mood changes in the direction of aggression, anxiety, and sadness. Two subjects reported visual "hallucinationlike" phenomena.

In this country, only seven published reports of sensory-overload experiments have been found by the writer.[50-56] Ludwig[50,51] has reported preliminary results of ongoing studies with sensory overload produced by intense auditory and visual stimuli for 2½ hr. Two banks of 12 150-w floodlamps of assorted colors randomly lighted provided the visual stimuli. Auditory stimulation consisted of randomly delivered unpatterned and cacophonous sounds. The subjects were confined to a soundproof air-conditioned chanber of 9 × 12 ft. About 40% of the subjects reported "mild to profound distortions in reality testing," which Ludwig refers to as "psychedelic effects." They included illusions, hallucinations, increased visual imagery, disturbed time sense, distortions of body image, and paranoid ideation. Not all subjects experienced the whole gamut of these subjective effects. More recently, Ludwig reported results of exposing chronic schizophrenic patients to his sensory-overload design.[52] In comparison to normals and nonschizophrenic psychiatric patients, schizophrenic subjects displayed greater reactivity to sensory overload, and their behavior tended to be more disorganized.

Haer[53,54] and Gottschalk et al.[55] have set out to investigate if excessive and atypical auditory and visual stimulation ("sensory overload") could evoke transient psychopathological states. The experimental design used in this series of studies resembled that employed by Ludwig. Volunteers were confined in a chamber shaped like a geodesic dome, 6 ft high and 11 ft in diameter, upon whose white-painted interior walls and ceiling a movie film was projected. The film was composed of sequences of colored abstract images, followed by pictures related to themes of birth, death, violence, etc. Auditory stimulation was provided by extremely loud sounds of electronic music. Each experiment lasted 45 min. The psychological effects were tested with the social–alienation–personal–disorganization scale, believed to measure a psychological dimension of the schizoid–schizophrenic continuum and reflecting varying degrees of withdrawal and disorganized thinking, with the rod-and-frame test of space perception, which measures the perceptual style of field dependence–independence, and the cognitive–intellectual impairment scale. The results show that exposure to this particular variant of sensory overload produced an increase in the scores on the scale of social alienation–personal disorganization as well as in the cognitive–intellectual impairment scores. These findings imply that the experience elicited some degree of brain dysfunction and a tendency toward modes of thinking and behavior associated with schizophrenia. The degree of cognitive impairment was highest in field-dependent subjects, i.e., those who are generally more influenced by the conditions of the perceptual field. People characterized by the perceptual–cognitive style of field dependence appear to be susceptible to psychological disorganization by a variety of factors that interfere with their perceptual clarity and familiarity, be it sensory or sleep deprivation, or intake of deliriogenic drugs affecting brain function. Like Ludwig's subjects, those studied by Gottschalk and Haer reported illusions, hallucinations, delusional ideas, disturbance of time sense (subjective feeling that time is slowed down), and body-image distortions.

It would be premature to generalize from these early studies that differ in the details of experimental design and methods of assessment of psychological effects. The appearance of an altered state of consciousness in some of the experimental subjects is intriguing. It appears to confirm Lindsley's[2] neurophysiological speculation and his predictions based on it. He asserted that with excessive stimulation from two or more sensory modalities "blocking of the reticular formation may occur and behavioral immobilization and general confusion may result." Yet "excessive stimulation" is a coat of many colors; it involves more than the high intensity of stimuli. Wohlwill[57] distinguishes five aspects of the sensory–deprivation–overload dimension: level, diversity, patterning, instability, and meaningfulness. Diversity, complexity, or variation of stimulation tends to enhance and maintain autonomic and affective arousal and eventually leads to fatigue and withdrawal tendencies. Oswald[58] exposed male volunteers, whose eyes were glued widely open, to simultaneous, synchronized, rhythmic electric shocks, loud rhythmic music, and strong flashing lights. All his subjects went rapidly to sleep in this condition of overstimulation. This experiment suggests that extremely monotonous stimulation in subjects required to keep still or make only rhythmic movements leads to sleep, even though the stimuli are unusually intense. Oswald proposes that the monotony of the stimulation results in cessation of arousing responses of the reticular activating system. This effect could represent habituation or inhibitory corticofugal impulses in a person unable to escape stimulation. In either case the person would be prone to associative or dreamlike mentation characteristic of states of drowsiness, dreaming, and delirium. In all these states consciousness is reduced, reality testing impaired or suspended, and cognitive processes pervaded by personally significant autistic thoughts and imagery. It is possible that a similar sequence of events occurred in the experiments with sensory overload. The experimental design used by Ludwig and Gottschalk appears to maximize variation and unpredictability of stimuli, in contrast to Oswald's experiments. Their subjects did not apparently go to sleep, but the barrage of stimuli may have resulted in protective inhibition of the reticular activating system and thus a mild state of clouded consciousness.

Wohlwill[57] suggests that diversified stimulation lacking patterned information or structure would likely overtax the person's capacity to encode information and would be a source of stress. The experiments on sensory overload reported earlier do seem to have a relatively low degree of patterning, and this feature may contribute to their disorganizing psychological effects. Further, the stimulus conditions in these experiments are characterized by much movement in the visual stimulus field requiring constant attention to and tracking of the shifting stimuli. This feature may also contribute to the stress. Finally, the stimuli employed were mostly novel and, especially in Gottschalk's experiments, potentially capable of eliciting personally meaningful and disturbing associations. This aspect could have enhanced the affective arousal of the subjects and given rise to emotionally charged imagery.

It is clear that at this early stage the interpretation of the few studies on sensory overload is difficult and their relevance to the natural conditions uncertain. Few psychophysiological studies have been carried out in the overload experiments in humans. Chronic exposure of rats to combined auditory, visual, and motion overstimulation has resulted in their developing systolic hypertension, hypertrophy of the left ventricle of the heart, and histopathologic changes indicative of hyperfunction in the adrenal cortex.[59] The relevance, if any, of these animal studies for humans is uncertain. The human experiments do suggest that several aspects of the sensory overload have disorganizing and perhaps potentially psychotogenic effects. Conditions of modern, especially urban, life provide many stimulus conditions resembling those of sensory-overload experiments, even if not equal to them in the degree of overstimulation.

ATTRACTIVE-STIMULUS OVERLOAD

Most of the studies quoted so far have focused on stimuli that were aversive by virtue of their sheer quantity and intensity, or because subjects were required to respond to them in a manner and at a high pace imposed by the experimenter. Thus there was, especially in laboratory studies, either enforced confinement and passivity or, on the contrary, explicit expectation of speedy and flawless performance on more or less complex tasks. Such experimental designs are liable to reproduce only some aspects of naturally occurring stimulus conditions and related information overload. A different situation obtains when stimuli are deliberately selected on the basis of their *attractiveness* for the recipient.

Masserman et al.[60] carried out a series of experiments with monkeys exposed to a selection of nearly equally attractive foods. Food preferences of the animals were established prior to the main experiment in which each animal was starved for about 20 hr and then required to choose between its two most favored foods displayed in opposite compartments connected with the cage and visible from it. The first 20 of these trials were given daily; the next 30 occurred twice daily, with the animals receiving small feedings to maintain motivation. The monkeys displayed hesitation, extending to the point of refusal of all food for up to 2 days. After about 10 days in the difficult-choice situation, the monkeys displayed tics, agitation, distractibility, aggressive behavior, and fewer affiliation responses to experimenters and cagemates. Their behavior became indistinguishable from that of "neurotic" monkeys in which experimental neurosis had been induced by aversive conflicts.

While the focus of these experiments was on positive-choice conflicts rather than on overstimulation, they represent a provocative paradigm of a form of stimulus overload that appears to be particularly prevalent in the affluent societies. This writer has formulated a set of hypotheses comprising a theory of attractive-stimulus overload.[61-63] Attractive stimuli or information inputs are those that arouse appetitive and approach responses and tendencies in persons on whom they impinge. Attractiveness in this context is the result of an interaction between information and its recipient and is not an independent attribute of the information as such. Overload in this context refers to a state in which a person is exposed to more attractive stimuli than he is able to choose from and/or act upon because of psychological, temporal, or economic constraints. The main psychological impediment is an inner conflict related to choice from among attractive alternatives of nearly equal strength, or the approach–approach type of conflict.[61] Economic constraints prevent many from responding to attractive stimuli by goal-directed action and consummation. The writer contends that affluent societies expose their members to an overabundance of stimuli capable of arousing appetitive arousal in many individuals. These attractive stimuli pertain to both material and symbolic goals—that is, those related to things and to activities and life styles, respectively. This form of overload is a result of an economic system striving for creation of ever-new wants, the messages disseminated by advertising and the mass media of communication that arouse appetitive tendencies and urge people to act on them, and the related value system promoting ever-new wants. People are barraged by information inputs alerting them to an almost infinite number and variety of attractive options whose attainment promises pleasurable consummation. All this is based on the unspoken and questionable assumption that people have inexhaustible capacity for appetitive arousal and related striving and consummatory behavior.

Herman Kahn recently remarked that "the miseries of the future are likely to be due to the ambiguities of wealth, rather than to the pressures of poverty.... Wealth is not necessarily good for people.[64] Dubos[65] asserts that "affluence, like poverty, can constitute a cause of disease." Others speak gloomily of the malaise of affluence: "The more we feel we must have, the smaller the chance of gratifying all our wants and the greater the possibility of great expectations making for stress, tension, and anxiety."[66] These rather vague statements do not spell out in what ways affluence could have adverse effects on psychological and physical health. I would submit that behavioral effects of attractive-stimulus overload may have undesirable consequences related to the long-term effects of repeated appetitive arousal, its psychophysiological concomitants, and the maladaptive attempts at coping with the overload. These hypotheses are based on clinical impressions and await systematic studies.

The following coping strategies for attractive-stimulus overload are postulated: First, selective unresponsivity (that is, ability to ignore the bulk of attractive-stimulus input and not to respond to it with appetitive arousal). Second, reducing the number or impact of impinging stimuli by withdrawal or avoidance, or by the intake of chemical agents that alter consciousness, narrow the perceptual field, and reduce the pressure for choice and action. Third, repeated approach and attempts at consummation. This may take many forms, from overeating or excessive smoking to restless striving for abstract goals, such as ever higher social and economic status, recognition, etc., which may induce a person to work to the limits of his physical and psychological capacities. Others engage in binges of acquisitive behavior with short-lived satiety, followed by rising appetitive tension, a sense of emptiness, and renewed striving. Fourth, passive surrender, a state characterized by relative inaction, a sense of frustration, apathy, helplessness, and boredom. The person can neither withdraw from information inputs nor manage them. He tends to feel alienated, resentful, and quick to blame others for his predicament, but he feels unable to do anything about it. Such a state is painful and may end in violent acts against others or oneself.

To sum up, it is proposed that attractive-information overload is a common state in affluent societies and has potential adverse behavioral and social effects. It is apt to result in neurotogenic intrapsychic conflicts among incompatible approach tendencies and lead to maladaptive coping strategies that may take the form of behaviors inimical to health, psychological well-being, and social order. Here may lie one of the major sources of psychological limits to economic growth. More cogent, however, is the education of children for judicious coping with an overabundance of attractive stimuli and options.

The Information-Overload Concept in Psychopathology

In the past 15 years many clinical and experimental investigators have formulated the core psychological defect of schizophrenic patients in terms of a dysfunction of information processing. Lehmann[67] contends that the basic schizophrenic flaw consists in an inability to screen out irrelevant information effectively, with the result that the patient is flooded by both exteroceptive and interoceptive stimuli. This view has been inspired by Broadbent's[9] hypothetical selective device or filter, which is one of the mechanisms by which "systematic selection of information takes place at the entrance to the limited capacity system." The schizophrenic patient is believed to have a defective filtering mechanism, which makes him susceptible to information-input overload. This susceptibility is manifested by responsiveness to irrelevant stimuli, distractibility, overinclusive thinking, and subjective experience of being overwhelmed by environmental stimuli. In acute schizophrenia, stimuli of ordinary intensity are experienced as more intense, vivid, and compelling than normally.[68] This experiental state is acute schizophrenics has been called "psychedelic"[69] and appears to be similar to than reported by some normal subjects exposed to experimental sensory overload.[50] The critical difference between these two experientially similar conditions is that in acute schizophrenic patients a state of information overload is provoked by a level of stimulation that normal people experience as ordinary. Usdansky and Chapman[70] exposed normal volunteers to a forced-paced sorting task and reported that the subjects exhibited a type of error like those of schizophrenics performing without time pressure. This experiment has been recently repeated, in a modified form, by Grimes and McGhie.[71] They had schizophrenics, nonschizophrenic psychiatric patients, and normal subjects perform a sorting test under distraction stress in the form of simultaneous responding to a binary-choice task. The performance of normal subjects and nonschizophrenic patients was not different from that of schizophrenics under normal conditions. This finding was interpreted as supporting the hypothesis that schizophrenics are more readily overloaded with information than normals, presumably because of a dysfunction at the input level of information processing. Further, nonschizophrenic individuals who do not display such a dysfunction under normal conditions may perform in a manner characteristic of schizophrenics if forced to perform at fast pace under distraction stress. It is possible that the key variable in these experiments is not the information load as such, but the *time stress* accompanying paced tasks.[72]

Silverman[68] has recently reviewed a large body of clinical and experimental evidence supporting the hypothesis of dysfunction of the sensory-filter mechanism in the central nervous system in a whole range of psychiatric disorders. He claims that various lines of research, psychological, clinical, and electrophysiological, support the presence of an information-overload condition in the schizophrenias. Various schizophrenic symptoms, such as withdrawal, thought blocking, paranoid delusions, and reduced spontaneity of movement and speech, are, according to Silverman, protective strategies to reduce the experienced information overload. The result of pheonothiazine administration is to alleviate stimulus or information overload. The response to these drugs, however, is different in paranoid and nonparanoid schizophrenics. While both groups exhibit improvement of psychotic behavior, the phenothiazine-medicated paranoid patients show decreased thought disorder and improved attention, in contrast to the nonparanoid schizophrenics, whose thought disorder becomes more pronounced and attention more impaired. Silverman asserts that nonmedicated acute paranoids are in an overstimulated state because their sensory filter is faulty and because, in contrast to nonparanoid schizophrenics, they tend to habitually augment rather than reduce sensory stimulation. Psychedelic drugs, such as LSD, heighten sensitivity to low-intensity stimulation and increase arousal. These effects are probably defended against by reduction in responsiveness comparable to that of nonparanoid schizophrenics and hypersensitive normals. Silverman hypothesizes that this is a compensatory mechanism, one of neural inhibition in the diffuse sensory system and in cortico–cortical association pathways occurring as adjustment to marked excitation in the primary sensory pathways of the brain caused by ISD.

In summary, many of the behavioral and experiential characteristics of schizophrenics and individuals intoxicated with psychedelic drugs have been hypothetically explicated as representing manifestations of information overload and attempts at coping with it. In schizophrenic patients the overload is postulated to be due to a defective sensory filtering mechanism in the central nervous system. This defect allows hypersensitivity to ordinary stimulation and an experience of being flooded by stimuli from the environment and the body. Predictably, schizophrenics show increased disorganization under conditions of experimental sensory overload.[52] These are clinical observations suggesting that the brain-damaged and the elderly may be more susceptible to information overload and its disorganizing effects on cognitive processes. It is a common clinical observation, for example, that people over 60 years of age may become delirious on admission to hospital or transfer to other unfamiliar surroundings.[73] This cognitive disorganization may be, at least in part, the result of information overload in someone whose information-processing capacity is diminished by some degree of cerebral damage that allows adequate functioning in a familiar milieu.

DETERMINANTS OF INFORMATION OR SENSORY OVERLOAD

From the practical point of view the crucial questions are: Which environmental conditions are likely to result in information overloads for most individuals? Which persons are particularly vulnerable to experience overload under average conditions of information input? The diverse studies and methodological approaches discussed so far allow tentative answers to these questions. In addition, one has to take into account observations on the individual differences in the need for and tolerance of sensory stimulation. For the sake of clarity, I will discuss separately relevant enduring personality characteristics, attributes of the sensory and information input, and situational constraints.

All classes of studies reviewed here indicate explicitly or implicitly the existence of individual differences in susceptibility to information and sensory overload. Not all subjects are equally uncomfortable; not all show the same degree of psychological dysfunction, if any, when exposed to noise, forced-paced tasks, or experimental sensory overload. Studies in psychopathology have explicitly identified classes of individuals particularly vulnerable to information overload. Silverman[68] has received studies suggesting that some "normal" people are hypersensitive, i.e., hyperresponsive to minimal-intensity stimulation. Such hypersensitivity is apparently maximal in nonparanoid schizophrenic patients. Hypersensitive individuals, normal and abnormal, show less effective performance on many complex psychological tasks. Other normals as well as psychopathic personalities and manic–depressive patients appear to be hyposensitive to stimulation.[68]

Observations of neonates reveal individual differences in the responsiveness to sensory stimuli. Some infants become readily overwhelmed by stimuli of an intensity that appears optimal and pleasurable for other infants. Korner[74] postulates that the most enduring characteristics of an individual derive from his capacity to cope with sensory stimuli and his individual stimulus needs. Her observations suggest innate differences in sensory thresholds that may determine a person's enduring perceptual style, his optimal level of stimulation needed for best performance and subjective comfort, his tendency to seek or avoid strong stimulation, and his level of information and sensory input at which overload is liable to occur.

Petrie[75] has studied individual differences in stimulus-intensity control. She proposed that each person is characterized by perceptual reactance, i.e., an automatic tendency to decrease or increase perceived intensity of stimuli. Individuals whom she calls the reducers tend subjectively to decrease what is perceived, the augmenters to increase what is perceived, the moderates neither to reduce nor to augment. Thus the reducer and the augmenter represent extremes of a continuous variation. The reducers are relatively tolerant of pain but intolerant of sensory deprivation and social isolation. The augmenters show the opposite tendency. These two perceptual types represent contrastings needs for stimulation and tolerance of intense stimulation. As Petrie puts it, "The reducer begins right away to limit the amount of stimulation impinging on him; the augmenter lays himself wide open to it and increasingly so." In agreement with the main thesis of this article, Petrie states that pronounced unsought stimulation, such as noise, is increasing in our environment and that the sensibilities and skills of perceptual augmenters are the most threatened by such stimulation. Under conditions of sensory bombardment the augmenter tends to temporarily reduce the intensity of perceived stimulation as an apparent compensatory and protective mechanism. As Petrie emphasizes, however, bombardment with sound, light, heat, and the like is liable to cause suffering to the augmenters. Recent experiments show that augmenters prefer quiet, peaceful, and simple stimulus situations. On the contrary, reducers have a high need for complex, novel, and interesting situations.[76] It may be predicted that people identified as augmenters are particularly liable to experience sensory and information overload in stimulus situations that may be well tolerated, if not actually sought after and enjoyed, by the reducers.

Petrie's work represents one of a number of approaches to individual differences in the need for and tolerance of sensory stimulation or information input. Other investigators have developed related constructs, such as sensation seeking[77] and arousal seeking,[78,79] that designate relatively enduring personality traits. These traits are of critical importance for a person's subjective experience of and preference for a particular type of environment, work situation, leisure activities, etc. Zuckerman[80] has formulated an optimal level of stimulation theory whose key postulate asserts that every person has characteristic optimal levels of stimulation and arousal for effective cognitive performance, motor activity, and subjective sense of well-being or positive affective tone. Zuckerman asserts that identification of a person's characteristic optimal stimulation level helps one to understand the nature of his reactions to environments that produce understimulation or overstimulation. Further, it is postulated that people will tend to avoid both extremes of sensory input and to seek stimulus situations that they subjectively experience as pleasurable or at least free from discomfort. There is some correspondence between the levels of stimulation and of arousal. Arousal, indicated by various measures of autonomic-nervous system activity, secretion of pituitary, adrenocortical, and adrenomedullary hormones, and the EEG, is positively related to stimulus intensity, complexity, novelty, and associated affective meanings. Invididuals differ with regard to the level of these stimulus variables that produce subjectively comfortable or pleasurable levels of arousal, as well as in their tolerance of and need of high arousal levels. Very high level of arousal relative to the person's optimal level results in cognitive disorganization, impaired task performance, negative affective tone, irritability, and somatic cymptoms.

The second set of pertinent variables pertains to the environment. One needs to distinguish quantitative and qualitative aspects of sensory and information inputs. The former include intensity, duration, and rate of change. The latter pertain to sensory modality, novelty, complexity, incongruency, attractiveness, and subjective meaning. It is obvious that some of these qualitative dimensions depend on the recipient. Whether particular information is categorized as novel, incongruent, or attractive, and what subjective meaning it has for the individual, will depend on his previous learning, current affective state, and other subject factors. Welch's[16] concept of the mean level of environmental stimulation would gain in heuristic value if it were conceived as the sum total of the quantitative and qualitative aspects of stimuli or information inputs produced by a given environment. As the multifactorial mean level of environmental stimulation rises, it will eventually elicit overload state and its physiological concomitants in all individuals.

The third and final class of variables relevant to information overload pertains to situational constraints—that is, characteristics of the situation in which exposure to information occurs. The various studies discussed earlier point to the importance of such factors as the degree of predictability of and control over stimulation, freedom to withdraw from stimuli versus confinement, the presence or absence of imposed tasks to be performed and the related demand for vigilance and mental output, whether tasks are forced-paced and thus involve time stress, the need for choice and decisionmaking in response to the information input, and the subject's expectations and wishes regarding success or failure to experience certain psychic changes or to perform tasks demanded of him. This list is not complete. It may suffice, however, to highlight the complexity of this area of behavioral research.

Toward a Theoretical Integration

A unified theory of sensory and information overload needs to be related to hypotheses and constructs formulated over the past two decades to account for the phenomena of sensory deprivation.[1] Further, a basic assumption underlying the concept of information overload asserts that the human organism functions as an information-process system of limited channel capacity. This view, however, is too reductionist. As von Bertalanffy puts it, "Man is not a passive receiver of stimuli coming from the external world, but in a very concrete sense *creates* his universe."[81] This, he points out, is the universe of symbols, material and nonmaterial, whose creation makes man human. Man's symbolic activity has the following consequences relevant to our theme: First, he contributes symbolic stimuli that constitute information inputs. Second, symbolic stimuli are a class of physical stimuli originating in the social environment and giving rise to psychophysiological responses whose nature and intensity are determined by the subjective significance, or meaning, of the stimuli for the individual receiving them. Third, man's capacity for autonomous symbolic activity in thought and imagery, some of which is outside of his awareness, is itself a source of information input that may not only be released by but may also modify, supplement, and distract attention from external information inputs. Fourth, there is experimental evidence that the production of stimulus-independent thought decreases as a function of the rate at which information is presented to human subjects.[82]

Theories of sensory deprivation have attempted to account for behavioral and psychophysiological effects of relevant experiments. They have used concepts of arousal, optimal level of stimulation or information input, homeostasis, perceptual feedback, information processing, field orientation, and motivation.[1] Some of these concepts can be applied to a theory of information overload. This theory may be formulated as a set of postulates as follows:

1. Each individual is characterized by an optimal level of information input that he needs for optimal cognitive and motor performance and a sense of well-being.

2. Each individual will seek a level of information input that is consonant with his enduring and current need and tolerance. The latter are partly determined by innate and learned factors constituting relatively stable personality traits.

3. Every individual has a critical tolerance level beyond which increments in information input will result in a state of overload characterized by unpleasant feeling tone, some degree of cognitive disorganization, decrements in cognitive task performance, and evidence of arousal and fatigue.

4. The state of overload is facilitated by confinement, inability to control sensory inputs, demands for complex task performance, time pressure, and need for choice and decisionmaking.

5. Each environment is characterized by a mean level of physical and social stimulation that affects individuals according to their stimulus needs and tolerance.

6. High levels of stimulus and information input result in a high level of cerebral–cortical and autonomic-nervous-system arousal that tends to decrease with time as a result of adaptation, which implies reduced responsiveness.

7. Adaptation appears to extract psychological and physiological cost manifested by impaired performance and pathophysiological changes increasing susceptibility to disease.

8. Information overload is a category of psychosocial stress brought about by excess of symbolic stimuli relative to the individual's processing capacity.

9. Information overload elicits coping strategies aimed at reduction of or escape from information inputs and related distress. These strategies may take the form of behaviors inimical to health (e.g., intake of drugs) and social order.

10. Postindustrial society provides a wide range of conditions producing information and sensory overload for large segments of the population.

The foregoing hypotheses will require validation by multidisciplinary research. They have obvious social and medical relevance.

SUMMARY AND CONCLUSIONS

Sensory and information overloads are among the hallmarks of modern life; their influence on psychological and physical well-being of individuals as well as on social behavior appears to be far-reaching. It is a social and public-health problem no less grave than overpopulation, pollution, and the growing scarcity of natural resources. The experience of overload is contributed to by both man-made transformation of the physical environment and the mass production of symbols and messages facilitated by the growth of information technology. It is said that we are in the midst of a revolution in information that is having a profound impact on the quality of life, human consciousness, and social behavior.[83] This revolution promotes an accelerated rate of cultural change and related shifts in value systems that themselves contribute to the information overload and make formidable demands on human adaptive capacity. It has been postulated that the high prevalence of and mortality from essential hypertension and coronary heart disease in technological societies are at least partly related to accelerated social change and technological development and their related social effects and one's modes of coping with them.[15,35] Futurists predict that the data explosion and the growth of information technology will continue unabated.[84,85] These forecasts highlight the social importance of the issues discussed here. As the recently published report of the Working Party for Future Studies in Sweden states: "*Overstimulation* threatens to engulf ever larger parts of the social organism. Many men and women are chronically exposed to sensory overstimulation (e.g. noise), cognitive overstimulation (e.g. information flow from the mass media), and social over-stimulation (e.g., congestion in cities). . . . Overstimulation increases as a direct consequence of the accelerating pace of technological advance. That also increases the risk of faster wear and tear on the human organism. It is therefore an imperative mission for interdisciplinary research to shed light on man's reactions to overstimulation."[86] Will the scientific community rise to this challenge?

REFERENCES

1. Zubek JP (ed): Sensory Deprivation: *Fifteen Years of Research.* New York, Appleton-Century-Crofts, 1969.
2. Lindsley DB: in Solomon P, Kubzansky PE, et al (eds): *Sensory Deprivation.* Cambridge, Harvard University Press, 1961, pp 174-194.
3. Rossi AM: in Zubek JP (ed): *Sensory Deprivation: Fifteen Years of Research.* New York, Appleton-Century-Crofts, 1969, pp 16-43.
4. Neisser U: *Cognitive Psychology.* New York, Appleton-Century-Crofts, 1966, p 7.
5. MacKay DM: *Information, Mechanism and Meaning.* Cambridge, M.I.T. Press, 1969.
6. Jones A: in Zubek JP (ed): *Sensory Deprivation: Fifteen Years of Research.* New York, Appleton-Century-Crofts, 1969, pp 167-206.
7. Mucchielli R: *Introduction to Structural Psychology.* New York, Equinox, 1970, p 80.
8. Miller JG: in Waggoner RW, Carek DJ (eds): *Communication in Clinical Practice,* Boston, Little Brown, 1964, pp 201-224.
9. Broadbent DE: *Decision and Stress.* London, Academic Press, 1971, p 9.
10. Milgram S: *Science* 167:1461, 1970.
11. Stokols D, Rall M, Pinner B, Schopler J: *Environ Behav* 5:87, 1973.
12. Desor JA: *J Person Soc Psychol* 21:79, 1972.
13. Calhoun JB: *Sci Am* 206:139, 1962.
14. Henry JP, Ely DL, Stephens PM: in: *Physiology, Emotion and Psychosomatic Illness.* Ciba Foundation Symposium 8. Amsterdam, 1972, pp 225-251.
15. Henry JP, Cassel JC: *Am J Epidemiol* 90:171, 1969.
16. Welch BL: in: *Symposium on Medical Aspects of Stress in the Military Climate.* Washington, DC, Walter Reed Army Institute of Research, 1964, pp 39-99.
17. Zlutnick S, Altman I: in Wohlwill JF, Carson DH (eds): *Environment and the Social Sciences.* Washington, DC, American Psychological Association, 1972, pp 44-58.
18. Galle OR, Gove WR, McPherson JM: *Science* 176:23, 1972.
19. Cozby PC: *J Res Person* 7:45, 1973.
20. Goldsmith JR, Jonsson E: *Am J Public Health* 63:782, 1973.
21. Glass DC, Singer JE: *Urban Stress.* New York, Academic Press, 1972.
22. Kryter KD: *Am J Public Health* 62:389, 1972.
23. Cameron P, Robertson D: *J Appl Psychol* 56:67, 1972.
24. Gattoni F, Tarnopolsky A: *Psychol Med* 3:516, 1973.
25. Elliott CD: *Br J Psychol* 62:375, 1971.
26. French JRP, Caplan RD: In Marrow AJ (ed): *The Failure of Success.* New York, AMACOM, 1972, pp 30-66.
27. French JRP, Caplan RD: *Industr Med* 39:383, 1970.
28. Sales SM: *Admin Sci Quart* 14:325, 1969.
29. Danev SG, Wartna GF, Bink B, et al: *Ned Tijdschr Psychol* 26:23, 1971.
30. Ettema JH, Zielhuis RL: *Ergonomics* 14:137, 1971.
31. Zwaga HJG: *Ergonomics* 16:61, 1973.
32. Wilkinson RT, El-Beheri S, Gieseking CC: *Psychophysiology* 9:589, 1972.
33. Frankenhaeuser M, Nordheden B, Myrsten AL, Post B: *Acta Psychol* 35:298, 1971.
34. Miller JG: *Am J Psychiatry* 116:695, 1960.
35. Rosenman RH, Friedman M: *Med Clin North Am* 58:269, 1974.
36. Kitamura S, Tada H: *Toh Psychol Fol* 28:69, 1970.
37. Hatayama T, Takayama T, Komatsu H: *Toh Psychol Fol* 28:73, 1970.

38. Kikuchi R, Kikuchi T, Kawaguchi M, et al: *Toh Psychol Fol* 28:84, 1970.
39. Sato S, Murai N, Kinebuchi C: *Toh Psychol Fol* 28:93, 1970.
40. Kitamura S, Hatayama T, Maruyama K: *Toh Psychol Fol* 29:45, 1970.
41. Takayama T, Hatayama M: *Toh Psychol Fol* 29:53, 1970.
42. Saito S, Tada H: *Toh Psychol Fol* 29:59, 1970.
43. Sato S, Kinebuchi C, Murai N: *Toh Psychol Fol* 29:65, 1970.
44. Kitamura S, Maruyama K, Tada H: *Toh Psychol Fol* 30:1, 1971.
45. Hatayama T, Komatsu H: *Toh Psychol Fol* 30:5, 1971.
46. Komatsu H, Ota H, Kato T: *Toh Psychol Fol* 30:10, 1971.
47. Saito S: *Toh Psychol Fol* 30:15, 1971.
48. Shimada M, Kawata N, Okabe S: *Toh Psychol Fol* 30:24, 1971.
49. Komatsu H, Kawata N, Shimada M: *Toh Psychol Fol* 31:11, 1972.
50. Ludwig AM: *Am J Psychiatry* 128:1294, 1972.
51. Ludwig AM: *Arch Gen Psychiatry* 25:413, 1971.
52. Ludwig AM: *J Nerv Ment Dis* 157:210, 1973.
53. Haer JL: *Percept Mot Skills* 33:192, 1971.
54. Haer JL: *J Study Conscious* 3:161 1970.
55. Gottschalk LA, Haer JL, Bates DE: *Arch Gen Psychiatry* 27:451, 1972.
56. Zuckerman M, Persky H, Miller L, Levin B: *Proceedings 77th Annual Convention, American Psychological Association*, 1969, pp 319–320.
57. Wohlwill JF: Paper presented at American Psychological Association meeting, Washington, DC, Sept 5, 1971.
58. Oswald I: *Br Med J* 1:1450, 1960.
59. Smookler HH, Buckley JP: *Fed Proc* 29:1980, 1970.
60. Masserman JH, Aarons L, Wechkin S: *Am J Psychiatry* 115:481, 1963.
61. Lipowski ZJ: *Am J Psychiatry* 127:273, 1970.
62. Lipowski ZJ: *Behav Sci* 16:467, 1971.
63. Lipowski ZJ: *Soc Sci Med* 7:517, 1973.
64. *Humanist*, Nov/Dec 1973, p 47.
65. Dubos R: *Man, Medicine and Environment.* New York, New American Library, 1969, p 103.
66. Katona G, Strumpel B, Zahn E: *Aspirations and Affluence.* New York: McGraw-Hill, 1971.
67. Lehmann HE: in Freedman AM, Kaplan HI (eds): *Comprehensive Textbook of Psychiatry.* Baltimore, Williams & Wilkins, 1967, p 626.
68. Silverman J: *Psychopharmacologia* 24:42, 1972.
69. Bowers MB, Freedman DX: *Arch Gen Psychiatry* 15:240, 1966.
70. Usdansky G, Chapman LJ: *J Abnorm Soc Psychol* 61:143, 1960.
71. Grimes C, McGhie A: *Can J Behav Sci* 5:101, 1973.
72. Danev SG, Winter CR, Wartna GF: *Activ Nerv Sup (Praha)* 14:1, 1972.
73. Lipowski ZJ: *J Nerv Ment Dis* 145:227, 1967.
74. Korner AF: *Am J Orthopsychiatry* 41:608, 1971.
75. Petrie A: *Individuality in Pain and Suffering.* Chicago, University of Chicago Press, 1967.
76. Sales SM: *J Person Soc Psychol* 19:124, 1971.
77. Zuckerman M, Bone RN: *J Consult Clin Psychol* 39:308, 1972.
78. Schubert DSP: *Int J Soc Psychiatry* 11:221, 1965.
79. Mehrabian A, Russell JA: *Environ Behav* 5:315, 1973.
80. Zuckerman M: Zubek JP (ed): *Sensory Deprivation: Fifteen Years of Research.* New York, Appleton-Century-Crofts, 1969, pp 407–432.
81. von Bertalanffy L: *General System Theory.* New York, Braziller, 1968, p 194.
82. Antrobus JS: *Br J Psychol* 59:423, 1968.
83. Gerbner G: *Sci Am* 227:153, 1972.
84. McHale J: *Ekistics* 35:321, 1973.
85. Henry N: *Futures* 5:392, 1973.
86. *To Choose a Future.* Stockholm, Kungl Boktryckeriet, 1974, p 99.

Psychosomatic Medicine in the Seventies 4

An Overview

Psychosomatic medicine as a scientific discipline and an approach to medical practice has staged a spectacular comeback. After seeming to be dormant, if not extinct, for almost two decades, it is once more in the mainstream of contemporary medicine and thought. The problem of assessing the relative contribution of psychological, biological, and social factors to the development, course, and outcome of physical and psychiatric disorders has regained a dominant position in both medicine and psychiatry. Psychosomatic medicine has provided them with a relevant set of theoretical assumptions and a long tradition of addressing the mind–body problem in research and clinical practice. The field has grown rapidly in breadth, complexity, and diversity. It has attempted to answer very old questions about human health and disease with the aid of modern investigative methods. Its current revival seems to mark the twilight of the golden age of reductionism, of an intolerant and narrow approach to the study and treatment of disease from a purely biological, psychological, or social viewpoint.

It is significant that the 27th World Health Assembly, held in May 1974, endorsed a holistic and ecological approach to medical research, practice, and training.[1] The participants urged all nations to support research on the role of psychosocial factors in health and disease. They contended that these factors can precipitate and counteract physical and mental illness and are thus crucially important in the prevention and management of all disease. This historical resolution vindicated the traditional psychosomatic viewpoint.

Knowledge of these developments is not general. Confusion about the current state of psychosomatic medicine is widespread. Semantic ambiguities abound and impede meaningful communication. Old stereotypes and outdated viewpoints linger on. Some psychiatrists and other physicians view psychosomatic medicine as "an improbable hybrid of clinical thinking, physiological speculation and psychoanalytic theory"[2] or as a doctrine of "well-meaning but ill-defined humanism."[3] These views betray deplorable ignorance of the current state of the field. It is time to set the record straight. Three recent books[4-6] should help in this regard.

It is difficult to give a balanced account of a subject that is so broad, diversified, and vigorously evolving. Bias in the choice of topics and in emphasis is unavoidable. My objective is to survey selected themes in theory, research, clinical applications, and training, which together comprise psychosomatic medicine in the seventies.

Reprinted from *American Journal of Psychiatry* 134(3):233–244. 1977 Copyright © 1977 by the American Psychiatric Association. Reprinted by permission.

Definition of Psychosomatic Medicine

Psychosomatic medicine has three interrelated facets that jointly define its scope. (1) It is a scientific discipline concerned with the study of the *relationships* of biological, psychological, and social determinants of health and disease. (2) It is a set of postulates and guidelines embodying a holistic approach to the practice of medicine. (3) It encompasses consultation–liaison psychiatry.[7]

This tripartite definition includes both the scientific and the clinical aspects of the field, which have always been its integral constituents.[8] As a scientific discipline, psychosomatic medicine has focused on the reciprocal relationships between psychological and physiological variables and has attempted to correlate them with specified conditions and changes in the person's social environment. To do so it has had to simultaneously employ research methods, explanatory concepts, and languages belonging to three distinct levels of abstraction—social, psychological, and physiological. The principal scientific task has been to elucidate the precise role of defined social and psychological factors in maintaining health and codetermining the development and course of disease. A complementary task has involved the study of the influence of specified physiological variables on psychological functioning in all of its principal aspects—information processing, motivation, emotions, and psychomotor behavior, both normal and abnormal.

From its inception psychosomatic medicine has been more than a scientific discipline. It has also represented a point of view on the nature of man and a reformist movement in, as well as an approach to, medicine. It has predicated a view of mind and body as abstractions derived from a more concrete entity—a person. It has affirmed that to achieve comprehensive knowledge of people it is necessary to study them as individual mind–body complexes ceaselessly interacting with the social and physical environment in which they are embedded. Thus the psychosomatic conception of man is integrative, holistic, and dynamic. Psychosomatic medicine advocates a unified concept of health and disease. This advocacy and the related guidelines for clinical action justify the connotations of psychosomatics as a reformist movement in medicine and a distinct approach to the prevention, diagnosis, and management of disease. It is an approach antithetical to reductionism, one that affirms the uniqueness, complexity, and the systems view of man.[7]

Ambiguity has clouded the concept of psychosomatic medicine, and widespread fallacies about it need to be corrected. It is erroneous to regard it as an affirmation of metaphysical dualism, an advocacy of psychological causation of physical illnesses, and a study of the so-called psychosomatic disorders. The concept of psychogenesis of organic disease is as reductionistic as the germ theory of it, against which psychosomatic pioneers inveighed. This concept is no longer tenable and has given way to the doctrine of multicausality of *all* disease, one that fits the facts best. It is consonant with this doctrine to view social and psychological factors as codeterminants of health and illness and thus as elements having etiological and modifying significance in human morbidity. The relative contribution of these factors varies from disease to disease, from person to person, and from one episode of the same disease in the same person to another episode. It is one of the tasks of psychosomatic research and of every physician to try to determine the extent of this relative contribution in various disorders and in individual patients. Clinical management should be based on such assessment.

If the foregoing arguments are accepted, then it becomes clear that to distinguish a class of diseases as "psychosomatic disorders" and to propound generalizations about "psychosomatic patients" is misleading and redundant. Concepts of single causes and of unilinear causal sequences—for example, from psyche to soma and vice versa—are simplistic and obsolete. The dynamic interaction of multiple factors occurring in varying constellations and time sequences, and modified by feedback effects, underlies all changes in health. To break down this complexity into testable hypotheses and validate them, to formulate integrative theories, and to develop effective preventive and therapeutic methods are the chief objectives of psychosomatic medicine today.

Critics complain that psychosomatic medicine is an undefinable, overinclusive, and scientifically useless concept. On the contrary, the discipline, as here defined, meets the need for an integrative and overarching science of man as a biological organism, a self-aware person, and a social being. More specifically, it is a body of empirical knowledge and practical precepts regarding the role of symbolic processes and their emotional correlates and behavioral consequences in health and disease. The current revival of the field attests to the fascination it engenders and the intellectual challenge it poses.

A HISTORICAL PERSPECTIVE

Psychosomatic medicine in the seventies can be better understood if viewed against its historical background. In its present form as an organized field of scientific inquiry it is about 50 years old. However, its historical roots reach back to the origins of Western medicine and thought in Greece of the fifth century B.C.[8] It is sobering to find that many themes in psychosomatic research and theory today were formulated and recurrently addressed over the centuries. For example, Gaub, a professor of medicine in Leyden, wrote in 1747 that "the reason why a sound body becomes ill, or an ailing body recovers, very often lies in the mind. Contrariwise, the body can frequently both beget mental illness and heal its offspring" (cited in reference 9, p. 71). Gaub wrote of the harmful, even lethal, effects on the body of intense fear, rage, and joy as well as of unexpressed sorrow and suppressed anger.

In 1872 Tuke[10] compiled a vast body of observations and anecdotes recorded in Western medical literature and pertaining to the influence of the mind on the body in health and disease. That monumental book was a landmark since it presented in a coherent theoretical framework a mass of previously scattered and unorganized information. Thus the groundwork for a new science was laid. Yet it took another half-century for psychosomatic medicine to evolve as a recognized discipline. It is clear that the late nineteenth century provided an unfavorable climate for empirical study of the mind–body problem. Three independent developments made such study possible. Freud, Pavlov, and Cannon offered new methods of research and explanatory concepts that propelled the mind–body problem into prominence again.

By the 1920s the stage was set for psychosomatic medicine to emerge from the background of philosophy and medical folklore. What had started as a cluster of hunches, clinical anecdotes, and imaginative speculations became a subject of scientific investigations. Both conceptual and research tools were at last available. For the next 30 years or so the field followed two major directions—psychodynamic and psychophysiological, respectively. The former was inspired by psychoanalytic theory and relied on psychoanalytic concepts and methods of making observations. The most influential representative of that trend was Alexander.[11] His specificity theory, which linked in a causal chain specific unresolved unconscious conflicts with specific somatic disorders, dominated the field until about 1955.

Alexander formulated many of the core assumptions of psychosomatic medicine.[11] He postulated the decisive role of unconscious conflicts and related emotions in the development of such disorders as bronchial asthma, ulcerative colitis, thyrotoxicosis, essential hypertension, rheumatoid arthritis, neurodermatitis, and peptic ulcer. His was an imaginative approach, one that stimulated much clinical research and raised hopes of effective therapy aimed at the resolution of the pathogenic conflicts. Yet this methodological approach had weaknesses. It causally linked variables of very different levels of abstraction, e.g., conflict and peptic ulcer, without due regard to the intervening psychophysiological mechanisms. Validation of Alexander's hypotheses proved predictably difficult.[12] The hoped-for efficacy of therapy based on them did not materialize despite some successes.[13] The hypotheses gained wide currency and were reduced by uncritical supporters to simplistic "psychosomatic formulae" that were applied indiscriminately to all patients suffering from one of the psychosomatic disorders. By about 1955 this approach had ground to a halt and left in its wake widespread disenchantment with psychosomatic medicine as a whole. The field suffered a sharp drop in popularity and credibility and seemed to be heading for the annals of medical history.

The second major direction in psychosomatic research and theory, the psychophysiological one, was concurrently developed with less fanfare by Wolff and his many collaborators at Cornell University over a period of 30 years, i.e., until his death in 1962. It was marked by careful scientific and experimental design, quantification of the studied variables, focus on conscious and thus more readily elicited psychological factors, and concern with the mechanisms mediating between symbolic stimuli and processes on the one hand, and peripheral physiological changes on the other. Wolff developed a theory of psychological stress and applied it to a wide range of somatic diseases.[14] He and his co-workers carried out ingenious psychophysiological studies and employed epidemiological methods in research on the role of social and psychological factors in disease. His work has had a decisive influence on psychosomatic research during the past 15 years.

This brief historical sketch may lend a sense of continuity to the following survey of the current psychosomatic scene.

Current State of Psychosomatic Theory

The influence of psychoanalysis on psychosomatic medicine has waned in the past 20 years. It has been difficult to validate the proposed primacy of unconscious psychological factors, such as conflicts, in the pathogenesis of various somatic disorders. Alexander's specificity theory still has a few adherents, and attempts to validate its hypotheses continue.[12] Although the theory has some value for clinical prediction and the therapy of patients suffering from one of the seven "psychosomatic disorders,"[13] it has failed to generate new research and clinical applications. Other psychoanalytic concepts, such as conversion, somatization, physiological regression, repressed affects, and psychogenesis, continue to be used by some workers to account for various somatic disorders. There is much less of a tendency, however, to claim that these concepts can adequately explain the occurrence of any of the major diseases prevalent today. They are more helpful for understanding certain somatic complaints not based on demonstrable pathology.[7] The tendency to psychologize bodily functions has been tempered.

Psychoanalytic concepts and methods of observation continue to be important for psychosomatic medicine. They contribute knowledge of the unconscious significance of all information for the person, of the symbolic meaning of body parts and functions, and of unconscious motivation and conflicts. All of these factors influence a person's psychophysiological responses to life events and situations and susceptibility and psychological reactions to illness. Thus they codetermine the timing of onset, course, and outcome of disease. Yet unconscious factors are merely one class of relevant variables that must be studied in relation to all of the other classes to achieve comprehensive knowledge.

Current psychosomatic theory has been influenced by general systems and information theories, the doctrine of multicausality of somatic functions and behavior, notions of psychophysiological response specificity and activation, the theory of operant conditioning and self-control of visceral functions, the hypothesis of object loss as an antecedent of disease, and by the concepts of psychosocial stress, cognitive appraisal and meaning, individual susceptibility to disease, adaptation, coping, and feedback.[4,5,7] The most influential theoretical formulations have been generated by Wolff,[14] Grinker,[15] Engel,[16] and Lazarus,[17] among others.[8]

In contrast to the first phase of psychosomatic medicine (between about 1925 and 1955), the present phase is marked by relatively less emphasis on individual psychodynamics and more on psychophysiological responses to environmental stimuli. Theoretical perspectives have broadened to include the effects of social factors on health. Family interaction and disruption, conditions and relationships on the job, urbanization, poverty, migration, and rapidly changing value systems and lifestyles are some of the social variables whose impact on psychophysiological functioning and health is generating hypotheses and research.[5] This trend has complemented, not supplanted, traditional psychodynamic and psychophysiological approaches. The individual has not been lost sight of. Yet a *social* and *ecological* dimension has enriched the previously two-dimensional psychosomatic theories that focused on psychophysiological interactions but disregarded the social milieu.[18] As Dubos[19] reminds us, "The understanding and control of disease require that the body–mind complex be studied in its relations to external environment."

Another major shift in focus is shown in the current concern with conscious emotions and cognitive processes and their anatomical substrate and physiological concomitants. These psychological variables are more easily elicited and quantified than the unconscious ones and are thus more amenable to scientific study. Their physiological concomitants and consequences must be identified if we are to move beyond vague talk about the mysterious leap from the mind to the body. Without knowledge of the mediating mechanisms, hypotheses of psychosomatic etiology would remain inspired speculations.

Thus current psychosomatic theories are more complex and holistic than ever. They reflect the scientific zeitgeist marked by acceptance of complexity, by attempts to study and relate multiple variables, and by striving for theories straddling interdisciplinary boundaries.

Dominant Theoretical Concepts and Formulations

Psychosomatic hypotheses and research are attempting to answer several deceptively simple questions. Why does a person respond to particular social situations and specific life events with a given pattern of psychological and physiological changes? Which psychological variables may help predict when an individual will become ill and what illness he or she will develop? Through which pathways and mechanisms do symbolic stimuli bring about changes in susceptibility to somatic illness? Which kinds of social situations and events are most likely to predispose to and precipitate illness in a given person or group? Which behaviors, attitudes, and social conditions are most conducive to health and to adaptive coping with illness? What are the psychological characteristics of people who most readily become ill or complain of bodily symptoms, or both?

Current psychosomatic theories and research revolve around these questions. Answers to them are sought to advance control over disease and suffering. The main goal is to identify those psychosocial variables which increase susceptibility to illness as well as those which enhance resistance to and adaptive coping with it. Such knowledge is needed as a basis for social and psychological measures that will help to prevent and ameliorate diseases causing chronic disability and premature death. There is accruing evidence that this goal may be achieved by modifying specific behaviors, attitudes, and emotional responses and improving social supports.

It is worth attempting to outline the general framework of current psychosomatic theory against which the more specific explanatory concepts and hypotheses may be viewed. A core assumption asserts that man's symbolic activity, subserved by the cerebral structures and functions, influences organismic processes at all other levels of organization down to the cellular level. Thus the realm of conscious and unconscious perceptions, thoughts, memories, imagery, and fantasy constitutes a set of factors affecting homeostasis, adaptation, and health. In turn, symbolic activity is influenced by environmental stimuli and by bodily processes that directly affect cerebral functions. Symbolic processes are responsive to information inputs from the following three sources: the environment, the body, and the partly autonomous symbolic activity itself. Social situations and events are obviously the most significant source of information for the person. Information can affect the individual insofar as it is appraised, consciously, unconsciously, or both, and endowed with subjective meaning. The latter is a condition for activation of emotions. In turn, emotions have physiological concomitants and cognitive and behavioral consequences, all of which can bring about changes in health.[18] These propositions will be further discussed in the section on psychosocial stress.

The second set of core assumptions pertains to the role of enduring psychological and physiological tendencies to react to specific stimuli with individually specific patterns of cognitive, emotional, behavioral, and physiological responses. These tendencies codetermine which life situations and changes are most likely to result in a given illness in the person. They are partly inborn and partly learned and are subject to modification and self-control.[20] Developmental factors and the kinds, timing, duration, and intensity of environmental, especially social, stimuli during the early development of the organism and personality help shape future psychophysiological response patterns. They codetermine individual susceptibility to disease.[21]

The following three currently influential sets of concepts and hypotheses reflect the preceding assumptions: *psychosocial stress, psychophysiological response specificity,* and *individual susceptibility to disease.*

PSYCHOSOCIAL STRESS

This concept has been methodologically fertile despite its weaknesses.[14,16,17,22,23] It implies that social situations and events as well as such psychological states as conflicts and frustrated strivings may disturb homeostasis and impose adaptive demands on the organism. This class of variables is usually referred to as "stressors,"[22,23] "stressful life events,"[24] or "life changes."[25]

Ambiguity has resulted from three meanings of the term "stress." For different writers it connotes a state of the organism; the stressors; or an area of study including stressful stimuli, an organism's responses to them, and the totality of intervening variables.[14,27,22,23] Controversy also persists regarding the relative specificity versus nonspecificity of physiological changes evoked by various stressors[23] I propose the following definition: psychosocial stress refers to external and internal stimuli that are perceived by and are meaningful to the person, activate emotions, and elicit physiological changes that threaten health and survival.

Psychosocial stress may be, indirectly, as injurious as extremes of temperature, pathogenic microorganisms, and physical trauma.[7,14,16] It is distinguished from these other categories of stress or stressors by virtue of its dependence on symbolic activity and emotions. Psychosocial stress is not necessarily pathogenic and may be beneficial. Its effect on health depends on the person's coping capacity, social support, and other factors. The key intervening variables in psychosocial stress are information, its cognitive appraisal and subjective meaning, and emotions.

The following five major categories of subjective meaning of information may be distinguished: threat, loss, gain or relief, challenge, and insignificance.[26] Information that signifies threat, loss, or both for the person is particularly liable to evoke dysphoric emotions of fear, anxiety, anger, grief, depression, guilt, and shame. Such emotions play a crucial role in mediating the adverse effects of such information on the functions of the body and on illness behavior. They activate one of the following three defensive behavioral tendencies: fight, flight, or immobility (conservation-withdrawal).[27] Subjective meaning of information has sociocultural, personality, and experiential determinants. On it depends what constitutes stress for the individual.

Emotions are viewed as intervening variables between meaning of information and bodily changes elicited by it.[28,29] They may also be activated by direct stimulation of the limbic–hypothalamic system. They have physiological concomitants (cardiovascular, respiratory, glandular, musculoskeletal, and so forth) that may have one or more of the following effects: (1) be perceived and augment, reduce, or change the quality of the emotion; (2) predispose to, precipitate, make manifest, exacerbate, or ameliorate a pathological bodily process; (3) motivate behavior inimical or conducive to health; (4) set in motion ego mechanisms of defense and coping strategies aimed at relief of distress; and (5) be communicated as somatic symptoms and foster adoption of the sick role.[26]

Psychophysiology of emotions has been one of the foci of stress research and theory.[28,29] Neuroendocrine mechanisms are of key importance. Efforts continue to identify those social and psychological variables which constitute the most common forms of stress by virtue of the emotions that they arouse. It is postulated that the more disturbing an event or situation is for the person, the higher the probability that it will lead to bodily dysfunction and disease. The kind, intensity, and duration of the evoked emotions are the decisive variables.

Bereavement,[30] loss of job,[31] disturbed family interaction,[32,33] specific work conditions,[34] and sensory and information overloads[35] are examples of common psychosocial stressors. There are two major approaches to the study of psychosocial stress, qualitative and quantitative. Proponents of the former approach are exemplified by Engel (cited in reference 36) and Schmale.[36] They have proposed that *object loss* is a common antecedent of illness. According to this hypothesis, actual, anticipated, or fantasied loss of a valued person, possession, body part, or life style is likely to lead to a psychological state called the giving up–given up syndrome and its associated emotions of helplessness or hopelessness. Thus the quality, or subjective meaning, of a life change is postulated to be correlated with onset of illness. The quantitative approach, represented by Holmes and Masuda[37] and Rahe,[25] asserts that the magnitude of recently accumulated life changes is predictive of near-future illness and its severity. These two approaches should be viewed as mutually complementary rather than exclusive.

The value of the concept of stress has been challenged lately.[22] Semantic ambiguity has detracted from is usefulness. It is difficult to distinguish between stress-induced illness and illness behavior.[38] Despite these methodological flaws the concept of stress has heuristic value. It has helped to bring together in a coherent framework a mass of observations on the relationship of social factors, the individual's symbolic activity, and changes in health. It has prevailed in the face of criticisms and modifications and is likely to be with us for a long time to come.[23]

PSYCHOPHYSIOLOGICAL SPECIFICITY

As recently revised,[39] this concept pertains to the probability that a person will respond to a given stimulus situation with a predictable set of psychological and physiological changes. Such a prediction must be based on the following three sets of variables.

1. The nature, intensity, and duration of the stimulus situation. If the latter is known to evoke similar responses in many individuals, then one talks of *stimulus response specificity* or stereotypy.

2. The enduring psychological and physiological response characteristics of the person, or *individual response specificity*. These variables are critically important for the prediction of individual differences in response to the same type of stimulus situation, be it the death of a close person, loss of a job, or public speaking. This issue has generated the bulk of psychosomatic hypotheses and research. Personality, genetic factors, developmental history, past exposure to illness, unconscious conflicts and modes of defending against them, behavior patterns, attitudes, and operant conditioning have all been invoked to account for individual psychophysiological response characteristics and for susceptibility to illness in general and to specific diseases in particular.[7,8,40] Mirsky's formulation[41] of the etiology of duodenal ulcer exemplifies a multifactorial hypothesis postulating individual response specificity.

3. The *current psychophysiological state* of the person. Current emotional state, fatigue, level and pattern of autonomic arousal, presence of physical illness, and state of consciousness are some of the variables subsumed under this heading.

This concept highlights current attempts to study the interactions of multiple variables influencing psychophysiological functioning in health and disease. It is broader than that propounded by Alexander[11,12] and applicable to both normal and pathological responses. It is less ambiguous and more general than the concept of stress and free of value judgments of what is stressful. Its weakness lies in its low explanatory power. One must study the various variables in a given person to be able to predict with reasonable probability how he or she will react. The concept is valuable as a blueprint for psychosomatic research and a construct linking many interacting variables.

INDIVIDUAL SUSCEPTIBILITY TO DISEASE

Psychosomatic theories of etiology fall into the following two classes: *specificity* and *generality*. Both assert that social and psychological variables contribute to morbidity; however, they differ in regard to the proposed nature of the causal links and pathogenesis. Specificity theories postulate that specific psychological variables have a predictable relationship to specific physiological variables, somatic disorders, or both. Specific psychological characteristics such as particular emotions; unresolved unconscious conflicts over sexual, dependent, or hostile strivings; personality style; temperament; attitude; behavior pattern; and mode of communicating distress have been correlated with specific physiological characteristics, both normal and abnormal. Causal links have been claimed or implied between some of these psychological variables and specific disorders, especially the psychosomatic ones. A well-known example of proposed specificity is the relationship between Type A behavior pattern and the development of coronary heart disease and is complications.[43] Thus it is postulated that specific psychosocial factors contribute to specific, or individual, susceptibility to disease.

The generality theories hold that a wide range of life events may increase the probability that the person will become ill. A postulated state of general susceptibility to disease is thought to be the intervening variable.[43] It is not implied that this state is a nonspecific and unitary one like Selye's concept of stress (cited in reference 3). This is indeed unlikely. Epidemiological studies, however, have consistently demonstrated a positive correlation between the magnitude of life change and the subject's near-future ill health and its severity.[24] A lowered resistance of the host to all kinds of pathology is postulated.[44]

In my opinion, the generality and specificity theories complement each other neatly. The former theories have identified conditions in a person's life whose occurrence increases the probability of imminent illness. The latter theories allow a measure of prediction of which events are potentially hazardous for a given person or class of people sharing one or more psychological characteristics and which illness is most likely to follow exposure to such events. Combined, the two theories enhance our ability to predict illness and to identify persons at risk. They do not prove that life events or specific psychological characteristics are causally related to disease rather than being statistical correlates of it. In any case, however, the theories provide a much-needed basis for social and psychological preventive measures for individuals whom they help identify as vulnerable.

Psychosomatic medicine has progressed thanks to imaginative theorizing, methodological advances, and systematic observations in the clinic and laboratory. Both theory and data gathering are necessary. In the following section the growing empirical basis of the field is reviewed.

CURRENT TRENDS IN PSYCHOSOMATIC RESEARCH

A diversity of studies and methods of investigation characterizes psychosomatic research today. Adherence to the scientific method has improved the quality of this research. Gone are the days of sweeping generalizations from the clinical studies of a few individuals. Many relevant studies are not labeled as "psychosomatic" by the investigators. Their inclusion here follows logically from the definition of the field as a whole. Thus any study that focuses on correlations among social, psychological, and physiological variables may be designated "psychosomatic." Furthermore, such studies usually relate to issues of health and illness.

The following five major groups of studies comprise psychosomatic research in the seventies:

1. Study of the role of specified social and psychological factors in the etiology of a wide range of human diseases.

2. Study of mediating mechanisms, that is, of neuroendocrine, neurophysiological, and immune processes intervening between the central nervous system activity expressed in psychological terms and the physiological functions, both normal and abnormal, of organs and tissues.

3. Study of psychosocial responses to physical illness and their effects on its course and outcome.

4. Study of the influence of specified somatic processes on psychological functioning.

5. Study of the effectiveness of behavior-modifying therapies on somatic disorders.

Psychosomatic research is of necessity multidisciplinary and multifactorial. Its methodology encompasses the following three general approaches: psychophysiology, i.e., laboratory and experimental work using human and animal subjects; epidemiology; and clinical studies.[5]

A brief survey of examples of the subjects studied and the methods employed may give the reader a glimpse of the vast scope and clinical relevance of this research.

ETIOLOGICAL STUDIES

Attempts to identify psychological and social factors that might prove to be causally related to bodily disorders have never ceased. However, as Susser[45] has pointed out, the most common etiological factors are neither sufficient nor necessary but only contributory. This comment should temper the zeal to postulate psychogenesis of any somatic disorder. As Engel[16] has urged, we should revise our simplistic concepts of etiology. It is most appropriate to conceive of it in terms of the dynamic interaction of several sets of factors, including psychosocial ones, of different weight and temporal relationships that together enable the development of a given disease. This modified concept of etiology is particularly applicable to the most prevalent diseases today.[44,46,47]

Medicine's main efforts are currently directed at unraveling the etiology of the chronic diseases responsible for the highest rates of premature mortality and the greatest burden of disability, suffering, and cost. Coronary and cerebrovascular diseases, respiratory disorders, cancer, diabetes, essential hypertension, rheumatoid arthritis, multiple sclerosis, and epilepsy head the list. Psychosomatic studies have focused on these diseases. Psychosomatic research has been directed at all of the major diseases since psychosocial factors are generally believed to have a direct bearing on their incidence, course, and outcome.[44,46] This vindicates Engel's insistence that psychosomatic investigators should move beyond their compulsive preoccupation with "psychosomatic disorders."[48]

Immense efforts are being made to elucidate the precise role of social and psychological factors in the etiology of coronary heart disease.[49-52] Some evidence suggests that these factors do play a role in the genesis of the disease and certainly in predisposing an individual to and precipitating acute cardiac events, i.e., myocardial infarction, arrhythmias, angina pectoris, and congestive heart failure.[53] Behavior related to eating habits, smoking, exercise, and work may affect coronary heart disease by means of the so-called risk factors.[53] Particular attention, however, has been paid to hypotheses that specific personality characteristics manifested by a recognizable behavior pattern and rewarded by affluent societies may have a direct pathogenic effect through chronic or repeated activation of specific neuroendocrine mechanisms.[42,49,50]

The concept of the coronary-prone, the so-called Type A, behavior pattern continues to be investigated.[49,50] This pattern features competitiveness, aggressiveness, restlessness, a tendency to speed up all activities, impatience, a sense of being under time pressure, marked dedication to work, and ceaseless striving for achievement. Retrospective and prospective studies[49,50] indicate that people displaying these characteristics have a higher than expected probability of developing coronary heart disease and myocardial infarction and of dying prematurely. Considering the fact that about 650,000 people die of coronary artery disease in this country every year and that 25% of them are 35 to 64 years old,[53] the practical importance of identifying psychosocial factors of etiological and prognostic significance is obvious. The results to date are promising and may soon be applied in preventive programs.[42,49,50] Behavior modification is particularly relevant to this area, since millions of individuals are at risk and traditional psychotherapeutic methods are obviously inapplicable on such a scale, even if they proved to be effective.

Essential hypertension is another condition that has spawned a vast number of psychosomatic studies.[53] Their results are not conclusive but have already provided a number of suggestive clues. It is believed that emotional and autonomic arousal induced by a variety of stressful stimuli in genetically predisposed people will provoke repeated pressor responses that may lead to chronic hypertension.[53] Studies of this condition have employed clinical,[54,55] epidemiological,[55] and experimental animal methods.[56] Henry and collaborators[56] induced hypertension and cardiovascular pathology in mice by altering their cages so as to maximize their encounters and to disrupt their social organization. An epidemiological study by Cobb and Rose[55] found a high incidence of hypertension in air traffic controllers. Clinical studies have focused on repressed hostility as a predisposing factor to the disease,[54] and on the effects of biofeedback[57] and relaxation[58] in lowering high blood pressure. These are but a few selected examples of psychosomatic research in this area. The findings to date support the hypothesis that certain social conditions and personality characteristics combine to increase the probability of a person's developing hypertension. No single factor is decisive, and it makes no sense to label essential hypertension a "psychosomatic disorder."

Even such "organic" diseases as cancer are being investigated from the psychosomatic viewpoint. Both clinical and animal studies are in progress.[59,60] Psychological clinical studies have focused on two variables—personality characteristics and emotional antecedents of cancer. Studies of patients with breast and lung cancers[59,60] show that they are characterized by a marked tendency to repress experience or suppress expression of certain emotions, especially anger. A second group of studies[61,62] has attempted to relate onset of cancer to recent object loss, but the results are contradictory. Current knowledge of immune mechanisms allows one to hypothesize that events at man's symbolic level of organization and their emotional correlates may modify, i.e., enhance or inhibit, the body's immune defenses, whose role in the genesis of neoplasia is postulated.

The animal studies by Riley[63] are relevant. He found that mice carrying the Bittner oncogenic virus had a different latency time for development of mammary carcinoma. After 400 days, 92% of the mice subjected to much handling and other stress had developed tumors, compared with only 7% of the undisturbed, nonstressed animals. Riley proposed that stress leads to increased adrenal cortical activity and consequent deficiency of T cells, impairment of host defense system, and thus increased individual susceptibility to cancer.

A different approach to etiology is one focused on the relationship between *stressful life changes* and *general morbidity* rather than on specific disease.[64] This epidemiological approach is prominently represented by Hinkle (cited in reference 64), Holmes and Masuda,[37] and Rahe.[25] Hinkle claimed that exposure to social change may lead to a major change in health if the former is subjectively important, if there is preexistent illness or susceptibility to it, and if there is a significant change in the subject's activities, habits, ingestants, exposure to pathogens, or in the physical characteristics of his environment. Thus a confluence of variables is necessary for a life event or situation to contribute to morbidity.[24] Holmes and Masuda[37] have asserted that the magnitude of life change is related to the time of disease onset and the seriousness of the resulting chronic illness. They postulated that life changes may contribute to causation of disease by lowering resistance to it. Rahe[25] proposed that exposure to life change may lead to perception of physical symptoms and reports of near-future illness, but that several intervening variables modify its impact on health. These variables consist of the subject's past experience, psychological defenses, coping style, and degree of physiological activation. The protective role of adequate social supports is increasingly recognized.[44,64,65]

Dozens of life change studies have provided evidence that the onset of illness is more likely to occur after a person has experienced an event that made adaptive demands on him or her. Events signifying a loss for the person are more likely to be followed by illness. Intensive studies of individuals, such as those carried out by the Rochester group,[36] support this contention. Epidemiological studies can only indicate statistical correlations and need to be supplemented by clinical research. The methodology of life change studies is constantly being refined to increase their sensitivity.[24,25] A life change is a relatively discrete event of brief duration. However, social situations that are of long duration and devoid of dramatic change, such as a frustrating marital relationship or job, may also affect health.[66]

There is evidence that members of the lower socioeconomic classes have generally higher rates of morbidity, mortality, and disability.[67] What are the psychosocial factors associated with poverty that have etiological significance? Low status integration is viewed as a major form of social stress contributing to disease.[47] Most chronic diseases, such as coronary heart disease or cancer, have a long preclinical phase. Life changes may be predictive of the onset of clinical manifestations but may reveal nothing about the etiology of any disease.[68] Thus we still need to study personality variables and enduring behavior patterns as well as chronic life situations and social conditions for clues to etiology. Work on the Type A behavior pattern and on personality correlates of cancer and other major chronic diseases must continue to help identify who is at risk, from what disease, and when. Longitudinal studies are already yielding intriguing data.[69]

STUDIES OF MEDIATING MECHANISMS

In order to establish causal links between social and psychological factors on the one hand and physiological and pathological changes on the other, one needs to identify mediating physiological processes and pathways. This is the domain of clinical and laboratory psychophysiological research employing human and animal experimental subjects.[70] Current research focuses on neurophysiological,[71] neuroendocrine,[72] and immune[73,74] mediating mechanisms.

Mason[75] has done some of the most important work in this area over the last 20 years. His research on the psychoendocrinology of emotions has involved concurrent assays of about ten hormonal responses to a variety of psychosocial stimuli.[75] The subject's emotional state, psychological defenses, developmental history, and current psychosocial situation have to be taken into account to allow prediction of the pattern of hormonal responses to a given stimulus. Levels of cortisol, adrenaline, noradrenaline, thyroxine, insulin, growth hormone, and testosterone are found to respond concurrently, sensitively, and relatively specifically to the emotion-arousing stimuli. Mason concluded that psychological influences profoundly alter hormonal balance in the body on both a short- and long-term basis and thus may affect all metabolic processes. He endorsed the psychosomatic concept of disease as a disordered integration of the dynamic steady state.

A related area of psychophysiological research has focused on catecholamine secretion in response to both laboratory analogues of "natural" stress and to the daily streses, such as commuting.[76,77] Studies by Frankenhaeuser and collaborators[77] have shown that an increase in catecholamine levels in the blood occurs in response to both pleasant and unpleasant situations and during both understimulation and overstimulation. Thus increased catecholamine secretion accompanies emotional arousal elicited by ubiquitous environmental stimuli.[77] Repeated and protracted increases in adrenaline and noradrenaline secretion occasioned by recurrent emotional arousal evoked by noise, crowding, appetitive stimuli provided by the media, driving in heavy traffic, and other common stimuli provided by the contemporary affluent environment may contribute to the high prevalence of cardiovascular diseases.[54] Novel, discrepant, and unpredictable stimuli and information tend to elicit intense and prolonged and thus potentially injurious arousal.[35,53]

Psychophysiological research has not been confined to the laboratory. For example, Taggart and associates' ingenious studies of public speakers[78] have shown that they exhibited tachycardia, changes in the ECG, and increased levels of plasma noradrenaline, triglycerides, and free fatty acids. This is but one example of a large number of recent studies of psychophysiological responses to social stimuli. Use of telemetric recording apparatus allows the monitoring of several physiological indices in people engaged in their daily activities. This is a highly promising approach to the study of physiological mediating mechanisms. It helps to identify the nature and psychophysiological consequences of common stressful situations.

In general, the vast volume of psychophysiological studies carried out in the last two decades has advanced our knowledge of the pathways and processes interposed between social stimuli and psychological responses to them and of the changes in a wide range of physiological functions and indices. These changes provide links in the sequence of events leading from psychosocial factors to bodily disease.

Studies of Psychosocial Responses to Disease

This area of research, sometimes referred to as somatopsychology, has flourished lately after years of neglect.[79] The influence of psychosocial factors on the course and outcome of all kinds of physical illness has been convincingly demonstrated.[26,79,80] The subjective meaning of illness-related information has been shown to be more important for the occurrence of maladaptive responses to disease than the latter's severity.[26] The concepts of coping, illness behavior, and the sick role have become widely accepted.[26,81] These factors are influenced by the patient's personality and family interactions and by the conscious and unconscious meaning for him or her of the diseased organ, dysfunction, and diagnostic label.[26] The kind and intensity of the emotional responses to personal illness are related to the meaning of the illness and affect its course and outcome. Anxiety, for example, is extremely common among cardiac patients and may precipitate every major complication of heart disease.[52-54,82] It can also contribute to psychogenic invalidism following myocardial infarction.[83]

Recent studies[79] show that psychiatric complications are common among the physically ill and that medical and psychiatric disorders coexist in 25 to 50% of the patients studied in every type of treatment setting. These findings highlight the necessity for *integrated* medical and psychiatric health care and for continued growth of liaison psychiatry.

Numerous studies[80,84] have focused recently on psychological responses to and psychiatric complications of modern medical and surgical treatments and therapeutic environments. Open-heart and coronary bypass surgery, chronic renal hemodialysis, and organ transplantation have brought both benefits and psychiatric casualties.[85,86] Finally, the vast recent increase of research in thanatology represents a logical extension of the psychosomatic approach to medicine.[26]

Psychosomatic etiological studies aimed at primary prevention have had limited success to date.[87] By contrast, somatopsychic research has already contributed to more effective prevention and amelioration of psychiatric complications of somatic disease and disability. This area of research has had a profound effect on current medical practice and training. Interested readers are referred to several recent reviews.[5,26,79,80]

STUDIES OF THE INFLUENCE OF SOMATIC PROCESSES ON BEHAVIOR

This research logically belongs to the domain of psychosomatic medicine. It comprises studies of the psychological aspects of cerebral function and dysfunction. Recent research on brain–behavior relationships is indispensable for the understanding of psychosomatic processes.[88] There is a renewed interest in psychopathological manifestations of cerebral disorders[89]; a new classification of the organic mental disorders reflects this.[89] Limitation of space precludes discussion of recent developments in this field.

STUDIES OF BEHAVIOR-MODIFYING THERAPIES

One of the most striking developments of the past decade is the application to somatic disorders of treatments aimed at modifying behavior, attitudes, and emotional responses. Advances in this area have followed developments in psychopharmacology and behavior modification. Inspired by learning theory, studies on biofeedback,[90,91] behavior modification,[92] and various relaxation techniques[93] have opened up new therapeutic vistas. The rapidity with which these studies have led to therapeutic applications in medicine reflects implicit acceptance of basic psychosomatic assumptions. Current widespread interest in meditation and biofeedback reflects the belief that man has a measure of volitional control over visceral functions which may be used to counteract potentially injurious physiological arousal elicited by the stresses of modern life. Psychotropic drugs,[94] individual and group psychotherapies,[95,96] and hypnosis[97] complete the list of a growing number of therapies applied to modify physiological functions and somatic disorders by means of effects on psychological functions and behavior. Stunkard[98] is right in stating that "the development of increasingly effective therapeutic techniques has changed the emphasis in psychosomatic medicine from understanding to action."

TEACHING PSYCHOSOMATIC MEDICINE

The transmission of information about advances in this field has lagged behind developments in theory, research, and clinical applications. Consultation–liaison psychiatry has carried the brunt of clinical teaching. Liaison psychiatry, a clinical component of psychosomatic medicine, has been extensively reviewed recently[99] and cannot be discussed here. There is an urgent need for guidelines on the teaching of all aspects of psychosomatic medicine to medical students and residents, psychiatric trainees, and other health professionals.[100] This overview is intended as a conceptual framework and resource for this teaching. Psychiatrists and other physicians cannot be considered adequately trained unless they have been exposed to at least some of the material discussed in this article. Several English-language journals contain much of the pertinent information and should be available in every medical library. They include *Psychosomatic Medicine, Journal of Psychosomatic Research, Journal of Human Stress, International Journal of Psychiatry in Medicine, Psychosomatics,* and *Psychophysiology.* Several fairly recent books fill the need for reference sources on all aspects of the field.[4–6,24,28,80]

CONCLUSIONS

I have tried to present a balanced overview of the broadly conceived field of psychosomatic medicine in the seventies. Theoretical, investigative, clinical, and teaching aspects have been touched upon. Key theoretical postulates and concepts have served me as a core around which major research and clinical developments could be meaningfully arranged. I have documented the contention that the field is expanding rapidly and that ignorance of it would mean that one is out of touch with one of the most vital areas of contemporary science, thought, and medicine. The relevance of psychosocial factors to health is compelling in these times of rapid social change demanding adaptation.[46] It is at the *interface* between the various disciplines concerned with man, with health and disease, that foremost intellectual challenge faces science today.

Psychosomatic medicine in the seventies is far more diversified, scientifically rigorous, methodologically resourceful, and therapeutically relevant than ever before. Its hallmarks include a multifactorial approach to the study of health and disease, formulation of testable hypotheses and their careful validation, concern with the clinical applicability of research, and development of integrative theories to harness complexity. It is unlikely that this is a passing fad. The implications of the current advances in the field for medicine, psychiatry, and the behavioral sciences are too far-reaching to permit doubt that its continued growth is inevitable.[101,102] The scientific and clinical issues that this discipline has addressed have a bearing on man's survival and its quality.

REFERENCES

1. World Health Organization: Technical Discussion 6, 27th World Health Assembly. Geneva, WHO, 1974.
2. Shepherd M: Book review of OW Hill (ed): *Modern Trends in Psychosomatic Medicine 2. J Neurol Neurosurg Psychiatry* 34:207, 1971.
3. Lipowski, ZJ: Psychosomatic medicine (letter to editor). *Lancet* 1:175, 1974.
4. Reiser MF (ed): *Organic Disorders and Psychosomatic Medicine. American Handbook of Psychiatry*, ed 2. Arieti S, (ed-in-chief). New York, Basic Books, 1975, vol 4.
5. Lipowski ZJ, Lipsitt DR, Whybrow PC (eds): *Psychosomatic Medicine: Current Trends and Clinical Applications.* New York, Oxford University Press, 1977.
6. Hill OW (ed): *Modern Trends in Psychosomatic Medicine 3.* London, Butterworths, 1976.
7. Lipowski ZJ: Review of consultation psychiatry and psychosomatic medicine: theoretical issues. *Psychosom Med* 30:395–422, 1968.
8. Wittkower ED: Historical perspective of contemporary psychosomatic medicine. *Int J Psychiatry Med* 5:309-319, 1974.
9. Rather LJ: *Mind and Body in Eighteenth Century Medicine.* Berkeley, University of California Press, 1965.
10. Tuke DH: *Illustrations of the Influence of the Mind upon the Body in Health and Disease.* London, Churchill, 1872.
11. Alexander F: *Psychosomatic Medicine.* New York, WW Norton & Co, 1950.
12. Alexander F, French TM, Pollock GH (eds): *Psychosomatic Specificity.* Chicago, University of Chicago Press, 1968.
13. Kellner R: Psychotherapy in psychosomatic disorders. *Arch Gen Psychiatry* 32:1021-1028, 1975.
14. Wolff HG: *Stress and Disease.* Springfield, Ill, Charles C Thomas, 1953.
15. Grinker RR: *Psychosomatic Research.* New York, WW Norton & Co, 1953.
16. Engel GL: A unified concept of health and disease. *Perspect Biol Med* 3:459–485, 1960.
17. Lazarus RS: *Psychological Stress and the Coping Process.* New York, McGraw-Hill, 1960.
18. Lipowski ZJ: Psychosomatic medicine in a changing society: Some current trends in theory and research. *Compr Psychiatry* 14:203-215, 1973.
19. Dubos R: *Man, Medicine, and Environment.* New York, American Library, 1968.
20. Shapiro D, Surwit RS: Operant conditioning: A new theoretical approach in psychosomatic medicine. *Int J Psychiatry Med* 5:377-387, 1974.
21. Ader R: The role of developmental factors in susceptibility to disease. *Int J Psychiatry Med* 5:367-376, 1974.
22. Hinkle LE: The concept of ''stress'' in the biological and social sciences. *Int J Psychiatry Med* 5:335-357, 1974.
23. Mason JW: A historical view of the stress field. *J Hum Stress* 1:6-12, 1975.
24. Dohrenwend BS, Dohrenwend BP (eds): *Stressful Life Events: Their Nature and Effects.* New York, John Wiley & Sons, 1974.

25. Rahe RH: Epidemiological studies of life change and illness. *Int J Psychiatry Med* 6:133-146, 1975.
26. Lipowski ZJ: Physical illness, the patient and his environment: psychosocial foundations of medicine, in Reiser MF (ed): *American Handbook of Psychiatry*, ed 2, Arieti S (ed-in-chief). New York, Basic Books, 1975, vol 4, pp 3-42.
27. Engel GL, Schmale AH: Conservation withdrawal: A primary regulatory process for organismic homeostasis, in *Physiology, Emotion & Psychosomatic Illness*. Ciba Foundation Symposium 8 (new series). Amsterdam, Elsevier, 1972, pp 57-87.
28. *Physiology, Emotion & Psychosomatic Illness*. Ciba Foundation Symposium 8 (new series). Amsterdam, Elsevier, 1972.
29. Levi L (ed): *Emotions—Their Parameters and Measurement*. New York, Raven Press, 1975.
30. Clayton PJ: The clinical morbidity of the first year of bereavement: A review. *Compr Psychiatry* 14:151-157, 1973.
31. Kasl SV, Gore S, Cobb S: The experience of losing a job: Reported changes in health, symptoms and illness behavior. *Psychosom Med* 37:106-122, 1975.
32. Minuchin S, Baker L, Rosman BL, et al: A conceptual model of psychosomatic illness in children. *Arch Gen Psychiatry* 32:1031-1038, 1975.
33. Meissner WW: Family process and psychosomatic disease. *Int J Psychiatry Med* 5:411-430, 1974.
34. McLean A (ed): *Occupational Stress*. Springfield, Ill, Charles C Thomas, 1974.
35. Lipowski ZJ: Sensory and information overload: behavioral effects. *Compr Psychiatry* 16:199-211, 1975.
36. Schmale AH: Giving up as a final common pathway to changes in health, in Lipowski ZJ (ed): *Psychosocial Aspects of Physical Illness*. Basel, S Karger, 1972, pp 20-40.
37. Holmes TH, Masuda M: Life change and illness susceptibility, in Dohrenwend BS, Dohrenwend BP (eds): *Stressful Life Events: Their Nature and Effects*. New York, John Wiley & Sons, 1974, pp 45-72.
38. Mechanic D: Stress, illness, and illness behavior. *J Hum Stress* 2:2-6, 1976.
39. Roessler R, Engel BT: The current status of the concepts of physiological response specificity and activation. *Int J Psychiatry Med* 5:359-366, 1974.
40. Miller NE: Application of learning and biofeedback to psychiatry and medicine, in Freedman AM, Kaplan HI, Sadock BJ (eds): *Comprehensive Textbook of Psychiatry*, ed 2, Baltimore, Williams & Wilkins Co, 1975, vol 1, pp 349-365.
41. Mirsky IA: Physiologic, psychologic and social determinants in the etiology of peptic ulcer. *Am J Dig Dis* 3:285-313, 1958.
42. Friedman M, Rosenman RH: *Type A Behavior and Your Heart*. New York, Alfred A Knopf, 1974.
43. Thurlow HJ: General susceptibility to illness: A selective review. *Can Med Assoc J* 97:1397-1404, 1967.
44. Cassel J: The contribution of the social environment to host resistance. *Am J Epidemiol* 104:107-123, 1976.
45. Susser M: *Casual Thinking in the Health Sciences*. New York, Oxford University Press, 1973, p 124.
46. Psychosocial factors and health. *WHO Chron* 30:337-339, 1976.
47. Dodge DL, Martin WT: *Social Stress and Chronic Illness*. Notre Dame, Ind, University of Notre Dame Press, 1970.
48. Engel GL: Selection of clinical material in psychosomatic medicine. *Psychosom Med* 16:368-373, 1954.
49. Jenkins DC: Psychologic and social risk factors for coronary disease. *N Engl J Med* 294:987-994, 1976.
50. Jenkins DC: Recent evidence supporting psychologic and social risk factors for coronary disease. *N Engl J Med* 294:1033-1038, 1976.
51. Eliot RS (ed): *Stress and the Heart*. Mount Kisco, NY, Futura Publishing Co, 1974.
52. Gentry WD, William RB (eds): *Myocardial Infarction and Coronary Care*. St Louis, CV Mosby Co, 1975.
53. Lipowski ZJ: Psychophysiological cardiovascular disorders, in Freedman AM, Kaplan HI, Sadock BJ (eds): *Comprehensive Textbook of Psychiatry*, ed 2. Baltimore, Williams & Wilkins Co, 1975, vol 2, pp 1660-1668.
54. Pilowsky I, Spalding D, Shaw J, et al: Hypertension and personality. *Psychosom Med* 35:50-56, 1973.
55. Cobb S, Rose RM: Hypertension, peptic ulcer and diabetes in air traffic controllers. *JAMA* 224:489-492, 1973.

56. Henry HP: The induction of acute and chronic cardiovascular disease in animals by psychosocial stimulation. *Int J Psychiatry Med* 6:145-158, 1975.

57. Goldman H, Kleinman KM, Snow MY, et al: Relationship between essential hypertension and cognitive functioning: Effects of biofeedback. *Psychophysiology* 12:569-573, 1975.

58. Stone RA, De Leo J: Psychotherapeutic control of hypertension. *N Engl J Med* 294:80-84, 1976.

59. Greer S, Morris T: Psychological attributes of women who develop breast cancer: A controlled study. *J Psychosom Res* 19:147-153, 1975.

60. Abse DW, Wilkins MM, Van de Castle RL, et al: Personality and behavioral characteristics of lung cancer patients. *J Psychosom Res* 18:101-113, 1974.

61. Schonfeld J: Psychological and life experience differences between Israeli women with benign and cancerous breast lesions. *J Psychosom Res* 19:229-234, 1975.

62. Schmale A, Iker H: The psychological setting of uterine cervical cancer. *NY Acad Sci* 125:807-813, 1966.

63. Riley V: Mouse mammary tumors: Alteration of incidence as apparent function of stress. *Science* 189:465-467, 1975.

64. Rapkin JG, Struening EL: Life events, stress, and illness. *Science* 194:1013-1020, 1976.

65. Cobb S: Presidential address—1976: social support as a moderator of life stress, *Psychosom Med* 38:300-314, 1976.

66. Gersten JC, Friis R, Langner TS: Life dissatisfactions, job dissatisfaction and illness of married men over time. *Am J Epidemiol* 103:333-341, 1976.

67. Syme SL, Berkman LF: Social class, susceptibility and sickness. *Am J Epidemiol* 104:1-8, 1976.

68. Goldberg EL, Comstock GW: Life events and subsequent illness. *Am J Epidemiol* 104:146-158, 1976.

69. Thomas CB, Greenstreet RL: Psychobiological characteristics in youth as predictors of five disease states: Suicide, mental illness, hypertension, coronary heart disease and tumor. *Johns Hopkins Med J* 132:16-43, 1973.

70. Johnson LC: Psychophysiological research: aims and methods. *Int J Psychiatry Med* 5:565-573, 1974.

71. Kiely WF: From the symbolic stimulus to the pathophysiological response: neurophysiological mechanisms. *Int J Psychiatry Med* 5:517-529, 1974.

72. Whybrow PC, Silberfarb PM: Neuroendocrine mediating mechanisms: from the symbolic stimulus to the physiological response. *Int J Psychiatry Med* 5:531-539, 1974.

73. Amkraut H, Solomon GF: From the symbolic stimulus to the pathophysiologic response: immune mechanisms. *Int J Psychiatry Med* 5:541-563, 1974.

74. Stein M, Schiavi RC, Camerino M: Influence of brain and behavior on the immune system. *Science* 191:435-440, 1976.

75. Mason JW: Emotion as reflected in patterns of endocrine integration, in Levi L (ed): *Emotions—Their Parameters and Measurement*. New York, Raven Press, 1975, pp 143-181.

76. Patkai P: Laboratory studies of psychological stress. *Int J Psychiatry Med* 5:575-585, 1974.

77. Frankenhaeuser M: Experimental approaches to the study of catecholamines and emotion, in Levi L (ed): *Emotions—Their Parameters and Measurement*. New York, Raven Press, 1975, pp 209-234.

78. Taggart P, Carruthers M, Somerville W: Electrocardiogram, plasma catecholamines and lipids, and their modification of oxprenolol when speaking before an audience. *Lancet* 2:341-346, 1973.

79. Lipowski ZJ: Psychiatry of somatic diseases: epidemiology, pathogenesis, classification. *Compr Psychiatry* 16:105-124, 1975.

80. Lipowski ZJ (ed): *Psychosocial Aspects of Physical Illness*. Basel, S Karger, 1972.

81. Twaddle AC: The concepts of the sick role and illness behavior, in Lipowski ZJ (ed): *Psychosocial Aspects of Physical Illness*. Basel, S. Karger, 1972, pp 162-179.

82. Cay EL, Vetter N, Philip AE, et al: Psychological status during recovery from an acute heart attack. *J Psychosom Res* 16:425-435, 1972.

83. Cay EL, Vetter N, Philip AE, et al: Return to work after a heart attack. *J Psychosom Res* 17:231-243, 1973.

84. Aitken C, Cay EL: Clinical psychosomatic research. *Int J Psychiatry Med* 6:29-41, 1975.

85. Howells JG (ed): *Modern Perspectives in the Psychiatric Aspects of Surgery*. New York, Brunner/Mazel, 1976.

86. Abram HS: Psychiatry and medical progress: Therapeutic considerations. *Int J Psychiatry Med* 6:203-211, 1975.

87. Hurst MW, Jenkins CD, Rose RM: The relation of psychological stress to onset of medical illness. *Annu Rev Med* 27:301-312, 1976.

88. Karczmar AG, Eccles JC (eds): *Brain and Human Behavior.* New York, Springer-Verlag, 1972.

89. Lipowski ZJ: Organic brain syndromes: overview and classification, in Benson DF, Blumer D (eds): *Psychiatric Aspects of Neurological Disease.* New York, Grune & Stratton, 1975, pp 11-35.

90. Hauri PP: Biofeedback and self-control of physiological functions: clinical applications. *Int J Psychiatry Med* 6:255-265, 1975.

91. Birk L (ed): *Biofeedback: Behavioral Medicine.* New York, Grune & Stratton, 1973.

92. Price KP: The application of behavior therapy to the treatment of psychosomatic disorders: Retrospect and prospect. *Psychother Theory, Res Pract* 2:138-155, 1974.

93. Benson H, Greenwood MM, Klemchuk H: The relaxation response: psychophysiologic aspects and clinical applications. *Int J Psychiatry Med* 6:87-98, 1975.

94. Solow C: Psychotropic drugs in somatic disorders. *Int J Psychiatry Med* 6:267-282, 1975.

95. Kinston M, Wolff H: Bodily communication and psychotherapy: a psychosomatic approach. *Int J Psychiatry Med* 6:195-201, 1975.

96. Stein A: Group therapy with psychosomatically ill patients, in Kaplan HI, Sadock BJ (eds): *Comprehensive Group Psychotherapy.* Baltimore, Williams & Wilkins Co, 1971, pp 581-601.

97. Frankel FH: Hypnosis as a treatment method in psychosomatic medicine. *Int J Psychiatry Med* 6:75-85, 1975.

98. Stunkard AJ: Presidential address—1974: From explanation to action in psychosomatic medicine: the case of obesity. *Psychosom Med* 37:195-204, 1975.

99. Lipowski ZJ: Consultation-liaison psychiatry: Past, present, and future, in Pasnau RO (ed): *Consultation-Liaison Psychiatry.* New York, Grune & Stratton, 1975, pp 1-28.

100. Reichsman F: Teaching psychosomatic medicine to medical students, residents and postgraduate fellows. *Int J Psychiatry Med* 6:307-316, 1975.

101. Engel GL: Memorial lecture: the psychosomatic approach to individual susceptibility to disease. *Gastroenterology* 67:1085-1093, 1974.

102. Freyhan FA: Is psychosomatic obsolete? A psychiatric reappraisal. *Compr Psychiatry* 17:381-386, 1976.

Holistic–Medical Foundations
of American Psychiatry

5

A Bicentennial

> *The cure of many diseases is unknown to the physicians of Hellas, because they disregard the whole, which ought to be studied also, for the part can never be well unless the whole is well.*
> PLATO, *Charmides*

> *Psychology which explains everything explains nothing, and we are still in doubt.*
> MARIANNE MORE

Much has been written in recent years about psychiatry's identity crisis. A historian summed it up well: "The field of psychiatry is now in a state of uncertainty and restlessness, unable to abandon the traditional theoretical models and unprepared to face the challenge of the great social issues at stake."[1, p. 71] I believe that the current malaise can be counteracted by a clear reaffirmation rather than an abandonment of those traditional models which have proven to be especially durable and effective. A historical perspective is indispensable to identify them. A look back at 200 years of American psychiatry reveals a conceptual model that is truly its foundation and hallmark. I shall refer to it as the holistic–medical model or approach. It is the purpose of this paper to retrace that model's evolution and the achievements that it made possible and to underscore its fitness as an organizing principle to serve psychiatry in the 1980s and beyond.

DEFINITION OF TERMS

The word "holistic," derived from the Greek *holos*, or whole, was introduced by Smuts[2] in 1926, and it has been used with increasing frequency but varying clarity since. Smuts used the term "holism" in two senses: to refer to the "fundamental factor operative towards the creation of wholes in the universe" (p. 86), and to desig-

Reprinted from *American Journal of Psychiatry* 138:888–895, 1981. Copyright © 1981 by the American Psychiatric Association. Reprinted by permission. This work was supported in part by GP Special Training Grant MH-13172 from NIMH.

nate the philosophical doctrine embodying the holistic conceptions. According to Smuts, both matter and life consist of unit structures whose synthesis produces natural wholes or organisms. A whole is always more than the sum of its parts; it is not something added to the parts but constitutes the parts in their synthesis. Personality, the highest and most evolved structure in the universe, encompassses mind and body as its constituent elements or aspects. The science of personality should unify and integrate all of the sciences dealing with the human mind and the human body.

In a strict sense, the word "holistic" refers to the theory of holism as formulated by Smuts. As the term became adopted by psychologists, physicians, and laymen, it lost its metaphysical connotation. Goldstein,[3] for example, spoke of the "holistic approach" to man, one whose hallmark is the concern with the study of the human organism *as a whole*. That approach is antithetical to the atomistic one, which focuses on sections isolated from the whole. Global or unified theories of human behavior have been called holistic, biopsychosocial, general systems theory, and unified theory.[4] Von Bertalanffy's organismic conception and general system theory[5] represent the most elaborate and sophisticated formulation of holistic conceptions in biology and the behavioral sciences. However, that author dismissed Smuts' holism as a "philosophical speculation, hardly supported by any facts in our present knowledge."[5, p. 198]

In psychiatry Adolf Meyer is the foremost representative of the holistic approach. He advocated the importance of an integrated approach to the study of man and respect for the "data which are in the mind of the holist, to use General Smuts' term."[6] The holistic approach was adopted by psychosomatic writers, especially Dunbar.[7]

In medicine, "holistic" designates an approach that advocates the view of "the whole person in the context of the total environment."[8, p. 16] The holistic approach to health and disease contrasts with the reductionistic, biomedical, or mechanistic approach, which affirms mind–body dualism rather than unity and ignores the psychosocial aspects of man's functioning. Most recently, "holistic medicine" emerged as a vague catchword for an antiscientific and antimedical approach to health and illness; that perverted use of the term must not be confused with its traditional meaning.[8]

The following definition is proposed: "holistic" refers to an approach to the study of man in health and illness and to health care that focuses on the person as a whole, that is to say, a mind–body complex embedded in a social field. The holistic approach calls for an integrated use of data, concepts, and tehniques derived from biologic, psychologic, and social modes of abstraction to explain human behavior and to study and treat all deviations from health in individuals. As Hegel put it, "The true is the whole."[9, p. 11]

"Medical" in the present context refers to the viewpoint that psychiatry is an integral part of medicine, with which it shares the concern for the scientific study of disease and treatment of the sick. As a distinguished British observer noted in 1930, "It is not better buildings or maintenance that constitute the real difference of American psychiatry. The difference depends upon the medical spirit dominating it, and consequent preoccupation with treatment and research."[10, p. 851] I submit that this still applies.

THE PRECURSORS

Benjamin Rush (1745–1813), the author of the first American textbook of psychiatry[11] and the man generally regarded as the father of American psychiatry,[1,12] inaugurated its holistic-medical tradition in the 1780s. A professor of medicine, he not only lectured on diseases of the mind but stressed psychologic aspects of all diseases. In an introduction to his lectures he proposed that "the knowlege of the human mind is the most *important* branch of all the sciences," one eminently useful to physicians as they may "draw many active and useful remedies from this course, for the cure of diseases which belong exclusively to the body."[12, p. 10] Elsewhere Rush spoke of the reciprocal influence of the body and mind and of man as a "single and indivisible being, for so intimately united are his soul and body, that one cannot be moved, without the other."[13, p. 256]

Rush's teachings failed to prevent psychiatry's isolation from the rest of medicine in this country, an isolation that lasted for over a century after his death. Yet the holistic conceptions did not die. In 1832 Amariah Brigham (1798–1849), the founder and first editor of the *American Journal of Insanity,* now the *American Journal of Psychiatry,* published his *Remarks on the Influence of Mental Cultivation upon Health.*[14] He emphasized "intimate connexion between the mind and body" (p. 11). The mind depends on the healthy state of the body, particularly of the brain; and it influences the functions of the body in health and disease. Insanity is a disease of the brain that may be caused by either physical factors or moral ones such as "violent excitement of the mind." According to Brigham, the influence of the mind in producing disease is neglected by physicians, yet it is exemplified by dyspepsia and other bodily disorders.

The year 1844 was the turning point for American psychiatry for two reasons: the *American Journal of Insanity* began to appear, and several months later the forerunner of the American Psychiatric Association was formed. Psychiatry, or rather, "psychological medicine," as it was called then, emerged as a specialty. From then on the *Journal* and the presidents of the Association provided the leadership for the specialty. One of their first efforts was to bring the teaching of medical psychology to the medical schools, a goal that proved to be elusive. In 1863 Pliny Earle was appointed professor of psychological medicine at the Berkshire Medical Institute in Pittsfield, Massachusetts, probably the first such chair established in this country.[15] He lamented that the treatment of insanity had been "transferred from the doctors to the turners of the key" and argued eloquently in favor of making psychological medicine a part of the medical curriculum. Earle's views were endorsed by John Gray,[17] then editor of the *Journal,* who called for making psychological medicine a required part of medical teaching and practice. A struggle to end the separation of psychiatry and the rest of medicine had begun.

Between 1867 and 1873 several clinics for the treatment of nervous disorders and insanity were opened in Philadelphia, New York, St. Louis, and Boston.[15] Toward the end of the 19th century some leaders of psychiatry began to press for the development of psychiatric outpatient departments in the general hospitals to provide for the treatment of early and mild cases of mental illness and to offer proper instruction for medical students. Concurrently, others clamored for the establishment of "psychopathic" wards in the general hospitals.[18] The first general hospital psychiatric unit was organized by Mosher at the Albany Hospital, Albany, New York, in 1902.[18]

Thus, in the second half of the 19th century American psychiatrists initiated a movement to bring psychiatry into medical education and into general hospitals. Those developments helped shape American psychiatry in the 20th century. Meanwhile, Hughes,[19] a psychiatrist,was expounding remarkably holistic notions about health and disease. He predicted, overly optimistically, that an era was approaching when the whole patient would be treated. He argued that "in a newer, broader, truer sense than ever before, do we recognize the monism of man. . . . In estimating the causes, concomitants and sequences of his diseases, we consider the whole man in his psychoneurophysical relations."[19, p. 902] Hughes expressed other innovative views: organs affected by repeated or prolonged hysterical disorder may at times develop organic disease; a breakdown in the central nervous system by which its resistance is lessened makes possible and precedes all cases of cancer as well as phthisis and other bacterial diseases; secretion of bile may be interfered with by prolonged mental anxiety, worry, and exertion; and leukemia may result from profound nervous exhaustion or emotional shock. As the mind through the mediation of the central nervous system has such a profound influence on the body's resistance to disease, there is a physiologic basis for all forms of psychotherapy and for the importance of the physician's attitude toward the patient.

The growing reformist ferment in late-19th-centruy American psychiatry was catalyzed by S. Weir Mitchell's memorable address to the American Medico–Psychological Association in 1894.[20] An eminent neurologist, he roundly criticized psychiatrists for isolating themselves from the rest of medicine, failing to study mental disorders scientifically, and condoning abject conditions of asylum patients. His sharp critique helped accelerate the trends aimed at ending the isolation of psychiatry from the rest of medicine and from science and at bringing psychiatric services physically closer to other medical ones. Research at last got under way, pioneered by van Gieson and Adolf Meyer. The former wrote a blueprint for it that called for scientific, multidisciplinary, laboratory-based investigations of mental disorders.[21] Such research required "cooperation of all the medicobiological and psychological sciences."[21] Meyer succeeded van Gieson as director of the Pathological Institute of the New York State Hospitals in New York City in 1902. He was to become the greatest single influence shaping 20th-century American psychiatry according to the holistic–medical model.

THE AMERICAN SCHOOL: PSYCHOBIOLOGY

The holistic–medical viewpoint was advanced by two men who dominated American psychiatry in the first 40 years of this century: Adolf Meyer and William A. White. They shared a common conceptual ground that is best subsumed by Meyer's term "psychobiology."[22] The holistic conceptions and premises of the latter have influenced psychiatry in this country in all of its major aspects: theory, clinical practice, organization of services, training, and research. Because of its distinctive features and the degree to which it has influenced American psychiatry, one is justified in referring to psychobiology as the American school. White[23] argued that an American school of psychopathology could be distinguished from various European schools by its characteristic assumptions, such as the belief in the unity of the organism and in the absence of the metaphysical distinction between mind and body. White and Meyer, who were both immensely erudite and prolific writers, spelled out the holistic conceptions of the American school of psychiatry.

White's core views,[23] germane to my theme, may be summarized as follows: The basic philosophical premise, essential to the progress of psychiatry, is that the mind and body are not separate entities acting on one another but only two distinct yet integral aspects of the human organism as a whole. Study of the parts of the organism cannot result in the knowledge of the whole, since the organism is not merely an aggregation of parts but something more: *an integrated whole,* a psychobiologic unity. The psyche represents a higher form of integration, one evolved in response to a complex environment. Mental reactions are total and not partial reactions of the organism. Psychology, the study of the mind, must be regarded as a biologic science. Disease is a manifestation of the dynamic interplay between organism and environment. It is always both somatic and psychic, but in any given patient it may be predominantly either one or the other. There is a psychologic factor is all disease. Since man is a member of the social group and must somehow fit into it, he can be fully understood only if his relationships to his social environment are taken into account. Mental illness occupies the borderland between the individual and the social group. Psychiatry is that medical specialty which "approaches the problem of the whole individual."[23, p. 111]

Meyer's conceptions [22,24,25] were no less holistic than White's. His psychobiology was to be the study of man *as a person* in health and disease. As Lidz[24] observed, Meyer was primarily concerned with issues of the mind–body unity and the integration of the person. He spoke of the "medically useless contrast of mental and physical"[25, p. 38] and asserted that mental activities were functions of the total organism. Focus on the scientific study of the person, the unique biologic unit capable of symbolization or mentation, was the hallmark of psychobiology. "Psychiatry" designates the study and treatment of all abnormal conditions involving man's behavior and mentation. Meyer contrasted a genetic–dynamic, pluralistic, empirical, nondogmatic, and commonsense psychiatry with that governed by "theory-inspired imperialism of fixed doctrine."[25, p. 57] The psychiatrist must be primarily a physician, one specially trained to study and treat personality functions. Psychobiology should be an integral part of medical training.

Meyer's teachings have had a profound influence on all of the major aspects of American psychiatry and have given it its distinctive holistic–medical stamp. His eclectic, comprehensive, multifactorial approach to the study of man in health and disease, to medicine and psychiatry, offers a conceptual framework of enduring clinical usefulness. Meyer and White influenced psychiatric training and research, the organization of psychiatric services and psychiatry's role in medical practice and teaching. The interrelated development of psychosomatic medicine and liaison and general hospital psychiatry, as well as the marked expansion of the amount of psychiatric teaching in medical schools, represented the implementation of the medical–holistic postulates of the leaders of the American school of psychiatry. Because those postulates advocated the integration of psychiatry and the rest of medicine, it was logical to try to bridge the gap between the two areas in education, delivery of health care, and research. I will review briefly those key developments because they reflect most directly the impact of the holistic–medical viewpoint on American psychiatry and the rest of medicine during the past 50 years and because they continue to challenge us today.

PSYCHOSOMATIC MEDICINE: A HOLISTIC APPROACH TO HEALTH AND DISEASE

Psychosomatic medicine was one of the main trends in American psychiatry to emerge between the two World Wars. It comprised a systematic, scientific approach to the study of the role of psychologic and social factors in human disease, as well as an advocacy of the treatment of the whole patient. Its emergence had been spurred by four major new approaches to the study of man: Gestalt psychology, psychoanalysis, Pavlovian conditioning, and Cannon's psychophysiology.[7] In this country the writings of psychobiologists, primarily Meyer, White, and Jelliffe,[26] had prepared the ground for the psychsomatic movement to enter the stage in the early 1930s. Powell[7] has shown the links between those older psychobiologists and Dunbar, who played a key role in the American psychosomatic movement beginning in 1934. Her painstaking review of the literature on psychosomatic relationships[27] was a landmark that launched psychosomatics in America and popularized the word "psychosomatic." She was the founder of the American Psychosomatic Society and of its journal, *Psychosomatic Medicine,* in 1939 and a pioneer in the application of a holistic approach to medical practice and public health. She represented the holistic, psychobiologic viewpoint in psychosomatics, whose influence is still felt today despite the failure of most historical accounts of psychosomatic medicine to do justice to its importance.[7]

Dunbar emphasized correlations between psychosocial and biologic variables rather than supposed psychologic causation, or psychogenesis, of physical illnesses. Her main concern was the study and treatment of *the patient as a whole.*[7] That approach contrasted with the two other major theoretical trends—the psychoanalytic and the psychophysiologic—that dominated psychosomatic medicine in the first phase of its development, i.e., between 1934 and 1955. The psychoanalytic (dynamic) approach stressed psychic forces, conflicts, unconscious factors, and specificity of psychologic etiology (psychogenesis) of certain physical disorders. The psychophysiologic approach, inspired largely by Cannon's work and most prominently represented by Wolff, focused on the study of psychophysiologic mechanisms in disease, the etiologic role of psychologic stress and defenses against it, and on rigorous experimental and clinical research.[7]

The holistic or psychobiologic approach of Dunbar and the psychophysiologic one of Cannon and Wolff had been largely eclipsed by the dynamic school of Alexander[28] and his followers until about 1955. In the past 25 years, however, psychosomatic medicine in this country has reaffirmed its original holistic stance. It has abandoned the search for the psychogenesis of ever more somatic disorders, an effort that reflected a reductionistic view of disease causation, one analogous to the germ theory and thus incompatible with the contemporary doctrine of multifactorial causality of all disease.[29] Psychosomatic research has moved far beyond the early focus on a handful of disorders of multifactorial origin misnemed "psychosomatic."[29] The idea that all physical illnesses have a psychosocial aspect in their causation, course, and outcome has gaimed wide acceptance. Engel's recent formulation of the biopsychosocial concept of disease[30] reflects a holistic approach to medicine by a leader in the psychosomatic field. The application of that approach to the practice of medicine has advanced concurrently under the label of consultation–liaison psychiatry.

CONSULTATION–LIAISON PSYCHIATRY: A BRIDGE BETWEEN MEDICINE AND PSYCHIATRY

It followed logically from psychobiologic and holistic postulates that psychiatry ought to play a part in the everyday practice of medicine. It was no accident that it was a pupil of Meyer's, Henry,[31] who in 1929 wrote a pioneering paper on psychiatric liaison with medicine in a general hospital. Meyer[25] himself recommended that "liaison activity" be part of psychiatric training.

Liaison psychiatry is that subdivision of clinical psychiatry which involves consultation to and collaboration with nonpsychiatric physicians in all types of medical settings, but especially in general hospitals. It is primarily concerned with problems of diagnosis, management, study, and prevention of psychiatric morbidity in the physically ill and those who manifest their psychologic distress in the form of somatic complaints.[32] Its goal has been to enhance psychosocial and psychiatric aspects of medical care. The term "liaison" in this context connotes a psychiatrist's efforts to sensitize physicians and other health workers to the psychosocial dimension of illness, to teach them to identify and manage psychopathology, and to improve communication between patients and staff. "Liaison psychiatry," a term first used in the literature by Billings,[33] refers to the whole area of psychiatric clinical work, education, and research at the borderland between psychiatry and all of the other medical specialties.

By 1940 a number of general hospitals featured an active psychiatric consultation or liaison service that offered teaching of medical students and physicians in addition to clinical service in the form of consultation.[34] Liaison departments flourished between 1934 and the late 1940s. Psychiatric liaison teaching was acclaimed as "one of the most valuable means of emphasizing the total aspect of the patient and of breaking down the barriers between psychiatry and other clinical subjects."[34, p. 229] The rise of liaison psychiatry was soon followed by its relative dormancy until the 1970s.[35] Its decline was symptomatic of psychiatry's drift away from the rest of medicine and the holistic concepts in the 1950s and 1960s.

The past 10 years have seen a striking revival of liaison psychiatry.[35] Changing trends in health care delivery, marked by emphasis on primary care, resulted in a decision by the Education Branch of NIMH to give high priority to the funding of consultation–liaison services in general hospitals, with a view to strengthening the education of medical students and physicians in psychosocial and psychiatric aspects of medicine. Epidemiologists estimate that about 15% of the American population is affected by mental disorders in 1 year and that about 60% of these individuals are identified and/or treated in the primary care sector.[36] These figures highlight the key role of primary physicians as providers—for better or worse—of mental health care, and thus the need to train these physicians in the diagnosis, treatment, and proper referral of mentally disturbed patients. Liaison psychiatrists have been given a major part in such training. Liaison services have grown rapidly in number, staff, and prestige that they lacked until recently. Despite continuing obstacles to its growth and goals related to the indifference and even hostility to it on the part of some psychiatrists and other physicians, liaison psychiatry is likely to continue playing a key role in the slow process of integrating psychiatry into the rest of medicine.

GENERAL HOSPITAL PSYCHIATRY

The remarkable growth of general hospital psychiatry in America over the last 50 years, and especially in the last 20, represents one of the most far-reaching developments in psychiatry's history. More than any other organizational change, that development has helped to raise the standards of psychiatric patient care, training, and research and to reduce the isolation of psychiatry from progress in the rest of medicine. It took much effort and many years to get that development under way.

Attempts to develop general hospital psychiatry in this country began at the turn of this century. Mosher[37, 38] published a blueprint for the first general hospital psychiatric unit that was to open at the Albany Hospital in 1902 and formulated the following goals for general hospital psychiatry: (1) providing psychiatric care for cases of acute mental illness, "whether idiopathic or complicating medical or surgical disease"; (2) providing care whose standards would match those available to general medical patients; (3) allowing the patient to be treated in close proximity to his or her community and without the stigma of commitment; and (4) training interns and nurses in psychiatric care. These goals are still valid today.

In the 1920s general hospital psychiatric units began to spread. By 1932, of a total of 4309 general hospitals in the United States, 112 provided a department for mental patients; in 1939 there were 153.[39] In some hospitals no beds were specifically set aside for psychiatric patients, but a consultation or liaison service was established instead.

General hospital psychiatry offered an unprecedented opportunity to study and manage psychiatric problems encountered in medical and surgical patients. Psychosocial and psychiatric aspects of physical illness and injury were highlighted as never before. Psychiatric patients could benefit from modern medical diagnostic and therapeutic methods. Techniques of crisis intervention helped many such patients to be restored to premorbid functioning and community expeditiously. The general hospital provided an appropriate setting in which psychiatrists, medical students, and all types of health workers could learn to apply holistic concepts of health care. Yet unforeseen obstacles and problems began to interfere with general hospital psychiatry's original goals.[40]

Closer contacts between psychiatrists and other physicians brought into sharper relief their different approaches to illness and its management. As Kubie[41] warned. "Thus a rivalry is bound to arise, sometimes hidden, sometimes outspoken, sometimes friendly, sometimes bitter: a rivalry which may produce good or evil" (pp. 255–256). Nonpsychiatric physicians often felt incompetent in the face of psychiatrists' comments and recommendations. Such reactions fostered resistance against the latter. Psychiatrists were inclined to be defensive and eager to prove their competence in an unfriendly milieu. Establishment of psychiatric units often gave rise to conflicts over space, funds, and influence, and sharpening of territorial and conceptual boundaries followed. Paradoxically, despite their hard-won physical proximity in the general hospitals, psychiatry and the rest of medicine began to drift apart, and the holistic–medical approach was given little more than lip service. The original goals of the pioneers of general hospital psychiatry were becoming diluted and perverted.

Despite these obstacles and problems, a rapid increase in the number of general hospital psychiatric units took place in the 1960s and 1970s. By 1970 there were 750 and in 1978, 1,203.[42] In 1975, nonfederal general hospitals accounted for 16.3% of total psychiatric patient care episodes.[43] Clearly, general hospitals have become a major sector in the psychiatric care delivery system. Their role is expected to grow in the coming years, since psychiatric and other medical care will likely become increasingly integrated for economic reasons.

Psychiatry in Medical Education

Benjamin Rush was the first known teacher of psychiatry in this country. About 100 years later, in 1895, Adolf Meyer began to teach it and became the most influential driving force behind efforts to bring it once more into medical education. Those two holistic thinkers pioneered psychiatric education in America. Progress was slow. Ebaugh[44] called the period prior to 1914 "psychiatry in isolation" and that between 1914 and 1931 "the breakdown of isolation." In 1931, almost one-half of the medical schools still had no clinical facilities for teaching psychiatry, yet by 1940 all schools offered such teaching, with an average of 92 hours of instruction per school.[44] The next 30 years brought further expansion of psychiatry's place in the medical curriculum. Teaching of behavioral sciences and psychiatry in the preclinical years increased dramatically, with almost four times more hours devoted to it in 1960 than in 1940.[45] The time spent teaching psychiatry and behavioral sciences in the medical curriculum as a whole rose from an average of 92 hours in 1940 to an average of 362 hours in 1966.[45]

While these figures show quantitative progress, they say nothing about the effectiveness of quadrupled hours of teaching in influencing medical students' attitudes and physicians' actual practice. There is some evidence that success in those areas falls far short of expectations. The original purpose of bringing psychiatry into the medical curriculum was to prepare students to appreciate and manage ubiquitous psychosocial aspects of disease, to properly identify and treat or refer patients with psychiatric disorders, and to adopt a holistic approach to patients.[44] There is reason to doubt that these goals have been accomplished to a degree commensurate with the expansion of psychiatric teaching.[35, 46] The decline in the proportion of medical students choosing psychiatric careers, from 7% in the period 1945–1964 to between 2% and 3% in 1980, raises questions about the effectiveness of current psychiatric teaching.[47] Psychiatry itself, riven by dissension and given to insupportable claims by competing theoretical and therapeutic approaches, has hardly offered an exemplary model of a holistic approach in recent years. If our teaching is to carry conviction, we have to do more than pay lip service to the holistic conceptions in both the theory and practice of psychiatry.

HOLISTIC–MEDICAL APPROACH TODAY

Holistic–medical conceptions have brought American psychiatry closer to medicine and science and have constituted the dynamic force behind the expansion of psychiatric services and education. They are still a vital force today.

Psychiatrists increasingly recognize that no single theoretical approach—psychodynamic, behaviorist, sociologic, or biologic—can fully account for the phenomena of human behavior or for the occurrence of mental illness. Reductionism will not do. A holistic, comprehensive, multifactorial theoretical framework is needed for the science of man in health and illness and for psychiatry.

One of the major current trends is the renewed interest in psychiatric diagnosis and classification. For about three decades that aspect of psychiatry was disparaged in this country. Interpretation of behavior in terms of psychodynamic hypotheses rather than its careful description and classification was emphasized. Yet description and classification presuppose observation, and all three are among the cardinal procedures of empirical sciences, including psychopathology.[48] *DSM-III*, a multiaxial classification, reflects a trend toward a more holistic approach to psychiatric diagnosis. Furthermore, the emphasis on diagnosis reaffirms psychiatry's link with the rest of medicine, since it stresses one of the key medical procedures. Classification's main purpose is heuristic, namely, to generate testable hypotheses about causal relationships.[49] *DSM-III* should stimulate a multifactorial approach to the study of causes of mental disorders. Only such an approach can do justice to the complexity of schizophrenic, affective, and organic mental disorders.

One of the principal current directions of psychiatric research is the study of brain–behavior relationships. Psychopharmacology and the rapid advances in the neurosciences have combined to propel that investigative approach into prominence. Latest developments, such as positron emission tomography, may spell a new era in psychiatric research.[50] We must be careful, however, to avoid regression to the 19th century's "brain mythology," the naive belief that human behavior and mental disorders can be fully explained by neurophysiology and other neurosciences. The holistic approach can help us avoid slipping into such reductionism.

In psychiatric treatment the holistic–medical approach provides an organizing framework of practical usefulness. It encourages the use of that form of therapy (or combination of therapeutic modalities) which is most likely to benefit an individual patient. That approach combines respect for data of observation and their comprehensive evaluation with a humanistic concern for the uniqueness of the person and his or her history, liabilities and assets, and personal ways of experiencing the world and coping with it. It is this last aspect that makes psychodynamic conceptions indispensable for the understanding and management of every patient. Equally indispensable is the medical evaluation of psychiatric patients, since there is a well-documented positive association between physical and mental illness.[51] According to the holistic–medical viewpoint, psychiatric and other medical health care are inseparable. Continuing development of general hospital psychiatry reflects, in part, that contention.

Psychiatric training by and large continues to be based on holistic conceptions derived from psychobiology and is likely to become even more firmly anchored in both the biologic and the behavioral sciences.[52] To confine training to either of them would effectively destroy psychiatry's legitimate claim on being recognized as a distinct specialty and profession. The holistic approach to psychiatric training cultivates an open, eclectic mind rather than one held captive by a single theory or therapy.

CONCLUSIONS

The holistic–medical tradition and conceptions that distinguish American psychiatry have endured, despite changing fortunes, for 200 years. That tradition was clearly reaffirmed in both Masserman's 1979 presidential address[53] and Stone's response.[54] Masserman proclaimed our adherence to the medical model. Stone predicted that in the future psychiatry would draw even closer to medicine, since both psychiatrists and other physicians shared the commitment to helping "the whole person." Rush and Meyer would have approved. Now the words will have to be translated into concrete actions or they will remain empty slogans.

Effective integration of psychiatry and medicine is an elusive and unfulfilled goal, one to strive for in the coming years against continuing obstacles alluded to in this paper. Currently the economic, social, political, and scientific forces that influence the directions in health care delivery and research seem to favor a holistic approach. Psychiatrists are reappraising their role in the health care system. We now have the crucial advantage of possessing *organizational structure*, in the form of general hosptial psychiatry, availability of teaching hours, and research facilities, that barely existed 50 years ago.

"Concrete actions" now imply reform of the existing structure rather than its erection from scratch. Such reform is needed in the areas of clinical service and education. If the medical–holistic postulates are to be more fully implemented, better collaboration will have to develop between psychiatrists and other physicians in health care delivery both in general hospitals and in private practice in the community. This implies not only greater availability of consultation–liaison services in all health care facilities, including primary practice, but also increased readiness by psychiatric inpatient units to accept the physically ill.[40] Psychiatric training should emphasize more than heretofore the psychosocial aspects of physical illness, psychopathology related to the latter, brain–behavior relationships in health and disease, psychogeriatrics, and holistic conceptions—subjects that are neglected in at least some training programs. Unless psychiatrists learn to appreciate those issues during their training, they will not be able to teach medical students and help other physicians effectively.

As a participant Canadian observer of the American scene, I have been impressed by the ease with which new trends in psychiatric theory and therapy, sometimes modestly referred to as "revolutions," rise in this country, to be followed by disenchantment and decline. The implied promise of a millennium of positive mental health is raised by each successive revolution and then wanes in the face of critical reappraisal. Yet after the enthusiasm has subsided and exorbitant claims have been debunked, a sediment of usable knowledge, concepts, and therapy remains, and the specialty grows. Psychobiology and the holistic conceptions it espoused promised neither solutions to the riddles of human behavior nor remedies for its disorders. That was both its strength and weakness—its strength since it provided a conceptual framework for integrating the various theoretical approaches, research findings, and therapies without being exclusively committed to any of them and thus, like them, vulnerable to obsolescence; and its weakness in that it could not provide a rallying cry or incentive for passionate allegiance. Its legacy lies in the organizational structure, mentioned earlier, and in the unbroken tradition of thought that can provide our profession with identity and direction in the years to come.

Holistic–medical conceptions provided a vital, inspirational, and organizing force for American psychiatry during its formative period in the first 40 years of this century and assured its current preeminence. Insistence on using concepts, methods, and theories derived from biologic, behavioral, and social sciences for the study of man in health and disease and for treatment has been the hallmark of the holistic approach, one that is both humanistic and scientific. It has withstood assorted fads, revolutions, and crises in American psychiatry and offers an effective and unifying force for it as it enters the 1980s. It is an approach that could only flourish in a pluralistic, open, and democratic society, since it is the product of the liberal mind. It challenges any theory or doctrine that claims to explain fully human behavior and illness, for it insists that the true is the whole.

REFERENCES

1. Mora G: Historical and theoretical trends in psychiatry, in Freedman AM, Kaplan HI, Sadock BJ (eds): *Comprehensive Textbook of Psychiatry*, ed 2. Baltimore, Williams & Wilkins Co, 1975, vol 1.
2. Smuts JC: *Holism and Evolution*. New York, Macmillan Publishing Co, 1926.
3. Goldstein K: *Human Nature in the Light of Psychopathology*. New York, Schocken Books, 1963.
4. Grinker RR Sr (ed): *Toward a Unified Theory of Human Behavior*, ed. 2 New York, Basic Books, 1967.
5. Von Bertalanffy L: *Problems of Life*. New York, John Wiley & Sons, 1952.
6. Meyer A: Presidential address: Thirty-five years of psychiatry in the United States and our present outlook. *Am J Psychiatry* 85:1–31, 1928.
7. Powell RC: Helen Flanders Dunbar (1902–1959) and a holistic approach to psychosomatic problems, I: The rise and fall of a medical philosophy. *Psychiatr Q* 49:133–152, 1977.

8. Sobel DS (ed): *Ways of Health*. New York, Harcourt Brace Jovanovich, 1979.
9. Hegel GWF: *Phenomenology of Spirit*. Oxford, England, Clarendon Press, 1977.
10. Mapother E: Impressions of psychiatry in America. *Lancet* 1:848-852, 1930.
11. Rush B: *Medical Inquiries and Observations upon the Diseases of the Mind*. Philadelphia, Kimber and Richardson, 1812.
12. Farr CB: Benjamin Rush and American psychiatry. *Am J Psychiatry* 100:3-15, 1944.
13. Rush B: *Sixteen Introductory Lectures*. Philadelphia, Bradford and Innskeep, 1811.
14. Brigham A: *Remarks on the Influence of Mental Cultivation upon Health*. Hartford, Conn, Huntington, 1832.
15. Hall JK (ed): *One Hundred Years of American Psychiatry*. New York, Columbia University Press, 1944.
16. Earle P: Psychologic medicine: its importance as a part of the medical curriculum. *Am J Insanity* 24:257-280, 1867.
17. Gray JP: Insanity, and its relations to medicine. *Am J Insanity* 25:145-172, 1868.
18. Sweeney GH: Pioneering general hospital psychiatry. *Psychiatr Q Suppl* 36:209-268, 1962.
19. Hughes CH: The nervous system in disease and the practice of medicine from a neurologic standpoint. *JAMA* 22:897-908, 1894.
20. Mitchell SW: Address before the fiftieth annual meeting of the American Medico-Psychological Association, held in PHiladelphia, May 16th, 1894. *J Nerv Ment Dis* 21:413-437, 1894.
21. van Gieson I: *Correlation of Sciences*. Utica, NY, State Hospitals Press, 1899.
22. Meyer A: *Psychobiology: A Science of Man*. Springfield, Ill, Charles C Thomas, 1957.
23. White WA: *Foundations of Psychiatry*. New York, Nervous and Mental Disease Publishing Co, 1921.
24. Lidz T: Adolf Meyer and the development of American psychiatry. *Am J Psychiatry* 123:320-332, 1966.
25. Winters EE (ed): *The Collected Papers of Adolf Meyer*. Baltimore, Johns Hopkins Press, 1951, vol 3.
26. Jelliffe SE: *Sketches in Psychosomatic Medicine*. New York, Nervous and Mental Disease Monographs, 1939.
27. Dunbar H: *Emotions and Bodily Changes, A Survey of Literature on Psychosomatic Interrelationships: 1910-1933*. New York, Columbia University Press, 1935.
28. Alexander F: *Psychosomatic Medicine*. New York, WW Norton & Co, 1950.
29. Lipowski ZJ: Psychosomatic medicine in the seventies: An overview. *Am J Psychiatry* 134:233-244, 1977.
30. Engel GL: The need for a new medical model: A challenge for biological science. *Science* 196:129-136, 1977.
31. Henry GW: Some modern aspects of psychiatry in general hospital practice. *Am J Psychiatry* 86:481-499, 1929.
32. Lipowski ZJ: Consultation-liaison psychiatry: An overview. *Am J Psychiatry* 131:623-630, 1974.
33. Billings EG: Liaison psychiatry and intern instruction. *J Assoc Am Med Coll* 14:375-385, 1939.
34. Ebaugh FG, Rymer CA:*Psychiatry in Medical Education*. New York, Commonwealth Fund, 1942.
35. Lipowski ZJ: Consultation-liaison psychiatry: Past failures and new opportunities. *Gen Hosp Psychiatry* 1:3-10, 1979.
36. Regier DA, Goldberg ID, Taube CA: The de facto US mental health services system. *Arch Gen Psychiatry* 35:685-693, 1978.
37. Mosher JM: The insane in general hospitals. *Am J Insanity* 57:325-329, 1900.
38. Mosher JM: A consideration of the need of better provision for the treatment of mental disease in its early stage. *Am J Insanity* 65:499-508, 1909.
39. Heldt TJ: Psychiatric services in general hospitals. *Am J Psychiatry* 95:865-871, 1939.
40. Greenhill MH: Psychiatric units in general hospitals: 1979. *Hosp Commun Psychiatry* 30:169-182, 1979.
41. Kubie LS: the organization of a psychiatric service for a general hospital. *Psychosom Med* 4:252-272, 1942.
42. American Hospital Association: *Hospital Statistics, 1979*. Chicago, AHA, 1979.
43. Taube CA, Redick RW: *Provisional Data on Patient Care Episodes in Mental Health Facilities, 1975*. Washington, DC, US Department of Health, Education, and Welfare, 1977.
44. Ebaugh FG: The history of psychiatric education in the United States from 1844 to 1944. *Am J Psychiatry* 100:151-160, 1944.

45. American Psychiatric Association: *Teaching Psychiatry in Medical School*. Washington, DC, APA, 1969.

46. Markham B: Can a behavioral science course change medical students' attitudes? *J Psychiatr Educ* 3:44–54, 1979.

47. Nielsen AC: Choosing psychiatry: The importance of psychiatric education in medical school. *Am J Psychiatry* 137:428–431, 1980.

48. Lipowski ZJ: Psychopathology as a science: Its scope and tasks. *Compr Psychiatry* 7:175–182, 1966.

49. Sokal RR: Classification: Purposes, principles, progress, prospects. *Science* 185:1115–1123, 1974.

50. Images of brain function (editorial). *Lancet* 2:725–726, 1979.

51. Lipowski ZJ: Psychiatry of somatic diseases: Epidemiology, pathogenesis, classification. *Compr Psychiatry* 16:105–124, 1975.

52. Bowden CL, Humphrey FJ, Thompson MGG: Priorities in psychiatric residency training. *Am J Psychiatry* 137:1243–1246, 1980.

53. Masserman JH: Presidential address: The future of psychiatry as a scientific and humanitarian discipline in a changing world. *Am J Psychiatry* 136:1013–1019, 1979.

54. Stone AA: Response to the presidential address. *Am J Psychiatry* 136:1020–1022, 1979.

The Holistic Approach to Medicine $\quad 6$

> . . . as you ought not to attempt to cure the eyes
> without the head, or the head without the body,
> so neither ought you to attempt to cure the body
> without the soul. And this, he said, is the reason
> why the cure of many diseases is unknown to the
> physicians of Hellas, because they disregard the
> whole, which ought to be studied also, for the
> part can never be well unless the whole is well.
> PLATO, Charmides

THE HOLISTIC CONCEPTIONS IN A HISTORICAL PERSPECTIVE

The above quotation from Plato spells out the holistic approach to medicine and bears witness to its ancient roots. The term "holistic," which derives from Greek *holos*, or whole, is of more recent vintage, having been introduced by Smuts in 1926.[1] It connotes an approach to the study of man in health and in disease, and to medical practice, marked by the concern with the individual *as a whole*, as a person and a psychophysiological organism interacting with the social and physical environment. A core assumption of the holistic approach, one that Plato[2] expressed so concisely, asserts that the whole is more than the sum of its parts. Thus, to understand man fully, one needs to study him as a mind–body complex, a biopsychosocial unit. Study of parts of that unit can never result in complete knowledge of the unit as a whole.

The holistic approach, with its roots in ancient Greece, has challenged medicine for centuries.[3,4] It suffered a far-reaching setback in the seventeenth century when Descartes formulated the doctrine of the essential duality of body and mind. The body was to be the object of scientific investigation, whereas the mind or soul was to be the province of religion and philosophy. Ryle[5] called this view "the dogma of the Ghost in the Machine" or the Cartesian myth. That "dogma" has exerted a profound influence on the development of the science of man and of medicine. As Cassell put it, "physicians, in company with other scientists, were given the (technical) body, while philosophers and theologians were assigned the (moral) mind. Obviously this controversy has not cooled."[6,p.112] To use Ryle's metaphor, in the view of many physicians, the human machine and its malfunction belong to medical science; the Ghost or the mind, or psyche, is the hunting ground of the "soft" sciences such as psychology and psychiatry. That conceptual split has influenced clinical practice and medical research to this day, yet attempts to counteract the doctrine of mind–body dualism and its influence on medicine have never ceased. The most systematic and organized movement advocating holistic conceptions emerged in Europe and the United States in the 1920s and early 1930s and was labeled "psychosomatic medicine."

Psychosomatic medicine, or psychosomatics, has been based on the assumption that mind and body are but convenient abstractions derived from an integrated psychosomatic or biopsychosocial unit, that is to say, a person. Psychosomatics was to promote research as well as a clinical approach that regarded biological, psychological, and social aspects of man, and their complex interactions, as determinants of health and deviations from it. The emergence of psychosomatic medicine had been facilitated by a new wave of interest in studying human behavior in all its aspects that followed in the wake of the research and writings of Gestalt psychologists, Freud, Pavlov, Cannon, and the American psychobiologists such as Adolf Meyer. Those precursors had inspired the emergence of three main trends in psychosomatic research and theory: the psychoanalytic, the psychophysiological, and the psychobiological. Each of the trends emphasized a different methodological approach to the study of man and of disease.[7,8]

The psychoanalytic approach utilized the method of observation and the theoretical concepts developed by Freud and his followers. Franz Alexander[9] became the main representative of that approach and one of the most influential figures in psychosomatics in the period between 1932 and 1955. Alexander and his fellow psychoanalysts focused on the postulated causal role of unconscious factors, such as unresolved intrapsychic conflicts, in bringing about one of the so-called psychosomatic disorders. That term was often used to designate those physical illnesses in which psychological factors were believed to play a major, if not a decisive, causal role. Bronchial asthma, essential hypertension, rheumatoid arthritis, ulcerative colitis, duodenal ulcer, thyrotoxicosis, and neurodermatitis were the main diseases and disorders most consistently referred to as "psychosomatic." Alexander postulated that the presence of a specific constellation consisting of an unconscious psychological conflict and the emotions engendered by it, as well as the defenses against them, results in a specific psychosomatic disorder.[9] His specificity theory proved to be difficult to validate. It emphasized psychological causation, or psychogenesis, of bodily diseases and thus represented a psychological counterpart to the germ theory. Like the latter, it postulated a linear causal chain leading from a specific single cause to a specific disease. It is not surprising that Alexander's approach bogged down and may be considered obsolete.[4,10,11] The most valuable and lasting contribution of the psychoanalytic approach to psychosomatics has been to make us aware of the influence of unconscious motives, conflicts, defenses, symbolic meanings, and fantasies upon how a person interprets and reacts to information, thinks, feels, and acts. The unconscious variables need to be taken into account both in the theories of causation of illness and in explanations of a person's normal and abnormal reactions to a physical illness or injury.

The psychophysiological approach to psychosomatics, one derived from Cannon's work on the physiology of emotions, focused on the study of correlations between selected psychological, physiological, and pathophysiological variables. This approach has relied largely on experimental design, using both human and animal subjects, but has also employed clinical and epidemiological research methods. The most prominent pioneer of the psychophysiological approach to psychosomatic studies was Harold

G. Wolff.[12] He and his students developed the theoretical concept of psychological stress and initiated studies on the impact of stressful life events on health. It should be pointed out that those studies were in some measure inspired by the writings of the founder of psychobiology, Adolf Meyer.[12]

Finally, the psychobiological approach to psychosomatic medicine, one derived form Meyer's conceptions and most prominently represented by Helen Flanders Dunbar,[13] has been truly holistic.[7,8] As such, it has consistently emphasized the notion of multifactorial etiology of disease and hence the need for a comprehensive, biopsychosocial view of man in health and illness. This viewpoint provides the foundation for a holistic-medical practice, one combining biomedical knowledge and modern technology with a humanistic concern for an individual and his or her personality and relationships with others.

Thus, for the past 50 years, psychosomatic medicine has stood in the forefront of the struggle to promote a holistic approach to medicine. It achieved considerable popularity, especially in the United States, immediately after World War II and then suffered relative eclipse in the 1950s and 1960s. Its diminished appeal was the result of several factors. Medical technology advanced rapidly and seemed to offer promise of successful conquest of many diseases causing premature death and chronic disability. Biomedical advances occurred independently of any psychosocial considerations, and many physicians and lay people grew skeptical of the need for a holistic approach. Extravagant claims and promises made by some enthusiastic partisans of psychosomatic medicine failed to be supported by concrete gains in disease prevention and treatment. Disenchantment and cynical denigration of the field followed in the wake of the initial uncritical acceptance of psychogenetic hypotheses and their implied potential to advance effective therapies based on psychological understanding. It seemed for a while that psychosomatic medicine and the holistic approach were to be relegated to the realm of the history of failed medical ideas, like mesmerism, for example.

In the past 20 years, the climate of opinion has changed substantially. Writers such as von Bertalanffy,[14] Dubos,[15,16] and Engel[17,18] have helped turn the tide and stimulated renewed interest in holistic conceptions. Concurrently, dissatisfaction with the growing depersonalization of medical practice and the skyrocketing cost of biomedical technology began to spread. It became increasingly clear that despite its impressive advances, biomedicine had failed to prevent the high prevalence of chronic diseases, which became the main public health problem once the infectious diseases had been largely controlled. The importance of the life-style and human behavior as factors contributing to morbidity and premature mortality, could no longer be denied. Moreover, the role of psychosocial factors in the course and outcome of all diseases came to be increasingly acknowledged. Concurrently, psychosomatic research and theory have changed drastically.[10,11] Instead of focusing on postulated psychogenesis of certain chronic diseases of unknown etiology and on the unconscious psychological factors, psychosomatic research has shifted its focus to elucidation of the mediating psychophysiological mechanisms and processes interposed between the impact of life events on the individual, on the one hand, and the subsequent pathological changes in his organism, on the other. At the same time, public discontent with the conduct of medical care and its cost has prompted a search for alternatives and correctives to the biomedical–technological approach, a trend that has proved favorable to a more holistic approach to medical research and practice.

The term "holistic" has recently been adopted by various groups claiming to provide medical care mindful of man's biological, psychological, and spiritual aspects.[19-21] Holistic medicine, as its advocates call it, is being promoted as an *alternative* rather than a *corrective* to biomedicine. It is unfortunate that the word "holistic" has been chosen by a health movement that is in many respects antiscientific and regressive. The credibility of the holistic approach, one boasting ancient heritage and impressive intellectual tradition, could suffer a setback as a result. This provides an added reason for the need to restate its key postulates and assumptions as they pertain to health, disease, and medical practice. It is germane to discuss, at this point, the evolution of the meanings of the concepts of health and disease, to be followed by discussions of the doctrine of multifactorial etiology and the role of psychosocial factors in disease, respectively.

HEALTH, DISEASE, AND ILLNESS

These concepts have undergone repeated changes over the centuries, as has been documented by medical historians such as Sigerist.[22] He points out that the ancient Greek physicians viewed health as a perfectly balanced condition of the body. The Romans broadened that concept by adding a new dimension to it, namely that of mental health. Juvenal's dictum *mens sana in corpore sano*, healthy mind in a healthy body, reflected that expanded view of health. With the advent of Christianity, the concept of health underwent another fundamental change in that it stressed the primacy of the spiritual health, the health of the soul, over that of the body. The body could be diseased yet the person could remain healthy, provided that his soul was pure. That concept did not, however, disparage the concern with bodily health during the Middle Ages; the body was considered to be the vessel of the soul and God's creation to be cherished and protected.

Towards the end of the seventeenth century, John Locke reaffirmed the earlier, Roman, view of health: "A Sound Mind in a sound Body, is a short, but full Description of a happy State in this World." The eighteenth century brought a renewed emphasis on both physical and mental health as an important value for the individual and society. In the nineteenth and twentieth centuries the concept of health was given an added dimension, the social one. Health came to be viewed not as simply the absence of disease, but as a positive state: a healthy person was one who was well balanced in body and mind and well adjusted to his or her physical and social environment.[22] The World Health Organization proposed an ideal definition of health as a state of complete physical, mental, and social well-being. Dubos[15] observed that the concept of perfect and positive health is utopian, in that man would never be perfectly adapted to his environment and be able to live without stress, struggle, and suffering. Criteria of health will differ, argues Dubos, depending on the environmental conditions and on the social norms and the individual's values. Dubos offers a relativistic definition of health as a "physical and mental state fairly free of discomfort and pain, which permits the person concerned to function as effectively and as long as possible in the environment where chance or choice has placed him."[15, p.351]

Thus, the prevailing contemporary conceptions of human health tend to be *relativistic* rather than idealistic; *positive* rather than simply negative, that is, implying nothing more than the absence of disease; *holistic*, in the sense of including both physical and mental well-being and functioning; and *ecological* or adaptational in that they emphasize the individual's mode of adaptation to his or her environment. These conceptions of health disavow the notion of a sharp boundary between health and disease, between what is normal and what is not.

The concept of *disease* has undergone changes over the centuries no less than that of health. Two major conceptions of disease have vied for supremacy since 400 B.C. down to our times: the *physiological* and the *ontological*.[6] The ancient physiologists, such as Hippocrates, held that disease resulted from an imbalance of the humors of a person and reflected a disturbed relationship between man and his environment. By contrast, the ontologists regarded diseases as entities or things having independent existence and invading the victims. The ontological viewpoint was given a powerful boost in the nineteenth century with the formulation of Virchow's doctrine of the cellular basis of disease and, later, Koch's and Pasteur's germ theories of disease. The doctrine of cellular pathology asserted that anatomical lesions invariably preceded and determined the type of clinical manifestations. The germ theory of disease postulated that diseases were entities featuring structural changes and caused by specific or unique pathogenic agents. More recent concepts, such as those of biochemical lesion or molecular pathology, may be seen as extensions of the doctrine of cellular pathology and specificity of etiology. The ontological conceptions of disease eschewed concern with the sick person. The ontologists have been mostly preoccupied with structural and chemical changes in the body whose occurrence they have sought to explicate without taking into account the person and his social environment. Modern biomedicine may be viewed as a direct descendant of the nineteenth-century ontological doctrines that came to dominate Western medical thought. Those doctrines and the research they inspired have resulted in spectacular medical advances in the last 100 years. Yet, the psychosocial and the ecological dimensions of disease and medical practice have become severely neglected in the process. A reaction against the reductionism of biomedicine has grown gradually and has promoted the development of alternative concepts and definitions of disease.

A number of attempts to define disease have been made lately. However, no generally accepted definition has yet been proposed. Some writers speculate that the concept of disease might have evolved historically as an explanation for suffering or disability experienced by people in the absence of obvious injury.[23] Diseases came to be conceived as things or entities that were thought to be responsible for the symptoms, that is the illness, of the afflicted person. Such a *realist* concept of disease stands in contrast to a *nominalist* view of it held by some medical scientists. The nominalists regard diseases as arbitrary concepts and as convenient names given to specified clusters of observable phenomena. They also reject the realist notion of diseases as causes of illness and deny the validity of a unified concept of disease. A representative nominalist definition of disease asserts that "In medical discourse, the name of a disease refers to the sum of the abnormal phenomena displayed by a group of living organisms in association with a specified common characteristic or set of characteristics by which they differ from the norm of their species in such a way as to place them at a biological disadvantage."[24]

Some medical theorists make an explicit distinction between disease and *illness*. For example, Feinstein[25] defines disease as those data about a patient which are formulated in impersonal terms, that is to say, morphological, chemical, physiological, and other related terms. By contrast, illness refers to data of a personal nature, namely, subjective symptoms and objective signs. Susser[26] views disease as a process that elicits a state of physiological and psychological dysfunction that is confined to the individual. "Illness" signifies, for that author, a subjective state of psychological awareness of dysfunction. Proponents of such sharp distinction between the concepts of disease and illness tend to view the former as a biological event, one involving a disruption of the structure or function, or both, of a part or system of a person's body.[27] By contrast, they conceive of illness as a human event, which comprises subjective distress and psychosocial consequences resulting from the interaction between a sick person and his environment. Disease constitutes, according to this view, but one type of environmental stimulus that may give rise to an illness. Other such stimuli include stressful life events or situations having disturbing emotional significance for the person.[27]

Antithetical to the preceding conceptions are those advanced by writers such as Engel, Brody, and Fabrega, who have formulated a holistic concept of disease, one that includes illness, and have referred to it as a "unified,"[17] "systems,"[28,29] or "biopsychosocial"[18] concept. These holistic formulations have been influenced by von Bertalanffy's general system theory[14] and represent a departure from, and a challenging alternative to, the biomedical, dualistic, and reductionistic concept of disease that has dominated Western medical thought for the past 100 years. Furthermore, these new conceptions may be seen as reaffirming and extending, "in modern dress," the tenets of Hippocratic medicine which proclaimed the dependence of man's health and disease on the interplay between the whole person and his environment.[15]

For the proponents of the unified or systems conceptions, disease is a *biopsychosocial* and not merely a biological event. The human, or experiential, aspect of disease is the illness.[18] There is no sharp dividing line between health and disease, as these two concepts are relative and their definitions are influenced by sociocultural and psychological, and not just by purely biological, considerations. Disease represents adaptive failure or disturbances in the growth, development, or homeostasis of the organism as a whole or of any of its systems.[17] Disturbance or failure at any one level of the hierarchical organization of man, be it the molecular, cellular, tissue, organ, cognitive, or symbolic level, is liable to spread to and affect some or all of the remaining levels. Thus, *disease involves the organism as a whole*. It comprises experiential, behavioral, and social dimensions that constitute its integral aspects or components. Disease has no existence apart from the experiencing person, the patient. The holistic conceptions of disease do away with the dualistic distinction between mind and body, soma and psyche. Mind and body are only abstractions that refer to distinct levels of human organization and are so inextricably linked together, in both health and disease, that one cannot be disturbed without involving the other.

The holistic conceptions have important implications for the theories of disease etiology and for the management of patients. They imply that the psychosocial dimension is an integral part of every disease or illness (the author uses these two terms as synonyms). Furthermore, the unified concept of disease leads logically to the notions of multiple causality and of the psychological and social factors as a class of causal factors in human disease.

MULTIFACTORIAL ETIOLOGY

The germ theory of disease asserted that every infectious disease was primarily caused by a microorganism that was transmissible from one host to another. The theory spurred the search for specific agents that caused specific diseases. That causal model was successful up to a point but had considerable limitations. It obscured the fact that one-to-one causal relationships are rare in biology and that complex relationships between causes and effects prevail.[26] Where causation in medicine is invoked, it usually turns out that event A is neither necessary nor sufficient to bring about event B.[30] Even in the case of infection, the germ theory proved to be an oversimplification in that it neglected to take into account various factors that play a part in determining whether the host–germ–environment interaction will lead to clinical evidence of disease.[31] Those factors include susceptibility, genetic constitution, human behavior, and socioeconomic variables. Just as pregnancy does not necessarily follow insemination, so infection is not invariably produced by access of a germ.[31]

The inadequacy of the germ theory in accounting for the occurrence of infection has provided impetus for the search for more adequate causal models. Growing prevalence and incidence of chronic diseases in recent decades have necessitated formulations of multifactorial etiology that fit observations better than the notions of a linear causal chain and of a single specific cause necessary and sufficient to bring about a particular disease. As Susser[26] points out, the most common types of causes or determinants of disease are those that are neither necessary nor sufficient but can be contributory. Such a causal factor may be clinically established by demonstrating that the postulated cause precedes the effect and that altering the cause alters the effect.[32] A known contributory cause may not be present in every case and not all individuals who possess the contributory cause will experience the effect. For example, cigarette smoking may be considered to be a contributory cause of lung cancer. Determinants have many possible effects, and effects have many determinants.[26] Most diseases are the consequence of a set of determinants acting simultaneously or sequentially. In other words, in medicine we are usually dealing with *multiple causality*.

Thus, in the last few decades, the notions of etiology have moved beyond the germ theory and the concepts of specificity of causal agents and of simple causal sequences. The new models are *ecological* and *multicausal*. The ecological model calls for the study of the agent, host, and environment in their processes of reciprocal interaction.[26] The understanding of disease and its adequate prevention require that the host, conceived of as the body–mind complex, be studied in his or her relationship to the physical and social environment.[16] That model is *dynamic* in the sense that it stresses processes rather than static relations and emphasizes reciprocal relationships involving feedback effects: action is succeeded by reaction, which feeds back into the situation.[26] Multicausality permits inclusion of the psychological attributes and states of the host, as well as the host's interactions with his social environment and its characteristics, among the contributory determinants or causes of any disease. In turn, the latter may be viewed as a determinant of the sick person's mentation and behavior, that is, of his mental health.

PSYCHOSOCIAL FACTORS IN ETIOLOGY

Psychosocial factors may be regarded as a class of contributory causes of disease. The term "psychosocial" is a rather awkward hybrid, but it has achieved a good deal of currency since Halliday[33] used it as a title for his book in 1948. "Psychosocial" refers to psychological and social, or interactional, aspects of man's functioning. As those two aspects are inextricably linked, so the language reflects the link by joining them together into one word.

The notion that psychological factors play an important role in the causation of physical illness has been around since the beginning of recorded Western medical thought.[4,34] Medical writings from the sixteenth century onward are replete with statements and clinical anecdotes attesting to the belief that a person's emotional state plays a causative role in disease. For example, Archer,[35] a seventeenth-century medical writer, expressed that belief explicitly when he wrote that "the observation I have made in practice of physick these several years, hath confirmed me in this opinion, that the origin, or cause of most men and womens sickness, disease, and death is, first, some great discontent, which brings a habit of sadness of mind. . . ."[35, p.120] Similar views were held by many medical writers of the eighteenth century and were particularly well spelled out by the famous Dutch physician Gaub.[36] An English psychiatrist, Tuke,[37] compiled and organized a large number of clinical observations and anecdotes reported over the span of several centuries, illustrating the alleged influence of the mind on physical health and illness. It is only in this century, however, that such sporadic observations and anecdotal reports have been formulated as testable hypotheses and subjected to systematic observation and, to some extent, experiment.

During the past 60 years, a sustained and widespread research effort has focused on attempts to identify those personality variables, psychological states, behaviors, and life events and situations that might prove to contribute to the development of a wide range of human diseases. As a result, observations have accrued that support the contributory role of psychosocial factors in the causation of all types of human morbidity. This statement, however, must not be misconstrued as implying psychogenesis of disease, that is, the notion that psychological variables are either a necessary or a sufficient condition for it to occur. No adequate empirical support for psychogenesis of any type of physical illness has been offered so far. The most readily demonstrable and accepted contributory role in disease causation is assigned to behavior. Specific habits pertaining to eating, exercise, risk taking, smoking, substance abuse, sexual practices, and so forth exemplify psychological factors whose contributory etiological role is no longer contested nowadays. Controversy begins, however, when various personality variables, emotional states, and life events or changes are postulated to contribute to physical morbidity in general, or to specific diseases processes in particular. Review of that research and of the related controversies is outside the scope of this chapter. On the other hand, theoretical assumptions underlying that whole area of investigation are germane to the writer's topic and will be summarized presently.

A distinguishing and defining characteristic of man is his ability to create, and use for communication, symbols in thought and language. That symbolic activity is enabled by the structure, function, and organization of the human brain and can be viewed as an aspect of cerebral function, one that can influence bodily processes at all levels of organization down to the cellular level.[10] Symbolic activity is influenced by cerebral processes, which are in turn affected by the functioning of the whole organism and by the dynamic state of its constituents and its *milieu intérieur*. Symbolic activity, or the mind, that is, the realm of conscious and unconscious perceptions, thoughts, memories, images, and action tendencies, is partly autonomous and partly responsive to the information inputs from the body and the external environment. Since man is a social creature, his interactions with and information inputs from his social environment constitute the most important, since personally the most meaningful, source of information. That information is likely to influence the person's symbolic activity and to elicit emotional correlates of the latter. Emotions may be viewed as variables intervening between symbolic or cognitive activity, on the one hand, and bodily changes induced by the latter, on the other.[10] Information that is novel to the recipient, or is interpreted by him in terms of subjective meaning signifying threat, loss, or gain, appears to be particularly effective in arousing intense emotions. The latter have physiological concomitants (e.g., cardiovascular, respiratory, glandular, musculoskeletal) that may have several effects relevant to the person's health: (1) they may be perceived and augment, reduce, or change the quality of emotional arousal; (2) they may motivate the person to behave in a manner injurious or conducive to his or her health; (3) they may set in motion various psychological defenses and coping strategies whose aim is to reduce emotional distress; (4) they may be communicated to other people in the form of symptoms or complaints and foster adoption of a particular socially sanctioned role, the so-called sick role; and (5) they may predispose to, precipitate, help make manifest, exacerbate, or ameliorate a disease process in any body part or system.[10]

It is meaningless to say that emotions cause disease; they cause nothing. It is equally incorrect to propose that any other psychological variable causes disease; it can only influence susceptibility to disease through the mediation of neuroendocrine processes controlled by the brain. The quality, intensity, and duration of evoked emotions are important factors determining the impact of symbolic activity and information inputs on susceptibility to disease.

The way in which a person interprets particular events and reacts to them emotionally and behaviorally is in part determined by his enduring personality dispositions or traits, which reflect his history and genetic endowment, and experiences retained in memory. All those factors codetermine which life situations and changes will be meaningful for the person, how he will appraise them, and what specific emotions they will elicit in him. An individual's susceptibility to a particular physical illness and the timing of its onset are likely to be influenced by these variables. They may be viewed as individual predispositions that precede and codetermine a person's total response to a given event or situation.

A construct that is often invoked in discussions about the postulated effects of the various psychosocial variables on health is that of psychological or *psychosocial stress*.[10] Derived from the work of Cannon, Selye, and Wolff, this concept has achieved considerable currency despite its ambiguity,[38-40] which is the result of three distinct connotations of the term "stress" proposed by various writers. Thus, stress may connote a state of the organism exposed to certain stimuli or stressors; the stressors, that is stimuli which evoke stress responses in the organism; and an area of study that includes stressful stimuli or stressors, an organism's responses to them, and the totality of intervening variables.[41] Despite this semantic ambiguity, the concept of psychosocial stress has considerable heuristic value as an organizing construct for a whole set of psychological and social variables that evoke physiological responses and are relevant to issues of health and disease.

Despite frequent proclamations that psychosocial stress is an important etiological factor, attempts to document its causal role in disease have led to conflicting results. It is a fallacy to state that psychosocial stress is *directly* pathogenic. Rather, it appears to influence, that is, enhance or reduce, a person's susceptibility to disease by altering the balance of the body's neuroendocrine and immune mechanisms.[42] Psychosocial stress may be defined as *those social interactions and events as well as those psychological states that impose a burden on the organism by virtue of the emotions and the disturbances of body homeostasis that they elicit.*

Numerous attempts have been made to identify those psychological and social variables which could be regarded as psychosocial stressors. Engel,[17] for example, distinguished three categories of phenomena that may bring about psychological stress: (1) loss or threat of loss of psychic objects, that is, persons, ideals, body functions or parts, or other values; (2) injury to the body; and (3) frustration of drives. Other investigators have focused on stressful life events or changes.[43] Bereavement, loss of job, disturbed family interaction or family disruption, work overload, migration, and a host of other events and situations have been proposed to represent psychosocial stressors. There is some evidence that they may actually increase the probability of a near-future impairment of health. Whether such impairment does actually take place appears to depend on additional conditions that may be termed moderator variables,[26] namely, those which modify, that is, increase or reduce, the strength of association between psychosocial stressors and morbidity. Individual predisposition, the psychophysiological state of the person at the time of exposure to stressful stimuli, availability of social supports, and the presence of or exposure to specific physicochemical or microbiological disease agents represent moderator variables that modify the effect of stress on the organism. Their configuration in a given case codetermines the occurrence and form of illness.

Clearly, simple, linear notions of causality cannot do justice to the complex effects of psychosocial stressors on health. Such complexity has no doubt contributed to the contradictory findings reported in the literature and to the skepticism of those who seek relatively clear-cut cause-and-effect relationships comparable to those obtained in laboratory experiments. Complexity, however, is a fact of life and has to be accepted. To deny the role of psychosocial stress in disease etiology would be tantamount to denying any validity to the countless clinical observations accumulated over the centuries. Psychosocial stress may be viewed as an independent variable, one comprising a set of etiological factors in human morbidity that are predicated on the fact of man's capacity for symbolic activity which enables him to appraise and communicate information, to endow it with subjective meaning and respond to it emotionally, and to anticipate future events. Symbolic activity is a facet of cerebral function that can, by means of neuroendocrine pathways and mechanisms, profoundly affect homeostasis as well as the body's defenses against noxious factors introduced from without or arising from within the body. By such indirect means, symbolic activity can enhance the organism's susceptibility or resistance to disease.

Etiological versus Reactive Factors

Medical writers tend to distinguish between etiological or causative factors, on the one hand, and the reactive ones, on the other. The reactive factors refer to a person's psychosocial responses and to symptoms of disease. The distinction between etiological and reactive psychosocial factors must not be viewed as a hard and fast one. For example, a loss and the emotions it engenders may in a given person contribute to the onset of a physical illness and then continue to influence his psychological state and behavior throughout his illness. Yet the distinction is heuristically and clinically useful. Physical illness or injury, regardless of its causation, may be viewed as an independent variable or stimulus that leads to psychosocial responses. As Engel[17] proposed, injury to the body constitutes a major form of psychological or psychosocial stress, one that may be studied in its own right. One may also regard illness as a source of personally meaningful information inputs for the sick individual which elicit cognitive, emotional, and behavioral responses.[44] Such responses can be identified, described, and classified.

Thus, when one speaks of psychosocial aspects of physical illness and injury, one is referring to the ubiquitous psychological and social responses to manifest disease.

These responses may be continuous with those that had contributed to its development in the first place. One need not postulate discontinuity between the premorbid etiological and the disease-reactive psychosocial factors. Those factors may increase or reduce the intensity of disease and thus infuence its course and outcome.

In summary, the holistic approach is as old as the history of Western thought and medicine. It advocates the view of man as a unified, biopsychosocial organism in ceaseless interaction with the social and physical environment. It insists that to treat a patient adequately, the physician needs to take into account the sick person as a whole rather than focus entirely on a diseased organ or system. The holistic approach has been systematically propagated for the past half century by a movement called "psychosomatic medicine," which, after a period of enthusiastic reception, suffered temporary eclipse in the 1950s and 1960s, only to be revived in the past 20 years or so.

The holistic approach to medicine influences the manner in which the states of

health and disease are defined. It postulates that both these states have biopsychosocial determinants and hence that the etiology of all diseases is bound to be multifactorial. Psychosocial variables constitute a class of etiological factors whose relative contribution varies from disease to disease but is never absent. They influence to some
extent not only the very occurrence and the timing of onset, but also the course and
outcome of every disease.

REFERENCES

1. Smuts JD: *Holism and Evolution*. New York, Macmillan Publishing Co, 1926.
2. Hamilton E, Cairns H (eds): *The Collected Dialogues of Plato*. New York, Bollingen Foundation, 1961, p 911.
3. Rather LJ: *Mind and Body in Eighteenth Century Medicine*. Berkeley, University of California Press, 1965.
4. Lipowski ZJ: What does the word "psychosomatic" really mean? A historical and semantic inquiry. *Psychosom Med* 46:153-171, 1984.
5. Ryle G: *The Concept of Mind*. London, Hutchinson, 1949.
6. Cassell EJ: *The Healer's Art*. Philadelphia, JB Lippincott Co, 1976.
7. Powell RC: Helen Flanders Dunbar (1902-1959) and a holistic approach to psychosomatic problems. I. The rise and fall of a medical philosophy. *Psychiatr Q* 49:133-152, 1977.
8. Powell RC: Helen Flanders Dunbar (1902-1959) and a holistic approach to psychosomatic problems. II. The role of Dunbar's nonmedical background. *Psychiatr Q* 50:144-157, 1978.
9. Alexander F: *Psychosomatic Medicine*. New York, Norton, 1950.
10. Lipowski ZJ: Psychosomatic medicine in the seventies: An overview. *Am J Psychiatry* 134:233-244, 1977.
11. Lipowski ZJ: Review of consultation psychiatry and psychiatry and psychosomatic medicine. III. Theoretical issues. *Psychosom Med* 30:395-422, 1968.
12. Lipowski ZJ: Holistic-medical foundations of American psychiatry: A bicentennial. *Am J Psychiatry* 138:888-895, 1981.
13. Dunbar S: *Emotions and Bodily Changes: A Survey of Literature on Psychosomatic Interrelationships: 1901-1933*. New York, Columbia University Press, 1935.
14. Bertalanffy L von: *General System Theory*. New York, Braziller, 1968.
15. Dubos R: *Man Adapting*. New Haven, Yale University Press, 1965.
16. Dubos R: *Man, Medicine, and Environment*. New York, The New American Library, 1968.
17. Engel GL: A unified concept of health and disease. *Perspect Biol Med* 3:459-485, 1960.
18. Engel GL: The need for a new medical model: A challenge for bio-medicine. *Science* 196:129-136, 1977.
19. Berliner HS, Salmon JW: The holistic alternative to scientific medicine: History and analysis. *Int J Health Serv* 10:133-147, 1980.
20. Svihus RH: On healing the whole person: A perspective. *West J Med* 131:478-481, 1979.
21. Sobel DS (ed): *Ways of Health. Holistic Approaches to Ancient and Contemporary Medicine*. New York, Harcourt Brace Jovanovich, 1979.
22. Sigerist HE: *Medicine and Human Welfare*. New Haven, Yale University Press, 1941.
23. Editorial: The concept of disease. *Br Med J* 2:751-752, 1979.
24. Campbell EJM, Scadding JG, Roberts RS: The concept of disease. *Br Med J* 2:757-762, 1979.
25. Feinstein AR: *Clinical Judgement*. Baltimore, Williams & Wilkins, 1967.
26. Susser M: *Causal Thinking in the Health Sciences*. New York, Oxford University Press, 1973.
27. Barondess JA: Disease and illness—A crucial distinction. *Am J Med* 66:375-376, 1979.
28. Brody H: The systems view of man: Implications for medicine, science, and ethics. *Perspect Biol Med* 17:71-92, 1973.
29. Fabrega H Jr: *Disease and Social Behavior: An Interdisciplinary Perspective*. Cambridge, Mass, MIT Press, 1974.

30. Murphy EA: *The Logic of Medicine.* Baltimore, Johns Hopkins University Press, 1976.
31. Stewart GT: Limitations of the germ theory. *Lancet* 1:1077-1081, 1968.
32. Riegelman R: Contributory cause: Unnecessary and insufficient. *Postgrad Med* 66:177-179, 1979.
33. Halliday JL: *Psychosocial Medicine. A Study of the Sick Society.* New York, Norton, 1948.
34. Kaplan HI, Kaplan HS: An historical survey of psychosomatic medicine. *J Nerv Ment Dis* 124:546-568, 1956.
35. Archer J: *Every Man His Own Doctor.* London, Printed for the Author, 1673.
36. Rather LJ: *Mind and Body in Eighteenth Century Medicine.* Berkeley, University of California Press, 1965.
37. Tuke DH: *Illustrations of the Influence of the Mind upon the Body in Health and Disease.* London, Churchill, 1872.
38. Hinkle LE: The concept of "stress" in the biological and social sciences, in Lipowski ZJ, Lipsitt DR, Whybrow PC (eds): *Psychosomatic Medicine. Current Trends and Clinical Applications.* New York, Oxford University Press, 1977, pp 27-49.
39. Mason JW: A historical view of the stress field. *J Hum Stress* 1:6-12, 1975.
40. Wolff HG: *Stress and Disease.* Springfield, Ill, Charles C Thomas, 1953.
41. Lazarus RS: *Psychological Stress and the Coping Process.* New York, McGraw-Hill, 1960.
42. Cassel J: Psychosocial processes and "stress": Theoretical formulation. *Int J Health Serv* 4:471-482, 1974.
43. Dohrenwend BS, Dohrenwend BP (eds): *Stressful Life Events: Their Nature and Effects.* New York, John Wiley & Sons, 1974.
44. Lipowski ZJ: Psychosocial aspects of disease. *Ann Intern Med* 71:1197-1206, 1969.

What Does the Word "Psychosomatic" Really Mean?

Really Mean?

A Historical and Semantic Inquiry

7

INTRODUCTION

Students, colleagues, and lay people have often asked me: "What is psychosomatic medicine? What does the word 'psychosomatic' really mean?" To try and answer these questions with reasonable clarity I have reviewed the literature and given the matter a good deal of thought. The literature, however, reveals a lack of consensus with regard to the meaning of these terms, and it actually addresses the issue infrequently. Journals and societies calling themselves "psychosomatic" exist in various countries, and are presumably based on the assumption that their professed field of interest is a distinct and clearly delimited one. Discussions with concerned colleagues reveal, however, that ambiguity and controversy persist, and that some individuals would gladly bury the word "psychosomatic" altogether, replacing it with some other, hopefully less ambiguous term, such as "biopsychosocial," for example. Yet, as a historian of psychosomatic medicine shrewdly observed years ago, even though the word "psychosomatic" is unsatisfactory, it is "so deeply entrenched in the literature that it will never be eradicated."[1, p. 402] Indeed, so far it has resisted all attempts to eliminate it, as indicated by the fact that both this journal and the Society of which it is an organ continue to be called "psychosomatic." This being so, another attempt to trace the roots of and to define the terms in question is called for, so as to provide a basis for a wider discussion.

Having proposed a definition of psychosomatic medicine in the past,[2,3] I was challenged to return to this subject by a recently published account of the history of this field written by Ackerknecht,[4] a medical historian. He argues that if one defines psychosomatic medicine in terms that convey the "recognition of a partial, or sometimes total, *psychogenesis of disease*" (emphasis added), then its origins reach back to ancient Greece. Ackerknecht ends his article with a conclusion that "the basic element of psychosomatic medicine represents a dialogue between doctor and patient, their cooperation.... The psychosomaticist seems above all to be the physician who specializes in listening to the patient.... we may be glad to have retained a specialist of this type."[4, p. 23]

Thus, in the eyes of the historian just quoted, psychosomatic medicine constitutes an ill-defined area, one concerned with demonstrating psychogenesis of disease, and a medical specialty distinguished by listening to patients. If this view of the field is correct, then the contents of the current psychosomatic journals, for example, are largely irrelevant to its proper scope. If it is not, then a rebuttal and clarification are called for in order to put the matter straight and to avoid the spread of misleading conceptions. It appears that a disturbing gulf exists between a historian's conception of what psychosomatic medicine is about and the interpretation endorsed by most workers who are active in this field and identify themselves with it. This discrepancy may well have arisen because of the historical development of psychosomatic concepts and the coexistence of several connotations of the word "psychosomatic" in the literature. In an attempt to clarify this issue I propose to review in this article some of the representative dictionary definitions as well as the historical development and roots of the terms "psychosomatic" and "psychosomatic medicine." I will also formulate a set of definitions that will prove, hopefully, acceptable to the majority of workers in the discipline.

DICTIONARY MEANING OF "PSYCHOSOMATIC"

The Oxford English Dictionary lists the word "psychosomatic" for the first time in a supplement published in 1982, and offers a set of its definitions. It defines the adjective "psychosomatic" as one "involving or depending on both the mind and the body as mutually dependent entities."[5, p. 888] The term has been used to refer to the following: (1) *physical disorders*, those caused or aggravated by psychologic factors, and, less often, to mental disorders caused or aggravated by physical factors; (2) the *branch of medicine* concerned with the mind–body relations; and (3) the *field of study*, one sometimes designated "psychosomatics," concerned with the relationship between mind and body.

It is noteworthy that the above definitions hightlight two distinct connotations of the word "psychosomatic," viz, concern with *mind–body relationship* and the *psychogenesis* of physical disorders, respectively. By emphasizing the mind–body issue the Dictionary gives the term "psychosomatic" a strong philosophic stamp, one that workers in psychosomatic medicine have tried to stay away from, as I will show later on. Moreover, to speak of mind and body as "entities" implies dualism and hence invites controversy. Writers on psychosomatics have traditionally, if not always logically and consistently, affirmed their antidualistic stance and tended to opt for some form of monism, arguing that mind and body are one or are merely separate aspects of a person, or of the organism as a whole. Nevertheless, this connotation of the word "psychosomatic" may be referred to as the *holistic* one, in the sense that it presupposes the inseparability of mind and body as well as their mutual dependence. Yet to state, as the Dictionary does, that the chief concern and the object of study of psychosomatic medicine is the relationship between mind and body strikes me as a misleading assertion, because it is too abstract and too far removed from what workers in this field actually try to accomplish. Thus, the Dictionary definitions highlight and compound the ambiguity of the word "psychosomatic."

A representative psychiatric dictionary offers an even narrower and more contentious definition of the word "psychosomatic."[6] It states that the latter may be used only in a "methodological sense," to refer to "a type of approach in the study and treatment of certain disturbances of body function."[6, p. 613] Furthermore, it deplores the tendency to use the word "psychosomatic" to refer to a class of disorders whose causation is believed to implicate emotional factors, and thus to imply a dualism that does not really exist, since no disease is free from the influence of psychologic factors. Such a criticism of this particular connotation and usage of the term has been voiced by many authors.[2] The Expert Committee of the World Health Organization, for instance, has deplored the common use of the term "psychosomatic disorders" as one reaffirming mind–body dichotomy and undermining a much-needed holistic approach to the practice of medicine.[7] The Committee wisely recommended that efforts should be made to work out generally acceptable terms and definitions that would be useful for teaching and research. The present article represents one such effort.

One may conclude that representative dictionary definitions of the terms "psychosomatic" and "psychosomatic medicine" are unsatisfactory, since they fail to reflect adequately the connotations of these words contained in psychosomatic literature. The sources of this semantic confusion might become clearer as one traces the historic development of these terms.

History of the Word "Psychosomatic"

Margetts[1, 8] is to my knowledge, the only writer to make a serious effort to trace historic development of the term "psychosomatic." He asserts that the latter was first used in 1818 by the German psychiatrist Heinroth, in a rather cryptic sentence, "As a general rule, the origin of insomnia is psycho–somatic, but it is possible that every phase of life can itself provide the complete reason for insomnia.[1, p. 403] Margetts points out that Heinroth regarded the body and soul as one, but the quoted passage gives little indication of the real implications of his use of the word "psychosomatic." This compound word appears to reflect a fashion, common in German literature of the early 19th century, for the usage of such terms as psycho–physical or somato–psychic.[1] That tendency was adopted by some English writers, such as the eminent psychiatrist Bucknill,[9] who in 1857 argued that one could distinguish three theories of insanity, that is the somatic, the psychic, and the somato–psychic. Bucknill went on to say that "The psychosomaticists find in the liability of the cerebral instrument to disease, a reasonable basis for the irresponsibility of the insane."[9, p. 15] Gray,[10] editor of the *American Journal of Insanity,* misquoted Bucknill to say that one of his three proposed theories was "psycho–somatic." This may have been the first time that the term appeared in America. In the same article, Gray asserts that "the reciprocal influence of body and mind is a fact constantly before the physician" (p. 155).

A curious early example of the use of the word "psychosomatic" turns up unexpectedly in the novel *Hard Cash,* written in 1863 by a prolific English writer, Charles Reade.[11] The major theme of that novel is the abuse of psychiatric commitment in England for the purpose of getting rid of offensive relatives. A devious asylum doctor tries to persuade a father to commit his son by extolling the virtues of the asylum under his directorship, and promises to provide "the nocturnal and diurnal attendance of a psycho–physical physician, who knows the psycho–somatic relation of body and mind...."[11, p. 405]

Apart from the above scattered examples, the word "psychosomatic" was used infrequently in the literature of the 19th century and prior to the 1930s.[8] It is absent from the unusually comprehensive *Dictionary of Psychological Medicine* edited by Tuke,[12] which lists only the term "psychosomatiatria," one defined as "a medicine for mind and body" (p. 1034). Nor does it appear in Tuke's classic compilation of works illustrating the influence of the mind on the body, first published in 1872, in which he uses related terms such as "psycho–physical phenomena" and "psycho–physiology."[13, p. 455]

Felix Deutsch, in 1922, was probably the first author to introduce the term "psychosomatic medicine."[14] The 1920s may be generally viewed as a period during which the ground was prepared for the emergence of psychosomatic medicine in the following decade. In 1925, a book was published in Vienna presenting philosophic arguments as well a clinical observations from several areas of medicine supporting the notion that medicine has neglected to consider the role of psychologic factors in the etiology of disease and in the treatment of patients.[15] The several contributors, including Paul Schilder, cited the work of Gestalt psychologists, Freud, Pavlov, and Cannon to bolster their contention that the proper subject of medicine should be the organism as a structural and functional unity, one that includes the psyche. The publication of that comprehensive treatise paved the way for an encyclopedic compilation of the relevant literature to appear 10 years later.[16]

The heyday of the term "psychosomatic" and the true beginning of psychosomatic medicine were both launched by the publication in 1935 of Dunbar's *Emotions and Bodily Changes: A Survey of Literature on Psychosomatic Interrelationships: 1910–1933*.[16] Dunbar seemed to have some misgivings about her choice of the term "psychosomatic interrelationships," which, she remarked, was "inadequate to express the conviction that psyche and soma are...two aspects of a fundamental unity."[16, p. 427] She could not think of a better term, however, and her legacy is, for better or worse, still with us today. However one might regret Dunbar's choice of the word "psychosomatic," which she helped to popularize, the appearance of her book marked the emergence of psychosomatic medicine as an *organized* field of scientific inquiry and a movement aimed at propagating a holistic approach to medical practice. Until then psychosomatic conceptions had been sustained by conviction and clinical anecdotes, rather than based on systematic observations applying scientific methodology to demonstrate their empirical validity.

An event of singular importance for the development of psychosomatic conceptions and medicine was the appearance, in 1939, of the first issue of the journal, *Psychosomatic Medicine*. It was inaugurated by an Introductory Statement,[17] in which its editors tried to come to grips with the definition of the new field and offered the following: "Its object is to study in their interrelation the psychological and physiological aspects of all normal and abnormal bodily functions and thus to integrate somatic therapy and psychotherapy."[17, p. 3] The editors took pains to spell out what psychosomatic medicine was *not:* (1) equivalent with psychiatry, (2) restricted to any specific area of pathology, (3) a medical specialty, (4) concerned with the "metaphysics" of the mind–body problem. On the positive side, they emphasized that the new field's attributes: (1) concern with the psychologic approach to general medicine and all of its subspecialties, (2) interest in the interrelationships between emotional life and all bodily processes, (3) based on the premise that there is no "logical distinction" between mind and body, (4) involving research on correlation of psychologic and physiologic processes in man, and (5) both a special field and an integral part of every medical specialty.

Insofar as the Statement represents the views of the early leaders of psychosomatic medicine, it is in a sense authoritative, and since, to my knowledge, it has never been formally repealed, it presumably expresses the "official" position of this journal. For these reasons alone it deserves critical scrutiny. The proposed definition of the field rightly encompasses both its *scientific* and *clinical* aspects. The editors define the scope of psychosomatic medicine, and hence the object of its scientific interests, as the interrelation of psychologic and physiologic aspects of the functions of the *body* rather than of the *person*. Moreover, by stressing that psychosomatic medicine is distinct from psychiatry, which, as they put it, is concerned with the "diseased mind," they appear to unwittingly affirm mind–body dualism, a position they explicitly disavow. By emphasizing the distinction between the two disciplines, the editors convey the impression that psychosomatic conceptions do not apply to psychiatry. This is an unfortunate implication, one that contradicts the holistic viewpoint and deepens the deplorable gap between medicine and psychiatry. Had the editors referred in their definition to the dual functions or aspects of the person rather than the body, they would have reaffirmed their otherwise implied holistic stance.

Another major flaw of the Statement is the absence of any mention of the environmental, and especially the social, factors. Thus, the impression is conveyed that psychosomatic medicine is concerned exclusively with psychophysiologic phenomena occurring, as it were, in a social vacuum. This is a serious omission that may have resulted from the strong psychoanalytic orientation of some of the editors, and their consequent preoccupation with intrapersonal rather than interpersonal issues. In view of that bias, it is remarkable that the Statement makes no direct reference to the concept of psychogenesis, one that plays a prominent role in the writings of such psychosomatic pioneers and editors as Alexander.[18] That concept has attracted considerable criticism over the years and will not be missed.

The editors emphatically dissociate themselves from philosophic ("metaphysical") concerns, yet by asserting lack of logical distinction between mind and body they betray their distinct monistic, that is, metaphysical, bias. It cannot be gainsaid that many writers on psychosomatics have concerned themselves, explicitly or not, with the mind–body problem and have taken a strongly antidualistic position.[18] To deny this fact would be intellectually dishonest. One can, however, understand the reluctance of researchers and clinicians to define their area of interest in terms of highly abstract and perennially controversial philosophic concepts. Yet, the latter lurk in the background of many psychosomatic theoretical statements and are often implicit in them. This may be the reason underlying the definitions of the Oxford English Dictionary quoted earlier, which put the emphasis squarely on the mind–body problem as the major concern of psychosomatic medicine. The historical roots of psychosomatic conceptions, to be discussed later, may help clarify this contentious issue.

On the clinical side, the Statement stresses that psychosomatic medicine designates a method of approach to the problems of etiology and therapy, one applicable to all medical specialties, but fails to specify what this should imply in practice. They only allude vaguely to the understanding of the "psychic component of disease process," call for integration of somatic therapy and psychotherapy without saying how this can be done, and mention the doctor–patient relationship. Equally vague are the references to emotional "tensions" and "life," which appear to reflect the one-sided emphasis on emotions as the principal psychologic factors influencing and correlating with physiologic changes.[15,18]

All in all, the Introductory Statement represents an important historic landmark in the development of psychosomatic conceptions and medicine. It may be viewed as a bench-mark and starting point for the more recent attempts to define the field. Looked at from the perspective of over 40 years, it was a bold effort to launch and delimit the scope of a new field, yet one with ancient antecedents. The editors' Statement may be criticized for its errors of omission and commission touched on above, and should be revised and reformulated to reflect recent developments in the field and to serve as a point of reference for historians, teachers, and investigators.

It would be neither feasible nor profitable to try and review all the variants of the definition of psychosomatic medicine having appeared in the literature since 1939. It must suffice to say that the authors who have bothered to define the field at all have on the whole tended to stress its holistic or biopsychosocial connotation.[2,18,19] Some writers have insisted that the term "psychosomatic" should be used only to designate a method of approach to both research and clinical work, one that features concurrent and integrated use of biologic and psychosocial methods, concepts, and languages.[18,19] The writers holding this latter view object to the notion that psychosomatic medicine be considered a distinct scientific discipline with a defined object of study.

There is an inherent problem with the link-up of the words "psychosomatic" and "medicine," since they belong, at least in part, to two distinct levels of abstraction and discourse. Medicine is concerned with issues of health and disease. "Psychosomatic," however, has a broader and more abstract connotation, one that touches on the problem of mind and body, and hence pertains to views on the nature of man. When by somebody's whim those two words became linked, confusion and ambiguity that perplex us to this day resulted. What has come to be designated "psychosomatic medicine" constitutes a recent phase in the long history of efforts to apply a set of premises and precepts, which may be called "psychosomatic," to the issues of health and disease, and to the care of patients. At the same time, however, the word "psychosomatic" may be used to refer to certain philosophic concepts that are part of Western intellectual history, one that has a broader scope than the history of Western medicine, and, in fact, encompasses it. I will try to develop this thesis further with a brief outline of the history of psychosomatic conceptions.

My discussion is not to be viewed as an aborted attempt to present a comprehensive history of the subject, a task for which I posses neither the requisite competence nor space; that is the task of a historian. To my knowledge, such a history has never been published and is badly needed. What follows is merely a selective historic sketch germane to my thesis.

PSYCHOSOMATIC CONCEPTIONS: HISTORICAL PERSPECTIVE

Historians tell us that what we call "psychosomatic medicine" represents, in part, continuation in modern dress of conceptions whose origins go back to the beginning of Western thought and medicine.[1,4,16,20,21] In other words, these ideas antedate the coining of the word "psychosomatic" and the emergence of psychosomatic medicine as a discipline by over 2000 years. A brief review of some of those historic antecedents may help us appreciate not only a remarkable continuity of the conceptions under discussion, but also the roots of the contemporary connotations of the word "psychosomatic" and its puzzling ambiguity. I submit that the modern meaning of that term incorporates two old conceptions, namely the *holistic* and the *psychogenic,* which are not usually clearly distinguished and thus contribute to its ambiguity. I will try to support this contention with selected historical references and quotations.

THE HOLISTIC CONCEPTION

The word "holistic" is derived from the Greek *holos,* or whole, and was introducd into the literature by Smuts[22] in 1925. Though of recent vintage, this term may be applied to postulates about the nature of man and to precepts about medical care that can already be found in the writings of Greek philosophers, such as Plato and Aristotle. The core postulate of the holistic viewpoint is that the notions of mind and body refer to inseparable and mutually dependent aspects of man. As Drabkin observes, "A sense of inseparability of the psychic and the somatic life grows out of basic human experience, and ancient literature, medical and nonmedical, has no end of examples of the somatic effects of emotional changes and the emotional effects of somatic changes."[20, p. 227] Applied to the practice of medicine, the holistic conception afirms the need for physicians to take into account both the mental or psychologic and the physical or physiologic aspects in the study of disease and the treatment of patients. In his much-quoted passage in the dialogue Charmides, Plato[23] argues: "The cure of many diseases is unknown to the physicians of Hellas, because they disregard the whole, which ought to be studied also, for the part can never be well unless the whole is well." Plato seems to imply that attention to the person as a whole, a mind–body complex, is the best approach a physician can adopt in treating patients.

Plato's observation suggests that a holistic attitude was by no means predominant in medicine of his time, and whether it has ever dominated the medical scene since is an open question. Western medicine from Hippocrates on has tended to be staunchly naturalistic and somatic, or physiologic, although this has not prevented many medical writers from emphasizing the need to treat the whole person. Regardless of the philosophic views, if any, a physician may hold about the mind–body problem, he or she can apply a holistic approach in clinical work. Many medical writers from the Roman times onward have explicitly or implicitly advocated such an approach. Even the formulation of a radical dualism by Descartes in his Discourse on Method in 1637 did not result in the disappearance of holistic conceptions from the medical literature. This is especially well exemplified by the work of the 18th century Dutch physician Gaub, who wrote that "the reason why a sound body becomes ill, or an ailing body recovers, very often lies in the mind. Contrariwise, the body can frequently both beget mental illnesses and heal its offspring."[21, p. 71] Hence, argues Gaub, "should the physician devote all of his efforts to the body alone, and take no account of the mind, his curative endeavors will pretty often be less than happy and his purpose either wholly missed or part of what pertains to it neglected."[21, p. 70] As Rather,[21] the translator of Gaub's remarkable Essays published in 1747 and 1763, comments, the Dutch writer's views were neither original nor isolated, as they had been expressed by many medical authors before him. For that reason Gaub, argues Rather, cannot be regarded as a true forerunner of psychosomatic medicine. It was only the advent of cellular pathology, founded by Virchow in the 1850s, that largely resulted in "wiping out recollection of the attention traditionally accorded to mind–body relationships. Hence, psychosomatic medicine in our time has appeared to many as a new and almost unprecedented movement in medical thought."[21, p. 15]

Another 18th century medical writer, Benjamin Rush (1745–1813), the most prominent American physician of his time and the man officially declared the father of American psychiatry, expressed holistic conceptions no less clearly than Gaub.[24] As a professor of medicine at the College of Philadelphia and later at the university of Pennsylvania, Rush taught the importance of viewing the patient as a whole and was concerned with psychosomatic relations[25] In one of his lectures, for example, he spelled out the holistic approach to medicine in these memorable words, "Man is said to be a compound of soul and body. However proper this language may be in religion, it is not so in medicine. He is, in the eye of a physician, a single and indivisible being, for so intimately united are his soul and body, that one cannot be moved, without the other."[26] It is justified to consider Rush as a true forerunner of American psychosomatic medicine, as Binger,[27] his biographer, has suggested.

In the 19th century, the holistic conceptions in medicine suffered considerable decline but did not vanish.[28] Outstanding examples of their survival are provided by the writings of Henry Holland,[29] Physician Extraordinary to Queen Victoria, and of Daniel Hack Tuke,[13] who in 1872 published an extraordinary compilation of anecdotal clinical evidence illustrating the influence of psychologic factors on bodily functions. Tuke, however, was not just a compiler. He tried to provide a theoretical framework for his anecdotal illustrations based on physiologic principles, and to offer physicians an empirical justification to use "psycho–therapeutics" in a deliberate, methodical manner in the treatment of physical illness. At the end of the 19th century, Sir William Osler reviewed the holistic statements of Plato as they pertain to medical practice, and saw in them a foreboding that "in the medicine of the future the interdependence of mind and body will be more fully recognized, and that the influence of the one over the other may be exerted in a manner which is not now thought possible."[30]

Osler made the above prediction in a talk given in 1893. Within only 1 year appeared an article by Hughes in which he not only spelled out the holistic conception with clarity, but also offered a remarkable corollary to Osler's forecast. Hughes, editor of the journal *Alienist and Neurologist,* foresaw, perhaps too optimistically, that "We are approaching an era when the whole patient is to be treated, no more only a part or organ solely."[31, p. 902] He asserted that "In estimating the causal concomitants and sequences of his diseases, we consider the whole man in his psychoneurophysical relations." Hughes proposed that all bodily functions are influenced by emotions, both in health and disease, through the mediation of the central and vegetative nervous systems. For example, he asserted that a "breakdown in the central nervous system by which trophic and resisting powers are greatly lessened, makes possible and precedes all cases of cancer."[31, p. 901] He argued that if the mind has, through the agency of the neural mechanisms, such a widespread influence on bodily processes, this fact provides "physiologic basis of all forms of psychotherapy," and the latter should be employed by physicians as a powerful therapeutic tool. Hughes' article may be considered a landmark in the development of the holistic approach to medicine, even though it is seldom quoted.[24]

In the first 30 years of this century, the holistic conceptions became elaborated and propagated by the psychobiologic school of psychiatry, notably by Meyer and White.[24, 32] The basic premise of the psychobiologists was that mind and body are not separate entities acting on one another, but only two distinct yet integral aspects of the human organism, a psychobiologic unit, as a whole interacting with the environment. Disease should be viewed as a product of this interaction, and it always encompasses both somatic and psychologic aspects. Powell,[32] in one of the few scholarly recent papers on the history of psychosomatic medicine, points out that the holistic conceptions of the psychobiologists were adopted by Dunbar, and through her writings became one of the three principal theoretical positions in psychosomatic medicine. The other two viewpoints were the psychoanalytic and the psychophysiologic.[32] The holistic approach was also prominently represented by Goldstein[33] in his book *The Organism* published in 1939, and many other writers, not necessarily identified with psychosomatic medicine, since then.

In the view of this writer, the holistic conception has been most concisely stated by Woodger,[34] A British biologist and philosopher of science, in his book *Biology and Language:*". . .the notions of body and mind are both reached by abstraction from something more concrete. For these more concrete objects we have the convenient and familiar word persons. But even the notion of person is abstract in the sense that every person is a member of some community of persons, upon which the *kind* of person he is, and even his continued existence as a person, depends." This statement may be regarded as an expression of a *methodologic* and *linguistic* approach to the mind-body problem rather than a metaphysical one, and hence it appears to be most appropriate for psychosomatic medicine and for clinical work generally. For Woodger, the person, a member of a social group, is the starting point and an indivisible unit, one from which the notions of mind and body are abstracted for the purpose of study, and hence as a methodologic strategy. These two abstrations require separate languages with which to formulate descripive and theoretical statements about the functioning and behavior of persons, both in health and disease. This type of formulation eschews the concept of mind and body as *entities,* whose mutual relationship is the subject of philosophic speculation and is expressed in terms of competing metaphysical view-points, be they dualistic or monistic.

I have tried to present in this section some of the historic antecedents as well as the core meaning of the connotation of the word "psychosomatic," which I propose to call "holistic." This connotation lies at the heart of what many writers have referred to as the "psychosomatic approach" to issues of health and disease, and to the treatment of patients. As Dubos[35] states it, "The understanding and control of disease requires that the body–mind complex be studied in its relations to external environment." He points out, however, that the holistic (or psychosomatic) approach refers to an abstract ideal that cannot be fully attained in actual practice and that does not lend itself to the acquisition of exact knowledge. Other critics have asserted that adoption of the holistic approach is not a necessary condition for humane patient care.[36] Be that as it may, it is not the purpose of this article to defend the merits of holistic conceptions or approach, but merely to elucidate their semantic and historic relation to the word "psychosomatic." In the next section I propose to discuss the second major connotation of that term, that is, the psychogenic.

THE PSYCHOGENIC CONCEPTION

The second core connotation of the term "psychosomatic" may be referred to as equivalent to "psychogenic," in the sense that it implies an etiologic hypothesis about the role of psychologic factors in human disease. In other words, the psychogenic conception asserts that certain attributes or functions of the organism, those that be called "psychologic" or "mental," constitute a class of causative agents in morbidity. This conception, as I propose to illustrate by selected examples, has a lineage as old as the holistic one.

According to Lewis,[37] the word "psychogenic" was introduced into psychiatry by Sommer, a German psychiatrist, in 1894, to refer to hysteria. The term has been variously defined and applied since. Originally, authors used it only in reference to certain mental disorders that were thus implied to be of psychologic origin.[37] In the 1920s, however, the words "psychogenic" and "psychogenesis" came to be applied by some writers to bodily disorders in which psychologic factors were believed to play a major causal role.[15] Lewis[37] concluded his review of the term "psychogenic" with the wry comment that this vague word touched on unresolved issues of causality and dualism, and should best be buried. In the following discussion I will use "psychogenic" to imply psychologic causation.

From Hippocrates onward, countless medical writers have postulated that *emotions* influence body functions and may cause disease. He himself is quoted as saying. "Fear, shame, pleasure, passion . . . to each of these the appropriate member of the body responds by its action. Instances are sweats, palpitations of the heart. . . ."[38] A similar statement can be found in Aristotle's work "On the Soul."[16] For centuries after Hippocrates, emotions, or rather "passions" as they were called then,[16,39,40] were viewed not only as having an effect on the functions of the body, but also as causative, pathogenic factors. Galen,[41] one of the most influential medical writers of all times, included the passions among the causes of bodily disease. He referred to grief, anger, lust, and fear as "diseases of the soul" to be diagnosed and cured. Rather[21] asserts that, as a result of Galen's influence on European medicine down to the 19th century, physicians had devoted a great deal of attention to the psychologic causation of disease, and especially to the role of emotions as etiologic factors in a wide range of diseases, including some of the contagious ane epidemic ones. A typical illustration of this statement is provided by this passage from Archer's *Every Man His Own Doctor*, published in 1673,[42] "The observation I have made in practice of physick these several years, hath confirmed me in this opinion, that the original, or cause of most men and womens sickness, disease, and death is, first, some great discontent, which brings a habit of sadness of mind...." As Ackerknecht[4] comments, "It is not clear why it has never been fully realized that for 1700 years there has been in existence a continuous tradition of psychosomatics under the label of 'passions'."[4, p. 18]

In 1637, a book appeared which was to have a profound influence on Western thought, that is, Descartes' *Discourse on Method*, in which the problem and antithesis of mind and body were formulated more explicitly and radically than ever before.[21, 43, 44] Descartes separated mind (res cogitans), the thinking entity, from the nonthinking, machine-like body. This was a turning point in the development of modern medicine and in the ancient debate on the mind–body issue. While Cartesian dualism dealt a blow to the holistic conceptions in medicine, it did not, paradoxically, prove detrimental to psychogenic conceptions. On the contrary, the latter flourished in the 17th and 18th centuries. Descartes himself regarded the passions as bodily phenomena that could influence other somatic functions, and even have a pathogenic effect.

Despite the spread of a mechanistic approach to medicine in the 17th century, the greatest physicians of that age and the true founders of modern medicine, Harvey, Willis, and Sydenham, paid considerable attention to emotional factors in disease. Of particular interest in view of the recent concern with the role of psychologic factors in the development and course of cancer is the following comment by a German physician, Pechlin, made in 1691, and quoted by Rather,[45] "Indeed, I have never seen a cancer of the breast so thoroughly removed, even after extirpation, that would not, in consequence of fear and sorrow, rather suddenly once again slowly recrudesce and, after long difficulties, at length put an end to life."

In the 18th century, a systematic account of the influence of emotions on bodily function and disease can be found in Gaub's Essay of 1763.[21] He speaks of the harmful effects on the body of overt as well as suppressed anger, grief, terror, unrequited love, and excessive joy. His comments have a remarkably modern ring, as when he says of grief, for example, that when it is not "discharged in lamentation and wailing, but instead remains seated firmly within and is for a long time repressed and fostered, the body no less than the mind is eaten up and destroyed."[21, p. 140]

Other 18th century medical writers, notably Stahl, developed elaborate, philosophically based, psychogenic conceptions.[21,46] Two works that appeared at the end of that century offer a systematic presentation of contemporary views of the influence of the mind on the body.[47, 48] In his monograph, Corp discusses both the pathogenetic and the beneficial effects of the "mental faculties," including thoughts, attention, and emotions, such as hope, joy, anger, fear, grief, and anxiety, and proclaims "the dependence of mind and body on each other.'' Speaking of anger, for example, Corp lists among its potential harmful effects "palsy, apoplexy, and sudden death."[47, p. 56] He asserts that prolonged anxiety may injure the brain, resulting in failure of memory. Of grief, he says that it can lead to any bodily disorder. Persons who are afflicted with fear or dread of disease, claims Corp, have long been known to be the first to fall victim to plague during an epidemic of it. Hope, by contrast, may help protect against plague, and has generally curative powers, which physicians ought to promote.

The above selected examples, to which many others could readily be added, have to suffice as illustrations of the widespread interest in the influence of emotions on bodily functions and the occurrence of disease among 17th and 18th century medical writers. Friedreich,[49] an early historian of psychiatry, wrote that one of the dominant themes in 18th century medical literature was the reciprocal relationship between body and soul, including the influence of passions and affects on the former. He quotes numerous authors who dealt with that topic. In America, Rush[26] wrote at length about how useful the knowledge of the actions of the mind on the body should be to physicians, since those actions "influence many of the functions of the body in health. They are the causes of many diseases; and if properly directed, they may easily be made to afford many useful remedies."[26, p. 256]

It is notable that those psychogenic conceptions were not held by mavericks but, on the contrary, were presented as a matter of fact by the leaders of the medical profession and by the most influential medical writers of the 17th and 18th centuries. Furthermore, those views were expressed by authors who held opposed opinions on the nature of the mind and its relationship to the body. Dualists and monists, materialists and idealists all seemed to find such views congenial regardless of their own philosophic positions. That trend waned to some extent during the 19th century not so much because of a major shift in philosophic views, but rather because medicine was becoming more technologic, specialized, and focused on the body to the exclusion of mental factors. Virchow's theory of cellular pathology, followed by the discoveries of Pasteur and Koch in bacteriology, propelled medicine in the direction of the Cartesian mechanistic approach to the body and towards the doctrine that for every disease there is a single specific cause.[50] That very trend provoked, in this century, the rise of a counterreformation which came to be labelled "psychosomatic medicine."

During the 19th century, psychogenic conceptions still continued to be represented in medical literature, if on a lesser scale than previously.[28] An event of especial importance was the appearance, in 1833, of Beaumont's study of a man with exposed gastric mucosa.[51] That work was a landmark, as it reported the first *systematic* and prolonged observations of the influence of emotional states on the functions of an interal organ. The study of psychophysiologic relations was becoming scientific in the hands of Beaumont, a "backwood physiologist," as Osler[52] called him. Almost a whole century had passed before such studies, having been given impetus by the work of Pavlov[53] and Cannon,[54] became in the 1930s an integral component of psychosomatic medicine.[32] Psychosphysiologic studies have focused on mechanisms mediating between psychologic variables on the one hand, and normal and abnormal body functions on the other. As such, they have been concerned with processes and correlations rather than with issues of disease etiology, which are implied by the word "psychogenesis." Psychophysiology may be viewed as that outgrowth of the ancient concern with the impact of emotions on the working of the body that has been most consistently "scientific" in its approach to that subject, in the sense of relying on the experimental method and eschewing sweeping generalizations. Today, psychophysiologic research continues to be one of the most vital and indispensable divisions of psychosomatic studies,[3] but it would be incorrect to equate all of psychosomatic medicine with psychophysiology; a part is not identical with the whole.

A very different approach to the study of the influence of emotions on the body, one concerned with their precise nature and role in the etiology of disease, took its inspiration from psychoanalysis.[55] Freud's technique of free association afforded access to unconscious mental processes, while his concepts of unconscious conflict, repression, and conversion provided conceptual tools which could be applied to hypotheses about psychosomatic relationships. For Freud, hysterical symptoms appeared when affect associated with an idea strongly conflicting with the ego, and consequently repressed, became discharged in somatic innervation and symptoms. Freud used the term "conversion" to refer to the process whereby psychic excitation was transmuted into somatic symptoms, but he confined this hypothesis to hysteria and did not extend it to organic disease.

By contrast, some followers of Freud, such as Groddeck, Deutsch, and Jelliffe, advanced propositions about the etiology of organic disease, modeled on his formulations about the origin of hysterical symptoms.[55] Groddeck,[56] for example, asserted that every illness served the purpose of symbolically representing an inner conflict and aimed at resolving it, repressing it, or preventing that which was already repressed from becoming conscious.[56] His was the most radical formulation of psychogenesis to emerge as an offshoot of psychoanalytic theory, and drew sharp critiques from some of his psychoanalytic colleagues, such as Alexander, who advanced his own, more moderate, conceptions of psychogenesis.

Alexander,[18, 55] one of the pioneers of psychosomatic medicine, embarked in 1932 on a series of studies designed to elucidate the putative causal role of emotional factors in several chronic diseases of unknown etiology. His was an attempt to apply psychoanalytic technique and concepts to the ancient ideas about psychogenesis.[18] He distinguished sharply between conversion symptoms as symbolic expressions of psychologic issues in the form of somatic symptoms on the one hand, and organic diseases, which he viewed as vegetative responses to chronic emotional states, and, hence, devoid of any symbolic meaning, on the other. He called the latter disorders "vegetative" or "organ" neuroses, and referred to them as psychogenic organic disorders. Alexander postulated that every emotional state had its own physiologic syndrome, and both could be induced together by appropriate emotional stimuli. He maintained that fear, aggression, guilt, and frustrated wishes, if repressed, would result in chronic "emotional tensions" and consequent dysfunction of body organs.[18] The repression of wishes and emotions would occur if they gave rise to inner conflicts. Such conflicts, believed Alexander, displayed a predilection for, and hence tended to disturb the function of *specific* internal organs, by analogy to the affinity of certain microorganisms for specific body parts.[18] He termed his hypothesis "specificity theory," asserting that a specific "dynamic constellation" consisting of a nuclear conflict, the defenses against it, and the emotions engendered by it, tended to correlate with a specific "vegetative" response. Alexander applied these conceptions to such diseases as essential hypertension, rheumatoid arthritis, thyrotoxicosis, and peptic ulcer, and formulated complex psychogenic hypotheses to account for their occurrence.

Alexander took pains to stipulate that his theory of psychogenesis implied no more than that those physiologic processes in the brain that could preferably be studied by psychologic methods because they were subjectively experienced as emotions, ideas, or wishes, could, in some cases, constitute the first links in a causal chain leading initially to disturbance of function and ultimately to structural organic disease. Psychogenesis could not, however, fully account for the development of any such disease, since available evidence on the whole pointed to multicausality of all diseases. It was only the coexistence of specific emotional and somatic factors that could result in disease such as peptic ulcer, for example. Alexander explicitly disavowed the concept of "psychosomatic disease" as one incompatible with the doctrine of multifactorial etiology,[18, p. 52] but nevertheless he spoke of "psychogenic organic disorder"[18, p. 44] as an acceptable concept.

Alexander's hypotheses represent the most elaborate formulation of psychogenesis of organic disease ever advanced. They constitute, therefore, an important landmark in the history of the development of that conception, and of psychosomatic medicine generally. His views exerted, for better or worse, widespread influence for some 25 years, between about 1935 and 1960, and were clearly much more moderate than Groddeck's extreme panpsychologism. Despite their relative moderation, however, his theory of specific psychogenesis of selected diseases, those referred to by many writers as "psychosomatic," encountered growing criticism and suffered gradual eclipse.[2,57-60] The very notion of psychogenesis has come under attack as one seeming to imply that psychosomatic medicine is concerned with the role of the psyche as a "morbific agent," and promotes a simplistic notion of a linear causal chain leading from emotions to disease.[59] Such linear cauality has come to be regarded as inadequate to account for the development of most of human morbidity.

Alexander's hypotheses may be seen as a sophisticated modern reformulation of the idea expressed in a rudimentary form by Galen in the second century A.D., that passions can have a harmful effect on the body and may actually cause disease. Over the centuries, it was mostly the passions or emotions that were, for some reason, singled out from the whole repertoire of psychologic variables as potential etiologic agents. The most recent variation of this theme is represented by the concept of alexithymia, proposed in 1972 to refer to persons having difficulty in describing their emotions and exhibiting stunted fantasy life.[61] This ill-defined clinical construct has been misapplied by some writers as an explanatory concept in hypotheses about the origin of the so-called psychosomatic disorders.

The proposition that emotions "cause" disease is largely viewed today as arbitrary and invalid. Rather, they are considered to be intervening variables interposed between the meaning for the individual of the information impinging upon him or her on the one hand, and somatic responses that follow, on the other.[60] Indeed, the entire notion of psychogenesis, one incompatible with the currently prevailing doctrine of multicausality of disease, is no longer tenable, hence, the psychogenic connotation of the word "psychosomatic" should be explicitly discarded. As one writer put it succinctly, "To equate psychosomatic with psychogenetic is indeed pointless and obsolete.[62] The word "psychosomatic" should not be used to imply causality in any sense or context, but only to refer to the reciprocal relationships between psychosocial and biologic factors in health and disease.[63] Concern with the nature and role of the interplay of those factors in the development, course, and outcome of all diseases remains one of the central issues in psychosomatic medicine, but it can be adequately subsumed under the holistic or biopsychosocial connotation of the word "psychosomatic."[64] I propose that the latter connotation is the only one acceptable today.[3,65]

PROPOSED DEFINITIONS

Ackerknecht's article[4] as well as the Oxford English Dictionary's definition of the word "psychosomatic" quoted earlier in this paper attest to the need to define once more the core terms relevant to psychosomatic medicine, and to delineate this field. A recent connent by a psychologist highlights this need, "The field of psychosomatic medicine suffers from definitions and concepts that have emerged, over time, without the adequate forethought and structure to remove ambiguity and ensure that the field is properly delineated."[66] The ambiguity to which that author alludes appears to have two major sources: (1) the dual connotation of the term "psychosomatic," which I have tried to emphasize in this article from a historical persective; and (2) the fact that psychosomatic medicine has focused on the study of relationships among phenomena that cut across several branches of science and make sharp delineation of the field difficult if not actually undesirable. The problem of the complex relationships among psychologic, social, and biologic aspects of health and disease has puzzled interested observers for over 2000 years and remains a riddle. No wonder that a relatively recently organized scientific discipline concerning itself with that tangled knot has been beset by semantic confusion, false starts, and ambiguity. These obstacles related to the very subject matter of psychosomatic medicine should not, however, discourage periodic efforts to define it with reasonable clarity. Having tried to do so several times over the past 15 years,[2,3,61] I propose to try once more in the hope that my effort will stimulate discussion and facilitate teaching.

"Psychosomatic" is a term referring or related to the inseparability and interdependence of psychosocial and biologic (physiologic, somatic) aspects of humankind. (This connotation may be called "holistic" as it implies a view of the human being as a whole, a mind–body complex embedded in a social environment.)

"Psychosomatic medicine" (psychosomatics) refers to a discipline concerned with (1) the study of the correlations of psychologic and social phenonomena with physiologic functions, normal or pathologic, and of the interplay of biologic and psychosocial factors in the development, course, and outcome of diseases; and (2) advocacy of a holistic (or biopsychosocial) approach to patient care and application of methods derived from behavioral sciences to the prevention and treatment of human morbidity. (This aspect of the field is currently represented by liason psychiatry and behavioral medicine.)

As a field of study, or scientific discipline, psychosomatic medicine is concerned with observation and description of the phenomena that are its object of interest, and with the formulation of testable hypotheses and theories about biopsychosocial relationships, both in health and disease. While all this activity may be regarded as being highly relevant to the debate about the mind–body problem, the latter cannot be viewed as the subject matter of psychosomatic medicine, which is an empirical and not a philosophic discipline. As an operational working approach, mind and body may be regarded as abstractions derived for methodologic purposes for the study of persons. "Mind," in this view, refers to those aspects of man that are most conveniently studies of using methods of the behavioral sciences and described in the language of psychology. "Body," by contrast, is that aspect to which the investigative methods, concepts and language of biology are applied.

As organized advocacy of a holistic approach to health care, psychosomatic medicine propagates the folliwing premises and precepts:

1. Man is a biopsychosocial organism; one that receives, stores, processes, creates, and transmits information, and assigns meaning to it, which in turn elicits emotional responses. The latter, by virtue of their physiologic concomitants, may affect all body functions, both in health and disease.
2. Health and disease are more or less arbitrarily defined states of the organism and are codetermined by psychologic, social, and biologic factors, and always possess biopsychosocial aspects.
3. Study, prevention, diagnosis, and treatment of disease should take into account the varying contribution of all of the above three classes of variables.
4. Etiology is as a rule *multifactorial.* The relative weight of each class of causative factors, however, varies from disease to disease and from case to case; some are necessary and some only contributory.
5. Optimal patient care requires that the above postulates be applied in actual clinical practice.

"Psychosomatic disorder" (or illness or symptom) is a term still unfortunately used by some writers to refer to any somatic disease or dysfunction in which psychologic factors are postulated to play a necessary or sufficient causal role. This term has given rise to pointless and misleading polemics as to whether a given disease or disorder was or was not eligible for inclusion in the "psychosomatic" class. The continued use of this term should be discouraged, as it tends to perpetuate the obsolete notion of psychogenesis, one incompatible with the doctrine of multicasuality, which constitutes a core assumption of psychosomatic medicine. Like many other writers, this author has repeatedly urged that this term be discarded.[2,61]

SUMMARY AND CONCLUSIONS

Semantics and history of psychosomatic medicine are not popular topics nowadays, if they ever were; yet both of them constitute indispensable facets of any discipline that lays claim to a separate identity, as psychosomatics does. The latter, being an inchoate and inherently complex field of study, is especially in need of repeated efforts to clarify the meaning of its key terms, to delineate its scope, and to chart its development over time. Such efforts should pay off in improved teaching of this subject and in more effective communication with workers in other disciplines and with the general public.

I have tried in this paper to sketch the historic development of psychosomatic conceptions and address some relevant semantic issues. It appears that early in this century, the convergence of two ancient conceptions, the holistic and the psychogenic, prepared the ground for the emergence in the 1930s of psychosomatic medicine as an organized scientific discipline and a counterreformation against the mechanistic view of man and medicine. Those two conceptions came to be subsumed by the word "psychosomatic" and thus contributed its two distinct connotations. The latter have not usually been clearly distinguished; hence, the ambiguity of the term. I have argued that only the holistic connotation should be retained, as it properly conveys the contemporary viewpoint.

It is unfortunate that the word "holistic" has been appropriated recently by an antiscientific and antiintellectual so-called "holistic health movement,"[67] with resulting increment in semantic confusion and, in the eyes of many, loss of credibility for the misappropriated term. However, to retain it has merit as it is short, simple, and derived from the Greek—as were the very conceptions it has come to connote. Moreover, "holistic" has been part of the basic vocabulary of psychosomatic medicine from the beginning and conveys its core premises and purpose faithfully. As a historian aptly put it, the historic function of the psychosomatic movement has been to "vitalize the whole of medicine, psychiatry no less. . .with the holistic and ecologic viewpoint."[59, p. 9]

Eric Wittkower,[68] one of the earliest psychosomatic investigators, and my recently deceased former teacher, predicted in 1960 that in the future, psychosomatic medicine would be likely to follow one of three directions: (1) become a narrow specialty dominated by psychoanalysts, (2) confine itself to psychophysiologic research, or (3) develop into a holistic approach to medical problems. Looking back at the past two decades I would argue that the field has become an inseparable blend of psychophysiology and the holistic approach.[60,65]

REFERENCES

1. Margetts EL: The early history of the word "psychosomatic." *Can Med Assoc J* 63:402–404. 1950.
2. Lipowski ZJ: Review of consultation psychiatry and psychosomatic medicine. III. Theoretical issues. *Psychosom Med* 30:395–422, 1968.
3. Lipowski ZJ: Modern meaning of the terms "psychosomatic" and "liason psychiatry," in Creed F, Pfeffer JM (eds): *"Medicine and Psychiatry: A Practical Approach.* London, Pitman, 1982.
4. Ackerknecht EH: The history of psychosomatic medicine. *Psychol Med* 12:17–24, 1982.
5. Burchfield RW (ed): *A Supplement to the Oxford English Dictionary.* Oxford, Clarendon Press, 1982, vol III.
6. Hinsie LE, Campbell RJ (eds): *Psychiatric Dictionary,* ed. 3. New York, Oxford University Press, 1960.
7. *Psychosomatic Disorders.* Wld Hlth Org Techn Rep Ser No. 275, 1964.

8. Margetts EL: Historical notes on psychosomatic medicine, in Wittkower ED, Cleghorn RA (eds): *Recent Developments in Psychosomatic Medicine*. London, Pitman, 1954, pp 41–68.

9. Bucknill JC: *Unsoundness of Mind in Relation to Criminal Acts*. London, Longman, Brown, Green, Longmans & Roberts, 1857.

10. Gray JP: Insanity, and its relations to medicine. *Am J Insanity* 25:145–172, 1868–1869.

11. Reade C: *Hard Cash*. Boston, Dana Estes & Co., 1863, vol I.

12. Tuke DH (ed): *A Dictionary of Psychological Medicine*. Philadelphia, Blakiston, 1892, vol II.

13. Tuke DH: *Illustrations of the Influence of the Mind upon the Body in Health and Disease*, ed 2. Philadelphia, Henry C. Lea's Son & Co., 1884.

14. Stokvis B: Psychosomatik; in Frankl VE, Gebsattel VE, Schultz JH (eds): *Handbuch der Neurosenlehre und Psychotherapie*. München, Urban & Schwarzenberg, 1959, vol 3, pp 435–506.

15. Schwarz O (ed): *Psychogenese und Psychotherapie Körperlicher Symptome*. Vienna, Julius Springer, 1925.

16. Dunbar H: *Emotions and Bodily Changes: A Survey of Literature on Psychosomatic Interrelationships: 1910–1933*. New York, Columbia University Press, 1935.

17. Introductory Statement. *Psychosom Med* 1:3–5, 1939

18. Alexander F: *Psychosomatic Medicine*, New York, Norton, 1950.

19. Mirsky IA: The psychosomatic approach to the etiology of clinical disorders. *Psychosom Med* 19:424–430, 1957.

20. Drabkin IE: Remarks on ancient psychopathology. *Isis* 46:223–234, 1955.

21. Rather LJ: *Mind and Body in Eighteenth Century Medicine*. Berkeley, University of California Press, 1965.

22. Smuts JC: *Holism and Evolution*. New York, Macmillan, 1926.

23. Plato: Charmides, in *The Best Known Works of Plato*, translated by B Jowett. Garden City, NY, Blue Ribbon Books, 1942.

24. Lipowski ZJ: Holistic–medical foundations of American psychiatry: A bicentennial. *Am J Psychiatry* 138:888–895, 1981.

25. Shryock RH: *Medicine in America. Historical Essays*. Baltimore, Johns Hopkins Press, 1966.

26. Rush B: *Sixteen Introductory Lectures*. Philadelphia, Bradford and Innskeep, 1811.

27. Binger C: *Revolutionary Doctor, Benjamin Rush, 1746–1813*. New York, Norton, 1966.

28. Stainbrook E: Psychosomatic medicine in the nineteenth century. *Psychosom Med* 14:211–227, 1952.

29. Holland H: *Mental Physiology*. London, Longmans, Brown, Green and Longmans, 1852.

30. Osler W: *Aequanimatas*, ed. 2. London, H.K. Lewis & Co., 1928.

31. Hughes CH: The nervous system in disease and the practice of medicine from a neurologic standpoint. *JAMA* 22:897–908, 1894.

32. Powell RC: Helen Flanders Dunbar (1902–1959) and a holistic approach to psychosomatic problems. 1. The rise and fall of a medical philosophy. *Psychiatr Q* 49:133–152, 1977.

33. Goldstein K: *The Organism*, New York, American Book, 1939.

34. Woodger JH: *Biology and Language*. Cambridge, Cambridge University Press, 1952.

35. Dubos R: *Man, Medicine, and Environment*. New York, The New American Library, 1968.

36. Zucker A: Holism and reductionism: A view from genetics. *J Med Phil* 6:145–163, 1981.

37. Lewis A: "Psychogenic": A word and its mutations. *Psychol Med* 2:209–215, 1972.

38. Hippocrates: *Aphorisms*, translated by F Adams. London, William Wood, 1886, p. 143.

39. Rorty AO: From passions to emotions and sentiments. *Philosophy* 57:159–172, 1982.

40. Solomon RC: *The Passions*. Garden City, NY, Anchor Press, 1976.

41. Galen: *On the Passions and Errors of the Soul*, translated by PW Harkins. Ohio State University Press, 1963.

42. Archer J: *Every Man His Own Doctor*. London, 1673.

43. Lindeboom GA: *Descartes and Medicine*. Amsterdam, Radopi, 1979.

44. Wilson MD: *Descartes*. London, Routledge & Kegan Paul, 1978.

45. Rather LJ: *The Genesis of Cancer*. Baltimore, Johns Hopkins University Press, 1978.

46. Rather LJ: G.E. Stahl's psychological physiology. *Bull Hist Med* 35:37–49, 1961.

47. Corp: *An Essay on the Changes Produced in the Body by Operations of the Mind*. London, Ridgway, 1791.

48. Falconer W: *A Dissertation on the Influence of the Passions upon Disorders of the Body.* London, Dilly, 1796.
49. Friedreich JB: *Versuch einer Literaergeschichte der Pathologie und Therapie der psychischen Krankheiten.* Wuerzburg, Carl Strecker, 1830, p. 187–211.
50. Freymann JG: The origins of disease orientation in American medical education. *Prev Med* 10:663–673, 1981.
51. Beaumont W: *Experiments and Observations on the Gastric Juice and the Physiology of Digestion.* Plattsburg, NY, FP Allen, 1833.
52. Osler W: William Beaumont. A backwood physiologist. *JAMA* 39:1223–1231, 1902.
53. Pavlov IP: *The Work of the Digestive Glands,* translated by WH Thompson. Philadelphia, Lippincott, 1902.
54. Cannon WB: *Bodily Changes in Pain, Hunger, Fear, and Rage.* New York, Appleton, 1915.
55. Alexander FG, Selesnick ST: *The History of Psychiatry,* New York, Harper & Row, 1966.
56. Groddeck G: *The Book of the It.* New York, Vintage Books, 1961.
57. Grinker RR: *Psychosomatic Concepts,* revised ed. New York, Jason Aronson, 1973.
58. Lewis A: *Inquiries in Psychiatry.* New York, Science House, 1967.
59. Galdston I: Psychosomatic Medicine. *AMA Arch Neurol Psychiatry* 74:441–450, 1955.
60. Lipowski, ZJ: Psychosomatic medicine in the seventies: An overview. *Am J Psychiatry* 134:233–244, 1977.
61. Lesser IM: A review of the alexithymia concept. *Psychosom Med* 43:531–543, 1981.
62. Freyhan FA: Is psychosomatic obsolete? A psychiatric reappraisal. *Compr Psychiatry* 17:381–386, 1976.
63. Engel GL: The concept of psychosomatic disorder. *J Psychosom Res* 11:3–9, 1967.
64. Engel GL: The need for a new medical model: A challenge for biomedicine. *Science* 196:129–136, 1977.
65. Weiner H: The prospects for psychosomatic medicine: Selected topics. *Psychosom Med* 44:491–517, 1982.
66. Wright L: Conceptualizing and defining psychosomatic disorders. *Am Psychol* 32:625–628, 1977.
67. Kopelman L., Moskop J: The holistic health movement: A survey and critique. *J Med Phil* 6:209–235, 1981.
68. Wittkower ED: Twenty years of North American psychosomatic medicine. *Psychosom Med* 22:308–316, 1960.

Psychosocial Reactions to Physical Illness

II

The two articles in this section are concerned with the modes of people's psychosocial reactions to physical illness, injury and disability, and their proposed multiple determinants. The main purpose of this section is to provide a conceptual framework to serve as a basis for clinical assessment of the patient from the psychological and social viewpoints. Such an assessment is especially important in managing patients suffering from a chronic illness, deformity, or disability.

Psychosocial Reactions to Physical Illness 8

INTRODUCTION

A major illness or injury affects the patient's experience of his body and world. The quality of this experiential state is known directly only to the sufferer whose introspective account is the primary source of information. An outside observer has to rely on the sick person's verbal reports about how he feels in order to gain some understanding of the subjective experience. Empathy is needed to gain such understanding. Another source of data about the experience of illness is the observable behavior of the sick person, that is facial expression, posture, gestures, nonverbal vocalizations, physiological changes (e.g., respiratory, cardiovascular), and purposeful actions from which inferences can be made about inner experiential states. Students of the psychological aspects of physical illness, be they behavioral scientists or practicing clinicians, have to take into account both these sources of data for a proper evaluation of each patient.

A third aspect of a person's reaction to illness must also be taken into account, namely, the social or interactive aspect. To view the patient apart from the social context would leave out an essential aspect of the total experience of illness. Thus, it is more appropriate to speak of "*psychosocial*" rather than "psychological" reactions to illness and injury because the psychological and social aspects of it are for practical purposes inseparable. For the sake of study and clarity of exposition, however, one may break that total psychosocial response into three interlocked compenents: (1) the intrapsychic or experiential, (2) the behavioral, and (3) the social or interactive.

METHODOLOGY

For the purpose of research on psychosocial responses to illness one may employ several methodological approaches: (1) the phenomenological, concerned with the subject's conscious perceptions, cognitions, and feelings related to the illness; (2) the psychodynamic, focused on the unconscious symbolic meanings, fantasies, conflicting strivings, distortions, and misinterpretations related to the illness or injury; (3) the behavioristic, which confines itself to an analysis of the sick person's verbal and nonverbal publicly observable behavior; and (4) the sociological, concerned with the attitudes and behavior of the sick person as they are observed in social interactions and reflect values, norms, and beliefs held by other members of the social group and the culture to which the patient belongs.

Each of these approaches has a different focus, methods of study, terminology, and theories. Each aims at achieving knowledge on the basis of which an individual's behavior could be predicted and practical guidelines for preventive and therapeutic action could be developed. Each approach can provide valuable insights but none of them is sufficient to account for all facets of the experience and behavior of the physically ill. For this reason, and in an attempt to achieve an overview of the subject matter, I will try to integrate the diverse methodological approaches and give a composite account of the psychosocial responses to illness.

The methodological tools, or strategies, for collecting primary data in this complex field include the following: (1) autobiographical accounts of people suffering from various diseases; (2) health questionnaires; (3) psychological rating scales; (4) projective tests; (5) psychophysiological measurements; (6) opinion polls; and (7) analysis of dream contents and free associations.

Each of these research methods has its limitations and taps only a segment of the whole field. In the following discussion I will provide examples of and draw upon some of the various methodological approaches without attempting to review them exhaustively.

THE INTRAPSYCHIC EXPERIENTIAL ASPECT

And then suffering, bodily suffering such as I've known for three years. It has changed forever everything—even the appearance of the world is not the same—there is something added. *Everything has its shadow.*
KATHERINE MANSFIELD, Letter to J.M. Murray, October 18, 1920

The intrapsychic or experiential aspect of a patient's response to an illness or injury refers to his perceptions, thoughts, imagery, and emotions that compose subjective experience of illness. Every episode of painful, severe, life-threatening, or disabling disease or injury permeates the patient's experience of his body, self, and environment. Thus, an illness is first and foremost a private event.[1,2] It may be communicated to others in the form of autobiographical accounts, or conveyed more or less faithfully by an empathic outsider in the form of a clinical or literary history, or described using impersonal terms such as perception, cognition, emotion, and other scientific concepts.

Thus, three distinct ways of describing the intrapsychic dimension of illness response may be utilized: the autobiographical, the historical–literary, and the scientific–analytic. Whereas the first two types of description aim at capturing the totality of illness experience, the last type is deliberately analytic in that it isolates elements of the total experience for the purpose of psychological analysis and formulation of explanatory hypotheses.

THE TOTAL EXPERIENCE

Autobiographical accounts of illness have gained considerable popularity in recent years, as illustrated by the critical acclaim of books by Alsop,[3] Cousins,[4] and Sanes,[5] for example. The value of these works lies in their ability to inspire people to cope more adaptively with illness, or even overcome it. These autobiographical accounts also convey something of the uniquely personal, yet at the same time universally shared, human experience of anguish occasioned by a life-threatening or disabling illness. Of the many valuable autobiographical reports of illness published in recent years, those written by doctors are especially noteworthy.[5-9] Fiore[10] and Paoli[11] have written articulate and moving accounts of personal struggle with cancer, and Harrison[12] has described the experience of a heart attack and its impact on his life. Malraux[13] gives in *Lazarus* a poignant account of his own experience of an acute neurological disease and his encounter with "the god of dread," as he refers to his emotional response to attacks of vertigo, fainting, and delirium. The reader is encouraged to study these autobiographical accounts as they offer unusual insight into the personal reality of illness and thus supplement the impersonal and dreary descriptions of "clinical features" offered by medical textbooks.

Many novelists have written superb accounts of the experience of illness, which render admirably the subjective quality of various diseases and symptoms. An annotated bibliography is available for those interested in the links between literature and medicine.[14] Chekhov, Thomas Mann, Proust, Tolstoy, du Gard, Bernanos, Solzhenitsyn, and many other writters have contributed memorable descriptions of various illnesses as they are actually experienced. Reading these literary accounts is the most effective way, other than the firsthand experience, to develop empathy for how the sick feel. These accounts may be dismissed as anectdotal and unscientific, yet they convey the nuances of the existential state of being ill, which scientific analysis tends to depersonalize and divest of its essential human quality. The assorted autobiographical and literary accounts describe common features of illness experience which have also been observed by systematic students. Narrowing of interests, changed experience of time, a sense of discontinuity of one's existence, increased absorption in bodily functions and sensations, egocentric withdrawal, and a pervasive, unpleasant bodily feeling known as malaise are some of the common subjective concomitants of physical illness. Sense of insecurity, uncertainty about the future, and longing for human closeness are also often reported.[15-17]

A scientific approach to the psychosocial aspects of illness tends to be impersonal and atomistic. It breaks down a total subjective experience into its components that correspond to the currently accepted distinct mental functions. A brief account of this approach follows.

PERCEPTUAL–COGNITIVE RESPONSES

Cognitive processes are those whereby information is acquired, transformed, evaluated, stored, retrieved, and used.[18] Sensation, perception, attention, imagery, thinking, memory, concept formation, problem solving, and decision making are the major stages or aspects of cognition.[18,19] We are concerned here with the application of these concepts to the relatively narrow field of illness-related information and its effects on the patient's emotional and behavioral responses. A pathological change in the body constitutes the focal source of information. The relevant messages are of three main kinds: those arising from the body as a result of disordered function or altered structure, or both; those received from the social environment, for example, in the form of a doctor's statements; and those derived from the patient's memory in which information about diseases as well as about past illness experiences is stored. These three information inputs are endowed with conscious and unconscious meaning by the patient, and such meaning in turn elicits arousal of emotions consonant with it and influences the patient's behavior.

Perception of the sensory input related to physical illness or injury is influenced by the characteristics of the perceiving individual and of the perceived information and by the psychosocial situation of the patient. The quality, intensity, rate of onset, and source of the perceived stimuli are important as they influence the patient's overall response. For example, a sudden loss of consciousness, severe pain, massive bleeding, loss of balance, marked dyspnea, or paralysis of a limb—all are experiences that clamor for attention and decisions to act. Yet even such dramatic events are responded to differently by different persons. A striking example of such individual differences in response is provided by patients suffering from a heart attack. Some of them call for help immediately, whereas others try various home remedies and delay seeking medical help for hours.[20] These differences in behavior reflect in part the *perceptual-cognitive style* of the affected individual. Some people tend to habitually augment or reduce what they perceive and thus differ in what has been called perceptual reactance.[21] Repression–sensitization is a similar concept used by some psychologists to refer to a hypothetical polarity of perceptual reactivity.[22] Habitual augmentors or sensitizers are likely to perceive somatic sensations more keenly, appraise them more readily in terms of threat or harm, respond with more intense emotional and autonomic arousal, and report greater frequency and severity of bodily symptoms than reducers or repressors. These individual differences in perceptual–cognitive style color the patient's whole experience of illness and influence his emotional and behavioral responses to it.

People also differ with regard to their habitual cognitive coping sytle, and these differences tend to be brought out in the course of an illness. One may distinguish two major types of such style: *minimization* and *vigilant focusing*.[23] "Cognitive style" refers to a person's characteristic manner of dealing with information. In this discussion we are especially concerned with the habitual way in which a person responds to information that is threatening and disturbing. "Coping" in this context implies that challenge or threat to the person is involved.

Minimization may be regarded as a cognitive coping style characterized by a tendency to ignore, deny, play down, or explain away the personally threatening significance of internal or external information. When applied to illness and its symptoms, the manifestations of this cognitive style may range from a delusional denial of the very fact of being ill or having a particular disability to a selective misinterpretation of perceived bodily stimuli so as to reduce their threatening import. Tendency to such misinterpretation varies in extent from person to person. Some individuals display minimization of danger as a habitual mode of dealing with it. Delusional denial of the fact of illness or disability, that is, anosognosia, is the most extreme form of minimization and connotes disturbance of reality testing of psychotic proportions. It is encountered in the presence of widespread brain pathology, reversible or not, as in the cases described by Weinstein and Kahn,[24] or may be a manifestation of a severe dissociative disorder that occasionally follows surgery or accidental trauma. An autobiographical account of anosognosia following severe head injury has been written by a psychiatrist, LaBaw.[7]

The concept of denial, which many writers use instead of this author's more comprehensive term "minimization," has become ambiguous and abused. Its overinclusive usage has blurred the distinction between denial of clear-cut factual evidence of danger or damage to one's body (pathological denial) and the varying degrees of normal tendency to ignore unclear signs of threat.[25] One may deny an incontrovertible fact, or its personal significance, or the emotions it has evoked. A quantitative rating scale to estimate denial has been developed by Hackett and Cassem[26] and is a welcome attempt to grade the extent of denial instead of applying the concept in a global manner to a broad spectrum of attitudes toward threatening stimuli. Those authors define denial as the "conscious or unconscious repudiation of part or all of the total available meanings of an event to allay fear, anxiety, or other unpleasant affect." The term "denial" in respect to illness has acquired a negative conotation that is misleading and has encouraged zealous attempts to counteract it, disregarding the patient's values and perspective.[27] Some degree of denial of illness is common in the early phases of any sudden or severe illness or trauma and may be considered an adaptive response to a catastropic event.

To avoid the ambiguity and derogatory connotation of the concept of denial, the term "minimization" is offered here as preferable. It refers to a continuum of cognitive attitudes ranging from pathological denial at one extreme to underestimation of threat on the other. It may be adaptive or maladaptive, depending on the total situation. The actual extent of minimization may vary from person to person and at different stages of an illness in the same person. Some people, however, employ minimization as their preferred—if not consciously selected—mode of cognitive response to illness—related as well as any other personally threatening information.

Vigilant focusing connotes habitual readiness to respond to signals of danger with selective and sustained attention, and with attempts at clear understanding of the nature, source, direction, and personal implications of the danger. The person scans actively his store of knowledge as well as any available information for relevant clues, explanations, and predictions. Some individuals employing this style tend to have a low threshold for perception of bodily changes and exhibit a tendency to respond to any unfamiliar or intense stimuli as potentially threatening. This cognitive coping style is often seen in obsessional, suspicious, and anxiety-prone people. Their sense of security is readily undermined by a sense of lack of cognitive mastery over their stimulus input. To feel reasonably secure they must maintain perceptual clarity and intellectual mastery through knowledge and understanding, and a state of preparedness for novel or threatening information, both somatic and external to the body. When such a person becomes ill, he becomes alert for any clues that might help to understand what is happening, how to evaluate it, what to expect, and what course of action to take. The patient will not be satisfied unless he or she can find out what the doctor believes is wrong, how the diagnosis was arrived at, and what treatment is being planned. The patient is not satisfied with ambiguous or vague statements and is intolerant of ambiguity and uncertainty, which he tries to reduce to a minimum. The less explanation he receives, the more anxious and aroused is such a patient.

This style too is to be viewed as a continuum, with hypervigilance and excessive readiness to regard any perceived bodily change as having ominous significance at one extreme, and appropriate alertness to potential threats at the other. Between these poles should be placed obsessive brooding and worrying about perceived bodily stimuli and persistent rumination about what to make of them.

The two cognitive coping styles just described have been derived from clinical observation. They overlap with hypothetical personality and cognitive–perceptual styles postulated by other writers, such as field dependence–independence, repression-sensitization, reducing–augmenting, and sharpening–leveling. The two proposed styles stem from the author's observations of the attitudes and behavior of the physically ill seen in medical settings in his capacity as a psychiatric consultant to medicine and surgery for 25 years. Their practical value lies in the help they offer clinical workers in understanding their patients' behavior, recognizing their needs, and responding to their communications in a manner that enhances patient cooperation and reduces anxiety and irrational behavior. *Cognitive style influences the way a person appraises information and thus affects the meaning he imparts to it.*

PERSONAL MEANINGS OF ILLNESS

One way to conceptualize the psychosocial aspects of illness is to view them in terms of information that impinges on the person and is endowed with subjective significance, or *meaning*, by him. As suggested earlier, one may speak of three sources of illness-related information for each individual: somatic stimuli, messages from the social environment, and one's stored memories of acquired knowledge and experience. Somatic stimuli and environmental messages provide the ongoing information inputs that are evaluated by the person against the background of memories, values, beliefs, conflicts, needs, and expectations. The meaning of such inputs results from their subjective appraisal, both conscious and unconscious. Symptoms, doctors' statements, responses of significant others, media messages, and other information that the patient perceives and evaluates as pertaining to his state of health comprise illness-related information to which he imparts meaning.

The process of appraisal continues unabated throughout the duration of any illness. It may be set off by subliminal perception of bodily change, by conscious awareness of it, or by communications of others suggesting or declaring that one is ill. The appraisal may be true or false from the point of view of objective evidence that a demonstrable pathological process is present. Clearly, the vast majority of subjectively perceived bodily sensations do not signify disease in its current accepted sense. One may be uncomfortable or distressed without being ill and be ill without being aware of any discomfort. In our culture it is the physician's role and prerogative to be the proper judge as to whether a given complaint presented by a person signifies disease.

In a strict sense, one should speak of multiple, diverse, and changing information inputs that the sick person perceives, evaluates, and responds to. It is an ongoing, dynamic process, which we break down into segments to facilitate its analysis. It is legitimate and useful, however, to try to identify the dominant personal meaning of an illness for the given individual and study its determinants as well as consequences. The meaning of a given illness that the patient evolves will influence his emotions, decisions, communications, and actions. These consequences in turn feed back into and modify the meaning. Furthermore, the latter is also affected by the attitudes and behavior of others who respond to the patient's communications and actions. Thus, the evolved meaning influences and is in turn modified by the patient's emotional and behavioral responses as well as his or her social interactions. The dynamic interplay among these factors and the related feedback mechanisms contribute to the complexity of this subject, which is compounded by the fact that an illness may have different conscious and unconscious meanings for the patient, resulting in his inconsistent and perplexing attitudes and actions.

Categories of Meanings

On the basis of clinical observation I propose to distinguish five major categories of meaning of information pertaining to matters of health and illness[1,2]: (1) threat, (2) loss, (3) gain or relief, (4) challenge, and (5) insignificance

Threat implies anticipation of danger of harm or hurt to one's physical or psychic integrity, or both, and related expectation of suffering or even death. The threat may be clear or more or less ambiguous, depending in part on the clarity or ambiguity of the perceived information. There is some evidence that ambiguity of a situation or stimulus may be a threat factor in its own right, one likely to reduce the individual's coping ability.[28] A patient may interpret as threatening his bodily perceptions or a statement by another person, especially by a health professional, that a disease is present even if he is unaware of any symptoms, as may be the case in essential hypertension, for example. The readiness to interpret bodily or external stimuli as threatening tends to vary in degree from person to person and even in the same individual at different periods of life and in different situations. Thus, enduring predisposition, current emotional state, and the situational set all influence the tendency to view a change in one's somatic perceptions or a doctor's statements as threatening. Moreover, the features of the stimulus or information, such as its novelty or ambiguity, may also influence what meaning the person assigns to it.

Appraisal of any information as personally threatening may elicit psychophysiological consequences. Anxiety or fear is the emotion most likely to be experienced in the face of threat. For some writers, anxiety connotes anticipation of an unrealistic danger; fear, of a realistic one. These terms are inconsistently used in the literature, and it may be best to use them here interchangeably. If the meaning of threat is relatively ambiguous, perplexity may largely replace fear. Anxiety has a characteristic unpleasant feeling tone, ranging in intensity from vague uneasiness to dread and panic. That feeling tone is typically accompanied by physiological arousal and consequently by increased, decreased, or deranged activity of various organs and organ systems. Such changed activity, if perceived, gives rise to somatic symptoms such as palpitations, shortness of breath, muscle tension, chest pain, trembling, dizziness, and sweating. Every person is likely to possess a repertoire of such somatic concomitants of anxiety wich become activated in response to threatening information. He may in turn interpret them as threatening in their own right. Such a positive feedback effect tends to enhance the magnitude of the threat and the intensity of anxiety. One can often observe such a vicious circle in clinical practice. Intense physiological arousal concomitant with anxiety may have harmful effects on someone who suffers from coronary heart disease, for example. Increased sympathetic nervous activity and catecholamine secretion in a cardiac patient may precipitate angina, myocardial infarction, congestive heart failure, or a life-threatening cardiac arrhythmia.

At the psychological level, the experience of anxiety, with its physiological concomitants, is more or less distressing and aversive for the person, and he is motivated to counteract it. Such counteraction involves the deployment of both unconscious defense mechanisms and consciously motivated coping strategies aimed at relieving the emotional distress.[29,30] These defenses and coping strategies tend to vary widely in their adaptive value.

Verwoerdt[31] has proposed that a patient's attempts to cope with the threat posed by illness and the defense mechanisms he deploys in the process can be classified into three categories, according to their goal, which may be (1) to retreat from the threat and conserve energy, (2) to exclude the threat or its significance from awareness, or (3) to master the threat. The first goal is aimed at by deployment of the defense mechanism of regression, that is, by falling back on developmentally earlier modes of cognitive and behavioral coping. Clinically, regression may manifest itself as a constellation of self-centeredness, hypochondriasis, and exaggerated dependency. These are maladaptive and "deviant" responses to illness. They tend to be accompanied by feelings of depression, resentment, anxiety, and guilt. A variant of regression in the context of physical illness is withdrawal of interest, attention, and emotional charge from the affected body part or function. In its extreme form, withdrawal becomes a state of having given up, which represents capitulation to illness and lack of efforts to resist it. The related emotion is hopelessness.[32] It should be emphasized that withdrawal may be adaptive, when conservation of energy serves the cause of recovery and survival. It is maladaptive if it is carried too far and undermines recuperative powers of the organism and the patient's will to live.

The second goal is pursued by employing defenses such as suppression, denial, rationalization, depersonalization, projection, and introjection. Suppression connotes deliberate attempts to avoid unpleasant thoughts and feelings. Denial has been discussed earlier. Rationalization refers to a mode of reasoning aimed at accounting for a distressing fact so as to reduce its threatening significance. For example, some patients experiencing sudden chest pain of cardiac origin may misinterpret it as indigestion and thus diminish its personal importance. Depersonalization implies a subjective sense that what is being experienced is unreal, dreamlike, and alien. In this way anxiety may be temporarily alleviated and the ominous facts lose some of their impact. Projection connotes assignment of blame for one's predicament, thoughts, and emotions to other people or nonhuman external agents. This allows deflection of attention from disturbing information and focusing it on spurious external enemies and dangers. Anger usually accompanies the use of this defense and serves to reduce anxiety and sense of helplessness. Finally, introjection implies assigning to oneself disturbing information from external forces. A patient, cited by Verwoerdt,[31] had been told that biopsy of a lymph node revealed the presence of a metastasis. Subsequently the patient declared that the doctor never really said such a thing and that it was really the patient's own idea.

Defenses aimed at mastery of the threat, the third type of goal, include intellectualization, isolation of thoughts from emotions, counterphobic and obsessive-compulsive mechanisms, and acceptance and sublimation. The last two defenses are viewed as optimal modes of response to illness.[31] They are, however, appropriately applied to situations involving loss or disability rather than threat and anxiety.

Coping strategies deployed by people to deal with threat and anxiety also vary in their adaptive value. Ideally, the person responds to threatening information by seeking more information with which to further assess the magnitude and implications of the threat and to plan actions aimed at averting the threatened danger or reducing its impact. Other coping strategies commonly used to avoid or reduce anxiety include immersion in work or some other activity that distracts attention from anxiety-provoking information and suppression of symptoms of anxiety through the use of various relaxation techniques, sedatives, alcohol, and so forth.

It should be stressed that arousal of moderate anxiety may have salutary and adaptive effects. It may lead the person to take rational action to ascertain if a threat does exist, prompting him to seek timely medical consultation. Furthermore, anxiety may provide motivation to comply with the prescribed medical regimen, such as taking antihypertensive drugs or undergoing a needed operation. On the contrary, defenses and coping strategies aimed at reducing anxiety may succeed in their intended purpose but result in a grave problem, such as addiction, or in behavior incompatible with a rational and adaptive management of the threat. Thus, interpreting an information input as threatening may have either adaptive or maladaptive consequences depending on the intensity of the aroused anxiety and the nature and appropriateness of the modes of dealing with it.

Loss in this context refers to both concrete and symbolic losses occasioned by illness. In a concrete sense, we speak of loss of particular body parts, functions, and attributes caused by disease or injury. Symbolic losses include damage to self-esteem, security, satisfaction of needs, pursuit of valued goals, economic reverses, and the like. These two categories of loss overlap but are not identical. Actual loss of a limb or internal organ need not be followed by a sense of deprivation and related emotions. Nor is the objective extent or gravity of the concrete loss a sufficient condition for a proportionately intense subjective response. What to an outsider may seem to be a trivial impairment of function or change of bodily appearance may evoke a profound sense of loss in the affected person, which depends on the symbolic meaning and on the value of the impairment or change for the given individual. For example, some patients, expecially adolescents, treated by cancer chemotherapy are more disturbed by the loss of hair that often results than by the ominous implications of the fact of having cancer.[33] On the other hand, surgery as mutilating as hemicorporectomy need not result in a psychological disorder.[34]

The usual emotional response to a subjectively serious loss, concrete or symbolic, takes the form of *grief*, which may merge imperceptibly with a *depressive disorder* of some degree of severity. Grief may be regarded as a normal and adaptive step in the work of mourning, whose optimal outcome implies coming to terms with the fact of loss. Absence of grief after a personally significant loss is viewed by many psychiatrists as a manifestation of the defense mechanism of denial. It is then predicted that as a result loss will not be truly accepted and that a psychopathological reaction is likely to follow at some future time, even years after the event, on the anniversary of the loss, for example. The validity of this theoretical assumption has been challenged, however.[35] Lack of grief may mean that the given event was not perceived by the patient as a serious loss. More systematic investigation is needed to test the hypothesis that absence of grief is a harbinger of future psychopathology.

Other factors that may affect the subjective meaning of loss and the intensity of related grief are the degree to which the loss is viewed by the patient as irreparable and irreplaceable. Furthermore, the individual's psychological resources, and the availability of social support and economic security, may facilitate the process of adjustment, and the meaning of loss may give way to that of challenge posed by the disability.

Thus, many factors inherent in the person, the illness, and the environment codetermine whether a given illness or injury and its consequences are assigned the meaning of loss. They influence its depth, the intensity of the evoked grief or depression, and the duration of distress. Both the concrete and the symbolic losses give rise to an emotional response whose intensity tends to be proportionate to the *subjective value* of the lost body part, function, or attribute for the individual.

Loss of self-esteem may result from an illness or disability and seriously complicate the course of the latter. Such loss may occur when the patient views the illness as *punishment* for his or her real or imaginary misdeeds. Self-blame and feelings of guilt are at the core of that irrational attitude. The patient may blame himself or herself for having brought on the illness through carelessness or self-indulgence. He may become convinced that the disease signifies retribution or expiation for forbidden wishes or transgressions. Such a belief may appear in one of several variants, each of them giving rise to a different set of emotions and behavior. If the patient views the punishment as just and allowing atonement and forgiveness, he may bear it stoically and emerge from illness with a sense of elation and new beginning. Some people display considerable personality change and growth after an illness or operation that they view, consciously or not, as deserved punishment and atonement. If the patient regards the illness as a punishment both just and without hope of redemption, he is likely to submit to it passively and do nothing to get well. Such a given-up attitude may actually preclude recovery or, in any event, speed up death if the disease is incurable. If the patient regards the illness as punishment that is unjust or excessive, he is likely to feel resentful and ready to blame others for the predicament. Such patients may become frankly paranoid and turn their anger on physicians or family members.

Loss of self-esteem may also result from a view of the illness as a personal failing, moral weakness, or inexcusable loss of control over one's body. The usual emotional concomitant of such a view is shame. The patient's self-esteem is undermined, and he or she may try to conceal the illness or disability and minimize its seriousness, with possible adverse effect on its outcome. Some may try to make up for the shameful failure by acting the role of a compliant model patient.

Irrational views of one's illness like those cited may have far-reaching consequences for the patient's emotional state and behavior. They may lead to psychopathological reactions to illness, most often in the form of a depressive disorder of some degree of severity or of deviant illness behavior, or of both. Loss of self-esteem, with the related feelings of guilt or shame, engenders distress that magnifies the burden of the illness for the patient far beyond the objective losses occasioned by it.

Gain or relief is a meaning of illness or disability that connotes psychological, social, and/or economic advantage to the patient. Flaubert, who developed epilepsy at the age of 24, expressed such a meaning succinctly: "My illness has brought one benefit, in that I am allowed to spend my time as I like, a great thing in life."[36] The author of *Madame Bovary* made good use of that benefit.

An illness may provide a primary gain, implying that it facilitates subsidence, satisfaction, or avoidance of needs, impulses, and strivings that are a source of an intrapsychic conflict and related inner tension and distress. Aggressive, dependent, sexual, or power-seeking impulses are usually involved. Illness may reduce sexual drive, provide atonement for and thus allow its expression, or offer ready rationalization for the avoidance of sexual contacts that arouse inner conflicts. Dependent strivings may be given free expression and be gratified by someone who would disavow such impulses in the absence of illness. Power-seeking, competitive tendencies may become less of a personal problem if illness imposes and thus legitimizes their renunciation or, on the contrary, provides an opportunity for gaining power over others by virtue of being sick and disabled, by threats that unless the other complies, the patient may get worse or die, and by playing on the guilt feelings of others, usually members of one's family. Thus illness may provide rationalization for either avoidance or guilt-free expression of impulses that the patient could not face or express without an inner conflict. Another subjective gain or relief may be derived from a painful illness when the pain meets the patient's unconscious need for suffering to appease a sense of guilt for disavowed behavior, impulses, or fantasies.

The concept of the primary gain of illness has important practical consequences for clinical practice. It may help explain otherwise unaccountable behavior, as when a patient seeks relief and at the same time in various subtle ways resists treatment and recovery. Such a patient may decompensate psychologically when his illness is successfully treated. Examples of this apparent paradox are most often seen in chronic illnesses that have been woven into the patient's psychological defenses and life-style. This may happen after surgery for epilepsy[37] or chronic heart disease.[38] Such patients should have careful psychiatric assessment preoperatively if subsequent psychological complications are to be prevented. One should keep in mind that the concept of primary gain refers to psychodynamic factors of which the patient is unaware and cannot be blamed for their behavioral expression. Patients usually act in good faith when they seek treatment and clamor for relief, and one has to be alert for indirect verbal and nonverbal clues betraying an opposite, unconscious attitude.

Secondary gains from illness connote social and economic advantages accruing from it. Being sick may be seized upon by the patient as an excuse to avoid social roles and related responsibilities, to gain attention, and to secure social and economic support. Some patients derive considerable pride and satisfaction from suffering from a rare or undiagnosed disease that baffles doctors. Such distinction may be the only one that a particular patient has ever achieved, and he may be reluctant to give it up.

Thus, gain or relief is a global meaning of a given illness for the patient, one that influences his motivation to get well, or rather to remain sick. It may reflect the patient's childhood experiences with key family members who in various ways rewarded him for being ill.[39] Such learning experiences may predispose a child not only to conscious or unconscious simulation of physical illness in later life but also to seeking psychological gain from any type of illness.

A patient may simultaneously develop incompatible meanings of illness and thus exhibit contradictory and inconsistent behavior that may puzzle health care workers. The patient's conscious sense of loss may coexist with an unconscious meaning of the illness in terms of gain or relief, and inconsistent illness behavior is likely to ensue. When subjective gains, primary or secondary, derived from illness or disability outweigh the losses, the patient is likely to cling to his sickness and may develop emotional disturbances if recovery occurs.

Challenge is a meaning of illness as a set of tasks to be met and mastered. It is a common and perhaps the most adaptive meaning, one that leads to active, deliberate, and rational illness behavior. The patient is liable to seek medical advice with neither undue haste nor fateful delay, to comply judiciously with treatment and rehabilitation, to attempt to compensate to the utmost for permanent disability, and to work toward attainable recovery. He or she is likely to be free from disorganizing anxiety and other dysphoric emotional states, such as guilt, shame, anger, or depression. Threat and loss are viewed realistically and are tackled actively.

Insignificance implies a relative lack of subjective meaning assigned to illness or symptoms. This may be the result of low intelligence or lack of medical knowledge, or both. It may also be seen in people who are withdrawn, depressed, or apathetic, or in those who believe they are invulnerable. This weak cognitive appraisal of early symptoms of disease such as cancer may lead to fateful delay in seeking medical help or even to persistent avoidance of such help. The concept of denial may be erroneously invoked to account for the deviant illness behavior of such patients.

In summary, the concept of personal meaning of illness has considerable heuristic value and explanatory power for emotional and behavioral responses to illness, symptoms, and disability. The categories of meaning proposed here are based on personal clinical observations and have not been subjected to systematic research. They represent hypotheses awaiting validation, yet the author has found them clinically useful in helping to understand patients' attitudes and behavior, both normal and deviant. Evaluation of every patient should include inquiry into what meaning he or she imparts to his or her illness and symptoms. Such assessment may help the physician to understand the patient's attitude and behavior and to forestall the development of psychiatric complications and of deviant illness behavior such as noncompliance with the recommended treatment.

EMOTIONAL RESPONSES

The emotional responses to illness are inseparably linked to the cognitive-perceptual ones. Emotions may be viewed as intervening variables between cognitive appraisal of information and its subjective meaning, on the one hand, and the behavioral responses, on the other. The emotions evoked by physical illness or injury vary in quality, intensity, duration, and temporal sequence. They are often mixed and shifting.

Anxiety, sadness, grief, disgust, shame, guilt, anger, surprise, and *acceptance* are the most common emotions encountered and occur in various constellations.[40] Less often one observes *apathy, elation*, or *euphoria*. Each of these emotions has degrees of intensity and is not an either–or response. We have already discussed some of the main emotional components of the experience of illness in relation to the personal meaning of the latter. Emotional responses may also be influenced by cerebral disorders, primary and secondary, that alter the function or destroy the anatomical substrate of emotional experience. Furthermore, a patient's emotional responses are likely to be modified by his mood before the onset of illness. If the latter comes on, as it often does, in a setting of depressed mood, for example, then the patient's response is more likely to take the form of grief, guilt, or shame, and a depressive disorder. The quality of the patient's interpersonal relationships also influences his emotional responses to illness.

Whether one judges an individual's emotional response as normal or abnormal depends on its *appropriateness*, that is, its degree of correspondence to the objectively assessed severity of the danger, loss, and suffering. Such judgment is likely to be value-laden and to reflect the observer's bias. In clinical practice the most important issue is the way in which the evoked emotional responses enhance or hinder a patient's potential for recovery from physical illness and his capacity for adjustment to permanent disability.

THE BEHAVIORAL RESPONSE TO ILLNESS

Mechanic[41] has introduced the concept of "illness behavior" defined as "the ways in which symptoms may be differentially perceived, evaluated, and acted (or not acted) upon by different kinds of person." This definition subsumes, under the term "behavior," cognitive and perceptual responses to illness discussed in the preceding section, responses that are not usually referred to as behavior in psychology. For the sake of consistency, we will use the term "illness behavior" to designate only the observable responses, namely, *communications* and *actions* of the sick related to the illness and its symptoms.

COMMUNICATIVE BEHAVIOR

In this section I will focus on the patient's communications related to his or her illness. What the patient communicates about his perceptions, thoughts, and feelings, when, in what manner, and to whom are crucial aspects of his illness behavior. Communication is a two-way process, modified by the feedback from those at whom it is directed. In the case of illness-related communications, the responses of the doctor, patient's family, and other relevant persons influence the patient's readiness to communicate as well as the content and form of his messages. What and how a patient communicates has a bearing on the doctor's diagnostic reasoning.[42-54]

Medical sociologists have studied the variables that influence the patient's communicative behavior. Zola[52,53] and Zborowski[54] have explored the role of sociocultural factors on the manner in which patients communicate their symptoms. Zola[52,53] has studied patients attending outpatient clinics of a Boston general hospital and found that Irish and Italian patients presented their symptoms differently. The Irish tended to complain mostly of symptoms related to the eyes, ears, nose, and throat and understated complaints of pain. Italians, on the other hand, reported symptoms involving many parts of the body, complained in a dramatic language, and stated that their distress interfered with their social relationships. More Italian than Irish patients received a psychiatric diagnosis, which suggests that the manner of communicating symptoms influences doctors' diagnostic reasoning. Zola asserts that the physician's reaction to the patient's communication influences the amount and kind of information he is likely to obtain. When the doctor focuses selectively on some of the patient's complaints and discourages the reporting of others, he is likely to obtain skewed and misleading information and hence to make diagnostic errors.[52,55]

Zborowski[54] has investigated the manner in which patients of Old American, Jewish, Irish, and Italian origin communicate pain, both verbally and nonverbally. He found that Jews and Italians complained of pain with display of emotion, made no effort to understate their discomfort, and used freely nonverbal communication of distress by moaning, crying, and other emotional display. The Old Americans and the Irish, on the other hand, understated their complaints of pain and showed little expression of emotion. The Irish tended to describe pain in a generally vague manner. These two studies highlight the influence of ethnic and cultural background on the mode of reporting bodily distress.

Personality factors also influence the mode of the patient's communication. Individuals with a histrionic personality type, for example, are notorious for the dramatic flair of their complaints. A person's linguistic habits express his personality. Whereas some individuals tend to mislabel their bodily perceptions, others lack the ability to describe their emotional states and resort to somatic complaints and metaphors instead.[46] Obsessive–compulsive persons characteristically present their complaints with such a wealth of detail and with so many digressions that the doctor is likely to become inattentive, impatient, and confused. *Social* background is another significant variable. Patients from lower socioeconomic classes and from rural areas typically describe their emotional distress in terms of bodily discomfort.[56,57]

Patients tend to communicate selectively what they expect the doctors to be interested in, namely, bodily complaints. This social expectation may result in diagnostic errors and lead to unnecessary and expensive laboratory investigations to rule out physical illness when none is present. Some patients display a different variety of skewed communication: they complain of psychological distress but withhold crucial information about their somatic symptoms.[58] Patients with specific communicative disorders, such as aphasia or stuttering, present special problems. They may fail to make themselves understood by the doctor, especially one impatient to obtain information in the shortest possible time. A similar problem is often faced by a schizophrenic patient whose idiosyncratic and often bizarre mode of communication may preclude a meaningful verbal exchange with a physician.

COPING BEHAVIOR

The *actions* taken by a sick person in respect to his illness comprise what may be called coping behavior. The term "coping" has been variously defined and used by different writers.

Lazarus,[30] a psychologist, defines coping as the strategies for dealing with threat. He distinguishes two modes of coping: *direct actions*, that is, active preparation against harm; and *intrapsychic processes*, those aimed at withdrawing attention from threat, minimizing it, and seeking relief from it in fantasy. In a more recent publication Lazarus[59] equates intrapsychic forms of coping with what are usually called defenses. He explains that in coping, the person tries to "alter or master the troubled commerce with the environment." For example, if a student facing an important examination spends time in active preparation for it, he or she is engaged in coping activities, which may be effective or not.

Mechanic,[60] a sociologist, defines coping as the "instrumental behavior and problem-solving capacities of persons in meeting life demands and goals. It involves the application of skills, techniques, and knowledge that a person has acquired."

These two definitions are really complementary rather than mutually exclusive. Lazarus emphasizes threat and stress. Mechanic takes a broader view, an adaptational one, and underscores tasks and challenges, rather than dangers, with which people must deal. In the present context we are concerned with the application of the concept of coping to physical illness, which may be regarded as both a life crisis or stressor and an adaptive task or challenge.[61] I have proposed the following definition of coping in relation to illness, injury, and disability: *Coping refers to all cognitive and psychomotor activities that a sick person employs to safeguard bodily and psychic integrity, to recover reversibly impaired function, and to compensate for and adjust to permanent disability.*[23]

I have already discussed the principal cognitive modes of coping with illness. In this section I shall focus on the patient's behavioral *action* tendencies aimed at dealing with the threat, challenge, and specific tasks imposed by physical illness. Three major *styles of coping behavior* may be distinguished: (1) *tackling*, (2) *capitulating*, (3) *avoiding*.[23]

The *tackling* style of coping behavior refers to a disposition to display an active approach toward threat and challenges presented by illness or disability. In its extreme form this type of behavioral tendency manifests itself by confronting illness as if it were an enemy to combat and conquer. Such an attitude has been advocated recently as the best one for cancer patients to adopt. "Fighting back" has been deliberately encouraged as a means of prolonging survival of the cancer victim.[62] The patient may attempt to act as if he were healthy and try to perform routine activities as soon as, and at times before, the physician allows them. Postmyocardial infarction patients who return to full-time employment after the shortest interval, arthritics engaged in physical activities regardless of joint pain, and cancer patients continuing work until terminal illness are examples of this particular coping style. Such behavior may be adaptive or not, depending on its consequences. Some patients with rheumatoid arthritis, for example, continue full activity disregarding their pain and may bring about destructive changes in the joints, hardly an adaptive mode of coping from the point of view of its outcome. Less pronounced degrees of tackling, however, may be regarded as the most desirable and adaptive mode of coping behavior. Flexible and rational modulation of activity, timely recourse to medical advice, seeking of relevant information, judicious compliance with the recommended treatment regimen, attempting to achieve prompt recovery, collaboration with rehabilitative efforts, and developing satisfying substitutes for irreversibly impaired or lost functions are all manifestations of adaptive tackling.

Capitulating implies that the patient tends to give in passively to illness by either withdrawing from others or, on the contrary, becoming overly dependent on them. The withdrawing patient is likely to delay or neglect to seek medical help despite suffering painful or incapacitating symptoms. The passively dependent patient displays helplessness and expects to be taken care of. Capitulating patients are likely to remain disabled longer than their physiological condition warrants and to develop an undue dependence on doctors and hospitals. They show little or no willingness to conduct their affairs actively and assertively. The most extreme form of this behavioral tendency may be seen in those who have lost hope and given up resisting the illness. Such patients may die even though progression of the disease has been halted by medical intervention. Capitulating should not be confused with adaptive passivity during the acute phase of any life-threatening illness.

Avoiding pertains to active attempts to get away from the threat, demands, and challenges of illness. An overt suicidal attempt and self-destructive noncompliance with the treatment are extreme manifestations of this style. In a less pronounced form avoiding may be displayed by an intensely anxious patient who delays medical consultation for fear of being given a dreaded diagnosis. This coping style may be associated either with overt anxiety or with overt calm resulting from marked minimization of the threat of illness.

These coping styles may be viewed as reflecting three basic psychobiological defense tendencies in response to threat: fight, immobility (conservation–withdrawal), and flight, respectively. But such typologies should not be taken too literally. Undoubtedly, some individuals consistently display behaviors described here. Many, however, show mixtures of action tendencies or shift from one to another in the course of an illness. Furthermore, specific illnesses and disabilities present people with novel situations and tasks that may elicit a variety of specific *coping strategies* or techniques.[23] The coping styles described here represent relatively enduring personality characteristics. The actual strategies adopted by a patient to deal with pain, paralysis, incontinence, or aphasia, for example, are influenced not only by the patient's overall coping style but also by his specific disability and symptoms as well as by their severity, rate of onset, and degree of reversibility.[23-68] For example, an acute illness or trauma, such as myocardial infarction or burns, tends to elicit different coping strategies from those developed in response to a chronic illness.[61,68] Moreover, the mode of coping that a patient adopts appears to be influenced not only by his personality but also by such factors as the availability of empathic and skilled medical care as well as of adequate social supports.[69]

The concept of coping with illness and the impact of the assorted coping styles and strategies on a patient's adjustment to illness have become a subject of systematic studies only recently. Much of this research is still descriptive rather than devoted to the testing of specific hypotheses. The most recent investigations as well as clinical impressions do support the contention that the concept of coping has heuristic value in understanding how individuals adjust to illness.[64]

The Social (Interactional) Response to Illness

Under this heading I will discuss that aspect of the psychosocial response which involves interaction between the patient and his social environment, and especially the family members and doctors. This aspect has been studied mostly by medical sociologists, who have introduced such valuable concepts as those of the *sick role* and *sickness or sick-role behavior*.[70,71] These concepts can be discussed here only briefly, and interested readers are referred to textbooks of medical sociology and to Twaddle's[71] monograph for more detailed discussions.

The Sick Role and Sickness Behavior

The most influential theroretical construct relevant to the social aspect of the response to illness is that of the *sick role*, developed by Parsons.[72,73] The concept of any social role involves two kinds of expectations: (1) that the person will adopt certain prescribed attitudes and follow certain actions, and (2) that others should behave toward the person according to implicit and explicit rules. The sick role implies the following expectations: (1) exemption from the responsibilities and obligations of the premorbid social roles—such as wage earner, parent, and spouse—in relation to the nature and severity of illness; (2) obligation to seek the help of and comply with the advice of competent person; and (3) surrender of the sick role as soon as this is compatible with physiological recovery. Thus, it is expected that the person will play the sick role for a limited period of time and exert proper effort to achieve functional recovery and resume premorbid roles expeditiously. The sick role, according to Parsons, is deviant, yet one distinguished from other deviant roles by a crucial feature: the sick person is not held responsible for his deviant behavior.

A person may follow one of several courses with regard to the acceptance of, adherence to, and surrender of the sick role: (1) accept it only when the health condition warrants it and a qualified health professional recommends it, adhere to it as long as it is necessary for optimum recovery, and give it up when the recovery occurs; (2) adopt it readily and cling to it beyond physiological recovery and in disregard of medical advice that he is fit to give it up; (3) attempt to avoid its acceptance, then give in to it and try to hold onto it beyond recovery; (4) avoid it consistently until fully incapacitated or forced by others to accept it; or (5) adopt it in the absence of any demonstrable physical illness or injury and in defiance of professional opinion that he is healthy.

All these patterns of sick-role behavior are encountered in clinical practice, and it is important to identify that which the patient displays. One of the main problems facing doctors and other concerned individuals is to establish in any given case whether the person plays the sick role according to socially accepted rules or is delaying it unduly, or whether he uses it for psychological, social, or economic gains. The most extreme examples of misuse of the sick role are provided by those exhibiting one of the factitious disorders. In these cases, we may talk of *abnormal illness behavior*,[74] a form of deviant sick-role behavior. Patients displaying conversion symptoms or hypochondriasis, for example, may be viewed as players of the sick role in good faith and for largely unconscious motives.

The manner in which a person behaves with regard to the sick role is determined by personality, past experience with illness, the example set by family members, the health beliefs held by members of his social group, and the responses of the doctors and other interested people to the complaints. The family members may by their attitudes discourage or support acceptance of the sick role and its maintenance. The person's self-concept as a healthy, independent, and invulnerable individual may hinder acceptance of the sick role even at the risk of death. Some people refuse to consider themselves ill even though they show demonstrable pathology, others accept the fact of being ill but resist adopting the sick role, and others still play the role not for the purpose of getting well but for availing themselves of the privileges accorded by the society to its sick members.

The sick role has proved to be a heuristically fertile concept, even though its shortcomings have been criticized on both theoretical and practical grounds. The main criticisms have focused on the relative inapplicability of the concept to minor illnesses, to chronic and stigmatized diseases, and to illness behavior not involving contact with physicians.[71,75] Furthermore, the concept is flawed in that it fails to take into account sociocultural factors. There is no evidence to support the contention that people everywhere perceive the rights and obligations of the sick role in the same way as expressed in Parsons' original formulation. These and other criticisms, however, have not gainsaid the originality and heuristic value of his contribution.

Two aspects of the social response to illness, both of which influence (and are influenced by) the patient's sick-role behavior, are critically important: *interactions with the family* and *relationship between the patient and the doctor*.

Patients and Their Families

To view a sick person apart from his or her social environment is to deal with a truncated abstraction. Interpersonal relationships are crucially important in the experience of illness and in coping with it. Furthermore, these relationships are reciprocal, in that a patient's behavior is influenced by and in turn influences the so-called significant others, especially family members. As Litman[76] rightly stresses, the family provides the most important context within which illness occurs and is resolved. Only recently, however, has the dynamic interrelation between illness and the family been given systematic attention.[72]

The relationship between physical illness in one or more family members and the family dynamics has been stuided from several angles: (1) the influence of family interaction on the development of physical illness or injury, (2) the effects of the parental health behavior and attitudes toward illness on the learning of respective behaviors and attitudes by their offspring, (3) the impact of illness of a family member on the family interactions, and (4) the influence of the family on the patient's sickness behavior.

All these aspects of the reciprocal relationship between the physically ill or disabled member and his family are important for the studies of the course and outcome of disease, for preventive medicine, and for utilization and planning of health care delivery. Whether a patient's psychosocial responses are considered normal or pathological, assessment of family interactions is indispensable for the understanding of the patient's attitudes, mood, and behavior, for comprehensive diagnosis and management, and for the actions aimed at prevention of psychopathology in the family members.

A Theoretical Framework. Parsons and Fox,[77] in their classical paper entitled "Illness, Therapy, and the Modern Urban American Family," argued that the latter was particularly prone to the disorganizing effects of illness. A modern nuclear family is small, relatively isolated, close-knit, and characterized by intense emotional ties. As a result, the illness of one of its members is likely to upset all the others and to bring about a state of individual and collective imbalance. The consequences of this vulnerability depend in part on which member is sick. One general consequence is the tendency to relinquish the traditional care of the sick member within the family and delegate it to the hospital or nursing home. Another common tendency is for the relative to overreact to the sick member's readiness to adopt the sick role.

Illness of the *mother* of a small family is disturbing because of her unifying and emotionally supporting role. When she falls ill, her husband and children are likely to feel deprived of her accustomed affective support, and she herself is likely to experience an additional sense of burden and responsibility. Illness of the *husband-father*, as the main provider of economic security and the bearer of social status, tends to jeopardize the social and economic position of the whole family and to deprive the children of the mother's support, which becomes focused on the ill father. Illness of a *child* may bring to the surface, or increase, marital disharmony in the parents and intensify sibling rivalry by attracting special parental attention to the sick child. The delicately balanced intrafamily dynamics may be further disturbed if the sick member takes advantage of being ill to avoid customary roles and responsibilities. Since the sick role is a legitimate way of avoiding normal social demands and of inviting care-giving attitudes from others, it provides temptations related to the assignment of roles in the modern family. Thus, for the wife–mother, illness may offer welcome relief from the burden of her affectively supportive feminine role. For the husband-father, illness may offer a sanctioned rest from the internalized demands for achievement, competition, and independence of the masculine role. Not surprisingly, some men and women find these aspects of the sick role attractive enough to accept it too readily and prolong it unduly. As a result, serious strains may develop in the family relationships.

These influential theoretical formulations of Parsons and Fox were published 30 years ago and are badly in need of revision.[77] The American family has been changing. For example, recent studies indicate that the evolving patterns of conjugal roles characterized by shared responsibilities and tasks, and a high level of companionship, may lead to greater resilience in meeting the challenges and strains of illness.[78] The majority of all illness episodes are still being taken care of at home.[76] Nevertheless, the theoretical propositions of Parsons and Fox have not yet become replaced by formulations that reflect the impact of such far-reaching changes as the marked increase in the number of working women, childless couples, and single-parent families.

Family Relationships and Etiology of Illness. Investigators have attempted in recent years to identify those social factors which constitute psychological stresses for particular individuals and may contribute to the development of physical illness.[79] Family processes have come under scrutiny in this regard, and some evidence has accrued which suggests that certain types of family interaction could have etiological significance in disease. Such factors as marriage, divorce, and illness or death of a family member have been singled out as playing a potentially pathogenic role.[79] In the United States, mortality rates are higher for nonmarried people than married persons and are especially high for the formerly married.[80]

To establish that a particular type of intrafamily dynamics precedes the onset of physical illness does not establish a cause-and-effect relationship but makes it plausible. Meissner[81] hypothesizes that disruption of the family affective system due to any emotionally significant event may precipitate ''psychosomatic'' illness in vulnerable family members. He proposes that the intervening variable is a disturbed emotional state in such a vulnerable member which may lower his resistance to disease. An example of the contributory role of family dynamics to illness onset is offered by a study in which 16 families comprising 100 persons were followed up intensively for 1 year, with regular throat cultures for beta-hemolytic streptococci, periodic testing of antistreptolysin O titer, and clinical evaluation of all illnesses.[82] One of the factors that seemed to play an important role in determining host susceptibility to streptococcal illness was acute and chronic family stress. Much more research is needed, however, to establish the validity of the claim that family dynamics play a causative role in physical illness.

The Influence of Parental Attitudes on Children's Illness Behavior. Surprisingly little is known about this subject, and much that is written about it is anecdotal. Sperling,[39] for example, asserts that people who develop one of the so-called psychosomatic disorders, such as peptic ulcer, asthma, migraine, or ulcerative colitis, had been rewarded during childhood for being sick. According to this hypothesis, the mother of the ''psychosomatic'' patient rewarded him as a child for being sick, helpless, and dependent and rejected the child when he was healthy and striving for individuation. Such an early learning experience might result in a lifelong pattern of resorting to or exploiting illness as a strategy to control others and make them compliant.

Mechanic[83] has studied 350 children and their mothers to test the hypothesis that mothers influence health attitudes and illness behavior of their offspring. He found some support for this hypothesis, but the degree of inconsistency in the findings was too great to allow the conclusion that maternal influence was a significant factor. On the whole, children displayed remarkable resistance against the influence of people in their environment. For example, a mother's hypochondriacal attitude could not allow the prediction that her child would show either the same or the opposite attitude. There is some empirical evidence, however, that parents do influence the development of health attitudes and beliefs and the illness behavior of their offspring.[84] The extent and specific patterns of such influences, however, remain a matter of speculation.

Impact of Illness on Family Interactions. Illness in a *child* in relation to family dynamics has been the most studied topic in this generally underdeveloped area.[85-90] The nature of the child's illness and its characteristics, such as severity, duration, prognosis, and degree of disability, have emerged as some of the key independent variables. The impact of acute illness on family dynamics has been less studied than the consequences of chronic illness. From their study of the effects of acute illness, Green and Solnit[87] developed an influential concept of the vulnerable-child syndrome. They investigated a group of children who suffered a serious illness or accident prior to the age of 10 years and whose parents, usually mothers, expected them to die prematurely even after they had recovered. That belief resulted in a characteristic parent-child interaction, the so-called vulnerable-child syndrome. The children were found at follow-up to have marked problems with separation experiences, displayed many hypochondriacal complaints, underachieved at school, and showed poor impulse control. Their mothers persisted in overprotecting them and reacted with anxiety to the child's attempts at becoming independent. Levy[88] interviewed 750 parents of inner-city children while they were waiting in one of five general pediatric facilities. Parents' unwarranted fear that a particular child was vulnerable, that is, threatened by recurrence of an illness that had actually been resolved in the past, constituted a common reason for a medical visit. Vulnerable children made more visits per year and made many more of their visits to the emergency room than the children not viewed by their parents as vulnerable. Green[86] points out that symptoms in "vulnerable" children include difficulty with separation, sleep problems, abusive behavior toward the parents, and frequent absence from school. Parents' belief that a child is vulnerable results in excessive, and often needless, utilization of health facilities.

The impact of *chronic* or *fatal* illness in a child on family dynamics has been the subject of a number of recent studies.[85,89-100] Only a few selected examples of this research and several major hypotheses can be discussed here.

The response of the mother to a child's chronic illness has been shown to influence the child's attitudes and behavior. For example, when mothers of children with congenital heart disease overestimated its severity, the illness had a more disruptive impact on the family as a whole and on the affected child.[89] Maternal distortion of the facts of the illness as presented by the cardiologist as well as maternal anxiety were more influential in fostering the child's dependence and perceived own disability than the objectively estimated severity of the cardiac defect. Frydman[91] found that "distortion" of the severity of a child's illness correlated with parental psychiatric morbidity.

An adverse effect of a chronic illness in a child on the marital relationship of parents has been found in a study of 32 families of children with hemophilia, a disease marked by the occurrence of unpredictable episodes of bleeding that often require emergency treatment.[92] Nearly half the parents of intact families reported that hemophilia had a negative effect on their marriage. Some parents, however, reported that, on the contrary, coping with the child's illness had brought them closer together. The great majority of parents intimated that family relationships were negatively influenced by hemophilia.

Various patterns of disturbed family relationships have emerged from the studies of children with cystic fibrosis and their families.[93] Siblings of the affected children often complain of being neglected, and some of them attempt to attract attention by pretending to have symptoms of cystic fibrosis or some other somatic disease. Some siblings show poor school adjustment and delinquency, which appear to be causally related to the rivalries enhanced by the attention paid to the sick child. Mothers tend to complain of the fathers' lack of interest in the sick child, and this contributes to marital strain. The most serious disruption of family relationships was found in families showing lack of closeness and an inability to communicate feelings and to offer mutual emotional support. In such families the sick children tend to be ashamed of their illness and to cooperate poorly with treatment.

Ellenberger et al.[94] assert that the family of a child suffering from a chronic illness tends to go through several distinct, if overlapping, stages of adaptation to that stress: (1) early recognition of the possibility of illness; (2) warning, i.e., perception of the child's symptoms; (3) impact of discovery of illness, which is usually responded to calmly and rationally; (4) fragmentation of family organization during the acute phase of the child's illness; (5) recovery of the family interaction, marked by attempts to adapt to the fact of illness by trying to understand its genesis and treatment; (6) short-term adjustment (first 6 months after hospitalization) characterized by an atmosphere of warmth and sympathy; and (7) long-term adjustment, which may take one of three forms: focusing attention on the sick child, ignoring the child, or regarding him as a special member of the family unit.

The impact of *fatal illness* in a child on family dynamics has been the subject of numerous reports.[85,95-100] One of the studies focused on parents' reactions to a child's neoplastic disease, mostly leukemia.[97,98] A sequence of reactions could be observed, one beginning with a sense of shock at disclosure of the diagnosis, followed by a tendency to blame themselves, and ending with a degree of acceptance of the inevitable. The parents were observed to employ coping strategies that included the defense mechanisms of isolation of affect, intellectualization, and, less often, denial. The parents experienced conscious anxiety and depression when these defenses were failing. The investigators assessed selected physiological correlates of the parents' coping behavior and emotions.[98] They used excretion rates of 17-hydroxycorticosteroids (17=OHCS) as an indicator of psychological stress and found them to be relatively stable and low in those parents who were employing any type of defense mechanism effectively. Marked denial was associated with the lowest 17-OHCS excretion rates.

A different methodological approach and focus of inquiry are exemplified by a study of the impact of a child's leukemia on the child and his whole family.[99] Leukemic children over 4 years old communicated in various ways that they were aware of the seriousness of their disease and even of impending death. Older children were often aware of the diagnosis even though they had not been told what it was, and this tended to create a barrier to meaningful communication between the parents and the child. Mutual attempts at protection from emotional distress could be observed. The parents experienced pronounced anticipatory grief and persistent thoughts and fantasies about the child's expected death. Fathers tended to avoid involvement with their dying children, and this often left the mother with the burden of coping with the difficult situation. In about half the affected families one or more of the healthy siblings manifested distress by developing somatic symptoms, depression, anxiety, and a fear of becoming fatally ill themselves. Some of these behavioral disturbances seemed to be related to feelings of rejection by the parents, who were preoccupied with the leukemic sibling. The impact of the illness reached even the grandparents, some of whom were supportive, but many of whom were perceived by the child's parents as interfering and annoying. This study has shown that a fatal illness in a child is likely to have a disruptive effect on the whole family.

Chronic disease in an adolescent affects the family relationships differently in some respects than does the illness of a child.[101] A questionnaire study of a large sample of both healthy and chronically ill but not currently incapacitated adolescents has shown that history of a chronic illness in an adolescent does not as a rule elicit overprotective attitudes from their parents as long as no acute flareup of the illness occurs.[101] In that case, the parents tend to show more friendliness and solicitude toward the sick adolescent, especially a daughter, than at other times. Chronically ill adolescents do not seem to be appreciably different from their healthy peers in both their familial and extrafamilial interactions, such as dating and group social activities. Adolescents with a history of chronic illness are more likely than those lacking such history to feign physical illness as a means of obtaining various parental rewards.

The preceding study suggests that effective coping is the rule and that a chronically ill adolescent is not likely to be an isolated, lonely, and overprotected individual. A questionnaire survey, however, may miss the more subtle disturbances of family interaction which direct interviews with both the adolescent and his family could bring to light.

The impact of *parental illness* on the family dynamics has been the subject of much speculation but relatively few empirical studies.

The impact of an illness in the *mother–wife* on the family is likely to be disorganizing in view of her pivotal role.[77] The few reported studies tend to support this view.[76,102] One study has focused on the effects of the wife's severe disability, defined as physical impairment interfering with homemaking activities, on marital satisfaction.[103] Some of the women were bedridden. There was a striking lack of correlation between the severity of the wife's disability, on the one hand, and the marriage satisfaction of both partners, on the other. A severely disabled woman had a more unambiguous role and hence experienced less conflict over and pressure to meet her family obligations. Furthermore, her physical disability as such had little effect on marital sexual activity and satisfaction, which in turn were positively correlated with her marriage satisfaction. When the wife was more physically mobile, her role was more ambiguous, creating strains for her and leading to attempts to define her proper role in the marriage. Her greater mobility, however, tended to increase satisfaction of her need for safety and her husband's need for companionship. This study, though small in scope, highlights the complexity of the marital relationships of couples in which the wife is chronically disabled. Its findings challenge intuitive predictions to the effect that the greater the wife's disability, the less is the couple likely to be satisfied with their relationship.

Disability or illness of the *father–husband* tends to have different consequences for the family than that of the mother–wife. A role shift may result as the wife has to assume more responsibility for running the household.[104] She may have to take a job, and her absence from home deprives younger children of her attention and forces the older ones to assume more duties around the house. There are fewer social and recreational activities. The economic situation of the family tends to be undermined and lead to changes of accommodation and life-style, abandonment of plans for children's education, and debts. Marital discord tends to increase and shifts of roles between the partners may cause strains. The economic decline resulting from husband's illness is particularly marked for the disabled workers whose children have drastically reduced opportunities for educational, social, and economic advancement.[105,106] One study, however, has found that children of fathers disabled by spinal cord injury were well adjusted and emotionally stable.[107]

Disease in a marital partner may affect the marital interaction in a manner destructive for both partners. An example of such interaction is provided by a study of wives of diabetic men.[108] The wives tended to view their spouses' diabetes mellitus as a challenge for them to prove their usefulness by being indispensable for the husband. This tendency often gave rise to conflict and frustration when the husband insisted on minimizing his illness and neglected his treatment. The main dynamic interaction, however, revolved around the special diet and the husband's reduced sexual potency, a common complication of diabetes. The preparation of the special diet, and the food itself, served both partners as a way to express certain needs and feelings. The manner in which the wife handled the matter of the diabetic diet reflected her positive or negative feelings toward her husband. When the marital relationship was generally satisfactory, food presented no major problem. If the marriage was full of conflicts, the wife tended to sabotage and neglect the husband's special dietary needs. Food would then become a weapon used overtly or covertly to express resentment. In some cases the husband deliberately rejected his special diet and lashed out at his wife for offering it to him. In this way he could express his anger and hostility against the wife as well as his own self-destructive tendency. Impotence, partial or total, provided another major source of conflict in marital interaction. Some wives, for example, used the husband's impotence as a reason to criticize or ridicule him, whereas others saw it as willful rejection or else blamed themselves for having contributed to the sexual problem. In some cases the wife was relieved to be free from the performance of sexual intercourse, yet tended to blame her husband for depriving her of sexual satisfaction. This study illustrates the manifold ways, overt and covert, in which illness and its specific requirements can be drawn into marital interaction.

Myocardial infarction is a catastrophic event and strikes men more often than women. The impact of a heart attack on marital interaction has been the subject of a number of studies.[109–115] A husband's heart attack creates serious psychological stress for most wives, who tend to experience various psychological and somatic symptoms for as long as a year after the event. Depression and irritability exhibited by the husband may bring the marriage to a breaking point.[112] A wife's common fear that upsetting her husband could precipitate another, and possible fatal, heart attack may result in decreased communication and mutual estrangement.[114] The wife tends to blame herself, or be blamed by her husband, or both, for having brought on his heart attack; such guilt feelings do not foster intimacy and trust.[110] Both wives and children may feel put upon by and resent the demands for care and consideration for the patient.[114] The effect of the husband's sudden life-threatening illness on marital relations is influenced by their quality prior to his heart attack.[112,113] If the relationship had been poor, it tended to be even worse after the heart attack. Some couples, however, grow closer together in the face of a threat to the husband's life.[112] Fear and inhibitions regarding resumption of sexual activity on the part of the patient, his wife, or both are a common source of marital strain after myocardial infarction and make professional counseling mandatory before the patient is discharged from the hospital.[115]

Thus, illness in a family member tends to have manifold effects on the healthy members. Their mutual interactions as well as their attitudes and conduct toward the sick member reflect such factors as the nature of the illness and its severity, prognosis, and duration. The functioning of the family as a whole prior to the onset of the illness is an important modifying factor but appears to be a poor predictor of the impact of the illness on the family. A cohesive family, marked by marital satisfaction and family solidarity, is likely to be disrupted by the occurrence of physical illness in one of its members, whereas a more loosely tied and relatively poorly functioning family may be brought closer together.[76] Marital relationship is likely to be influenced for better or worse by any serious, especially chronic and disabling or disfiguring, illness. Companionship, social status, mutual affection and esteem, and sexual satisfaction may all be adversely affected.[103]

The effect of the illness of a spouse on family dynamics appears to be partly determined by the couple's manner of viewing and dividing conjugal roles. If the partners define such roles rigidly and are forced to shift them as a result of illness in one of them, then tension is likely to occur, both in the marriage and in the family as a whole. For example, if the husband sees his role as that of the undisputed head of the family, he may become distressed when illness forces him to transfer to his wife some of his prerogatives. Some husbands may unconsciously welcome this yet complain about it to save face. Others react with manifest resentment, hostility, anxiety, or depression. A wife may find a role shift to her liking and may be loath to give it up when the husband recovers and tries to reassert his previous authority. Conflict over dominance may be set in motion when the husband's illness forces him to give up an active role in sexual intercourse. Such a role shift brought about by the husband's paraplegia or severe backache, for example, could rekindle intrapsychic conflicts and doubts over sexual identity in one or both partners. However, recent surveys show that the marriages of paraplegics and quadriplegics are not likely to end in divorce and actually tend to be stable and satisfying.[116,117]

The Influence of the Family on Illness Behavior and Sick-Role Playing. Attitudes of the healthy members toward a sick member influence his attitude in regard to the sick role. The wife–mother appears to be particularly influential in this regard.[76] How she evaluates the symptoms complained of by her husband or children influences decisions whether to seek, delay, or forego medical consultation, to comply with the doctor's recommendations, and to adopt or avoid the sick role. These judgments and decisions have an effect on the timing of contact with health professionals and on the degree of utilization of health care facilities. The mother herself often tends to be reluctant to adopt the sick role and plays an important part as a judge of her children's and husband's grounds to adopt it. Mothers who are dissatisfied with their marriage and family life tend to recognize illness in their children and to use medical services more readily than those who are contented.[83] An unhappy mother may initiate a medical consultation for her child regardless of whether the child is sick.

Either spouse may encourage or hinder the adoption of the sick role by the other. Once such a role is adopted, adherence to it and timing of its surrender are also influenced by the family responses. A spouse or parent may derive gratification from caring for the sick family member and thus have a vested interest in encouraging him to maintain the sick role. Illness of a family member may help to stabilize a shaky family balance and give the healthy member who is most involved with the care of the sick one a sense of purpose and heightened self-esteem. If the sick member finds the sick role gratifying, an unspoken collusion with the care-giving family member may result and induce resistance to the surrender of the sick role by both partners. If the sick member recovers, the one who has cherished a caregiver's role may become emotionally disturbed. The dependency and other privileges of the sick role may arouse envy or resentment in one or more healthy family members who may try to force the sick member to give up the sick role prematurely. Finally, a sick or disabled family member may use the sick role as leverage to avoid certain demands and expectations of the healthy members or use the illness as a power-yielding strategy. A parent, for instance, may tie a child to him by using the child's illness to enforce compliance.

In summary, when a family member becomes ill or disabled, family relationships are affected, for better or for worse. The interactions that ensue influence the patient's mood, illness behavior, sick-role playing, and, ultimately, the course and outcome of the illness.

Interaction with Health Professionals: The Doctor–Patient Relationship

> I seldom consult physicians about the changes in my health, for these men take advantage of you when they have you at their mercy. They fill your ears with their prognostications. And formerly, when they took me unawares, weakened by my illness, they would come down on me with their dogmas and magisterial frowns, threatening me sometimes with severe pain, and sometimes with approaching death.
>
> Montaigne, *Essays*, 1595

The manner in which the patient interacts with the health professionals, especially doctors, influences his illness behavior as well as the course and outcome of the illness. The importance of the doctor–patient relationship as a framework within which therapeutic intervention takes place has long been recognized but only recently subjected to systematic scrutiny. Only a few representative conceptions and studies in this area can be touched upon here, and readers are referred to the relevant literature.[118–122]

The doctor–patient relationship may be viewed as a *social system*. Henderson[122] expressed this viewpoint succinctly: "A physician and a patient taken together make up a social system. They do so because they are two and because they have relations of mutual dependence." The patient depends on the doctor's expert knowledge and therapeutic skills, and the doctor depends on the patient for income and professional satisfaction. Parsons[72] elaborated that viewpoint further and proposed that the physician's social role centers around his obligation to facilitate the patient's recovery from illness to the best of his ability. The doctor's role involves the crucial prerogative to confer on a sick person the status of a "patient" and thus to legitimize the adoption of the sick role. Transactions within the doctor–patient system, however, are influenced not only by the ostensible and socially sanctioned features of the physician's social role, but also by the personal attributes, needs, and strivings of both participants. Thus, the doctor–patient relationship has two integral components: the *social* and the *personal*, including psychodynamic.

The doctor-patient relationship encompasses several major aspects, all of which have been the subject of much theorizing and some empirical studies:

1. The physician's professional values, standards, and attitudes.
2. The influence of personality and sociocultural variables on doctor–patient interactions.
3. The doctor–patient communication.
4. The patient's satisfaction with the doctor's attitude, performance, and provision of information.
5. The patient's compliance with the physician's recommendations.

Values and norms professed to guide physicians' behavior in regard to their patients are the subject of medical ethics. Lain-Entralgo[120] has pointed out that medical ethics is influenced by the changing religious and moral beliefs of the society in which medicine is practiced. He has traced the history of Western medical ethics to Hippocrates, whose major tenet consisted in accepting and implementing a postulated "instinct to help the sick." A physician was expected to have both friendship (*philia*) for the patient and love for the art of healing. This ideal has remained the cornerstone of medical ethics to the present day.

A contemporary concept of an ideal physician has been clearly formulated by the American Board of Internal Medicine: "A general internist is a physician who provides scientifically based, empathic care.... This care tends to be characterized by a mutual personal commitment between doctor and patient, by stability over time, by substantial breadth, by availability, and by an appropriate attention to elements of human support, sensitivity, and concern."[123]

Empathy, sympathy, concern for the patient, kindliness, integrity, warmth, genuineness, and compassion are qualities traditionally expected of physicians.[119] Yet, as a medical educator has wryly observed in regard to the United States, "Personal and compassionate care has always been a statistical rarity in this country." [124] This comment provides a realistic counterpoint to the idealistic pronouncements by drawing attention to the dissonance between the proclaimed ideal image of the doctor and hard facts. Nevertheless, the doctor's self-image and the lay person's expectations are likely to be influenced by the traditionally high-minded values and norms of the med-

ical profession. Failure to live up to them may provoke intense feelings of disappoint-
ment and righteous indignation in the patient, exemplified by Montaigne's scathing
remarks.

Three major models of the doctor–patient relationship have been proposed[125]: (1)
activity-passivity, in which the patient is relatively helpless and passive and the physician treats him in a manner similar to that of the parent of a helpless infant; (2)
guidance-cooperation, implying that the patient is able to follow directions and exercise his or her own judgment, but is nevertheless expected to comply with the advice
of the physician viewed as a competent guide; and (3) *mutual participation*, a model
most suitable for the management of the chronically ill patient who is largely responsible for his or her own care and needs to consult the doctor only infrequently. It is
a relationship befitting two adults, one of whom helps the other help himself or herself.

Each of these three models has features that make it appropriate for some, but not
all, situations. The first model is suitable when the patient is unconscious or otherwise severely cognitively impaired, or very young. The second model is appropriate
for cases of acute illness or trauma, for instance. The third model is fittingly applied
in most cases of chronic illness. Problems in the doctor–patient relationship may arise
when the doctor tries to follow rigidly a model that does not fit a particular situation.
For instance, physicians have traditionally tended to impose the second model, one
in which the doctor acts like a father who knows best and implicitly expects the patient to play the part of a compliant, trusting, and grateful child.[124] It is a common
custom for even a young doctor to call his patients by their first name, regardless of
their age. In some cases, a father–child type of relationship may be congenial for both
the doctor and the patient who then engage in it with mutual satisfaction. It is sometimes the patient who tries to involve an unwitting doctor in this type of relationship
and ends up resenting the doctor's refusal to play a fatherly role.

An inappropriately applied model may reflect the physician's or the patient's obsolete or distorted ideas about the nature of the doctor's social role and its prerogatives, or it may be a manifestation of the patient's *transference* or the doctor's *countertransference*. These terms imply a distorted perception by either the patient or the
doctor of the other's character and motives. The sources of such distortion are as a
rule unconscious. Transference or countertransference is probably at work when either
the patient or the doctor feels instant and intense liking or loathing, trust or suspicion,
attraction or revulsion, in regard to the other party. The concepts of transference and
countertransference should not be used loosely to refer to the ubiquitous positive or
negative emotional responses that one develops toward other people over time. Rather,
these terms should be reserved for the intense and irrational emotional responses that
cannot be readily accounted for in the light of the facts of the current encounter. A
patient may on meeting a particular doctor for the first time experience strong feelings of distrust and dislike, without being able to explain them. A closer inquiry is
likely to reveal that the patient associated some aspects of the doctor's physical appearance or manner with a frustrating figure, perhaps a parent, in his or her past. A
patient's transference and a doctor's countertransference are potentially disruptive factors in the doctor–patient relationship.[126]

Age, sex, physical appearance, personality, ethnic origin, and socioeconomic background are attributes of both the doctor and the patient that tend to influence their mutual relationship. Each participant brings into it his or her beliefs and prejudices as well as personal needs and expectations which may go beyond the explicitly professional character and constraints of a medical contact. Either the doctor's or the patient's needs for dependence, companionship, sexual gratification, or power may be stimulated by their encounter and result in attitudes likely to mar the quality and therapeutic efficacy of their relationship.

Characteristics inherent in the doctor's traditional social role may influence the doctor–patient relationship either positively or negatively. Lain-Entralgo[120] quotes Plato as saying that "the sick man loves the physician because he is sick." This type of love carries potential for marked *ambivalence*, which may be mutual. Montaigne's outburst of sarcasm quoted at the start of this section offers a poignant example of the negative feelings toward physicians. The doctor's role lends itself to such responses. He is an expert in matters of health, one expected to provide prompt relief and eventual cure. He judges if the particular person is to be declared sick. The doctor is a bearer of good or bad news for the patient, and his treatment may bring relief from suffering, or stave off death, or do neither. Expectations flowing from the doctor's role invest him in the patient's mind with power for good or evil. A patient's situation is marked by *uncertainty* and *dependence* on the doctor's competence, judgment, and good will. The doctor is usually aware of his professional obligation to provide relief and to heal, or at least not to do harm. This awareness is a challenge but also a potential burden. The doctor may feel repelled, or exploited, or imposed upon by a given patient, expecially one who is noncompliant, demanding, or hostile. A conflict between the doctor's sense of professional obligation to help and his wish to retaliate against or get away from such a patient may be intense. As any physician's knowledge and therapeutic efficacy are limited, he may experience a distressing sense of guilt, inadequacy, or failure. Such feelings may result in a negative attitude toward the patient. Thus, ambivalence may be mutual, being aided and abetted by the doctor's unique social role.

Communication is a key element of the doctor–patient relationship. As Lain-Entralgo[120] put it, "As soon as doctor and patient meet, they begin to communicate: they look at each other, talk and listen." Verbal and nonverbal communication between doctor and patient enables information to be exchanged and influences the patient's illness behavior for better or for worse. The importance of this subject is reflected in a growing body of literature.[60,121,127-133] The quality of the communication between doctors and patients is judged by many writers to be poor, and communication gaps are reportedly common.[121,129]

Studies have focused on two aspects of the doctor–patient communication: (1) the doctor's understanding of the patient's concern, and (2) the patient's satisfaction with the information about the cause, prognosis, and proper treatment of the illness given by the doctor.[130] Patients typically refer to doctors who understand them as warm and caring and tend to value these qualities more highly than the physician's ability to treat their illness effectively.[130] The degree of the doctor's understanding of what the patient is trying to communicate depends on such variables as the manner in which the patient presents his complaints, the length of time available for the interview, and the

manner in which the physician responds to the patient's verbal and nonverbal communication of distress.[130,132,133] Male physicians tend to take physical complaints of
men more seriously than those of women.[133] Many physicians are incompetent inter-
viewers and as a result elicit inadequate or skewed information about the patient's concerns and symptoms.

The patient's satisfaction with the illness-related information provided by the doctor
has been studied and permits several generalizations. The transmission of information
from doctor to patient influences the quality of medical care and course of treatment.
The physician's success in giving the patient adequate information about the illness
enhances the patient's ability to give a meaningful history and results in patient satisfaction. Patients' compliance with physicians' recommendations correlates positively
with the degree of satisfaction that the patients report in regard to the adequacy of information offered by the doctors. Insufficient, contradictory, or confusing information given by the doctor results in the patient's dissatisfaction and noncompliance.[121,129-131] A physician's response to a patient's communications and the degree
of emotional support he offers him has been shown to influence the patient's sense of
well-being and adjustment to chronic illness.[69]

SUMMARY AND CONCLUSIONS

I have reviewed major theoretical concepts and some representative studies in the
area of psychosocial reactions to physical illness. Somatic illness and injury constitute a form of stress to which an individual invariably responds subjectively, behaviorally, and socially. Three core components of psychosocial reactions are the personal meaning of illness, emotional responses elicited by such meaning, and modes
of coping behavior. These three components are postulated to influence a patient's adjustment to the illness, response to medical advice and therapy, and hence the course
and outcome of every illness. How a patient evaluates his illness in subjective terms,
responds to it emotionally, and copes with it may be judged by outside observers to
be adaptive and "normal" or maladaptive and thus "abnormal." Such judgments reflect the observer's knowledge, values, and bias. Maladaptive responses are likely to
be labeled in terms of the currently accepted classification and diagnostic criteria of
psychopathology. Adaptive or not, however, psychosocial responses may be viewed
as constituting an integral aspect of every illness episode, and as such call for evaluation as part of the clinical assessment of every patient. They should be taken into account in the planning and conduct of medical treatment.

Focus on the psychosocial reactions to illness respresents a relatively recent development and has been, in part, stimulated by people's discontent with the impersonality of medical care and by writings and research by psychosomatically oriented physicians and psychiatrists, medical sociologists, clinical psychologists, and other
concerned professionals and lay authors. Much of this literature is still descriptive and
speculative, but it also contains hypotheses and reports on research aimed at testing
them.There is an obvious need for more such research, especially on the impact of
the various patterns of psychosocial reactions on the course and outcome of specific

diseases, on the utilization and cost of medical care, and on the incidence of psychiatric disorders among the physically ill and their family members.

The present chapter focuses mainly on description of the various aspects and patterns of psychosocial reactions to physical illness and injury. In chapter to follow I will discuss the hypothesized determinants of those reactions (Chapter 9, this volume).

REFERENCES

1. Lipowski ZJ: Physical illness, the patient and his environment: Psychosocial foundations of medicine, in Reiser MF (ed): *American Handbook of Psychiatry*, ed 2, Arieti S (ed-in-chief). New York, Basic Books, 1975, vol 4, pp 3–42.
2. Lipowski ZJ: Psychosocial reactions to physical illness. *Can Med Assoc J* 128:1069–1072, 1983.
3. Alsop S: *Stay of Execution: A Sort of Memoir*, New York, JB Lippincott, 1973.
4. Cousins N: *Anatomy of an Illness as Perceived by the Patient: Reflections on Healing and Regeneration*. New York, Norton, 1979.
5. Sanes A: *A Physician Faces Cancer in Himself.* Albany, NY, State University of New York Press, 1979.
6. Greene R (ed): *Sick Docotrs*. William Heinemann Medical Books, 1971.
7. LaBaw WL: Denial inside out: Subjective experience with anosognosia in closed head injury. *Psychiatry* 32:174–191, 1969.
8. Pinner M, Miller BF (eds): *When Doctors Are Patients*. New York, WW Norton, 1952.
9. Van den Berg JH: *The Psychology of the Sickbed*. Pittsburgh, Duquesne University Press, 1966.
10. Fiore N: Fighting cancer—One patient's perspective. *N Engl J Med* 300:284–289, 1979.
11. Paoli P: *Determined to Live*. New York, Harcourt, Brace & World, 1968.
12. Harrison CY: *Thank God for My Heart Attack*. New York, Henry Holt & Co., 1949.
13. Malraux A: *Lazarus*. New York, Grove Press, 1978.
14. Trautmann J, Pollard C: *Literature and Medicine*. Philadelphia, Society for Health and Human Values, 1975.
15. Barker RG, Wright BA, Meyerson L, Gonick MR: *Adjustment to Physical Handicap and Illness: A Survey of the Social Psychology of Physique and Disability*. New York, Social Science Research Council, 1953.
16. Garnett JF, Levine ES (eds): *Psychological Practices with the Physically Disabled*. New York, Columbia University Press, 1962.
17. Shontz FC: *The Psychological Aspects of Physical Illness and Disability*. New York, Macmillan Publishing Co., 1975.
18. Neisser U: *Cognitive Psychology*. New York, Appleton-Century-Crofts, 1967.
19. Bourne LE, Dominowski RL, Loftus EF: *Cognitive Processes*. Englewood Cliffs, NJ, Prentice-Hall, 1979.
20. Lipowski ZJ: Cardiovascular disorders, in Freedman AM, Kaplan HI, Sadock BJ (eds): *Comprehensive Textbook of Psychiatry*, ed. 3. Baltimore, Williams & Wilkins Co., 1980, pp 1891–1907.
21. Petrie A: *Individuality in Pain and Suffering*, ed. 2 Chicago, University of Chicago Press, 1978.
22. Byrne D, Steinberg A, Schwartz MS: Relationship between repression–sensitization and physical illness. *J Abnorm Psychol* 73:154–155, 1968.
23. Lipowski ZJ: Physical illness, the individual and the coping processes. *Psychiatr Med* 1:91–102, 1970.
24. Weinstein EA, Kahn RL: *Denial of Illness*. Springfield, Ill., Charles C Thomas, 1955.
25. Janis IL: *Psychological Stress*. New York, Wiley, 1958.
26. Hackett TP, Cassem NH: Development of a quantitative rating scale to assess denial. *J Psychosom Res* 18:93–100, 1974.
27. Beisser AR: Denial and affirmation in illness and health. *Am J Psychiatry* 136:1026–1030, 1979.
28. Shalit B: Structural ambiguity and limits to coping. *J Hum Stress* 3:32–45, 1977.
29. Heim E, Moser A, Adler R: Defense mechanisms and coping behavior in terminal illness. *Psychother Psychosom* 30:1–17, 1978.

30. Lazarus RS: *Psychological Stress and the Coping Process.* New York, McGraw-Hill, 1966.
31. Verwoerdt A: Psychopathological responses to the stress of physical illness, in Lipowski ZJ (ed): *Psychosocial Aspects of Physical Illness.* Basel, Karger, 1972, pp. 119–141.
32. Schmale AH Jr: Giving up as a final common pathway to changes in health, in Lipowski ZJ (ed): *Psychosocial Aspects of Physical Illness.* Basel, Karger, 1972, pp. 20–40.
33. Holton CP: Psychological aspects of the management of adolescents with malignancy. *MCV Quarterly* 7:112–119, 1971.
34. Editorial: Mens sana in hemicorpore sano. *JAMA* 212:471–472, 1970.
35. Shontz FC: Physical disability and personality: Theory and recent research. *Psychol Aspects Disabil* 17:51–69, 1970.
36. Steegmuller F (ed): *The Letters of Gustave Flaubert 1830–1857.* Cambridge, Mass, The Belknap Press of Harvard University Press, 1980, p 23.
37. Horowitz MJ: *Psychosocial Function in Epilepsy.* Springfield , Ill, Charles C Thomas, 1970.
38. Kennedy JA, Bakst H: The influence of emotions on the outcome of cardiac surgery: A predictive study. *Bull NY Acad Med* 42: 811–849, 1966.
39. Sperling M: Transference neurosis in patients with psychosomatic disorders. *Psychoanal Quart* 36:342–355, 1967.
40. Plutchik R: *Emotion: A Psychoevolutionary Synthesis.* New York, Harper & Row, 1980.
41. Mechanic D: The concept of illness behavior. *J Chron Dis* 15: 189–194, 1962.
42. Abrams RD: The patient with cancer—His changing pattern of communication. *N Engl J Med* 274:317–322, 1966.
43. Charney E: Patient-doctor communication. Implications for the clinician. *Pediatr Clin North Am* 19:263–279, 1972.
44. Francis V, Lorsch BM, Morris MJ: Gaps in doctor-patient communication. *N Engl J Med* 280:535–540, 1969.
45. Hulka BS, Cassel JC, Kupper LL, Burdette JA: Communication, compliance, and concordance between physicians and patients with prescribed medications. *AJPH* 66:847–853, 1976.
46. Mechanic D: Social psychologic factors affecting the presentation of bodily complaints. *N Engl J Med* 286:1132, 1972.
47. Melzack R, Torgerson WS: On the language of pain. *Anesthesiology* 34:50–59, 1971.
48. Platt FW, McMath JC: Clinical hypocompetence: The interview. *Ann Intern Med* 91:898–902, 1979.
49. Stiles WB, Putnam SM, Wolf MH, James SA: Verbal response mode profiles of patients and physicians in medical screening interviews. *J Med Educ* 54:81–89, 1979.
50. Stoeckle JD, Davidson GE: Communicating aggrieved feelings in the patient's initial visit to a medical clinic. *J Health Hum Behav* 4:199–206, 1963.
51. Waitzkin H, Stoeckle JD: The communication of information about illness. *Adv Psychosom Med* 8:180–215, 1972.
52. Zola IK: Problems of communication, diagnosis, and patient care: The interplay of patient, physician, and clinic organization. *J Med Educ* 38:829–835, 1963.
53. Zola IK: Culture and symptoms: An analysis of patients' presenting complaints. *Am Sociol Rev* 31:615–630, 1966.
54. Zborowski M: *People in Pain.* San Francisco, Jossey-Bass, 1969.
55. Duff RS, Hollingshead AB: *Sickness and Society.* New York, Harper & Row, 1968.
56. Crandell DL, Dohrenwend BP: Some relations among psychiatric symptoms, organic illness, and social class. *Am J Psychiatry* 123:1527–1537, 1967.
57. Lowy FH: Management of the persistent somatizer. *Int J Psychiatry Med* 6:227–239, 1975.
58. Rosner BL: Use of valid psychological complaints to screen, minimize or deny serious somatic illness. *J Nerv Ment Dis* 143:234–238, 1966.
59. Lazarus RS: Psychological stress and ocping in adaptation and illness. *Int J Psychiatry Med* 5:321–333, 1974.
60. Mechanic D: *Medical Sociology,* ed 2. New York, Free Press, 1978.
61. Moos RH (ed): *Coping with Physical Illness.* New York, Plenum Medical Book Co., 1977.
62. Felton BJ, Revenson TA: Coping with chronic illness: A study of illness controllability and the influence of coping strategies on psychological adjustment. *J Consult Clin Psychol* 52:343–353, 1984.

63. Lazarus RS, Folkman S: Coping and adaptation, in Gentry WD (ed): *Handbook of Behavioral Medicine*. New York, Guilford Press, 1984, pp 282–325.

64 Felton BJ, Revenson TA, Hinrichsen GA: Stress and coping in the explanation of psychological adjustment among chronically ill adults. *Soc Sci Med* 18:889–898, 1984.

65. Hamburg D, Adams JE: A perspective on coping behavior. *Arch Gen Psychiatry* 17:277–284 1967.

66. Viney LL, Westbrook MT: Coping with chronic illness: Strategy preferences, changes in preferences and associated emotional reactions. *J Chron Dis* 37:489–502, 1984.

67. Viney LL, Westbrook MT: Coping with chronic illness: The mediating role of biographic and illness-related factors. *J Psychosom Res* 26:595–605, 1982.

68. Weisman AD: *Coping with Cancer*. New York, McGraw-Hill, 1979.

69. Ben-Sira Z: Chronic illness, stress and copng. *Soc Sci Med* 18:725–736, 1984.

70. Kasl SV, Cobb S: Health behavior, illness behavior, and sick role behavior. I. Health and illness behavior. *Arch Environ Health* 12:246–266, 1966.

71. Twaddle AC: *Sickness Behavior and the Sick Role*. Boston, GK Hall & Co., 1979.

72. Parsons T: *The Social System*. Glencoe, Ill, Free Press, 1951.

73. Parsons T: The sick role and the role of the physician reconsidered. *MMFQ (Health and Society)*, Summer 1975.

74. Pilowsky I: Abnormal illness behavior. *Br J Med Psychol* 42:347–351, 1969.

75. Segall A: The sick role concept: Understanding illness behavior. *J Health Soc Behav* 17:163–170, 1976.

76. Litman TJ: The family as a basic unit in health and medical care: A social–behavioral overview. *Soc Sci Med* 8:495–519, 1974.

77. Parsons T, Fox R: Illness, therapy, and the modern urban American family. *J Soc Issues* 8:31–44, 1952.

78. Pratt L: Conjugal organization and health. *J Marriage Fam* 34:85–95, 1972.

79. Grolnick L: A family perspective of psychosomatic factors in illness: A review of the literature. *Fam Process* 11:457–486, 1972.

80. Verbrugge LM: Marital status and health. *J marriage Fam* 41:267–285, 1979.

81. Meissner WW: Family process and psychosomatic disease. *Int J Psychiatry Med* 5:411–430, 1974.

82. Meyer RJ, Haggerty RJ: Streptococcal infections in families. *Pediatrics* 29:539–549, 1962.

83. Mechanic D: The influence of mothers on their children's health attitudes and behavior. *Pediatrics* 33:444–453, 1964.

84. Campbell JD: The child in the sick role: Contributions of age, sex, parental status, and parental values. *J Health Hum Behav* 19:35–51, 1978.

85. Anthony EJ, Koupernik C (eds): *The Child in His Family: The Impact of Disease and Death*. New York, J. Wiley & Sons, 1973, vol 2.

86. Green M: The "vulnerable child": Intimations of mortality. *Pediatrics* 65:1042, 1980.

87. Green M, Solnit A: Reactions to the threatened loss of a child: A vulnerable child syndrome. *Pediatrics* 53:58–66, 1964.

88. Levy JC: Vulnerable children: Parents' perspectives and the use of medical care. *Pediatrics* 65:956–963, 1980.

89. Offord DR, Cross LA, Andrews EJ, Aponte JF: Perceived and actual severity of congenital heart disease and effect on family life. *Psychosomatics* 13:390–396, 1972.

90. Travis G: *Chronic Illness in Children: Its Impact on Child and Family*. Stanford, Calif, Standford University Press, 1976.

91. Frydman MI: Perception of illness severity and psychiatric symptoms in parents of chronically ill children. *J Psychosom Res* 24:361–369, 1980.

92. Salk L, Hilgartner M, Granich B: The psyco-social impact of hemophilia on the patient and his family. *Soc Sci Med* 6: 491–505, 1972.

93. Tropauer A, Neal Franz M, Dilgard VW: Psychological aspects of the care of children with cystic fibrosis. *Am J Dis Child* 119: 424–432, 1970.

94. Ellenberger H, Saucier JF, Wittkower ED: Phases types de l'adaptation familiale à la maladie physique prolongée d'un enfant. *Can Psychiatr Assoc J* 9:322–330, 1964.

95. Easson WM: *The Dying Child: The Management of the Child or Adolescent Who Is Dying*. Springfield, Ill, Charles C Thomas, 1970.

96. Spinetta JJ: The Dying child's awarenes of death: A review. *Psychol Bull* 81:256–260, 1974.

97. Friedman SB, Chodoff P, Mason JW, et al: Behavioral observations on parents anticipating the death of a child. *Pediatrics* 32: 610–625, 1963.

98. Friedman SB, Mason FW, Hamburg D: Urinary 17-hydroxysteroid levels in parents of children with neoplastic disease: A study of chronic psychological stress. *Psychosom Med* 25:364–376, 1963.

99. Binger CM, Ablin AR, Feuerstein RC, et al: Childhood leukemia: Emotional impact on patient and family. *N Engl J Med* 280:414–418, 1969.

100. Sabbeth BF, Leventhal JM: Marital adjustment to chronic childhood illness: A critique of the literature. *Pediatrics* 73:762–768, 1984.

101. Peterson ET: The impact of adolescent illness on parental relationships. *J Health Soc Behav* 13:429–437, 1972.

102. Koos E: *Families in Trouble.* New York, King's Crown Press, 1946.

103. Fink SL, Skipper JK, Hallenbeck PN: Physical disability and problems in marriage. *J Marriage Fam* 30:64–73, 1968.

104. Marra J, Novis F: Family problems in rehabilitation counseling. *Personnel Guidance J* 38:40–42, 1959.

105. Crawford CO (ed): *Health and the Family.* New York, Macmillan, 1971.

106. Klein RF, Dean A, Bogdonoff MD: The impact of illness upon the spouse. *J Chron Dis* 20:241–248, 1967.

107. Buck FM, Hohmann GW: Personality, behavior, values, and family relations of children of fathers with spinal cord injury. *Arch Phys Med Rehabil* 62:432–438, 1981.

108. Katz AM: Wives of diabetic men. *Bull Menninger Clin* 33:279–294, 1969.

109. Croog SH, Fitzgerald EF: Subjective stress and serious illness of a spouse: Wives of heart patients. *J Health Soc Behav* 19:166–178, 1978.

110. Croog SH, Levine S: *The Heart Patient Recovers.* New York, Human Sciences Press, 1977.

111. Davidson DM: The family and cardiac rehabilitation. *J Fam Pract* 8:253–261, 1979.

112. Mayou R, Foster A, Williamson B: The psychological and social effects of myocardial infarction on wives. *Br Med J* 1:699–701, 1978.

113. Skelton M, Dominion J: Psychological stress in wives of patients with myocardial infarction. *Br Med J* 2:101–103, 1973.

114. Stern MJ, Pascale L: Psychosocial adaptation post-myocardial infarction: The spouse's dilemma. *J Psychosom Res* 23:83–87, 1979.

115. Papadopoulos C, Larrimore P, Cardin S, Shelley SI: Sexual concerns and needs of the postcoronary patient's wife. *Arch Intern Med* 140:38–41, 1980.

116. Crewe NM, Athelstan GT, Krumberger J: Spinal cord injury: A comparison of preinjury and postinjury marriages. *Arch Phys Med Rehabil* 60:252–256, 1979.

117. El Ghatit AZ, Hanson RW: Marriage and divorce after spinal cord injury. *Arch Phys Med Rehabil* 57:470–472, 1976.

118. Bloom SW: *The Doctor and His Patient. A Sociological Interpretation.* New York, Russell Sage Foundation, 1963.

119. Crisp AH: Therapeutic aspects of the doctor–patient relationship. *Psychother Psychosom* 18:12–33, 1970.

120. Lain-Entralgo P: *Doctor and Patient.* London, Weidenfeld & Nicholson, 1969.

121. Ley P, Spelman LS: *Communicating with the Patient.* London, Staples Press, 1967.

122. Henderson LJ: The patient and physician as a social system. *N Engl J Med* 212:819–823, 1935.

123. American Board of Internal Medicine: Clinical competence in internal medicine. *Ann Intern Med* 90:402–411, 1979.

124. Tisdale WA: The care of the patient: Ideal and illusion. *Yale J Biol Med* 42:385–393, 1970.

125. Szasz TS, Hollender MH: A contribution to the philosophy of medicine: The basic models of the doctor–patient relationship. *Arch Intern Med* 97:585–590, 1956.

126. Zabarenko RN, Zabarenko L, Pittinger RA: The psychodynamics of physicianhood. *Psychiatry* 33:102–118, 1970.

127. Bradshaw PW, Ley P, Kincey JA, Bradshaw J: Recall of medical advice: Comprehensibility and specificity. *Br J Soc Clin Psychol* 14:55–62, 1975.

128. Detmer DE, Conrad HH: Reflections upon directive language in health care. *Soc Sci Med* 9:553–558, 1975.

129. Freeman B, Negrete VF, Davis M, Korsch B: Gaps in doctor–patient communication: Doctor–patient interaction analysis. *Petiatr Res* 5:298–311, 1971.
130. Waitzkin H, Stoeckle JD: The communication of information about illness. Clinical, sociological, methodological considerations, in Lipowski ZJ (ed): *Psychosocial Aspects of Physical Illness.* Basel, Karger, 1972, pp 180–215.
131. Buchan IC: "Time and motion" in general practice. *Practioner* 221:298–301, 1978.
132. Hopkins P: *Six Minutes for the Patient.* London, Tavistock Publications, 1973.
133. Armitage KJ, Schneiderman LJ, Bass RA: Response of physicians to medical complaints in men and women. *JAMA* 241:2186–2187, 1979.

Determinants of Psychosocial Reactions to Physical Illness

9

INTRODUCTION

Many variables influence a person's reaction to physical illness or injury. Age, personality, past history, and current life situation; the nature and characteristics of the implicated disease or injury; and the quality of the patient's social and physical environment—all play a part.[1] It is clearly a *multifactorial process*. To list all the potentially relevant factors, without trying to select and integrate them in a clinically meaningful fashion, would result in a dreary and useless catalogue. Instead, I shall try to present the major determinants of psychosocial reactions to illness in a conceptually integrated manner, hoping that such a presentation will help the reader appreciate the complexity of this subject and its clinical relevance. In order to understand the meaning a sick person assigns to his illness, and how he reacts to it emotionally and copes with it, one needs to take into account the contribution of several categories of factors.

Everyone experiences physical illness in a unique manner. No single set of generalizations can do justice to all the individual, idiosyncratic features of subjective experience and observable behavior of a sick person. Yet generalizations are needed to serve as guidelines for clinical diagnosis and management. Furthermore, it would not suffice to confine oneself to the description of the various responses to illness, while failing to put forth hypotheses concerning the why and the how of the described reactions. Psychology and psychopathology of illness are empirical sciences which apply the usual scientific procedures, namely observation, description, classification, and formulation of testable explanatory hypotheses. The latter are evolved to account for the occurrence of the various patterns of psychosocial reactions encountered in clinical practice. To propose that a certain factor plays a causative or modifying role in the development of psychosocial and psychopathological reactions to illness amounts to formulating a hypothesis. Such hypotheses need to be validated before being accepted as facts.

CLASSIFICATION

The determinants of psychosocial reactions to physical illness, injury, or disability may be assigned to the following main classes[1]:

1. Intrapersonal factors
   A. Biological
      a. Age
      b. Sex
   B. Psychological
      a. Personality style and traits
      b. Past experiences with illness
      c. Intrapsychic conflicts and defense mechanisms
      d. Emotional state at the time of onset of illness
2. Sociocultural and economic factors
   a. Availability of social support
   b. Availability and quality of medical care
   c. Patient family's responses
   d. Health beliefs and attitudes
   e. Occupation and economic status
3. Disease-related factors
   a. Subjective significance of affected body part or function
   b. Spatiotemporal features of pathology
   c. Type and intensity of symptoms
   d. Severity of illness or disability
4. Physical environmental factors
   a. Characteristics of patient's physical environment such as hospital

This list of determinants is not exhaustive, yet it includes most of the major contributory causative factors. Their relative contribution may be expected to vary from patient to patient and from one episode of illness or injury in the same patient to another. All these factors, however, need to be evaluated for a thorough understanding of a given patient's psychological reaction to an illness or injury, for planning of treatment, rehabilitation, and prevention, and for research. Each of the proposed determinants may be viewed as an independent variable whose effects on patients' illness behavior, a dependent variable, can be the subject of research.

INTRAPERSONAL FACTORS—BIOLOGICAL

Age at which an illness or injury occurs is of major importance for the psychological responses to and consequences of the illness.

Psychosocial aspects of both acute and chronic illness occurring in *childhood* are the subject of voluminous literature.[2-8] This is no place to review these studies, and only a few of them will be quoted to illustrate the influence of age. Longitudinal studies that include healthy controls and provide data on the enduring psychological effects of illness suffered in childhood are particularly important. The largest such study involved more than 5000 children born in England, Wales, and Scotland during the first week of March 1946.[7] At age 15, all children who had experienced a *chronic* physical illness were examined and compared with the remaining, physically healthy children (89% of the total sample). It was found that 25% of the children with chronic illness had two or more abnormal behavioral symptoms at age 15, compared with 17% of the healthy group. Duration of the physical disorder rather than its severity was consistently related to the frequency of emotional symptoms. School underachievement, social isolation, and abnormal behavior were displayed by the chronically ill.

Studies of children stricken with a severe *acute* illness have shown that, compared to their healthy siblings, the formerly ill children had more conduct problems and a greater degree of psychological disturbance.[9,10] The ex-patients showed more problems with control of aggressive impulses than their well siblings. A study of preschool children's reactions to minor physical illness treated at home revealed two age-related behavioral patterns: Children 2 to 3 years old tended to display clinging dependence; the 4 to 6-year-olds showed, by contrast, a behavioral reaction characterized by withdrawal and self-contained, undemanding state.[11] More important than transient psychological reaction to a physical illness, however, is the impact of the latter on personality development and its legacy in the form of enduring tendency to deviant illness behavior and hypochondriasis in later life.

The impact of illness on a child and its possible long-range effects are related in part to the child's developmental stage at which the illness or injury has occurred.[5,12] Thus, illness and hospitalization in the first 3 years of life tend to heighten the child's sensitivity to separation as well as interfere with the development of autonomy and active self-expression. Illness in the 4- to 6-year-olds, at the height of the development of the conscience, may be interpreted by the child as punishment and predispose him to an excessive guilt-proneness. The preadolescent child tends to regard illness as a threat of mutilation and disfigurement, and hence to develop a sense of inferiority and inadequacy. The long-term psychological effects of illness are the result of complex interplay between the child's personality, level of cognitive functioning, and the developmental stage, the characteristics of the illness, and the nature of the family's responses to it. Despite the importance of this whole area for the understanding of illness behavior of adults, speculations and anecdotal accounts outnumber controlled longitudinal studies.

A related and important area of study concerns the development of the concepts of health, illness, and death in children.[2,13-19] Earlier studies indicated that the child achieves the concept of death as a universal and irreversible event only after the age of 9 years. More recent work suggests that although this finding is generally valid, it is not without exceptions. Childers and Wimmer,[16] for example, found that about 10% of children 4 years old responded positively to the question about universality of death, and from then on an increasing percentage of respondents in each age group gave a positive answer. All of the 9-year-olds in the sample answered positively. By contrast, awareness of the irrevocability of death was not elicited in children through 10 years of age. In another study, however, all children age 5½ to 14 years affirmed the finality of death.[17] There is reason to believe that early exposure to television may acquaint children with death earlier now than in the past, that they develop fear of death by observing the behavior of adults, and that they show no tendency (reported in earlier studies) to personify death.[17]

The studies cited have focused on the development of the concept of death in healthy children. Other investigators have been concerned with the awareness of dying in fatally ill children.[14,19] Recent work has shown that such children, aged 6 to 10 years, already express awareness of the seriousness of their condition and may experience intense anxiety related to it.[19] As an example, a study of leukemic children has concluded that most children more than 4 years old show evidence that they are aware of the gravity of their illness and some even entertain the idea of their premature death.[14]

Adolescence influences reactions to physical illness and hospitalization in a manner that renders them different from those of other age groups.[20-23] Physical illness or injury during this developmental phase intensifies the conflicts, uncertainties, and anxieties that typically accompany it. Adolescents grapple with issues of independence, separation–individuation, identity, self-concept, sexuality, body image, and impulse control. Their awareness of their own body is heightened, and they tend to fear physical damage and disfigurement as well as disability and death. These factors not only make adolescents exceptionally sensitive and vulnerable to the effects of bodily illness or injury but also predispose them to deviant illness behavior. The latter typically manifests itself as noncompliance with medical advice, minimization (or even true denial) of illness, and regression. The regressed adolescent behaves in a petulant, dependent, and demanding manner and may become withdrawn, sullen, and negativistic. Some adolescents deny illness, rebel against medical management, and regard doctors and nurses as authoritarian parental figures. Adolescent patients may express anger, anxiety, and despondency in quick succession and in various combinations. They tend to be particularly intolerant of pain, imposed passivity and dependence, immobilization, restrictions on physical activity and diet, and disfigurement of any type. These patients tend to cope with those challenges in ways that often interfere with their chances for recovery. Establishment of separate medical wards for adolescents in the general hospitals is a sign of the growing recognition of their special problems and ways of coping. Adolescent reactions to malignancy and diabetes tend to be particularly challenging for the medical staff and the patient's family.[23,24]

Middle age is another major phase of the human life cycle likely to influence psychological responses to physical illness. To my knowledge, no systematic research on this subject has been carried out to date, but clinical experience suggests that illness or injury may trigger or intensify the so-called midlife crisis. A middle-aged person who had always enjoyed good health and taken it for granted may react with a pervasive sense of the finality of life and an urgent need to reappraise his or her personal values, goals, and relationships with significant other people. Even relatively mild illness or injury may precipitate such a response and either serve as a stimulus to inner growth and creativity or trigger a prolonged depressive, anxiety, or somatoform disorder.

Old age is typically accompanied by lowered resilience and coping capacity, and hence by heightened proneness to psychological disorganization as a consequence of physical illness. Positive association between such illness and functional psychiatric disorders in the elderly has been documented.[25] Anxiety and depressive disorders are the most common psychopathological correlates of physical illness in the aged. The occurrence of one of these functional psychiatric disorders influences adversely the prognosis of physical illness in the elderly person. Some degree of brain damage is often present in people aged 65 years and older and predisposes them to delirium in response to a wide range of organic factors. Moreover, cognitive impairment, chronic, acute, or both, may influence an elderly patient's appraisal of physical illness or injury and consequently influence his emotional reaction to it and coping with it. Pathological grief or depression, helplessness, and maladaptive coping are common.

Thus, the age at which illness or injury occurs helps to determine the patient's psychosocial reaction. Being aware of this fact may allow the physician to look out for and try to prevent specific age-related psychopathological complications of physical illness.

Sex is another biological variable that appears to influence psychosocial responses to disease. Women report symptoms of both physical and mental illness, and utilize doctor and hospital services, at higher rates than men.[26] Three major hypotheses have been put forth to account for these differences: (1) women report more illness than men because it is culturally more acceptable for them to do so; (2) the sick role is more compatible with women's than with men's other social role obligations; and (3) women experience more stress because of their social position and hence suffer from more illness. None of these hypotheses has yet been validated. It does appear, however, that women's illness behavior is determined by the number and character of their social role obligations. The married, but *not* the unhappily married, women report less illness than the single, the widowed, or the divorced. Housewives report more symptoms than employed women, and women with preschool children report fewer symptoms than housewives with older or no children.

The influence of sex on reactions to illness may reflect either *biological* or *social* factors, or both. Disease that interferes with sexual or reproductive function, or alters secondary sex characteristics, may put a strain on the person of either sex by threatening his sense of sexual identity. The degree to which such disease signifies a threat for the given individual, however, is likely to reflect the prevailing concepts of the male and female social roles. One must beware of plausible, "common-sense" judgments in this area, as they may be quite misleading. For example, it is often asserted that mastectomy and hysterectomy are often followed by emotional disturbances, yet recent studies show that such disturbances are relatively uncommon.[27,28] Some body parts, such as the hair or the nose, may be endowed, consciously or not, with symbolic sexual significance, and their loss or injury may trigger abnormal psychological responses. Impotence resulting from diabetes or spinal cord injury, for example, may have the same effect. Disfigurement is likely to have a greater emotional impact on a woman than a man, reflecting the high value attached to attractiveness as part of the feminine role. Men are more likely than women to react emotionally to any illness or injury resulting in threat to or loss of social status and economic security. Their self-esteem and gratification, reflecting their own perception of the masculine role, tend to be undermined by inability to work at the premorbid level of efficiency, and an emotional disturbance is likely to result.

One may expect that since the sex-related social roles and stereotypes are currently undergoing profound changes, the influence of these factors on emotional and behavioral responses to illness is also likely to change.

INTRAPERSONAL FACTORS—PSYCHOLOGICAL

Personality, in the sense of relatively stable and and enduring dispositions to act and react in certain ways, may be expected to influence psychosocial responses to physical illness or injury. In an earlier chapter I have discussed briefly personality dimensions such as field dependence–independence, augmenting–reducing, repression–sensitization, and sharpening–leveling, in their relation to illness (chapter 8, this volume). These personality dimensions, usually referred to as cognitive or perceptual styles, influence the way in which the person processes and evaluates information and thus codetermine his response to somatic symptoms. The intensity of the subjective discomfort and related emotional distress as well as the patient's illness behavior appear to be influenced by his cognitive–perceptual style.

The cognitive style of *field dependence* or *independence*, has been the subject of extensive research.[29] A field-dependent person is relatively unable to perceive parts of a field as discrete, since his perception is dominated by the organization of the field as a whole. Such a person tends to have a poorly differentiated and integrated body image and self-concept; to use predominantly undifferentiated defenses of repression and denial; to show inappropriately high or low arousal in situations demanding vigilance; and to keep perceptions and emotions apart. A field-dependent individual's cognitive functioning can be readily disorganized by deprivation of sleep or sensory inputs, by sensory overload, and by deliriogenic drugs.[30-32] By contrast, the field-independent person tends to differentiate clearly parts of the perceptual field; to have a relatively well-differentiated and integrated image of his body and self; to use more adaptive psychological defenses such as intellectualization and isolation of affect; and to keep his thoughts and perceptions relatively separate from emotions.

Both field-dependent and field-dependent individuals tend to react to physical illness or injury in different ways. The former are more likely than the latter to minimize the significance of their illness and its symptoms, and either to avoid adopting the sick role or to embrace it too eagerly and to display excessive dependence.[33] Such dependence is typically manifested by displays of helplessness and by verbal appeals to be taken care of. Such patients often become overly attached to doctors, nurses, and hospitals.

Repression–sensitization is another proposed personality dimension reported to influence illness behavior.[34,35] This dimension is assessed by a 127-item scale derived from the Minnesota Multiphasic Personality Inventory and purports to measure a subject's psychological defensive style. The scale includes a continuum of psychological defenses ranging from anxiety–avoidant behavior (repression and denial) to anxiety–approach behavior (obsessive brooding and worrying). Studies have indicated that sensitizers have a lower tolerance for pain, report greater discomfort, complain more about their symptoms, and seek medical help more readily than repressors. The latter are more likely to receive a purely organic medical diagnosis than the sensitizers, whereas the former are likely to be given a psychological diagnosis.[35]

A related personality variable is that of *perceptual reactance*.[36,37] Its proponents assume that everybody has a tendency to habitually either augment or reduce what he perceives. Perceptual reactance represents a continuum, at one extreme of which one finds the augmenters, at the other the reducers. The former tend to experience pain and other somatic symptoms more keenly and to complain of them more readily than the latter. By contrast, the reducers habitually minimize the significance of their perceived bodily changes and consequently delay seeking medical care. Recent work suggests that perceptual reactance may have clinically and theoretically important physiological correlates. Johansson et al.[38] have observed that both healthy subjects and patients characterized by an augmenter response in the visual evoked potentials had relatively low endorphin levels in the cerebrospinal fluid (CSF). As such low endorphin levels have been shown to be associated with a low pain threshold, an association is hypothesized between the tendency to augment responses, on the one hand, and a low pain threshold and low CSF endorphin levels, on the other.

The personality characteristics discussed so far involve mostly perception. A more global approach to the study of personality in relation to physical illness has been proposed by Bibring and Kahana.[39,40] Their approach, based on psychodynamic conceptions and clinical observations, has not been as systematically investigated as the cognitive–perceptual style. Despite this obvious disadvantage, the psychodynamic approach has heuristic and clinical value. Bibring and Kahana have delineated seven *personality types* and their corresponding psychopathological variants (given in parentheses):

1. The dependent, overdemanding (oral)
2. The orderly, controlled (compulsive)
3. The dramatizing, emotionally involved, captivating (hysterical)
4. The long-suffering, self-sacrificing (masochistic)
5. The guarded, querulous (paranoid)
6. The superior-feeling, condescending (narcissistic)
7. The uninvolved, aloof (schizoid)

Each of these personality types is postulated to react to physical illness in a characteristic and predictable manner. For example, the orderly, controlled person is likely to view illness as a threat of loss of control over impulses. His personality type is believed to represent an attempt at overcompensation for childhood wishes to be disorderly, dirty, impulsively aggressive, and self-indulgent. The orderly, controlled personality evolves rigidly opposite character traits as an enduring strategy to keep disavowed impulses in check. Illness imposes a strain on these characterological defenses. It usually enforces a degree of dependence and thus encourages regression to childhood modes of dealing with the social environment. It may interfere with the patient's control over body functions, such as elimination, or impair his ability to sustain a self-disciplined and orderly behavior and life-style. Faced with the threat of the reemergence of the disavowed impulses and loss of control over their expression, the orderly, controlled patient begins to manifest predictable coping behavior. He redoubles efforts to maintain control by resorting to familiar strategies: intellectual mastery over the situation, increased orderliness and obstinacy, and obsessive doubting and indecision. Such a patient strives to know and understand as much as possible about the nature, cause, treatment, and prognosis of the illness and may either strive to be a good and compliant patient or, on the contrary, display rigidly obstinate and noncompliant behavior. An orderly or compulsive patient tends to search eagerly for information about all aspects of his illness and responds best to a doctor willing to provide it and to let the patient participate actively in decisions on treatment.

As these examples illustrate, this typology is not merely descriptive but is also based on psychoanalytic hypotheses about the development and early antecedents of personality. Regardless of whether one accepts such explanatory hypotheses or not, however, it offers clinically useful clues for the assessment and management of patients, provided that clinicians use it with due regard to the complexity and uniqueness of the individual. As Kahana and Bibring[40] rightly warn, in clinical work one must avoid an overly rigid application of a diagnostic classification as a substitute for observation of a patient's distinct characteristics.

Past experience with illness, both one's own and that of personally significant other people, tends to influence the subjective meaning of the current illness or injury. For example, someone who as a child experienced an illness that resulted in hospitalization and frightening separation from the mother is likely to view, consciously or not, any serious illness in adulthood as a threat of another painful separation and hence react to it with more intense anxiety than the objective facts of the current situation warrant. One's childhood experiences with illness, doctors, and hospitals leave enduring and often unconscious memories, which exert a powerful influence on one's responses as an adult. A child may learn to regard being ill as a prelude to parental disapproval, as a weakness to be ashamed of or feel guilty about, or, on the contrary, as a welcome opportunity to gain attention, affection, and loving care. Knowledge of the patient's subjective medical history may give the doctor some insight into an adult patient's idiosyncratic reaction to an illness.

Experience with illness in a significant other, such as a parent, may also be a influential factor. For example, witnessing a parent's epileptic seizure or heart attack may leave the child with an enduring notion that illness signifies frightening loss of control or intense pain. One's own, or a significant other person's, illness and symptoms may provide a model for conversion symptoms, as when the wife of a heart attack victim complains of chest pain imitating that of her husband's, or an epileptic patient develops pseudoseizures.

Intrapsychic conflict implies the presence of opposed action tendencies within the person. It may be conscious or not and is likely to exert a marked effect on the person's attitudes, emotions, and behavior. Such influence is likely to be most marked when the conflict is unconscious and involves disavowed impulses, on the one hand, and the opposing force of conscience and judgment, on the other. Any factor or situation that intensifies a person's specific inner conflict either by increasing the strength of the prohibited impulses or by weakening the established defenses against them is likely to be perceived as threatening and to evoke distressing emotions of anxiety, guilt, or shame. Illness provides a common type of situation likely to intensify any type of unresolved intrapsychic conflicts that the patient may harbor. Such conflicts usually revolve in our culture around impulses to violate social or personal prohibitions against the manifest expression of hostile, sexual, or dependent strivings. The more a patient's illness or injury intensifies his particular core intrapsychic conflicts, the more likely it is to acquire the meaning of a threat, to elicit excessive anxiety, and to lead to irrational illness behavior. For example, a person whose core conflict involves hostile impulses against others, and who had successfully kept such impulses at bay by routinely engaging in vigorous physical activity, may develop a crippling illness such as rheumatoid arthritis or paraplegia. His effective defensive strategy has now become curtailed or abolished, while at the same time the impulses may have become intensified in response to frustrations and hence anger engendered by the illness. Consequently, the intrapsychic balance is disturbed, conflict is intensified, illness acquires the meaning of an ominous threat, anxiety is triggered, and the patient faces a psychological crisis. A physician who appreciates the patient's predicament may be able to help him cope with it adaptively rather than by resorting to some form of irrational behavior or by developing a psychiatric disorder.

Finally, the predominant *emotional state or mood* of the patient at the time of onset of illness appears to be an important factor. When illness occurs in a setting of depressed mood or intense anxiety, the patient is likely to regard the illness as an added burden and to respond to it with a depressive or anxiety disorder.

SOCIOCULTURAL AND ECONOMIC FACTORS

A patient's reaction to an illness reflects not only his individual personality, experience, and current emotional state but also his family relationships, availability and quality of medical care, culture, and economic status. All these variables influence what meaning a particular illness will have for the patient and how effectively he will be able to cope with it.

Much attention has been paid in recent years to the postulated beneficial effects on health of *social support*.[41-43] This concept is still rather vague and its defining criteria have not yet been clearly formulated. Social support, in this context, refers to the availability of caring and emotionally supportive others. Some writers have hypothesized that such support provides a protective buffer against the deleterious effects of psychosocial stress on health.[42] On the contrary, loss of a close and emotionally supportive relationship with another person constitutes one of the most stressful life events. Recent loss of a personally highly valued relationship has been postulated to increase the risk of becoming ill.[44] Thus, an illness is more likely to occur after loss and hence in a setting of relative or complete lack of social support. Such lack, in turn, may predispose the patient to view his illness as an additional serious loss or threat of loss, and to respond to it with feelings of depression, anxiety, helplessness, or hopelessness. These emotions may make it more difficult for the patient to cope effectively with the challenge of a serious illness.

Not only recent loss of a close relationship can signify lack of social support. Its quality is no less important than its quantity. Marital discord, for example, can have the same effect. Medalie and Goldbourt[45] studied the development of angina pectoris in 10,000 Israeli men, aged 40 years and over, and followed them up intensively for 5 years. The investigators concluded that severe psychosocial problems, especially those involving the family, constitute an independent risk factor for the development of angina. On the contrary, the wife's love and support are factors that reduce the probability of the onset of angina, even when high levels of organic risk factors are present. It appears that family, and especially marital, discord may have a dual effect of increasing the probability that an illness will develop and of depriving the patient of social support needed for optimal coping with it.

The importance of the patient's *family responses* to his illness needs emphasis. The manner in which the spouse (or, in the case of a child, the parents) responds to the patient's communication of symptoms, as well as to his disability or disfigurement, may affect the patient's mood and behavior. It may spell the difference between adaptive coping with the illness on the one hand and the development of a psychiatric disorder or deviant illness behavior on the other.

Social support and family's response to the patient's illness are by no means the only social factors influencing his reaction to it. *Beliefs* and *attitudes* regarding health and various diseases that a person holds and shares with other members of his ethnic and socioeconomic group are also important. Research in this area has been carried out largely by medical sociologists, and the reader is referred to their works.[46,47]

Most people hold views about the likely causes and effects, prognosis, and social and economic consequences of the common diseases. Such beliefs range from the scientifically sound ones to the irrational and even delusional.[48] Medically sound or not, these beliefs influence the way in which the patient appraises the personal significance of a given illness, reacts to it emotionally, and acts. Patients display a general tendency to blame themselves or other persons, or nonhuman agents, for having caused the disease with which they are afflicted.[49] Many are found to believe that they have fallen victim to a given illness as either a result of excessive self-indulgence or of neglect of socially sanctioned precepts for a healthy and good life. Such beliefs may cause the patient to feel guilty, view his illness as punishment, and deal with it in a maladaptive manner. If the patient blames others, say the spouse, for having contributed to the development of the illness, the result is likely to be anger or resentment and accusations, which may sour the relationship with the accused person and possibly deprive the patient of a key social support. Croog and Levine[59] have found that one of five married men who had suffered a heart attack blamed marital problems for having contributed to it. In about 30% of all the married couples studied by those investigators, either the husband or the wife, or both, blamed their marital relationship for having caused the heart attack. Such beliefs about etiology may generate tensions in the marriage and interfere wiht adaptive coping. Some people believe that cancer is contagious and may fear to contract it or pass it on to others, as the case may be.

Certain diseases are *stigmatized* and to develop one of them may profoundly affect the patient's reaction to it because of this fact.[51-53] Sontag[52] has analyzed the stigmatized meaning assigned to tuberculosis and cancer in the Western societies. She points out that a disease that is dreaded and whose etiology is unclear is likely to be viewed as morally, if not literally, contagious. She argues that such a disease tends to become a metaphor for feared things such as decay, pollution, anomie, and weakness. Many cancer patients are being shunned by relatives and friends and are "the objects of practices of decontamination by members of their household, as if cancer, like TB, were an infectious disease."[52, p. 6]

Veneral diseases, epilepsy, tuberculosis, leprosy, and cancer are familiar examples of stigmatized illnesses. All of them are feared, and some of them carry a pejorative moral connotation or provoke aversion because of their repulsive outward main-festations.[53] To suffer from a stigmatized illness is to experience the added burden of avoidance by others, or their disapproval, or both. The sufferer is likely to respond to such opprobrium with feelings of shame and guilt, with loss of self-esteem, and with a sense of alienation and loneliness. He will tend to evolve strategies designed to conceal the disease so as to avoid the distress of being feared, shunned, or despised.[51,53]

Attitudes prevalent in the patient's social milieu toward the sick, disabled, and disfigured have an impact on his illness behavior. For example, the decision to seek medical help in response to symptoms is, in part, dependent on such attitudes.[46,47] Other relevant factors include the patient's actual symptoms as well as his knowledge and beliefs about diseases, attitudes toward and expectations from doctors and hospitals, and conceptions of what constitutes health and sickness.[1] All these variables are influenced by the patient's level of education and by his ethnic group and socioeconomic class. The patient's decision-making process has a bearing on timely seeking of medical consultation. Two undesirable patterns of this aspect of illness behavior have been identified: *excessive delay* in and *overhasty recourse* to seeking medical help.[46,47]

The manner in which a person evaluates his symptoms and acts, or fails to act, on them is partly determined by sociocultural and economic factors. Members of higher socioeconomic classes are more likely than lower-class members to see themselves as ill when they experience somatic symptoms. Lower socioeconomic status is one of the factors influencing excessive delay in seeking medical help for serious conditions such as cancer or heart disease.[1] Members of the lower socioeconomic classes tend to be wary of doctors and hospitals, to interpret symptoms as not indicative of disease, and to trust their own notions about health and sickness.[54] The poor from city slums and rural areas often hold beliefs about health and illness that are at variance with those held by members of the higher socioeconomic groups, including doctors. Such beliefs, coupled with the high cost of medical care, contribute to the medically deprived position of the poor.[54] Knowledge of scientific medicine varies considerably from one socioeconomic class to another and is generally lowest among the poor. Irrational health beliefs, attitudes, and practices are not confined to the members of the lower classes, however, and they are seen also among the affluent and well educated, some of whom have low opinions of health professionals and medical care and consequently tend to avoid them and to resort to folk medicine or self-medication.

The *high cost* of health care and illness influences the meaning of the latter for many patients, even those whose income is well above the poverty level. Delays in seeking medical advice and adopting the sick role as well as noncompliance with prescribed treatment are among the consequences of the common view that serious or prolonged illness amounts to a personal economic castastrophe.

Finally, major social or interactional factor of especial importance for the patient's psychosocial reactions to illness is his *relationship with the doctor* and other care-giving professionals, which I have discussed in Chapter 8. An equally important factor is the patient's experience of hospitalization.[1,55-58] Admission to a medical or surgical ward, or a specialized clinical unit, means exposure to a specific social milieu, one that includes physicians, nurses, and other personnel as well as other patients. It is a hierar-chically structured social setting, in which the dominant role is usually played by physicians, and which functions according to explicit and implicit rules of conduct, role definitions, and value system. As a patient one becomes a member of this social group and is expected to act *as a patient*. Members of the clinical team decide what is wrong with the patient, what investigations and therapy are required, and what kinds of behavior are acceptable. Accustomed to a measure of freedom, independence and privacy, the individual is expected, as a matter of course, to accept curtailment of these rights while he is hospitalized. He brings to this situation habitual attitudes toward and modes of coping with novelty, dependence, restrictions on freedom of choice and action, passive submission, and authority figures. Although most patients manage to adjust to this setting successfully, many find it distressing, and some cannot tolerate it without some form of protest.[55,56] Such protest may be expressed in a manner that the medical staff is likely to perceive as offensive and unacceptable. Those patients who express their protest, anger, or anxiety in the form of critical remarks or complaints about their care and caregivers, refuse to comply with ward routine or therapy, or demand better care are all likely to be viewed by the ward staff as "problem patients." Conflicts between such patients and staff readily arise, communication breaks down, and display of hostility by both sides may follow. The patient may sign out against medical advice, but even if he stays in the hospital, the situation is hardly conducive to his adaptive coping with illness and to optimal care.

Interactions between a patient and other members of the social group composing the ward community tend to affect his perception of illness and coping with it. Behavior of the doctors and nurses may have a therapeutic or countertherapeutic effect. The behavior and attitude of some physicians and nurses tend to elicit overly dependent, hostile, anxious, or sexually seductive responses in their patients more often than chance. The conduct of ward rounds may have an undesirable impact on some patients if it features uninhibited discussions of the patients' conditions within their earshot.[59] Appreciation of these various aspects of the hospitalization experience has led to attempts to create a *therapeutic social milieu* on medical and surgical wards.[58] Furthermore, a hospital provides not only a social but also a physical environment for the sick. The importance of that environment will be discussed in a later section.

DISEASE-RELATED FACTORS

The nature and characteristics of the disease or injury contribute yet another set of variables influencing the patient's psychosocial reactions. Factors such as the *site and extent of the lesion*; the *rate of onset* and the *progression* as well as the *duration* of somatic pathology; the kind and intensity of *symptoms and physiological dysfunction*; the severity of disability; and the *visibility* of pathological changes—all influence the patient's reaction.[1,58-76] These factors are personally important for the patient and hence tend to affect his or her perceptions, thoughts, emotions, communications, and behavior.

A given body organ or physiological function may have very different subjective significance and value for different individuals, one related to their unique life experience, body image, and chief defensive and coping styles.[1] Such personal significance and value, both conscious and unconscious, may have little to do with the issue of survival. For instance, loss of hair or a facial scar may be highly emotionally distressing for a given patient even though his life is not threatened. One may propose the following generalization: *The greater the subjective value of the body part or function affected by disease or injury is for the patient, the more intense and idiosyncratic is his or her emotional and behavioral reaciton likely to be.*

A given body part, organ, or function is likely to have special personal significance for its possessor when it plays one or more of the following roles[1]:

1. Constitutes a source of pleasure, high self-esteem, or economic security.
2. Helps maintain satisfying interpersonal relationships.
3. Enables effective coping with environment.
4. Prevents distressing emotions engendered by unresolved unconscious conflicts by bolstering defenses against them.
5. Enhances sense of personal identity and autonomy.
6. Has unconscious symbolic meaning that endows it with high personal value.
7. Helps preserve integrity of body image.

A few common clinical examples follow. Some persons set a high value on their physical prowess and activity as a source of pride and pleasure or as a means of discharging accumulated aggressive energy that might be directed against other people and thus intensify inner conflict over hostile impulses. A person who values and relies on regular physical activity, such as jogging, for such reasons is likely to respond with anxiety or sense of loss and grief, or even depression, to any illness or injury that precludes or seriously interferes with physical activity for a prolonged time. Depression is particularly likely to follow severe injury to a hand or the face.[60,61] The face is a highly visible part of the body and hence a particularly important component of one's body image having special implications for the person's social interactions. People for whom the face has a high personal value are likely to display an intense and often maladaptive psychosocial reaction when the face is injured or disfigured.[60] The hand is usually less significant than the face as a body part enhancing a person's attractiveness, but is likely to be highly valued for its role in ensuring enconomic security and as a source of pride and pleasure from its skillful and creative use. Adequate intellectual and perceptual functioning is highly valued in modern industrial societies. Impairment of these attributes by primary or secondary disease of the brain or of the special senses, whether reversible or not, is likely to be deeply threatening to individuals in our culture, especially to those with an obsessive-compulsive personality style, for whom intellectual activity and perceptual clarity are necessary not only as a source of security and self-esteem, but also as safeguards of control over repudiated impulses. A person with this personality style is also likely to react with intense psychological distress to the construction of a colostomy or to fecal or urinary incontinence, that is, to conditions interfering with his emphasis on cleanliness, and absence of bad body odor.[62] For many male patients colostomy signifies having become fragile and feminized.[63] Such a meaning of illness and its consequences may result in the patient's loss of self-esteem.

Population surveys provide factual information on the value that members of our society tend to attach to various body parts and organs. For example, 1000 men and women have been asked to rank 12 bodily parts according to degree to which they would be missed if removed or lost.[64] Men have ranked the penis, the testicles, and the tongue highest. Women up to the age of 70 have ranked the tongue first. In another study, the leg, the eye, and the arm were ranked as the most important.[64] It is a common belief that since the uterus and the breast are highly valued body parts for most women, the loss of either of them is likely to result in depression in a high proportion of patients. Recent studies, however, have shown that those beliefs are questionable and the mastectomy or hysterectomy is followed by depression much less frequently than is often believed.[27,28] Such studies are useful as they allow a measure of prediction of psychological response in specific clinical situations, yet they cannot replace direct inquiry into the value and importance of the lost, injured, malfunctioning, or disfigured body part for the individual patient. One may propose a second generalization: *A disease or injury that jeopardizes or destroys a body function or attribute that is highly valued by the patient is likely to evoke intense emotional responses and maladaptive coping.*[1]

The *temporal* characteristics of disease also tend to influence the patient's reaction to it. The rate of onset and the duration of the disease comprise its main temporal dimensions. A closely related feature of the disease process is its degree of *reversibility*. The view of disease as a process having a time dimension is reflected in terms such as *acute* and *chronic*. These terms, traditionally used in medicine, are ambiguous. There is no clearly defined boundary between acute and chronic illness. Within many diagnostic categories there are patients who are more disabled than ill, more acutely than chronically ill, and so forth.[65] The term "chronic illness," as commonly used, implies some degree of permanent disability. In many cases it is more appropriate to speak of acute or chronic *stage or phase* of illness rather than distinguish acute from chronic disease.[66]

The *acute* illness stage or phase implies relatively sudden onset of symptoms or injury intense enough to compel the patient to pay attention to it. Furthermore, by definition, the acute phase is time-limited, that is, the intense symptoms last a relatively short time, to be followed by full recovery, or by some degree of protracted or permanent ("chronic") illness or disability, or by recurrent acute episodes. A mild, commonplace acute illness, such as the common cold, is not likely to arouse an intense psychological reaction. If, however, the illness or injury is severe, painful, and incapacitating, it drastically interrupts a person's routine and readily evokes fears of disability, dependence on others, loss, and death.[1,59,70,71] Its personal meaning is liable to be that of threat, which triggers emotions of anxiety, or dread, or anticipatory grief. The patient is likely to respond with shock, disbelief, and sometimes futile attempts to escape into health.[67,68] The more the symptoms of an acute illness are unfamiliar, painful, or disabling, the more threatened and anxious is the patient likely to feel.[67] Sudden vertigo, dyspnea, paralysis, chest pain, or blindness, for example, usually arouses more or less intense fear and is particularly likely to motivate the sufferer to seek medical care. Some patients, however, tend to employ minimization or denial as a way of coping with an overwhelming threat and delay seeking help for symptoms of myocardial infaction, for example.[69] Other emergency coping strategies in response to acute and severe symptoms and illness include withdrawal, passive surrender, and regression.[70,71] Anxiety or fear aroused by the symptoms is usually accompanied by physiological concomitants, such as hyperventilation or tachycardia, which tend to aggravate the patient's physical condition and intensify the fear. A key aspect of an acute, severe illness is that the patient is as a rule unprepared for it, and hence the surprise, novelty, threat, dread, and psychophysiological arousal. Some patients respond initially to such a personal crisis with denial of its significance and with immobility.

Severe acute illness is usually followed by the *convalescent* or *rehabilitation* stage. Recovery from illness is expected to lead to the giving up of the sick role by the patient. This applies to all acute and fully reversible pathology as well as to those illnesses which leave little or no physical disability. The patient is expected to gradually surrender the sick role and return to his premorbid social roles. He is also expected to cooperate with rehabilitation whenever it is required. Psychosocial factors may interfere with these expected responses and lead to protracted disability or psychological invalidism. For example, a substantial proportion of survivors of a myocardial infarction fail to return to work despite a satisfactory recovery.[69]

The *chronic illness* stage implies a protracted course and, usually, the presence of some degree of irreversible pathology and of residual disability. Chronic illnesses, cardiovascular, neoplastic, degenerative, and respiratory, are the leading causes of morbidity in industrial societies. A chronic illness may follow an acute phase or develop insidiously and be punctuated by acute episodes. These temporal characteristics are important from the point of view of the patient's psychosocial reactions. For example, if an acute illness is followed by progressive, if incomplete, restitution to previous health, the patient is more likely to cope adaptively. If a stable disability occurs, the patient has time to adjust to it and develop adaptive coping strategies, such as satisfactory activities to replace those no longer feasible. On the other hand, a chronic disease or disability that is likely to worsen suddenly and unpredictably, such as multiple sclerosis or ulcerative colitis, adds an element of distressing *uncertainty* about the future.[72] Such uncertainty tends to impose a severe strain on the patient's emotional balance and coping resources. Many patients find it more difficult to cope with uncertainty than even with a severe but finite loss of function or body part. Similarly, inexorable *progression* of a disease process and disability tends to undermine the patient's hope and ability to cope.

Patterns of psychological adjustment to chronic illness and disability have been studied and described by many authors.[8,59,65,73-76] Chodoff[73,74] has described three such major response patterns: *insightful acceptance*, the *denial pattern*, and the *regressive pattern*. Insightful acceptance is characterized by relative lack of bitterness and hostility and of a sense of personal devaluation and defeat. The patient copes adaptively, cooperates with rehabilitation plans, tries to learn substitute skills, and looks for new sources of gratification. The denial pattern features minimization of the objective facts of illness and their personal significance as well as of one's emotional responses such as anxiety, depression, or anger. Such minimization varies in degree and may be explicitly expressed or only implied. It is not necessarily pathological or maladaptive, unless it concerns obvious facts and interferes with the patient's ability to cooperate with appropriate treatment or rehabilitation. The regressive pattern is characterized by marked dependence and passivity, which may be accompanied by overt or covert anger and hostility. Patients exhibiting this pattern tend to exaggerate their helplessness and disability and to demand exceptional attention and care from others. Some of these patients use chronic illness to manipulate family and health professionals by playing on their sympathy or feelings of guilt. This pattern is often displayed by patients with a histrionic personality and those who, although healthy, tend to overemphasize their independence and physical prowess.

The *terminal* phase of any illness signifies impending death. A sense of inescapable finality and closure replaces reasonable hope about the future.[1] It is the last stage of man's life cycle, one likely to evoke intense psychological responses in the patient who is sufficiently clear mentally to appreciate his predicament. Weisman and Kastenbaum[77] have described four general attitudes of patients facing impending death: *acceptance, apathy, apprehension,* and *anticipation* (i.e., acceptance accompanied by a conscious wish to die).

Thus, spatiotemporal, perceptual, and other features of a given illness or injury constitute a set of determinants of the patient's cognitive, emotional, and coping responses.

PHYSICAL ENVIRONMENTAL FACTORS

The influence of the physical environment in which the sick person lives on his reaction to illness is a seriously neglected subject. The only exception to this statement is provided by the relatively extensive literature concerned with the impact of the sensory environment in coronary and other intensive care units on patients' psychological well-being.[78,79] The features of the sensory environment can exert positive or negative effects on the patient's mood and cognitive functioning. Modern medicine has, on the whole, neglected this dimension of patient care. Sensory and aesthetic qualities of a typical hospital often leave much to be desired from the patient's point of view. A famous novelist–patient expressed it well: "The x-ray room was white-enameled, the corridor was white-enameled, my room is white-enameled. The flowers sent by my friends look out of place in this world devoid of wood or fabric, as alien as a planet on which only white paint, nickel, test tubes, glass objects, sheets—and invalids—could survive." [80, p. 59] Many hospitals provide an environment in which sensory monotony is broken unpredictably by noise or unpleasant odors, that is, by sensory inputs that for at least some patients are frightening or even cognitively disorganizing.

Some writers have proposed that sensory or perceptual deprivation and sensory overload contribute to the delirium manifested by a proportion of patients treated in coronary and surgical intensive care units.[78,79] The evidence for the deliriogenic effects of these clinical settings is inconclusive, however, but it does appear that sensory deprivation and overload could facilitate the onset of or intensify delirium in some patients, especially the elderly and the brain-damaged.[79]

An interesting recent study highlights the aversive characteristics of at least some coronary care units. The investigators had 17 healthy nurses spend one and a half hours in a coronary care unit under conditions imitating as closely as possible those to which patients were usually exposed.[81] The nurses reported experiencing distortion of time sense, in that time seemed to pass slowly and they had to make repeated efforts to maintain temporal orientation. They also experienced increasing restlessness, physical discomfort, loneliness, isolation, increased sensitivity to noise, and a sense of loss of control over self and environment. They were particularly disturbed by what the investigators regard as sensory overload in the form of auditory stimuli such as telephones ringing, monitor alarms, toilets flushing, conversations, intercom messages, noises from infusor pumps and suction equipment, and patients retching. The nurses felt assailed by a virtual cacophony which they found difficult to tolerate for what was only a fraction of the time that coronary care patients spend exposed to it. The importance of the physical environment on patients' psychological well-being is undeniable, and there is need for more research on this subject.

SUMMARY AND CONCLUSIONS

I have discussed the putative determinants of the ubiquitous psychosocial reactions to physical illness, injury, and disability. I have proposed that such reactions are codetermined by four broad classes of contributory factors and hence may be regarded as being of multifactorial origin. Rather than try to review in detail the theoretical and research literature on this subject, a task that would require a sizable book to do justice to, I have presented a conceptual schema for the integration of relevant theoretical concepts and empirical data. Interest in this whole area at the interface of medicine and behavioral sciences is of relatively recent origin. Indeed, the subject of psychosocial (or "somatopsychic" in the terminology of some writers) reactions to illness was severely neglected by researchers until 20 years ago or so. Psychosomatic investigators had been mostly interested in the postulated *etiological* role of the psychosocial factors in somatic diseases and tended to ignore the somatopsychic aspects. Rapid growth of liaison psychiatry, medical sociology, behavioral medicine, and health psychology in the past two decades has helped to focus attention on how the sick react to their illness psychologically, cope with it, and interact with their healthy family members and with the health professionals.

Adjustment to chronic physical illness and disability as well as response to acute physical illness or trauma has recently attracted a growing number of investigators from several disciplines. This multidiciplinary effort and the rapidly accumulating volume of published work have created problems for anyone trying to integrate current knowledge and thinking in this complex area. A schema such as that proposed in this paper will hopefully foster interdisciplinary communication and stimulate more research and efforts at conceptual integration. Meanwhile, it may serve as an introduction to this field for interested students and clinicians, and as a basis for psychosocial evaluation of patients.

I have avoided trying to draw a distinction between "normal" and pathological psychosocial reactions. The schema presented here may be readily applied to both of them, in that it comprises factors inherent in the host (patient), his disease, and his social and physical environment. In another chapter, I will focus on certain psychosocial and psychobiological variables that increase the probability that a patient will react to illness in a manner judged to be pathological and develop one of the currently recognized psychiatric disorders (chapter 11, this volume).

REFERENCES

1. Lipowski ZJ: Physical illness, the patient and his environment: Psychosocial foundations of medicine, in Reiser MF (ed): *American Handbook of Psychiatry*, ed 2, Arieti S (ed-in-chief). New York, Basic Books, 1975, vol 4, pp. 3–42.
2. Anthony EY, Koupernik C (eds): *The Child and His Family: The Impact of Disease and Death*. New York, Wiley, 1973.
3. Campbell JD: The child in the sick role: Contributions of age, sex, parental status, and parental values. *J Health Soc Behav* 19:35–51, 1978.
4. Geist RA: Onset of chronic illness in children and adolescents: psychotherapeutic and consultative intervention. *Am J Orthopsychiatry* 49:4–23, 1979.
5. Langford WS: The child in the pediatric hospital: Adaptation to illness and hospitalization. *Am J Orthopsychiatry* 31:667–684, 1961.
6. Mattson A: Long-term physical illness in childhood: A challenge to psychosocial adaptation. *Pediatrics* 50:801–811, 1972.
7. Pless IB, Roghman KJ: Chronic illness and its consequences: Observations based on three epidemiologic studies. *J Pediatr* 79:351–359, 1971.
8. Travis C: *Chronic Illness in Children: Its Impact on Child and Family*. Stanford, Calif., Stanford University Press, 1976.
9. Sigal JJ, Chagoya L, Villeneuve C, Meyerovitch J: Later psychological consequences of near-fatal illness (nephrosis) in early childhood: Some preliminary findings. *Laval Med* 42:103–108, 1971.
10. Sigal JJ, Chagoya L, Villeneuve C, Mayerovitch J: Later psychological sequelae of early childhood illness (severe croup). *Am J Psychiatry* 130:786–789, 1973.
11. Mattson A, Weisberg I: Behavioral reactions to minor illness in preschool children. *Pediatrics* 46:604–610, 1970.
12. Prugh DG, Staub EM, Sands HH, Kirschbaum RM, Lenihan EA: A study of the emotional reactions of children and families to hospitalization and illness. *Am J Orthopsychiatry* 23:70–106, 1953.
13. Bibace R, Walsh ME: Development of children's concepts of illness. *Pediatrics* 66:912–917, 1980.
14. Binger CM, Ablin AR, Feuerstein RC, et al: Childhood leukemia: Emotional impact on patient and family. *N Engl J Med* 280:414–418, 1969.
15. Brewster AB: Chronically ill hospitalized children's concepts of their illness. *Pediatrics* 69:355–362, 1982.
16. Childers P, Wimmer M: The concept of death in early childhood. *Child Dev* 42:1299–1301, 1971.
17. Gartley W, Bernasconi M: The concept of death in children. *J Genet Psychol* 110:71–85, 1967.
18. Natapoff JN: Children's views of health: a developmental study. *Am J Public Health* 68:995–1000, 1978.
19. Spinetta JJ: The dying child's awareness of death: A review. *Psychol Bull* 81:256–260, 1974.
20. Mechanic D: Adolescent health and illness behavior: Review of the literature and a new hypothesis. *J Hum Stress* 9:4–13, 1983.
21. Schowalter JE: Psychological reactions to physical illness and hospitalization in adolescence. *J Am Acad Child Psychiatry* 16:500–516, 1977.
22. Zeltzer L, Kellerman J, Ellenberg L, Dash J, Rigler D: Psychological effects of illness in adolescence. II. Impact of illness in adolescents—crucial issues and coping styles. *J Pediatr* 97:132–138, 1980.
23. Steinherz PG, Miller DR: The adolescent with cancer. *Adolescent Med Topics* 1:209–249, 1976.
24. Cerreto MC, Travis LB: Implications of psychological and family factors in the treatment of diabetes. *Pediatr Clin North Am* 31:689–710, 1984.
25. Kay DWK, Bergmann K: Physical disability and mental health in old age. *J Psychosom Res* 10:3–12, 1966.

26. Marcus AC, Seeman TE: Sex differences in reports of illness and disability: A preliminary test of the "fixed role obligations" hypothesis. *J Health Soc Behav* 22:174–182, 1981.

27. Meikle S, Brody H, Pysh F: An investigation into the psychological effects of hysterectomy. *J Nerv Ment Dis* 164:36–41, 1977.

28. Worden JW, Weisman AD: The fallacy in postmastectomy depression. *Am J Med Sci* 273:169–175, 1977.

29. Witkin HA, Dyk RB, Faterson HF, Goodenough DR, Karp SA: *Psychological Differentiation.* New York, Wiley, 1962.

30. Cartwright RD: Dream and drug-induced fantasy behavior. *Arch Gen Psychiatry* 15:7–15, 1966.

31. Cartwright RD, Monroe LJ: Individual differences in response to REM deprivation. *Arch Gen Psychiatry* 16:297–303, 1967.

32. Ludwig A: Sensory overload and psychopathology. *Dis Nerv Syst* 36:357–360, 1975.

33. Goldin GJ, Perry SL, Stotsky BA: *Dependency and Its Implications for Rehabilitation.* Lexington, Mass, DC Heath & Co., 1972.

34. Byrne D, Steinberg MA, Schwartz MS: Relationship between repression-sensitization and physical illness. *J Abnorm Psychol* 73:154–155, 1968.

35. Schwartz MS, Krupp NE: Repression-sensitization and medical diagnosis. *J Abnorm Psychol* 78:286–291, 1971.

36. Petrie A: *Individuality in Pain and Suffering,* ed 2. Chicago, University of Chicago Press, 1978.

37. Knorring L von, Monakhov K, Perris C: Augmenting-reducing: An adaptive switch mechanism to cope with incoming signals in healthy subjects and psychiatric patients. *Neuropsychobiology* 4:150–154, 1978.

38. Johansson F, Almay BGL, von Knorring L, Ternius L, Astrom M: Personality traits in chronic pain patients related to endorphin levels in cerebrospinal fluid. *Psychiatry Res* 1:231–239, 1979.

39. Bibring GL: Psychiatry and medical practice in a general hospital. *N Engl J Med* 254:366–372, 1956.

40. Kahana RJ, Bibring GL: Personality types in medical management, in Zinberg EN (ed): *Psychiatry and Medical Practice in a General Hospital.* New York, International Universities Press, 1964, pp 108–123.

41. Broadhead WE, Kaplan BH, James SA, et al: The epidemiologic evidence for a relationship between social support and health. *Am J Epidemiol* 117:521–537, 1983.

42. La Rocco JM, House JS, French JRP: Social support, occupational stress, and health. *J Health Soc Behav* 21:202–218, 1980.

43. Lin N, Simeone RS, Enselt WM, Luo W: Social support, stressful life events, illness: A model and an empirical test. *J Health Hum Behav* 20:108–119, 1979.

44. Lipowski ZJ (ed): *Psychosocial Aspects of Physical Illness.* Basel, Karger, 1972.

45. Medalie JH, Goldbourt U: Angina pectoris among 10,000 men. *Am J Med* 60:910–921, 1976.

46. Berkanovic E, Telesky C, Reeder S: Structural and social psychological factors in the decision to seek medical care for symptoms. *Med Care* 19:693–709, 1981.

47. Mechanic D: *Medical Sociology,* ed. 2. New York, Free Press, 1978.

48. Mabry JH: Lay concepts of etiology. *J Chron Dis* 17:371–386, 1964.

49. Bard M, Dyk RB: The psychodynamic significance of beliefs regarding the cause of serious illness. *Psychoanal Rev* 43:146–162, 1956.

50. Croog SH, Levine S: *The Heart Patient Recovers.* New York, Human Sciences Press, 1977.

51. Ablon J: Stigmatized health conditions. *Soc Sci Med* 15:5–9, 1981.

52. Sontag S: *Illness as Metaphor.* New York, Farrar, Straus & Giroux, 1977.

53. Gussow Z, Tracy GST: Stigma and the leprosy phenomenon. *Bull Hist Med* 44:425–449, 1970.

54. Suchman EA: Health attitudes and behavior. *Arch Environ Health* 20:105–110, 1970.

55. Volicer BJ, Isenberg MA, Burns MW: Medical-surgical differences in hospital stress factors. *J Hum Stress* 3:3–13, 1977.

56. Lipowski ZJ: Review of consultation psychiatry and psychosomatic medicine. 2. Clinical aspects. *Psychosom Med* 29:201–224, 1967.

57. Kaufman RM, Franzblau AN, Kairys D: The emotional impact of ward rounds. *J Mount Sinai Hosp* 23:782–803, 1956.

58. Janis IL, Leventhal H: Psychological aspects of physical illness and hospital care, in Wolman B (ed): *Handbook of Clinical Psychology.* New York, McGraw-Hill, 1965.

59. Westbrook MT, Viney LL: Psychological reaction to the onset of chronic illness. *Soc Sci Med* 16:899–906, 1982.
60. Chang FC, Herzog B: Burn morbidity: A follow-up study of physical and psychological disability. *Ann Surg* 183:34–37, 1976.
61. Cone J, Hueston JT: Psychological aspects of hand injury. *Med J Aust* 1:104–108, 1974.
62. Orbach CE, Bard M, Sutherland AM: Fear and defensive adaptations to the loss of anal sphincter control. *Psychoanal Rev* 44:121–175, 1957.
63. Orbach CE, Tallent N: Modification of perceived body and of body concepts. *Arch Gen Psychiatry* 12:126–132, 1965.
64. Lipowski ZJ: The importance of body experience for psychiatry. *Compr Psychiatry* 18:473–479, 1977.
65. Shontz FC: Severe chronic illness, in Garrett JF, Levine ES (eds): *Psychological Practices with the Physically Disabled.* New York, Columbia University Press, 1962.
66. Suchman EA: Stages of illness and medical care. *J Health Hum Behav* 6:114–128, 1965.
67. Hart LK, Reese JL, Fearing MO (eds): *Concepts Common to Acute Illness.* St. Louis, CV Mosby Co, 1981.
68. Peterson BH: Psychological reactions to acute physical illness in adults. *Med J Aust* 1:311–316, 1974.
69. Lipowski ZJ: Cardiovascular disorders, in Kaplan HI, Freedman AM, Sadock BJ (eds): *Comprehensive Textbook of Psychiatry,* 3 ed. Baltimore, Williams & Wilkins, 1980, pp 1891–1907.
70. Bracken MB, Shepard MJ: Coping and adaptation to acute spinal cord injury: A theoretical analysis. *Paraplegia* 18:74–85, 1980.
71. Visotsky HM, Hamburg DA, Goss MA, et al: Coping behavior under extreme stress. *Arch Gen Psychiatry* 5:423–448, 1961.
72. Mishel MH: The measurement of uncertainty in illness. *Nurs Res* 30:258–263, 1981.
73. Chodoff P: Adjustment to disability. Some observations on patients with multiple sclerosis. *J Chron Dis* 9:653–670, 1959.
74. Chodoff P: Understanding and management of the chronically ill patient. Part I. Who are the chronically ill? *Am Pract* 13:136–144, 1962.
75. Felton BJ, Revenson TA: Coping with chronic illness: A study of illness controllability and the influence of coping strategies. *J Consult Clin Psychol* 52:343–353, 1984.
76. Strauss AL: *Chronic Illness and the Quality of Life.* St. Louis, CV Mosby Co, 1975.
77. Weisman AD, Kastenbaum R: The psychological autopsy. *Commun Ment Health J,* Monograph 4, 1968.
78. Kornfeld DS: The hospital environment: Its impact on the patient. *Adv Psychosom Med* 8:252–270, 1972.
79. Lipowski ZJ: *Delirium: Acute Brain Failure in Man.* Springfield, Ill, Charles C Thomas, 1980, pp 135–144.
80. Malraux A: *Lazarus.* New York, Grove Press, 1978, pp 58–9.
81. Lindemuth JE, Breu CS, Malooley JA: Sensory overload. *Am J Nurs* 80:1456–1458, 1980.

Physical Illness and Psychopathology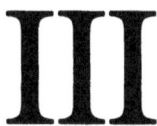

The chapters in this section deal with the association between physical, including cerebral, disease and psychopathology. Epidemiological and pathogenetic aspects of this relationship are reviewed. Six of the chapters deal specifically with psychiatric consequences of cerebral disease and dysfunction. They include a discussion of the *DSM-III* classification of organic mental disorders (organic brain syndromes), the psychopathology associated with brain disorders, and a detailed discussion of delirium and dementia—the two most important organic brain syndromes. Although these topics are not usually included in books on psychosomatic medicine, the author contends that they fall logically within its scope. Moreover, the diagnosis and treatment of the organic syndromes constitute a major portion of the work of liaison psychiatrists and of all health professionals concerned with the care of elderly patients. This practical consideration alone warrants the inclusion of this material.

III

Risk Factors and Psychopathology

Physical Illness and Psychiatric Disorder

Epidemiology

10

INTRODUCTION

During the past decade investigators have paid increasing attention to the association between physical illness and psychiatric disorders.[1] Several factors seem to have contributed to this welcome development. First, rapid development of consultation–liaison psychiatry has brought psychiatrists closer to the physically ill on a scale never known before. As a result, the types and frequency of psychiatric disorders in this patient population have come into focus and become a subject of a growing number of studies. Their aim has been to obtain data that could serve as a basis for estimating the extent of need for psychiatric services in the general hospitals and other medical health care facilities. Second, demographic trends in the Western countries and elsewhere have drawn attention to the growing number of the elderly, those aged 65 years and over, among whom the prevalence and incidence of both physical and psychiatric morbidity are high, and the two types of morbidity are frequently concurrent. In order to plan adequate health facilities for the elderly, it is important to establish how often psychiatric disorder complicates physical illness among them, which of these disorders are especially common, and what role the physical illness appears to play in their occurrence. Such information could lead to more effective prevention of psychiatric morbidity in the physically ill elderly patients. Third, the prevalence of chronic systemic diseases, cardiovascular, respiratory, neoplastic, musculoskeletal, and neurological, is high and may be expected to rise as the number of very old persons predictably increases in the coming decades. It is clearly important to have data about the frequency, types, and severity of psychiatric disorders in patients suffering from these diseases, as a basis for planning preventive and therapeutic measures. And fourth, medical progress has brought in its wake a host of psychiatric problems resulting from the side effects of new medical drugs and from such procedures as chronic renal hemodialyis, open-heart surgery, and intensive care. Psychiatric complications arising from these medical and surgical treatments increase the burden of illness for the patients and adversely affect their quality of life. To plan adequate psychiatric services as well as effective preventive and therapeutic measures it is necessary to collect data about the frequency and types of psychiatric disorders resulting from various forms of medical and surgical treatments.

Despite these cogent reasons to study the epidemiological and other aspects of psychiatric morbidity among the physically ill, and in spite of the recently increased research efforts in this direction, the body of accumulated data is still inadequate. Research has been hampered by methodological problems, to be discussed later, as well as ⊦ the lack of diagnostic criteria for the psychiatric disorders prior to the introduction of the new classification, the DSM-III, of mental disorders.[2] Moreover, few investigators have addressed the issue of the causal links between physical and psychiatric morbidity and of the related pathogenetic mechanisms.

In this chapter, I shall review some of the representative epidemiological studies of the association between physical and psychiatric ill health and discuss briefly the issues of classification and methodology. In a subsequent chapter I will focus on the pathogenetic mechanisms mediating between a physical illness or injury on the one hand and the ensuing psychiatric disorder on the other (chapter 11, this volume).

CLASSIFICATION

Psychiatric disorders judged to be causally related to physical illness may be divided into three major classes[1]:

1. Organic mental disorders (organic brain syndromes).
2. Reactive functional disorders.
3. Deviant illness behavior.

This classification implies some etiological assumptions that need to be made explicit. Traditionally, psychiatric disorders have been divided into those believed to be caused by demonstrable brain damage or dysfunction and those in which evidence of cerebral pathology is either lacking or is not considered to be causally related to the psychiatric disorder. The former class of disorders constitutes the organic mental disorders; the latter, the functional psychiatric disorders. This dichotomy has been preserved, albeit in a much attenuated form, in the currently official classification of mental disorders, or DSM-III,[2] adopted by the American Psychiatric Association in 1980, which continues to distinguish the organic from the functional mental disorders. In contrast to the previous two American classifications, however, DSM-III has markedly liberalized the concept of organic brain syndromes by including among them the personality, affective, and delusional syndromes whose descriptive features may be indistinguishable from those of the corresponding functional disorders, but which nevertheless are judged to be caused by cerebral damage or dysfunction. In the past the organic brain syndromes used to be defined entirely in terms of cognitive deficits or abnormalities, but this stricture no longer obtains.

The organic–functional dichotomy has certain practical advantages, provided that it is not viewed too rigidly. It provides a general direction for therapy, in that if the psychiatric disorder in a given individual is judged to be organic, then its treatment should aim first at removing or correcting, if possible, the putative organic pathogenic factor or factors. In the case of a functional disorder, the therapy is directed primarily at psychological and social factors believed to be implicated. Differentiation of organic from functional disorders does not imply that the latter are somehow independent of brain function. On the contrary, all that is implied here is that in some cases of mental disorders demonstrable cerebral pathology is a necessary condition for the occurrence of the disorder, whereas in other cases such an assumption has not yet been satisfactorily demonstrated. To say so does not, however, gainsay the premise that cerebral activity underlies all mental activity and behavior.

"Reactive" in the present context implies that a given physical illness or injury is believed to have contributed to the occurrence of the functional psychiatric disorder manifested by the patient. Neither cerebral damage nor dysfunction is believed to be responsible for the abnormal mental state, but rather the personal *meaning* of the illness-related information for the patient.[2] Physical illness or injury may be assumed to play a causal role of greater or lesser weight in some cases of every recognized form of psychopathology. Clinical observation indicates, however, that certain mental disorders are more often associated with somatic disease than others. Depressive and anxiety disorders appear to be by far the most common reactive psychiatric complications of physical illness.[1,3,4] Functional psychoses, somatoform disorders, and personality disorders appear to be less often implicated. It is likely that the bulk of the reactive disorders will eventually be found to fall into the category of adjustment disorder and its eight clinical types.[2, pp. 299-302] However, epidemiological studies in this area employing DSM-III diagnostic criteria remain to be carried out.

The current classification of mental disorders (DSM-III) is far from being a perfect instrument, owing to the limitations of our knowledge and because of conceptual limitations imposed by the complexity of human behavior and its causes. For example, it is not yet possible to delimit sharply the organic from the reactive functional mental disorders, and an element of arbitrariness in reaching a diagnostic decision is unavoidable at times. If the clinician is unable to decide in a given case whether a causal relationship obtains between a concurrent physical and psychiatric illness, then he should list the functional psychiatric disorder on Axis I (of DSM-III) and the physical disorder on Axis III[2] and thus leave open the issue of causality.

The category "deviant illness behavior" has been introduced by the writer to designate conduct of a physically ill or injured person that is incompatible with his optimal recovery.[1] Both overt and covert forms of illness-related self-destructive behavior fall into this category, which corresponds to noncompliance with medical treatment (a condition not attributable to a mental disorder) of DSM-III.[2, p. 333] Although it is not an accepted form of mental disorder, this category has been included here as it refers to psychological factors that may have an adverse effect on the course and outcome of any serious illness or injury, and one that constitutes a legitimate target for psychiatric therapeutic intervention.

METHODOLOGICAL PROBLEMS

Knowledge of the prevalence and incidence of the various psychiatric disorders assumed to be causally related to physical illness and injury is still rudimentary. A major reason for this unsatisfactory state of affairs is that epidemiological studies in this area have been plagued by semantic ambiguity and methodological errors.[1,4]

Key terms used by epidemiologists, such as "psychiatric," "physical," and "morbidity," are ambiguous. The most important studies in this area are said to explore the relationship between physical and psychiatric illness, or morbidity. What does this statement really mean? One way of resolving the issue of the meaning of these words would be to follow the nomenclature and definitions provided by the DSM-III, which represents an authoritative source of terms and diagnostic criteria pertaining to psychiatric disorders, but this is seldom done. The terms "physical" and "psychiatric" morbidity would then be understood to refer to the two respective classes of diseases or disorders included in the current international and American classifications. The term "psychiatric morbidity" encompasses both the organic and the functional psychiatric mental disorders. The category of organic mental disorders includes syndromes that are due to, and in some cases constitute the chief manifestation of, primary cerebral disease, as well as those caused by cerebral effects of systemic disease. Furthermore, brain diseases, such as primary degenerative dementia and multiinfarct dementia, have traditionally been included in the mental disorders section of the official classification. Logically, dementia and other organic brain syndromes due to these primary cerebral diseases should be considered to be instances of psychiatric distorders caused by organic disease.

The next major methodological problem concerns the complex and ambiguous issue of causality (see chapter 11, this volume, for further discussion). Most epidemiological studies in this area have focused on the *concurrence* of physical and psychiatric morbidity, rather than on the incidence of specific psychiatric disorders thought to be *caused by* physical illness and injury. Epidemiologists assert that we do not even know yet how often psychiatric disorder precedes physical illness and how often it is secondary to it.[3] Establishing the frequency of concurrence of these two types of morbidity does not, of course, say anything about the direction of casual relationships between them. In the case of organic brain syndromes, this issue is settled by definition, that is, one of them can be diagnosed only when it is judged to be a consequence of an organic disease, one arising in the brain or a systemic one affecting the brain secondarily. The problem is far more complicated in the case of a psychiatric disorder coexisting with a physical illness in the absence of any evidence of cerebral pathology. It is often difficult, or even impossible, to determine whether such a disorder is actually caused by the illness. Until adequate criteria to establish causal relationships have been formulated, the epidemiological studies in this area will continue to report only the frequency of the association between physical and psychiatric morbidity.

Ambiguities of terminology and of causal relationships are not the only methodological snags in this field.[4] Additional sources of error have been pointed out in a critical review of studies on psychiatric morbidity among patients suffering from systemic lupus erythematosus[5]: (1) biased selection of subjects; (2) lack of comparison groups; (3) dearth of prospective or experimental studies; and (4) unreliable recording of diagnostic data.

Sampling errors are well illustrated by the prevailing tendency on the part of researchers to investigate only patients admitted to hospital, or those referred for psychiatric consultation, rather than those attending outpatient clinics or those who have not received any treatment. Such biased patient selection can hardly provide reliable data on the incidence and prevalence of the various psychiatric disorders associated with the physical illness under study. Lack of comparison groups consisting of patients with a disease other than the index one is another source of misleading generalizations about the relative frequency of psychopathology associated with the given physical illness. It is meaningless to claim, for example, that patients with systemic lupus erythematosus are unusually prone to develop psychiatric disorders unless one has compared a representative group of such patients with a matched group of patients with another chronic disease such as rheumatoid arthritis.[6] Furthermore, the search for reliable epidemiological data has been confounded by the widespread predilection for cross-sectional or retrospective, rather than prospective, studies. Finally, variable methods of case identification and poor observational records have marred many studies, rendering them unreliable.[5] To obtain reliable data one needs to employ uniform investigative tools, unambiguous terminology, and explicit diagnostic criteria.

Methodological problems and errors just discussed suggest caution in interpreting and generalizing from published epidemiological data.[4] As most studies have focused on the concurrence of physical and psychiatric morbidity in various populations, they will be reviewed without an attempt to resolve the issue of the direction of their causal relationship, if any.

CONCURRENCE OF PHYSICAL AND PSYCHIATRIC MORBIDITY

The concurrence of physical and mental illness has been studied in the community as well as in medical and psychiatric inpatients and outpatients.[4] On the whole, these studies have found a *positive statistical association* between physical and psychiatric morbidity. As community studies have the advantage of dealing with relatively more representative samples, they will be briefly reviewed first.

COMMUNITY STUDIES

In the 1950s Hinkle and Wolff[7] carried out pioneering studies on the distribution of disease in several general population groups. Their findings prompted them to formulate several generalizations, or hypotheses, which amounted to a general theory of illness. They proposed that illnesses are not randomly distributed in the population but tend to *cluster* in such a way that, on an average, 25% of any group of people studied over a period of years account for about 50% of all illness episodes reported. Those persons who show the greatest susceptibility to physical ill health are also the ones displaying the greatest proneness to mental disorders. Furthermore, illnesses of all kinds tend to cluster not only in certain individuals but also in families and in time. The temporal "clusters" usually correspond to periods of psychosocial stress in the lives of the affected persons and are separated by periods of relative well-being. The average duration of a cluster is about 7 years. Hinkle and Wolff concluded that their studies demonstrated the concurrence of physical and mental morbidity.

Subsequent investigators have largely confirmed the findings of Hinkle and Wolff.[8] As an exception, one study of the distribution of psychiatric and organic disorders in a general practice population failed to show a postive correlation between them.[9] Eastwood and Trevelyan[10] have carried out one of the best designed studies. They screened a sample of 1471 men and women listed with a general practitioner in England, all of whom had been given both a medical and a psychiatric assessment. Those persons who had evidence of a psychiatric disorder (124 subjects) showed more physical morbidity than the psychologically healthy subjects. The researchers concluded that their findings supported the hypothesis of a positive statistical association between physical and psychiatric disorders. Schwab and co-workers[11] have studied, by means of an interview, a population sample in a Florida county and reported that the physically ill respondents had higher scores on all the mental illness scales than the physically healthy subjects. The investigators have proposed that low socioeconomic status is a major factor associated with high risk of both physical and psychiatric morbidity.

Introduction of the "general health questionnaire" (GHQ) by Goldberg[12] as a means of assessing suspected or probable psychiatric morbidity in the general population has provided epidemiologists with a useful screening device. Andrews and his collaborators[13] used the GHQ in a study of 863 persons living in a Sydney, Australia, suburb and found a positive association between the occurrence of physical and psychiatric illness in the representative suburban population sample.

The elderly, those aged 65 years and more, constitute the segment of the general population that shows high incidence and prevalence of both physical and psychiatric morbidity. A 4-year follow-up study of 297 elderly persons has found a positive association between physical illness and functional psychiatric disorders, especially the depressive ones.[14]

Community studies have conclusively demonstrated positive statistical association between physical and mental disorders. This finding suggests that an intimate relation between these two types of morbidity exists, but it does not resolve the issue of causality. Some writers have actually proposed that physical and mental disorders should be viewed as interrelated manifestations of people's ill health rather than as separate entities that could cause each other.[15] Eastwood[15] argues that to help settle this matter one needs to undertake prospective community studies. A cohort of randomly chosen subjects should be assessed medically, psychiatrically, and socially and be periodically reassessed on these parameters over a period of years. Only such prospective studies, employing strict diagnostic criteria and unambiguous terminology, could establish how often psychiatric disorders of various types follow physical illness and are causally related to it.

STUDIES OF HOSPITALIZED MEDICAL PATIENTS

Few studies of the prevalence of psychiatric morbidity among medical and surgical inpatients have been published to date.[4] Prevalence studies are designed to estimate the number of patients with a recognized mental disorder in a given population at one point in time. In actual practice, however, prevalence implies that the number was counted not at one instant but at any time during the period of survey.[16] A crucial problem in such studies is the choice of the case-finding technique and of the criteria for what constitutes a psychiatric case. Until recently researchers have used a variety of screening devices and widely differing diagnostic criteria. Psychiatric interview, self-administered questionnaires, and various personality scales have been employed for screening purposes.[17] In the past several years researchers have employed psychiatric screening tests and standardized diagnostic research interviews and used them to estimate the frequency of psychiatric illness among medical inpatients.[4,18]

As early as 1927, Heldt[19] estimated, on the basis of a retrospective chart review, that at least 30% of patients admitted to a general hospital may be expected to show either a primary psychiatric disorder or one secondary to physical illness. Moersch[20] reviewed records of 500 consecutive patients admitted to the Mayo Clinic around 1930 and found that 44% of them presented psychiatric problems, with or without an associated physical illness. It is remarkable that these earliest and methodologically primitive studies provided estimates of prevalence of psychiatric morbidity among medical inpatients that have been replicated by some more recent investigators using relatively sophisticated screening techniques.[17] One notes, however, that some studies have found substantially lower or higher prevalence.[17] The present writer reviewed reports published prior to 1967 and concluded that 30 to 60% of medical and surgical inpatients were likely to show psychiatric disorder sufficiently severe to create a problem for the treating physicians.[17]

Several recent studies have used new methods of psychiatric screening.[4,21-23] Knights and Folstein[21] have employed the GHQ to screen all patients admitted to three general medical wards over 1 month. They found that 46% of the patients scored greater than 4, suggesting the presence of an emotional disorder. Thirty-three percent of the patients showed cognitive impairment detected by the minimental status examination (MMSE). Maguire and his colleagues[22] have screened with GHQ all patients consecutively admitted to two medical wards during 2 months and concluded that 26% of their subjects were psychiatrically ill. These investigators have conceded that this percentage was probably an underestimate. Moftic and Paykel[23] found 36 cases (24%) of depression among 150 medical inpatients. Modestin[24] has carried out two studies of a total of more than 1000 medical inpatients in a Swiss district general hospital. In his first study he used a retrospective chart review; in the second, a psychiatric interview. He assigned a psychiatric diagnosis in about 70% of all the patients. De Paulo and his co-workers[25] screened patients on a neurological ward and found that 32% of them had cognitive deficits, whereas 50% scored 5 or more on the GHQ.

One recent study stands out as a model of careful design and critical evaluation of findings. Cavanaugh[26] has studied 335 randomly selected medical inpatients using three scales as screening devices, i.e., the MMSE, the GHQ, and the Beck depression inventory (BDI). She found that 28% of the patients had evidence of cognitive dysfunction on the MMSE, 61% showed emotional disturbance on the GHQ, and 36% were depressed as indicated by the BDI.

These studies have documented the high prevalence of psychiatric morbidity, much of it unrecognized and untreated, among medical and surgical inpatients. Psychiatric illness in hospitalized patients is often undetected.[26,27] Such patients are admitted to hospital because of known or suspected physical illness, and a proportion of them are likely to be discharged without any medical diagnosis. In the majority of the identified psychiatric cases, however, both a physical illness and a psychiatric disorder are found to coexist. Thus the studies of medical inpatient population lend support to the contention that these two types of morbidity are positively correlated. Among hospitalized medical patients the prevalence of psychiatric illness of some degree of severity has been variously reported to range between 26% and 72%.[4]

The marked discrepancy in the reported prevalence figures probably reflects several factors.[4,17] First, demographic characteristics of the patients studied may have differed. The elderly and the indigent medical inpatients are likely to show higher prevalence of psychiatric illness than the younger and the economically advantaged ones. Second, investigators have used different techniques of psychiatric case finding and different criteria of what constitutes a psychiatric case.[4] Third, the presence or lack of a psychiatric ward in the hospital under study may have resulted in a more or less selected patient population and hence a different prevalence of psychiatric morbidity.

Cavanaugh and Wettstein[4] have thoroughly reviewed the studies reported so far and conclude that "medical inpatient studies to date permit few inferences about the prevalence of psychiatric distress, symptoms, or diagnoses" (p. 203). Moreover, most prevalence studies have used screening tests to detect probable *psychiatric cases* and have not attempted to establish the prevalence of specific *psychiatric disorders* included in the official American classification of mental disorders.[4] It appears, however, that anxiety and depressive disorders (a large proportion of which may in fact be more appropriately classified as adjustment disorders) as well as organic brain syndromes constitute the bulk of psychiatric morbidity in the medical population.[4] This impression is supported by surveys of medical inpatients referred for psychiatric consultation.[28]

STUDIES OF PHYSICAL ILLNESS IN PSYCHIATRIC PATIENTS

Prevalence of physical illness has been studied in several kinds of psychiatric clinical settings. Patients hospitalized in general hospital psychiatric units and in state hospitals, as well as those attending psychiatric outpatient clinics, have been screened for evidence of physical illness.

Three representative studies of *general hospital psychiatric unit* patients reported a prevalence of physical illness of between 26% and 46%.[29-31] In a substantial proportion of cases such illness had not been recognized. Recent studies of various psychiatric patient populations have found the prevalence of physical illness to range from 33% to 60%.[32] Koranyi[33] has screened more than 2000 *psychiatric clinic patients* and found that 43% of them suffered from one or several physical illnesses, which in almost half the cases had not been recognized by the referring source. Barnes et al.[34] detected physical illness in 26% of chronic psychiatric outpatients.

Lansbury[35] found the average prevalence of physical illness among nearly 3000 patients at a *state hospital* to be 75.5%. Hall and co-workers[36] studied 100 state hospital patients consecutively admitted to a research ward and reported that 46% of them had an unrecognized physical illness which, in the investigators' opinion, either caused or exacerbated the concurrent psychiatric disorder. Allodi and Cohen[37] found major physical illness in 21% of a series of patients newly admitted to a psychiatric hospital. These physically ill patients had significantly longer hospitalization than the physically healthy ones.

Thus, studies of psychiatric patient populations also support the claim that physical and psychiatric disorders are positively associated, but in most cases fail to answer the question of how often the mental disorder may be regarded as a consequence of the concurrent physical one. Only several studies have addressed this issue. Hall and associates[38] screened 658 psychiatric outpatients and claim that 9.1% of them had a physical illness that was directly responsible for their psychiatric symptoms. Other investigators have postulated such a causal relationship to hold for from 12% to 42% of patients with concurrent physical and psychiatric illness.[32] It is not always clear, however, what criteria these authors have employed to arrive at the conclusion that a causal relationship does exist in a given patient. Kellner[39] attempted to establish how often psychiatric ill health follows physical illness. He studied 947 patients who were observed in a general practice for 2 years and found that 14% had an apparent inception of neurotic symptoms, such as depression and tension, after a physical illness or surgery. He concluded that at least minor psychiatric problems are more likely to occur after a physical illness than at other times. The issue of how often a psychiatric disorder is causally related to physical illness must still be regarded as unresolved.

STUDIES OF PSYCHIATRIC DISORDERS IN SPECIFIC ORGANIC DISEASES

The literature contains numerous reports on the frequency of various psychiatric disorders in specific organic diseases.[1,38,40] There is some evidence that neoplastic, cardiovascular, endocrine, pulmonary, and neurolgical diseases have relatively high statistical association with psychiatric morbidity.[1,38,41] It is not possible to review this literature here, as a whole monograph could be devoted to the subject. A recent study of the prevalence of psychiatric disorders among cancer patients deserves special mention since it was carefully designed and employed the DSM-III diagnostic criteria.[41] It found that 47% of the patients could be assigned a psychiatric diagnosis. About 69% of the psychiatric diagnoses consisted of adjustment disorders, and 13% involved major depression, 8% organic mental disorders. and 4% anxiety disorders. I predict that future studies of other common chronic diseases are likely to show a similar distribution of the DSM-III diagnostic categories. This statement does not, however, apply to the physically ill elderly, among whom the organic brain syndromes have been found to be far more common, especially in the community general hospitals.[42,43]

PHYSICAL DISEASES IN THE MAJOR PSYCHOSES

Tsuang et al.[44] have recently reviewed studies on the frequency of various physical diseases in schizophrenias and major depression. Cardiovascular and infectious diseases, as well as gastrointestinal cancer, show increased incidence in schizophrenics, whereas patients with major depression tend to have an increased incidence of circulatory, respiratory, and atopic diseases as well as of diabetes mellitus.

SUMMARY AND CONCLUSIONS

I have reviewed representative examples of epidemiological studies on the association between physical and psychiatric illness. With very few exceptions, these studies have found a positive statistical association between these two types of morbidity. This finding has important practical implications. It supports the arguments in favor of ready availability of medical diagnostic facilities for the psychiatric patients and of psychiatric consultations for the medical patients. No health facility could be considered to provide adequate patient care unless this requirement was fulfilled.

The issue of the frequency of a causal relationship between physical illness and the concurrent psychiatric disorder remains unresolved. It is possible that methods used in prevalence studies are not construed to resolve it. Longitudinal and prospective, rather than cross-sectional, studies, using more sensitive investigative methods, are needed to establish how often physical illness in general, and specific diseases in particular, result in psychopathology. Moreover, such studies should address the issue of the incidence and prevalence of specific psychiatric disorders among the physically ill. Such data are needed to plan realistically in the areas of prevention and availability of psychiatric services for this population.

In Chapter 11 I will address the issue of the putative pathogenetic mechanisms leading from a physical illness to injury to a psychiatric disorder.

REFERENCES

 1. Lipowski ZJ: Psychiatry of somatic diseases: Epidemiology, pathogenesis, classification. *Compr Psychiatry* 16:105–124, 1975.
 2. *Diagnostic and Statistical Manual of Mental Disorders*, 3 ed. Washington, DC, American Psychiatric Association, 1980.
 3. Cooper B, Morgan HG: *Epidemiological Psychiatry*. Springfield, Ill, Charles C Thomas, 1973.
 4. Cavanaugh S, Wettstein RM: Prevalence of psychiatric morbidity in medical populations, in Grinspoon L (ed): *Psychiatry Update*. Washington, DC, American Psychiatric Press, 1984, vol 3, pp 187–215.
 5. Gurland BJ, Ganz VH, Fleiss JL, Zubin J: The study of the psychiatric symptoms of systemic lupus erythematosus. *Psychosom Med* 34:199–206, 1972.
 6. Ganz VH, Gurland BJ, Deming WE, Fisher B: The study of the psychiatric symptoms of systemic lupus erythematosus. *Psychosom Med* 34:207–220, 1972.
 7. Hinkle LE, Wolff HG: The nature of man's adaptation to his total environment and the relation of this to illness. *Arch Intern Med* 99:442–460, 1957.
 8. Eastwood MR: Epidemiological studies in psychosomatic medicine, in Lipowski ZJ, Lipsitt DR, Whybrow PC (eds): *Psychosomatic Medicine. Current Trends and Clinical Applications*. New York, Oxford University Press, 1977, pp 411–420.
 9. Kreitman N, Pearce KI, Ryle A: The relationship of psychiatric, psychosomatic and organic illness in a general practice. *Br J Psychiatry* 112:569–579, 1966.
10. Eastwood MR, Trevelyan MH: Relationship between physical and psychiatric disorder. *Psychol Med* 2:363–372, 1972.
11. Schwab JJ, Traven ND, Warheit GJ: Relationship between physical and mental illness. *Psychosomatics* 19:458–463, 1978.
12. Goldberg DP: *The Detection of Psychiatric Illness by Questionnaire*. London, Oxford University Press, 1972.
13. Andrews G, Schonell M, Tennant C: The relation between physical, psychological, and social morbidity in a suburban community. *Am J Epidemiol* 105:324–329, 1977.

14. Kay DWK, Bergman K: Physical disability and mental health in old age. *J Psychosom Res* 10:3-12, 1966.
15. Eastwood MR: *The Relation between Physical and Mental Illness.* Toronto, University of Toronto Press, 1975.
16. Reid DD: *Epidemiological Methods in the Study of Mental Disorders.* Geneva, World Health Organization, 1960.
17. Lipowski ZJ: Review of consultation psychiatry and psychosomatic medicine. II. Clinical aspects. *Psychosom Med* 29:201-224, 1967.
18. Editorial: Psychiatric illness among medical patients. *Lancet* 1:478-479, 1979.
19. Heldt TJ: The functioning of a division of neuropsychiatry in a general hospital. *Am J Psychiatry* 7:459-481, 1927-1928.
20. Moersch FP: Psychiatry in medicine. *Am J Psychiatry* 11:831-843, 1932.
21. Knights EB, Folstein MF: Unsuspected emotional and cognitive disturbances in medical patients. *Ann Intern Med* 87:723-724, 1977.
22. Maguire GP, Julier DL, Hawton KE, Bancroft JHJ: Psychiatric morbidity and referral on two general medical wards. *Br Med J* 1:268-270, 1974.
23. Moftic HS, Paykel ES: Depression in medical in-patients. *Br Med J* 126:346-353, 1975.
24. Modestin J: Psychiatrische Morbiditaet bei intern-medizinisch hospitalisierten Patienten. *Schweiz med Wochenschr* 107:1354-1361, 1977.
25. De Paulo JR, Folstein MF, Gordon B: Psychiatric screening on a neurological ward. *Psychol Med* 10:125-132, 1980.
26. Cavanaugh S: The prevalence of emotional and cognitive dysfunction in a general medical population: Using MMSE, GHQ, and BDI. *Gen Hosp Psychiatry* 5:15-24, 1983.
27. Schuckit MA, Miller PL, Hahlbohm D: Unrecognized psychiatric illness in elderly medical-surgical patients. *J Gerontol* 30:655-660, 1975.
28. Lipowski ZJ, Wolston EY: Liaison psychiatry: Referral patterns and their stability over time. *Am J Psychiatry* 138:1608-1611, 1981.
29. Kerr WC: The importance of physical illness in psychiatric breakdown. *Aust NZ J Psychiatry* 8:269-271, 1974.
30. Maguire GP, Granville-Grossman KL: Physical illness in psychiatric patients. *Br J Psychiatry* 115:1365-1369, 1968.
31. Munoz RA: Mental, medical and social problems in a psychiatric population. *Psychosomatics* 17:194-196, 1976.
32. Koranyi EK: Somatic illness in psychiatric patients. *Psychosomatics* 21:887-891, 1980.
33. Koranyi EK: Morbidity and rate of undiagnosed physical illness in a psychiatric clinic population. *Arch Gen Psychiatry* 36:414-419, 1979.
34. Barnes RF, Mason JC, Greer C, Ray FT: Medical illness in chronic psychiatric outpatients. *Gen Hosp Psychiatry* 5:191-195, 1983.
35. Lansbury J: The prevalence of physical disease in a large mental hospital and its implications for staffing. *Hosp Commun Psychiatry* 23:148-151, 1972.
36. Hall RCW, Gardner ER, Popkin MK, Lecann AF, Stickney SK: Unrecognized physical illness prompting psychiatric admission: A prospective study. *Am J Psychiatry* 138:629-635, 1981.
37. Allodi F, Cohen M: Physical illness and length of psychiatric hospitalization. *Can Psychiatr Assoc J* 23:101-106, 1978.
38. Hall RCW, Popkin MK, Devaul RA, et al: Physical illness presenting as psychiatric disease. *Arch Gen Psychiatry* 35:1315-1320, 1978.
39. Kellner R: Psychiatric ill health following physical illness. *Br J Psychiatry* 112:71-73, 1966.
40. Hall RCW (ed): *Psychiatric Presentations of Medical Illness.* New York, Spectrum Publications, 1980.
41. Derogatis LR, Morrow GR, Fetting J, et al: The prevalence of psychiatric disorders among cancer patients. *JAMA* 249:751-757, 1983.
42. Lipowski ZJ: The need to integrate liaison psychiatry and geropsychiatry. *Am J Psychiatry* 140:1003-1005, 1983.
43. Lipowski ZJ: Transient cognitive disorders (delirium, acute confusional states) in the elderly. *Am J Psychiatry* 140:1426-1436, 1983.
44. Tsuang MT, Perkins K, Simpson JC: Physical diseases in schizophrenia and affective disorder. *J Clin Psychiatry* 44:42-46, 1983.

Physical Illness and Psychiatric Disorder

11

Pathogenesis

INTRODUCTION

Physical illness constitutes one of the major determinants of psychiatric morbidity. It may cause *recurrence, exacerbation,* or *inception de novo* of nearly every recognized psychiatric (mental) disorder (see reference 1 and Chapter 10, this volume). For example, myocardial infarction may trigger recurrence of a depressive disorder in one patient, markedly aggravate an anxiety disorder in another, or precipitate delirium in one who has never experienced it before. In all of these instances one may speak of psychiatric complications of the physical illness.

What are the causal links between somatic illness and psychopathology? Some writers have formulated stringent criteria for establishing a causal role of such illness in the development of the associated psychiatric disorder. For example, Eilenberg[2] has proposed the following criteria: (1) no past history of psychiatric illness; (2) no evidence of disturbed premorbid personality; (3) absence of psychologically or socially disturbing events preceding the illness; (4) unequivocal presence of mental illness; (5) resolution of the mental illness with specific treatment for the organic disease; and (6) relapse when such treatment is withheld, as may be the case with pernicious anemia, for example.

Strict criteria, like those cited, are based on obsolete conceptions of causality in biological systems. They presuppose the ubiquity of one-to-one causal relationships, which in real life are actually rare. Single-factor or specific-agent models of causality have been largely supplanted by the doctrine of multiple causes by the realization that the most common type of causal factor in human morbidity is neither necessary nor sufficient but rather contributory.[3] Physical illness or injury may play either a necessary or a contributory causal role in the occurrence of a psychiatric disorder. It constitutes a necessary, but not always a sufficient, condition for the occurrence of the so-called organic mental disorders. In all other cases its causal role may be considered to be *contributory.* This implies that some additional factor, or factors, must also be present to produce a psychiatric disorder. These factors may be subsumed under the general concept of *vulnerability* to develop a particular disorder. Both genetic and acquired predisposition may be implicated.

When a psychiatric disorder is found to be associated with a physical one, their mutual relationship may be one of three kinds: (1) coincidental, i.e., neither disorder has caused the other one; (2) psychiatric disorder has contributed to the occurrence of the physical illness; or (3) physical illness has played a causal role in the development or exacerbation of the psychiatric disorder. In the case of organic mental disorders, the necessary causal role of an organic cerebral factor is assumed by definition. In the case of all other types of psychiatric disorders associated with physical illness, its causal role may be postulated if at least two essential criteria are met: (1) physical illness or injury antedated the onset or exacerbation of the psychiatric disorder, and (2) psychiatric examination and history provide evidence for a causal connection.

Murphy and Brown[4] have proposed on the basis of their research that a depressive disorder may constitute an intermediate causal link between a personally important life event or change on the one hand and a near-future physical illness on the other. In such cases the depressive disorder will have antedated physical illness and may continue after its onset and complicate it without having been caused by it. For example, Lloyd and Cawley[5] found that of a group of 35 men showing a depressive disorder after their first myocardial infarction, 16 had suffered from depression *prior* to the infarct. Its occurrence, however, may have served to exacerbate the depression.

Physical illness or injury of any etiology may result in a psychiatric disorder by uncovering a latent, inherited or acquired, predisposition or vulnerability to the particular, say depressive, disorder. Furthermore, it may precipitate the recurrence of a disorder that the patient experienced in the past, or exacerbate a preexisting disorder, or bring about a disorder for which both past history and demonstrable predisposition are lacking. In all these cases the physical illness may be considered to have played a causal role in the development or exacerbation of psychopathology.

If one assumes that physical illness may play a causal role in at least some cases of psychiatric disorder that follows its onset, then one needs to address the question of putative *psychopathogenesis*. In other words, one needs to identify the intervening mechanisms, or factors, whereby physical illness or injury can give rise to psychopathology. Such identification could help physicians develop appropriate preventive and therapeutic measures. With this practical goal in mind, I will present a set of postulated pathogenetic mechanisms interposed between the onset of a physical illness or injury on the one hand and the development of a psychiatric disorder on the other.

PSYCHOPATHOGENETIC FACTORS

In several previous papers I have formulated a proposed taxonomy of psychosocial reactions to physical illness and a multifactorial schema of their determinants (see reference 1 and Chapters 8 to 10, this volume). That schema encompasses factors inherent in the patient, in his disease, and in his social and physical environment. It can be equally well applied to the normal as well as to the pathological reactions. In order to explain the latter, however, its explanatory power needs to be narrowed and sharpened. In other words, it is necessary to specify which particular factors appear to increase the probability that a given physical illness will result in the development of psychopathological, or psychiatric, complications.

For the purpose of this discussion one may consider a physical illness or injury to constitute an independent variable and a resulting psychiatric disorder—a dependent one. The pathogenetic factors or mechanisms may be regarded as intervening variables whose presence in a given case may help to explain why a psychiatric disorder had developed, and whose absence would make the occurrence of such a disorder unlikely. This issue constitutes the main focus of this paper. As the organic brain syndromes and depressive and anxiety disorders have been found to be the most common psychiatric consequences and complications of physical illness (see reference 1 and chapter 10, this volume), the proposed pathogenetic mechanisms would have to account for this observation in order to be clinically useful.

The whole area of psychopathogenesis of physical illness-related psychopathology has been neglected by researchers, and hence the body of established facts is quite modest. Speculation and theorizing still outweigh the relevant database. My purpose here is not to try to review in detail the research and theoretical formulations related to this topic, but rather to present a conceptual framework from which testable hypotheses could be derived and which may serve to bring together diverse lines of investigation and thought. Moreover, such a framework should have clinical usefulness by drawing attention to factors that may help predict and explain the development of psychopathology in a given case and thus have some value for its prevention and psychosocial management.

BASIC PSYCHOPATHOGENETIC FACTORS

One may distinguish two basic factors whose presence in a physically ill patient can result in the development of psychopathology (see reference 1 and Chapter 10, this volume): (1) cerebral damage or dysfunction, and (2) stressful personal meaning of illness for the patient.

"Cerebral damage" usually connotes destruction of some cerebral neurons. It may be focal or relatively widespread. "Cerebral dysfunction" refers to transient or permanent impairment of one or more brain functions as a result of cell loss, or metabolic derangement, or disordered neurotransmission, or a combination of these factors. The psychopathological manifestations that follow may be regarded as the consequences of direct interference with the cerebral substrate of a person's mental activity and/or manifest behavior. Depending on such variables as the nature, site, extent, rate of onset and spread, duration, and other features of the brain damage or dysfunction, the resulting organic brain syndrome may be either relatively circumscribed or global, in the sense that either one function is predominantly affected or more than one are impaired concurrently.[6] For example, in the amnestic syndrome memory is selectively impaired, whereas in delirium and dementia functions such as cognition, motivation, emotions, and psychomotor behavior may all be impaired or abnormal to some extent.

The psychopathology of the organic mental disorders will be discussed in Chapter 12. They are distinguished from other mental disorders on the assumption that cerebral damage or demonstrable dysfunction constitutes a necessary, if not always sufficient, condition for their occurrence (see Chapters 8 and 12, this volume).

The second basic pathogenetic mechanism proposed here differs fundamentally from the first one just discussed. It does not involve an insult to the brain but may be viewed as being mediated by *information* and its *appraisal* in terms of its personal significance and likely consequences for the individual. I discussed several categories of meaning of illness-related information in Chapter 8 and postulated its pivotal importance for the patient's emotional responses and coping behavior. Meanings, such as threat or loss, however, are extremely common consequences of appraisal of the personal significance of illness and in the majority of cases do not result in the development of maladaptive responses in the form of a psychiatric disorder. Clearly, additional conditions must be present in order for the particular meaning of illness to result in psychopathology. I shall call these modifying pathogenetic variables *auxiliary psychopathogenetic factors*. Their effect is to render a given meaning of illness, mostly threat or loss, *stressful*. This implies that the patient appraises his illness and its consequences to be so grave as to render him *helpless* to cope with it. In other words, he feels that the threat or loss is overwhelming, that is, exceeding, or at least taxing to the limit, his resources and capacity to exert control over his emotions, behavior, and environment.[7] Such a sense of helplessness and uncontrollability tends to engender intense dysphoric emotions of anxiety, depression, or anger and to lead to maladaptive behavior. Reported complaints as well as observable manifestations of this personal predicament constitute an anxiety or a depressive disorder.

AUXILIARY PSYCHOPATHOGENETIC FACTORS

I propose that the following psychosocial and psychobiological factors can modify the meaning of an illness for a patient in such a way as to make it stressful:

1. Frustration of drives and needs.
2. Increased intensity of intrapsychic conflicts.
3. Failure of defense mechanisms.
4. Loss of self-esteem.
5. Alteration of body image.
6. Disruption of normal sleep–wake cycle.
7. Social isolation and alienation.

This list is not meant to be exhaustive but, in this writer's view, does contain some of the major psychosocial and psychobiological factors contributing to the development of physical-illness-related anxiety and depressive disorders as well as of other nonorganic psychiatric conditions such as somatoform disorders and paranoid and transient reactive psychoses.

A disease may set off some or all of the proposed auxiliary factors or mechanisms in a given patient, and they may occur in various combinations, time sequences, and degrees of intensity. They overlap to some extent and represent different levels of abstraction and complexity; their respective psychopathogenetic potential is not likely to be the same. For instance, factors 1 to 3 on the list reflect psychodynamic conceptions, are relatively abstract and complex, and, taken together, appear to have a higher potential to elicit psychopathology than, say, alteration of body image. Disruption of the normal sleep–wake cycle may serve to disorganize some individuals quite readily, whereas others can tolerate it for considerable periods of time without showing signs of decompensation. Such clinical and laboratory observations impel us to postulate different *individual vulnerability* to the psychologically disruptive, and hence pathogenetic, effects of any of the proposed factors. Such vulnerability may be regarded as a personality attribute that acts as a modifier, in that it increases or reduces the probability that exposure to a given pathogenetic factor will actually result in a psychiatric disorder. Furthermore, the impact of a given set of pathogenetic factors may be expected to be modified, that is, facilitated or counterbalanced, by certain personality variables as well as by the quality of the *social supports*, if any, available to the patient at the onset of the illness and throughout its course. One may propose that the more of the pathogenetic factors are present in the given case, the more likely is psychopathology to ensue.

Frustration of Drives and Needs

Every disease involves some degree of deprivation of pleasure and fulfillment derived from satisfaction of biological drives and derivative needs. Such deprivation results in *frustration*, that is, failure to reach expected goals or rewards. Eating, drinking, sexual activity, physical activity, rest, intellectual or artistic performance, play, social intercourse, sense of security, capacity for independent living, aesthetic experience—any or all of them may be adversely affected or even precluded by illness or injury. The resulting frustration tends to elicit emotional and behavioral responses, both immediate and delayed. Anger and resentment are the most common emotional responses. The typical immediate behavioral response to frustration features tension, restlessness, and either direct or displaced aggression.[8] The latter may, but need not, be hostile. By contrast, some individuals do not respond with display of aggressive behavior, but with its opposite, i.e., a state marked by apathy, withdrawal, indifference, inattentiveness, and inactivity.[8]

In the case of illness, the source of frustration is within the patient's body, and hence outward aggression cannot get rid of it. Consummation of one or another desired goal may be thwarted because a necessary body part or function has become unavailable, or because goal-directed behavior elicits pain or some other distressing physical symptom. Furthermore, if the illness is chronic, then frustration of a given drive or need is likely to continue or be repeatedly experienced. Restrictions of diet or impotence in a diabetic male, for example, represent ongoing potential sources of frustration.

Most physically ill people cope with the inevitable frustrations in an adaptive manner, that is, without showing a psychopathological reaction. Many chronically ill patients harbor chronic resentment, which may be regarded as an undesirable but not necessarily a pathological emotional response. Those who do develop a psychopathological reaction to frustrations engendered by illness are likely to show one or more of the following features: (1) experience intense emotional arousal in the form of rage, envy, despondency, or hopelessness; (2) react to their rage, envy, or hostility with feelings of guilt; (3) exhibit tendency to withdraw and give up; (4) use defense mechanisms of projection, denial, or regression; (5) experience dysphoric emotions as somatic symptoms.

In each of these instances the frustration of drives and needs increases the probability of the development of a psychiatric disorder, be it depression, anxiety state, hypochondriasis, or conversion disorder.

Increased Intensity of Intrapsychic Conflicts

An intrapsychic conflict implies simultaneous existence of opposing and incompatible action tendencies within the person. Three main types of conflict may be distinguished: approach–approach, avoidance–avoidance, and approach–avoidance. The kind of conflict most likely to result in psychopathology is one that involves approach–avoidance. Such a conflict may or may not be conscious. The person experiences impulses to engage in some form of activity or pursue a particular goal which is countered by the opposing tendency. The impulses usually implicated in this type of conflict invoke some form of sexual, hostile, care-seeking, or power-seeking behavior. The opposing forces involve prohibitions emanating from the individual's conscience and social judgment. To act out the prohibited impulses would evoke feelings of guilt, or fearful anticipation of disapproval or punishment from other people, or both. Thus the impulses may be appraised by the person as dangerous to him, and mere awareness of them may be experienced as a serious threat to his well-being.

Such approach–avoidance conflicts are generally believed to result from learning experiences during childhood and, being usually unconscious, they tend to remain relatively unaffected by the individual's psychological maturation and expanded knowledge of the world. Conflicts are ubiquitous and as such are not to be viewed as pathological. Their potential to induce psychopathology stems from their capacity to elicit intense dysphoric emotions that the person is unable to control effectively, or to set in motion maladaptive defenses against the impulses or the unpleasant emotions or both. Such defenses are deployed for the purpose of reducing anguish, safeguarding self-esteem, and avoiding loss of control over disavowed and feared impulses. Unresolved intrapsychic conflicts may for long periods remain dormant, as it were, yet leave the person at risk for psychological decompensation and maladaptive behavior if certain life events or situations succeed in activating them. This may occur if either the impulses become strengthened, or the adaptive and effective defenses against them become weakened, or both.

Physical illness or injury is one of the factors that may intensify unresolved intrapsychic conflicts. It may do so by increasing the strength of the repudiated action tendencies, or by weakening the defenses against them, or by both these mechanisms. Frustration, discussed in the preceding section, may arouse hostile impulses, for example, and thus intensify the conflict between them and the opposing prohibitions. Anxiety attacks, or guilt feelings, or pervasive somatic symptoms may result and signalize a flareup of the conflict. In other cases, illness may heighten the wish to be taken care of and thus intensify the conflict over related action tendencies. For many people in our culture, being overly dependent on others represents a predicament to be avoided at any cost. Such persons are particularly likely to experience a conflict over dependent strivings elicited by the state of being physically ill. For others, it is sexual impulses of some type which are a source of conflict and which may be aroused by an illness or its treatment. For example, an older widow with strict prohibitions against sex outside of marriage may receive large doses of estrogens as a form of cancer chemotherapy and experience intense sexual drive as a result. In this case a side effect of the therapy may activate an intrapsychic conflict and its psychological consequences. Similarly, unconscious and feared homosexual tendencies may be aroused in a man who, because of a back injury, may be forced to adopt a passive role during sexual intercourse.

Failure of Adaptive Defense Mechanisms

Intensified and largely, or wholly, unconscious conflicts need not inexorably lead to psychopathology. Their outcome will depend on the patient's personality and social resources. Factors such as trait anxiety or a tendency to somatization are likely to increase the probability that a psychiatric disorder will develop. This probability is also greater if the heightened conflict results in one of the following: (1) arousal of intense and prolonged anxiety or guilt feelings; (2) shift to more primitive and less adaptive defense mechanisms; or (3) serious loss of self-esteem.

Verwoerdt[9] has proposed an explanatory model for the development of psychopathology in response to physical illness as a result of a shift to maladaptive mechanisms of defense. His formulation has been summarized in Chapter 8, this volume, and need not be repeated here. Failure to deploy defense mechanisms, adaptive or not, to counteract anxiety and other dysphoric emotions effectively is likely to result in a manifest anxiety or depressive disorder, or even a transient reactive psychosis. The consequences of loss of self-esteem will be discussed in the next section.

Loss of Self-Esteem

A common and important psychological consequence of physical illness is some degree of lowering or loss of self-esteem. When such a loss results from self-blame and a sense of personal failing or turpitude and thus guilt, the patient is at a high risk of developing a depressive disorder. Self-esteem, or self-regard, is a construct and a personality variable referring to the attitude toward and evaluation of oneself. It may be defined as the degree of acceptance or approval of one's attributes, actions, and character. For some writers, the concept implies the degree of congruence between a person's ideal and actual self.[10] Self-esteem cuts deeply into the life of every individual. Any serious threat to it constitutes a form of psychological stress and is likely to evoke stress responses. A major purpose of psychological defense mechanisms is to maintain, enhance, or restore self-esteem.[8]

A loss of self-esteem constitutes a pivotal psychological theme in, and a characteristic feature of, *depression*.[11-16] As Fenichel[13] put it, "Experiences that precipitate depressions represent either a loss of self-esteem or a loss of supplies which the patient had hoped would secure or even enhance his self-esteem" (p. 390). Physical illness exemplifies one of the many possible experiences that may result in lowering of self-esteem and hence preceipitate a depression. Several psychoanalytic writers, notably Bibring[12] and Jacobson,[15] have elaborated a theory of depression in which the construct of self-esteem plays a key role. According to Bibring, depression occurs when self-esteem becomes undermined after an experience, such as the development of a chronic physical illness, that thwarts the person's basic aspirations on whose fulfillment his self-esteem depends. Frustration of these aspirations, especially those to be loved and to be loving, causes a blow to and lowering of self-esteem. The aspirations may be divided into three groups, depending on the developmental stage from which they stem: (1) to be loved, worthy, independent; (2) to be loving, good, clean; and (3) to be admired, strong.

When a person comes to believe, rightly or wrongly, that he has failed to live up to those aspirations whose fulfillment is vitally important to his sense of own worth, the following consequences may follow: *loss of self-esteem*, a sense of *helplessness*, and a *depression*. According to Bibring, depression represents a manifestation of a state of helplessness resulting from failure to maintain adequate self-esteem. Such a failure may be caused by physical illness or injury. The state of helplessness that follows represents a reactivation of that experienced in childhood as a consequence of frequent or prolonged deprivation of vital needs, such as those to be taken care of, to be fed, and to be loved. Thus, early childhood deprivations are viewed by Bibring as factors predisposing to depression in later life. The strength of such predisposition in a given person is modified by such postulated variables as the tolerance for frustration, frequency and severity of the experience of helplessness in childhood, and the readiness with which the state of helplessness may be reactivated in later life.[14] It follows that considerable *individual differences* in predisposition and proneness to depressive illness must be postulated.

Although physical illness or injury results in a loss of self-esteem in some patients, only a proportion of them will develop a depressive disorder as a result. The severity of the loss and the degree of genetic predisposition to depression may be expected to codetermine whether or not a depressive disorder will develop. Furthermore, individuals characterized by chronically low or vulnerable self-esteem are also prone to respond with a further loss of it to a variety of life events and situations, including physical illness.

Illness or injury may lower self-esteem in one or more of several possible ways. It may serve to heighten intrapsychic conflict with consequent feelings of guilt, as we discussed in an earlier section. It may jeopardize, or even destroy, personal assets or strategies that had helped to safeguard the person's sense of own worth. It may cause rejection by personally important others on whose acceptance, love, and approval the patient's self-regard rested. And finally, it may lead to self-blame, that is, attribution of the illness to having transgressed or otherwise failed to live up to one's moral standards. In all of these instances the patient may evolve negative self-evaluations such as "I am bad," "I am weak," "I am unloved," "I am dependent," "I am ugly, dirty." Such disparaging self-evaluations lower the self-esteem and are a characteristic feature of *depressive illness*.[11]

Alteration of Body Image

Physical illness or injury alters to some extent the patient's body image, that relatively stable concept which everybody evolves about his own body. The most profound, and hence emotionally most disturbing, alteration is likely to follow an illness or injury that has caused a major change in the appearance of the body through disfigurement, mutilation, or dismemberment. Yet even invisible changes in body experience resulting from disease, such as various abnormal spontaneous sensations (paresthesias), or distorted sensory feedback, or disturbed body feelings such as malaise or fatigue, may also alter the person's body image. Such an alteration may be potentially psychopathogenetic, that is, play a contributory role in the development of disease-or injury-related psychiatric disorders.

The postulate that body image changes may play a causal role in psychopathology has been put forth by various writers but not yet adequately tested by empirical studies, and hence remains a plausible hypothesis. Its validity remains to be established by future research. A sizable body of clinical observation does, however, exist which justifies the use of the construct of body image in the discussion of the potentially psychopathogenetic mechanisms set in motion by bodily disease or injury.

The term "body image" (body schema, body percept, corporeal awareness) connotes the concept of, the attitudes toward, and the feelings about one's own body and its parts.[17-22] Schilder,[21] one of the foremost theoreticians in this area, defines body image as the "picture of our own body which we form in our mind, that is to say the way in which the body appears to ourselves" (p. 11). The word "picture" must not be taken to imply that the body image is merely a sort of visual mental representation of one's body. Schilder stresses that although visual impressions are crucial for the formation of the body image, tactile, postural, and indeed all of the senses also contribute to it. Sensory input constantly modifies the body image or schema, yet the latter is relatively stable and serves to modify the incoming sensory impressions. Furthermore, one's interactions with other people influence the body image and to a considerable extent determine one's attitudes toward and feelings about one's own body and its various parts. Brain disease involving the parietal lobe on the nondominant side can give rise to a whole range of body image disturbances, and this provides some support for the belief that the body schema has cerebral localization.[17] Recent research indicates that both parietal lobes as well as the sensorimotor cortex, the parietoccipital area, and the temporal lobe, all contribute to the elaboration of the body image.[22]

Extensive published research on the body image falls into two major categories[22]: (1) studies on body *perception*, which have largely employed the concept of body schema as a plastic model that everybody builds up from his somatic perceptions; and (2), studies of personality, which have employed the construct of body image as a personality variable, one closely linked with other aspects of personality. This research, in contrast to that on body perception, has been concerned with the body as a psychological, value-laden object, rather than with such issues as the accuracy and constancy of the perception of size and other objective body attributes. Personality-oriented research has tried to discover correlations between various measures of personality, on the one hand, and the various aspects of subjective body experience, on the other. Studies on body image boundary, body awareness, body language, and attitudes toward one's body and its parts—all fall into this category.[18,19,22]

The relevance of the concept of body image in the present context is suggested by the clinical observations that disturbances of the body image are caused not only by cerebral disease but also by a wide variety of physical illnesses and injuries that do not involve damage to or demonstrable dysfunction of the brain. Indeed, Schilder[21] claims that the body image is invariably changed by physical illness or injury: "Organic disease provokes abnormal sensations; it immediately changes the image of the body..." (p. 178). In turn, alteration of the body image increases the probability of the development of psychiatric symptoms or disorder. For example, hypochondriasis often follows a traumatic injury, a conversion disorder may be precipitated by disease of the nervous system, and a panic or depersonalization disorder may be induced by vertigo.

Two related hypotheses put forward by Schilder are also germane to this discussion: *unconscious symbolization* and *transposition*. Any body part may become endowed with unconscious symbolic meaning, which thus imparts to it special importance for the individual. For example, any body cavity or entrance to the body may unconsciously symbolize the female sexual organ. Similarly, any protruding part, such as the nose, hand, foot, or tooth, may unconsciously stand for the phallus. Different body parts, or elements of the body image, have different unconscious meaning and value for the given person, determined by his unique, especially childhood, body experience. Consequently, the emotional response to a physical illness or injury may be influenced by the unconscious symbolic meaning of the affected body part. For example, intense anxiety or depression may be elicited by changed sensory input from, damage to, or loss of the body part that has special unconscious significance for the person. Body parts may also become *transposed*, that is, one part may come to stand for another part. Schilder maintains that every round part, for example, can represent another—head, breast, buttock. Every open passage can be interchanged symbolically with another—mouth, ear, nostril, anus, vulva. Such unconscious transposition of parts of the body image may contribute to the occurrence of unexpected and baffling psychological and psychopathological reactions to illness and injury. For instance, loss of hair may trigger a depression of psychotic proportions in a man for whom the hair has come to unconsciously signify the phallus.

Certain parts of the body image are especially important for a given person. Such importance reflects both experiential and sociocultural factors.[20] Every person tends to focus on certain parts of his body and to disregard other parts. Research on *body awareness* has shown wide individual differences in the degree to which people are attuned to the sensory input from the body in general, and from specific body parts in particular.[18] One tends to be especially aware of those body parts which are subjectively highly valued or have become drawn into intrapsychic conflicts or defenses against them. Disease of or injury to a body part, one that the person has invested with especial emotional significance, and of which he or she is acutely aware, creates a high risk for the development of a psychiatric disorder. Injury to the hand or face, for example, is particularly likely to be followed by a depressive disorder.[23-26] Breast and gynecological cancers are postulated to have unique negative impact on body image of the affected woman and hence to constitute a serious risk of psychological decompensation.[27] Construction of a colostomy has been found to result in body image changes and, in some patients, a tendency to depression.[28] On the other hand, results of mutilating surgery, such as amputation, may be accepted with relative equanimity by the patient, suggesting that the *objective extent of body change does not correlate with the degree of body image alteration*, or at least with the intensity of psychological response.[29]

The preceding generalization is strikingly illustrated by the common occurrence of psychopathological, especially depressive, reactions to nondisabling, yet cosmetically disfiguring, chronic skin disorders such as vitiligo.[30] Injury to the nose, a body part often unconsciously equated with the penis, may cause emotional distress quite disproportionate to its severity.[31] On the contrary, a severe physical disability may not be followed by a correspondingly intense psychological reaction.[32]

Not only loss or mutilation but also *addition* of a body part may result in an alteration of the body image that is sufficiently emotionally disturbing to precipitate a psychosis, as exemplified by some cases of kidney and heart transplantation.[33] Moreover, any disease that causes major change in the patient's appearance, such as Cushing's syndrome, acromegaly, or Paget's disease, or any treatment that causes changes in secondary sex characteristics, for example, may induce a profoundly disturbing alteration of the body image and hence enhance a risk of psychopathology.

The concept of the body image has close links with other constructs related to the self such as self-concept, self-esteem, sense of separate identity, and sense of sexual identity. Devaluation of one's own body may undermine one's self-esteem. Poor integration and articulation of the body image tends to go hand in hand with a weak sense of separate identity. Disturbed or confused body image as one of a male or a female is likely to result in a blurred sense of sexual identity. If one accepts these postulated links, then it follows that disturbances of the body image occasioned by physical illness or injury can interfere with all major aspects of the noncorporeal self. Such disturbances may lower self-esteem and weaken one's sense of identity as a separate person and a member of a gender. Any of these consequences is potentially psychopathogenic.

Disruption of Sleep–Wake Cycle

Physical illness is one of the most common causes of insomnia.[34] About one third of Americans more than 18 years of age report having had some problems with sleep during a given year, but only about 2% define their unsatisfactory sleep as "insomnia."[35] In contrast, a study of male and female medical and surgical patients found that about 30% of the former and 40% of the latter suffered from "some form of insomnia."[36] About 70% of psychiatric inpatients suffering from severe insomnia had evidence of physical illness, compared to only 36% of the patients free from insomnia.[37] Ischemic heart disease, obstructive lung disease, and cancer appear to be particularly often associated with disturbed sleep.[38–43] Marked disorganization of sleep patterns has been observed after acute myocardial infarction.[39] Patients with chronic obstructive lung disease have frequent episodes of sleep apnea and oxygen desaturation, and hence nocturnal worsening of hypoxemia.[40,41] Some of these patients display excessive daytime sleepiness and reduced level of awareness.[41] In a pilot study, cancer patients reported a high frequency of disordered nocturnal sleep. Their insomnia correlated positively with anxiety and depression.[43]

Thus, findings reported to date suggest that sleep disorders are common in patients suffering from one of the three most prevalent chronic diseases. It remains to be established whether the observed disturbances of the sleep–wake cycle play a part in the development of psychiatric disorders among the physically ill. Experimental and clinical sleep studies indicate that such a role is indeed likely. An association exists between sleep disturbances and delirium.[44] Disruption of normal sleep patterns accompanies all cases of delirium as well as facilitating its onset and increasing its severity. Sleep deprivation has been suggested to be a major factor contributing to the occurrence of delirium in intensive care units, the so-called ICU syndrome.[45] Experimentally induced total sleep deprivation may produce psychotic symptoms in a vulnerable, if physically healthy, individual.[46] There is some evidence that such vulnerability may be exhibited by persons with the perceptual style of field dependence.[47]

Fragmentation of sleep, in contrast to its total deprivation, has not been found to affect the behavior and performance of physically healthy subjects.[46] It is likely, however, that fragmented sleep may be psychologically disruptive and demoralizing in a physically ill person. Anxiety and depression, which are often present in the physically ill, tend to correlate positively with insomnia, as suggested by our pilot study of cancer patients.[43] A vicious circle seems to develop, in that the emotional distress interferes wth sleep, while sleep loss enhances the distress. Furthermore, there is some evidence that anxiety and other dysphoric emotions increase the psychologically disorganizing effects of sleep deprivation.[48] Some writers have hypothesized that sleep loss constitutes an important factor in the development of acute psychoses.[48] Sleep disturbances often precede as well as accompany acute psychotic decompensation. Psychotic symptoms, such as thought disorder, confusion, hallucinations, and delusions, appear to be facilitated by the disorganization of the normal sleep–wake cycle.

Since few studies have focused specifically on the relationship between disturbed sleep and various forms of psychopathology occurring in the physically ill, one is left with circumstantial evidence of the type just referred to. Such evidence, coupled with personal and published clinical impressions, does suggest that disruption of the sleep–wake cycle plays a contributory role in the development of both organic and functional psychiatric disorders among the physically ill.

Social Alienation and Isolation

Physical illness or injury may result in the patient's becoming alienated and more or less isolated from his social environment. This undesirable outcome may be brought about by the nature of the disease and its symptoms, or by the patient's behavior induced by the illness. A disease that is stigmatized, or one that causes disfigurement or some form of visible disability, or one manifested by symptoms that other people consider revolting is likely to alienate the patient from others.(Chapter 8, this volume).

The following clinical vignette illustrates this problem. A middle-aged female patients had a colostomy constructed for colonic cancer. She was a single woman living with her sister, who was her only surviving close relative. The patient recovered well from surgery and seemed to respond adaptively to the fact that she had cancer and needed a colostomy. She was discharged from the hospital and returned home in a good emotional state. On the first day at home her sister remarked. "You stink." The patient responded with a rapidly deepening depression, which eventually necessitated her admission to a psychiatric unit.

This case illustrates how disease may elicit rejection of the patient by a key other person, with the consequent loss of self-esteem, unexpressed and self-directed rage, hopelessness, and depressive disorder. Any disfiguring disease, such as psoriasis, may have a similar effect. Stoughton[49] speaks of the "heartbreak of psoriasis" and describes some of the problems of patients suffering from that skin disease as follows: "Large, prominent red plaques on their skin are a source of constant embarrassment because of misunderstanding or even ridicule on the part of those who behold the marred skin surfaces of the carrier. Psoriasis is not just a skin disease; it is a high personal tragedy." Stoughton points out that of some five million victims of psoriasis in the United States, about 10% display very serious difficulties in adaptation which are due, in part, to the social reactions to the patient's visible skin lesions.

Visible disfigurement, such as that due to psoriasis, and disability tend to provoke aversive social responses. Such negative attitudes toward and the consequent avoidance of the victims have been studied by psychologists and sociologists.[50-52] The term "stigma" has been used by these investigators to refer to any physical attribute of a person that results in his being discredited and avoided. Stigmatized conditions are typically, but not exclusively, those which are visible.[50-53] To be stigmatized implies being to some extent alienated and isolated. In turn, alienation and isolation tend to have a damaging effect on the patient's body image and self-esteem, and thereby to contribute to the development of psychopathology, such as a depressive disorder.

Summary and Conclusions

I have proposed a multifactorial schema for the pathogenesis of psychiatric disorders occurring in the physically ill. Factors inherent in the patient, the disease, and the patient's social environment all contribute. Physical illness and injury may lead to psychopathology through one or both of two basic pathogenetic mechanisms: cerebral damage or dysfunction and stressful meaning of illness for the patient, respectively. Furthermore, the development of a psychiatric disorder may be facilitated by one or more of the postulated seven auxiliary mechanisms: frustration, intrapsychic conflict, failure of defenses, lowered self-esteem, altered body image, disturbed sleep-wake cycle, and social isolation and alienation. Individuals vary in their susceptibility to the psychologically disorganizing effects of these potentially pathogenetic factors. It is postulated that the most common psychiatric complications of physical illness, which include organic brain syndromes and anxiety and depressive disorders, result from the operation of one or more of the psychopathogenetic factors described in this chapter.

REFERENCES

1. Lipowski ZJ: Psychiatry of somatic diseases: Epidemiology, pathogenesis, classification. *Compr Psychiatry* 16:105–124, 1975.

2. Eilenberg MD: Psychiatric illness and pernicious anemia: A clinical re-evaluation. *J Ment Sci* 106:1539–1543, 1960.

3. Susser M: *Causal Thinking in the Health Sciences*. New York, Oxford University Press, 1973.

4. Murphy E, Brown GW: Life events, psychiatric disturbance and physical illness. *Br J Psychiatry* 136:326–338, 1980.

5. Lloyd GG, Cawley RH: Psychiatric morbidity in men one week after first acute myocardial infarction. *Br Med J* 2:1453–1454, 1978.

6. Lipowski ZJ: Organic brain syndromes: New classification, concepts and prospects. *Can J Psychiatry* 29:198–204, 1984.

7. Lazarus RS, Folkman S: *Stress, Appraisal, and Coping*. New York, Springer Publishing Co., 1984.

8. Hilgard ER, Atkinson RL, Atkinson RC: *Introduction to Psychology*, ed 7. New York, Harcourt Brace Jovanovich, 1979.

9. Verwoerdt A: Psychopathological responses to the stress of physical illness, in Lipowski ZJ (ed): *Psychosocial Aspects of Physical Illness*. Basel, Karger, 1972, pp 119–141.

10. Wylie RC: *The Self Concept*. Lincoln, University of Nebraska Press, 1961.

11. Beck AT: *Depression*. New York, Harper & Row, 1967.

12. Bibring E: The mechanism of depression, in Greenacre P (ed): *Affective Disorders*. New York, International Universities Press, 1953.

13. Fenichel O: *The Psychoanalytic Theory of Neurosis*. New York, WW Norton & Co., 1945.

14. Gill MM (ed): *The Collected Papers of David Rapaport*. New York, Basic Books, 1967.

15. Jacobson E: Contribution to the metapsychology of cyclothymic depression, in Greenacre P (ed): *Affective Disorders*. New York, International Universities Press, 1953.

16. Mendelson M: *Psychoanalytic Concepts of Depression*. Springfield, Ill, Charles C Thomas, 1960.

17. Critchley M: Disorders of corporeal awareness, in Wapner S, Witkin HA (eds): *The Body Percept*. New York, Random House, 1965.

18. Fisher S: *Body Experience in Fantasy and Behavior*. New York, Appleton-Century-Crofts, 1970.

19. Fisher S, Cleveland SE: *Body Image and Personality*. Princeton, NJ, Van Nostrand Co., 1958.

20. Lipowski ZJ: The importance of body experience for psychiatry. *Compr Psychiatry* 18:473–479, 1977.

21. Schilder P: *The Image and Appearance of the Human Body*. New York, International Universities Press, 1950.

22. Shontz FC: *Perceptual and Cognitive Aspects of Body Experience*. New York, Academic Press, 1969.

23. Cone J, Hueston JT: Psychological aspects of hand injury. *Med J Aust* 1:104–108, 1974

24. Macgregor FC: *Transformation and Identity. The Face and Plastic Surgery*. New York, Quadrangle, 1974.

25. Solnit AJ, Priel B: Psychological reactions to facial and hand burns in young men. *Psychoanal Stud Child* 30:549–566, 1975.

26. Steiner H, Clark WR: Psychiatric complications of burned adults: A classification. *J Trauma* 17:134–143, 1977.

27. Derogatis LR: Breast and gynecologic cancers. *Front Radiat Ther Oncol* 14:1–11, 1980.

28. Orbach CE, Tallent N: Modification of perceived body and of body concepts. *Arch Gen Psychiatry* 12:126–135, 1965.

29. Earle EM: The psychological effects of mutilating surgery in children and adolescents. *Psychoanal Stud Child* 34:527–546, 1979.

30. Porter J, Nordlund JJ, Beuf AH, Lerner AB: Psychological reaction to chronic skin disorders. A study of patients with vitiligo. *Gen Hosp Psychiatry* 1:73–77, 1979.

31. Book HE: Sexual implications of the nose. *Compr Psychiatry* 12:450–455, 1971.

32. Shontz FC: Physical disability and personality: Theory and recent research. *Psychol Aspects Disabil* 17:51–69, 1970.

33. Castelnuovo-Tedesco P: Organ transplant, body image, psychosis. *Psychoanal Quart* 42:349–363, 1973.

34. Kales JD, Kales A: Nocturnal psychophysiological correlates of somatic conditions and sleep disorders, in Lipowski ZJ, Lipsitt DR, Whybrow PC (eds): *Psychosomatic Medicine. Current Trends and Clinical Applications.* New York, Oxford University Press, 1977, pp 335-354.
35. Solomon F, White CC, Parron DL, Mendelson WB: Sleeping pills, insomnia and medical practice. *N Engl J Med* 300:803-808, 1979.
36. Johns MW: Factor analysis of subjectively reported sleep habits, and the nature of insomnia. *Psycho Med* 5:83-88, 1975.
37. Grumet GW: Severe insomnia in psychiatric inpatients. *Dis Nerv Syst* 29:256-258, 1968.
38. Johns MW, Egan P, Gay TJA, Masterton JP: Sleep habits and symptoms in male medical and surgical patients. *Br Med J* 2:509-512, 1970.
39. Broughton R, Baron R: Sleep patterns in the intensive care unit and on the ward after acute myocardial infarction. *Electroenceph Clin Neurophysiol* 45:348-360, 1978.
40. Guilleminault C, Lugaresi E (eds): *Sleep/Wake Disorders: Natural History, Epidemiology, and Long-Term Evolution.* New York, Raven Press, 1983.
41. Grant I, Heaton RK, McSweeney AJ, et al: Neuropsychologic findings in hypoxemic chronic obstructive pulmonary disease. *Arch Intern Med* 142:1470-1476, 1982.
42. Kinsman RA, Yaroush RA, Fernandez F, et al: Symptoms and experiences in chronic bronchitis and emphysema. *Chest* 83:755-761, 1983.
43. Beszterczey A, Lipowski ZJ: Insomnia in cancer patients. *Can Med Assoc J* 116:355, 1977.
44. Lipowski ZJ: *Delirium. Acute Brain Failure in Man.* Springfield, Ill, Charles C Thomas, 1980.
45. Helton MC, Gordon SH, Nunnery SL: The correlation between sleep deprivation and the intensive care unit syndrome. *Heart Lung* 9:464-468, 1980.
46. Johnson LC: The effect of total, partial, and stage sleep deprivation on EEG patterns and performance, in Bureh N, Altschuler HL (eds): *Behavior and Brain Electrical Activity.* New York, Plenum Publishing Co., 1974, pp 1-30.
47. Cartwright RD, Monroe LJ, Palmer C: Individual differences in response to REM deprivation. *Arch Gen Psychiatry* 16:297-303, 1967.
48. Gove WR: Sleep deprivation: A cause of psychotic disorganization. *Am J Sociology* 75:782-799, 1970.
49. Stoughton RB: The heartbreak of psoriasis. *JAMA* 229:334, 1974.
50. Goffman E: *Stigma: Notes on the Management of Spoiled Identity.* Englewood Cliffs, NJ, Prentice-Hall, 1963.
51. Kleck R: Physical stigma and nonverbal cues emitted in face-to-face interaction. *Hum Relations* 21:19-28, 1968.
52. Noonan JR, Barry JR, Davis HC: Personality determinants in attitudes toward visible disability. *J Personality* 38:1-15, 1970.
53. Ablon J: Stigmatized health conditions. *Soc Sci Med* 15:5-9, 1981.

Organic Mental Disorders

12

General Psychopathology

INTRODUCTION

The current official classification of mental disorders adopted by the American Psychiatric Association in 1980, or DSM-III,[1] distinguishes between organic mental disorders (OMD) and organic brain syndromes (OBS). The former term is used to designate a particular OBS whose etiology is known, for example, barbiturate withdrawal delirium or alcohol hallucinosis. "Organic brain syndrome" refers to a set of descriptive characteristics, or psychopathological symptoms and signs, without reference to etiology. This distinction implies that each OBS may be a manifestation of more than one possible etiological factor. If such a factor has been identified in a given case of an OBS, then the term "organic mental disorder" may be used.

OMD comprise psychopathological manifestations of brain damage or dysfunction, or both. These manifestations may include abnormalities or deficits in any aspect of mental functioning or behavior, be it personality, cognition, drives, emotions, attention, or psychomotor behavior. Clinical observation has led to the identification of several distinct clusters of such abnormalities or deficits, the so-called OBS, which are believed to be caused directly by cerebral disorders.[2] The latter may be primary, that is, having their origin in the brain, or secondary to systemic disease or exogenous poisons. The underlying cerebral disease may be diffuse, focal, or both, and constitutes a necessary condition for the occurrence of an OBS. Clearly, a great many potential causes of OBS exist. They may be divided into four main classes: (1) primary cerebral disease; (2) systemic diseases affecting the brain secondarily; (3) exogenous toxic agents; and (4) withdrawal from certain abused substances, such as alcohol.

OBS do not represent a homogeneous group in the sense that no single psychopathological feature characterizes all of them. It must be emphasized, however, that the most common, and hence clinically the most important, OBS, namely, delirium and dementia, feature deficits and abnormalities in all the major aspects of cognition.[2] This fact is no doubt responsible for the traditional, if erroneous, view that cognitive impairment is the invariable psychopathological manifestation of cerebral disease and hence the only identifying feature of OBS. DMS-III represents a departure from this view in that it includes among the OBS those in which cognition is not significantly affected.[1-4]

OMD have increasingly come into focus lately as a growing psychiatric, public health, and social problem, one closely related to the rising number of the elderly, those aged 65 years and over, who are especially prone to develop delirium and dementia.[2-4] A recent medical editorial speaks of dementia as an epidemic "casting a sombre shadow into the 2lst century."[5] More than 25 million Americans are currently aged 65 years or more, and this number is expected to double over the next 50 years.[6] This demographic trend justifies prediction that the incidence and prevalence of OBS will grow steadily, and that familiarity with them will be required of all physicians and not just psychiatrists, who incidentally have displayed remarkably little interest in them over the past three decades.[3] Apart from aging of the population, several factors contribute to a high incidence and prevalence of OMD: substance, especially alcohol, abuse; head injury; and diseases leading to cerebral hypoxia. Furthermore, advances in critical care medicine have enabled survival of many brain-damaged individuals, and new medical drugs include many that have cerebrotoxic side effects. All these factors conspire to ensure high frequency of OBS in the population, and especially in hospitals, in the years to come.

Etiology and Pathogenesis

OBS constitute psychopathological manifestations of brain damage or dysfunction. The underlying cerebral disorder may be primary, i.e., originating in the brain, or secondary, i.e., having its origin elsewhere in the body. Any form of pathology may be implicated: metabolic, traumatic, toxic, vascular, degenerative, infectious, or neoplastic. A given etiological factor may give rise to more than one OBS. For example, a brain tumor may induce delirium, dementia, amnesic syndrome, hallucinosis, or organic personality syndrome. The occurrence of one rather than another OBS appears to be influenced by such factors as the site and size of the brain lesion, its rate of growth or spread, the presence of raised intracranial pressure, and the degree of interference with cerebral blood flow, metabolism, and neurotransmission. What results is a set of psychological deficits or abnormalities reflecting some degree and pattern of disruption of the normal, integrated functioning of the cerebral substrate of mental activity and observable behavior.

One or more pathogenetic mechanisms may be brought into play by the etiological organic factors. *Cerebral neurons may be destroyed*, resulting in a loss of function dependent on their integrity or in a release from inhibition of other, sometimes even distant, brain structures. *Metabolism* of the brain as a whole, or of one of its parts, may become reduced or deranged, with resulting global or circumscribed functional failure. *Normal neurotransmission* may be disrupted, resulting in some form or degree of disorganization of the mental functions, such as memory or attention, or in an abnormal mood. Much remains unknown in this area despite remarkable recent progress in unraveling brain–behavior relationships in health and disease.

Although the presence of one or more organic factors listed in the introduction is considered to be a necessary condition for the occurrence of an OBS, *psychosocial factors* must also be taken into account. Behavior may play a causative role, as is the case in substance abuse, for example. Such variables as the personality, intelligence, educational level, coping style, and overall premorbid adjustment of the patient influence the form and severity of the psychopathology induced by cerebral disorders.

Subjective meaning of the perceived deficits in performance brought about by the organic disease may elicit a whole range of emotions, defensive strategies, and overt behaviors in the affected individual and serve to modify the presenting clinical picture. These psychological responses may take the form of a functional psychiatric disorder superimposed on, and at time increasing the severity of, the direct behavioral effects of cerebral pathology. Depression and anxiety, for example, are common emotional responses to subjective awareness of cognitive impairment and tend to magnify the latter, thus increasing the degree of disability. Social variables, such as bereavement or social isolation, may also influence the timing of manifest onset and the severity of cognitive impairment. Certain aspects of the sensory inputs impinging on the brain-damaged individual, such as their underload or overload, novelty, complexity, or ambiguity, may adversely affect his cognitive performance.

Thus, OMD should be viewed *holistically*, in that they represent the outcome of interaction of multiple factors, biological, psychological, and social. A biopsychosocial approach to these disorders is essential for the study and proper management of the individual patient.

GENERAL PSYCHOPATHOLOGY

OMD are no longer viewed as exclusively disorders of cognition. Not a single psychological impairment or abnormality may be regarded as an invariable or pathognomonic feature of cerebral damage or dysfunction. Heterogeneity of psychopathological manifestations of brain disorders has been formally acknowledged in DSM-III.[1,4] This recognition does not, however, gainsay the clinical observation that certain psychopathological manifestations are particularly likely to be associated with cerebral disease and hence provide valuable clinical clues to its diagnosis. These manifestations include the following impairments and abnormalities of psychological functioning[2]:

1. Impairment of cognitive functions.
2. Personality change.
3. Disorders of awareness, wakefulness, and attention.
4. Compensatory and protective strategies.

IMPAIRMENT OF COGNITIVE FUNCTIONS

Reception, processing, storage, and retrieval of information constitute the realm of cognition. Their optimal operation is indispensable for problem solving, action planning, decision making, and purposeful behavior and hence for adaptation to and coping with the environment. Perceiving, remembering, and thinking are the main cognitive functions, and all of them depend on intact and integrated function of the brain. When such function is impaired by relatively widespread damage to or metabolic derangement of the brain, the cognitive functions may be globally impaired. If brain structures subserving specific cognitive functions, such as memory, are damaged, then the corresponding function is likely to be *selectively* impaired. Disorders of cognitive functioning observed clinically include some constellation of the following deficits and abnormalities:

1. Overall decrement of intellectual functioning compared to the patient's premorbid performance.
2. Memory impairment, most often manifested as impaired recall of relatively recently acquired information or by ineffective formation of new memories and hence inadequate ability to learn. Remote memory is usually less likely to be affected.
3. Impairment of capacity for abstract thinking in all its aspects: concept formation, reasoning, calculation, problem solving, action planning, and judgment.
4. Impaired performance on novel and complex tasks as well as reduced ability to continue performing despite distractions by irrelevant stimuli.
5. Impaired spatiotemporal orientation.
6. Impaired grasp of the meaning of information inputs with resulting perplexity.
7. Impaired perceptual discrimination and/or experience of abnormal perceptions such as illusions and hallucinations, especially in the visual sphere.

In the OBS these impairments and abnormalities may occur in different temporal sequences and degrees of severity, singly or in various combinations. Impairments of memory and abstract thinking are the most common psychopathological manifestations of cerebral disease. The presence of such impairments in a patient provides an important clinical clue that brain damage or dysfunction exists and should prompt appropriate laboratory investigations. It should be kept in mind, however, that cognitive impairment may at times be manifested by patients free of demonstrable brain disorder and suffering from an affective disorder, for example.[2]

"Cognitive impairment" is an abstract concept, an inference from an individual's observed performance and subjective complaints. Cognitive or intellectual performance may be observed in a patient's everyday setting or in a neuropsychological laboratory. Work situation provides the most common "natural" setting in which cognitive deficits are likely to come to light first. The patient may draw disapproving attention to his occupational performance as a result of making unaccustomed errors or because of lapses of memory or judgment. The patient may display distractibility, perplexity, and fatigue.[7] Sustained mental effort tends to elicit fatigue and failing performance. Relatively novel and complex tasks are handled with growing difficulty, as are those which require vigilance and call for screening out of irrelevant information or for fine discrimination.[8] The patient may appear perplexed and flustered when faced with routine tasks and situations and may voice distrust in his ability to deal with them.[7] Customary efficiency and competence fall off, mistakes mount, and signs of deterioration of the habitual level of occupational performance multiply. It is important to recognize these relatively early and subtle manifestations of cognitive impairment, as such recognition should result in timely diagnostic investigations and proper treatment of the underlying brain disorder.[7,8]

The patient may not voice any complaints about, and actually deny awareness of, cognitive impairment. If he does complain about it, it is mostly in terms of forgetfulness, confusion, poor concentration, fatigue after mental effort, or difficulty meeting the demands of the job. Such complaints should always alert the clinician to the possibility that an OMD is present.

PERSONALITY CHANGE

A common manifestation of cerebral disease, both focal and widespread, is a change in the patient's characteristic ways of acting and reacting. This change may represent either an *accentuation* of the individual's personality traits or its true *alteration*, that is, emergence of attitudes and behaviors uncharacteristic for the patient. In the former case, the patient becomes more obessional, distrustful, impulsive, or histrionic than previously. His personality style may become accentuated to the point of caricature. On the contrary, a true alteration of the personality implies the appearance of behavior that prompts observers to remark that the patient is not himself but a changed person. Personality change may accompany demonstrable cognitive impairment or, less often, constitute the only or the most striking manifestation of cerebral disease. Organic personality syndrome is a designation for the OBS featuring personality change in the relative absence of cognitive deficits.

Aspects of personality that are most often affected by cerebral disease include expression and control of emotions, drives, and impulses.[2] Verbal and nonverbal expression of emotions becomes poorly modulated, precipitate, overly facile, and labile. The patient is likely to express any emotion with little restraint or consideration and to display so-called emotional lability, that is, cry, laugh, or show anger freely and switch from one emotional expression to another with undue ease. Some patients manifest mostly apathy, euphoria, or irritability. Outbursts of anger, sometimes leading to violence, may appear and result in criminal acts. Other patients display the atypical mawkish sentimentality and cry readily. This behavior is sometimes mistaken for depression, but closer observation reveals that the patient's emotions are shallow and transient and lack the depth and consistency of emotional expression of someone suffering from an affective disorder. Such emotional disinhibition and blunting are quite striking when displayed by a person who used to show emotions appropriately and selectively in the past. Patients suffering from an organic affective syndrome, however, provide an exception in that their expression of affective change tends to be indistinguishable from that of a sufferer from a corresponding functional disorder, depressive or manic.

Not only the expression of emotions but also that of drives and impulses is often affected by brain disease and contributes to personality change. A common change involves a general reduction in the intensity of drives, a falling off in manifest initiative, curiosity, and perserverance. Interests become narrower, and to outside observers the patient may appear strikingly dull and without zest. Some patients display unaccustomed lack of impulse control. They may act on any impulse, be it sexual, acquisitive, or hostile, with little restraint or concern for its impact on others or even on their own welfare. The patient may make inappropriate sexual advances, shoplift, offend others with coarse jokes or invidious comments, eat ravenously, or strike a person with little provocation. At the same time, expression of finer impulses and sentiments, aesthetic, charitable, ethical, or caring, tends to fade away, and the personality as a whole becomes impoverished.

DISORDERS OF AWARENESS, WAKEFULNESS, AND ATTENTION

Optimal levels of wakefulness, awareness, and attention are necessary for reception and processing of information, for selective recall, and for programming, regulating, and verifying mental activity and behavior.[9] An optimal level of cerebral activation or arousal as well as of the waking state of the cerebral cortex enables organized and purposeful mental activity and behavior to be initiated and to proceed. In states of reduced or excessive cerebral activation and abnormally diminished waking state, the person's awareness of environment and ability to attend to stimuli in a directed, selective, and sustained manner are impaired. As a result, cognitive processes tend to become disorganized and relatively ineffective, and purposeful mental activity and behavior become erratic or even impossible. The patient may find it difficult to distinguish imagery and dreams from true perceptions, to grasp the meaning of and register incoming information, and to think coherently.

Traditionally for the past century or so, many authors have used the concept of consciousness to encompass aspects of mental activity discussed in this section. Terms such as *clouding* or reduction of consciousness and mental confusion have been used to designate disturbances of awareness, wakefulness, and attention.[2,10] As no single definition of consciousness has been generally accepted to date, related terms, such as ''clouding of consciousness,'' remain ambiguous. For this reason, it is better to speak of *awareness* rather than consciousness. This term, in contrast to consciousness, is more descriptive than theoretical and hence relatively free of semantic ambiguity. One can be more or less aware of one's surroundings, or of one's self, or of one's commerce with the environment. Awareness is typically impaired in conditions of both reduced and abnormally heightened wakefullness, as in both these states the capacity for selective and sustained attention is diminished. Both states facilitate the occurrence of perceptual abnormalities, especially visual illusions and hallucinations.[10] Disorders of wakefulness, awareness, and attention are usually the consequence of relatively widespread disturbance of cerebral metabolism of acute onset, but they may also result from focal, especially vascular, lesions. They constitute the core psychopathology of delirium.[10]

COMPENSATORY AND PROTECTIVE STRATEGIES

Awareness of deficits in cognitive performance tends to motivate the patient to employ certain characteristic strategies aimed at compensation for the impairment and protection against anxiety, shame, and frustration triggered by failure to perform. As these compensatory and protective tactics are fairly stereotypical, they provide valuable clinical clues to the presence of cerebral disease, regardless of whether they are judged to be adaptive or not. Goldstein[11] made a pioneering study of these strategies in his large series of brain-damaged patients. He proposed that failure of a brain-damaged patient to perform a given task in a manner to which he was accustomed prior to the damage tends to elicit the so-called *catastrophic reaction*, that is, an intense and unpleasant emotional state similar to acute panic. The patient strives to avoid this distressing state by resorting to the protective and compensatory strategies, whose purpose is to ward off the experience of the catastrophic reaction.

Extreme orderliness, unawareness or denial of cognitive defect obvious to others, avoidance of testing situations in which defects could be exposed, evasion of performance by angry refusal or facetious excuses, perserveration, circumstantiality, and confabulation represent the most common forms of compensatory and protective strategies. The patient tends to employ them in various combinations so as to conceal, explain away, minimize, and make up for his defective performance.

The deficits and abnormalities discussed here comprise the main essential and associated features of currently recognized OBS and constitute the most common and important manifestations of cerebral damage or dysfunction. Relatively widespread brain pathology is manifested by more or less *global* impairment of cognitive funcitons, and hence by delirium or dementia. In contrast, focal brain lesions and various endocrine disorders and intoxication by certain exogenous poisons tend to induce a relatively *circumscribed* cognitive deficit or abnormality, represented by the amnestic syndrome and organic hallucinosis, respectively, or by an organic personality syndrome, or by an organic affective or delusional syndrome.[2]

REACTIVE PSYCHOPATHOLOGY

In addition to the symptoms of the various OBS, cerebral disorders often give rise to psychopathological manifestations that may be regarded as *reactive* to the awareness and personal meaning of the deficits and adnormalities for the patient. These reactive disorders may take the form of any type of functional psychosis, of neurosis, or of behavioral disorder and reflect the given patient's personality, conflicts, habitual defense mechanisms, quality of interpersonal relationships, and other variables. These reactive syndromes merge imperceptibly with the alteration of personality. It is impossible in clinical practice to distinguish sharply the direct effects of pathology on psychological functioning from the indirect ones occasioned by the response to the personal consequences of a cerebral insult by the *person as a whole*. As the reactive symptoms may initially be prominent in the patient's presenting clinical picture, it is important for the clinician to be aware of them.

Subjective awareness of the psychological deficits and abnormalities induced by cerebral disease may signify threat, or loss, or both, for the patient. Such meanings are likely to elicit more or less intense emotions of anxiety, grief, depression, anger, or shame. These emotions are experienced and manifested with varying degrees of intensity. Those persons for whom high-quality cognitive performance serves as a vital source of self-esteem, security, and gratification are especially likely to view intellectual deficits and perceptual distortions as a grave threat or less, and to react with correspondingly intense emotions. Some patients may commit suicide.[12] Others try to contain the painful emotions by employing various defense mechanisms such as projection, dissociation, regression, conversion, or somatization and manifest symptoms reflecting the choice of the particular mechanisms. Thus the patient may present with manifestations of a paranoid, or a somatoform, or a dissociative disorder. For example, an individual with a paranoid personality may begin to display a frank paranoid psychosis, featuring delusions of persecution, or jealousy, or somatic change. Many organic patients initially consult doctors for a variety of physical complaints, or symptoms of depression or anxiety, and may display marked hypochondriasis. When such complaints are voiced for the first time by a middle-aged or elderly person, one free of past history of psychiatric disorder, the clinician should carefully inquire into cognitive performance and medical history with a view to ruling out an early cerebral disorder, primary or secondary.

Summary and Conclusions

OMD constitute a clinical area of growing importance, largely owing to aging of the population and the high incidence and prevalence of these disorders in the elderly. A large number of organic factors can give rise to these disorders, which represent psychological, or psychopathological, manifestations of brain damage, or dysfunction, or both. Although impairment of some or all cognitive functions is a common and important feature of brain disorders, they may at times result primarily in abnormalities of personality or mood that are difficult to distinguish from the so-called functional mental disorders. Cognitive impairment as well as disorder of awareness, wakefulness, and attention may be viewed as psychopathological manifestations whose presence in a given individual offers presumptive, but not conclusive, evidence that a demonstrable brain disease or disorder is likely to be present. The same statement applies to personality change of the type described in this chapter.

Some of the manifestations of OBS are viewed as their essential and hence diagnostically crucial features. One needs to stress, however, that the psychopathology of cerebral disorders encompasses maladaptive, or pathological, reactions of the patient to the awareness and personal meaning of deficits and abnormalities brought about by deranged brain function. These reactions may take the form of any functional psychosis, or neurosis, or behavior disorder. It is essential to view an "organic" patient, that is, one suffering from a cerebral disorder, as a whole, and to adopt a biopsychosocial approach to diagnosis and overall management.

References

1. *Diagnostic and Statistical Manual of Mental Disorders*, ed 3. *DSM III*. Washington, DC, American Psychiatric Association, 1980.
2. Lipowski ZJ: Organic mental disorders: Introduction and review of syndromes, in Kaplan HI, Freedman AM, Sadock BJ (eds): *Comprehensive Textbook of Psychiatry*, 3. Baltimore, Williams & Wilkins, 1980, pp 1359–1391.
3. Lipowski ZJ: Organic brain syndromes: A reformulation. *Compr Psychiatry* 19:309–322, 1978.
4. Lipowski ZJ: Organic brain syndromes: New classification, concepts and prospects. *Can J Psychiatry* 29:198–204, 1984.
5. Editorial: Dementia: The quiet epidemic. *Br Med J* 1:1–2, 1978.
6. Siegel JS: *Demographic Aspects of Aging and the Older Population in the United States*. Special Studies Series P-23, Number 59. Washington, DC, US Department of Commerce, Bureau of Census, May 1976.
7. Lezak MD: Subtle sequelae of brain damage. *Am J Phys Med* 57: 9–15, 1978.
8. Chapman, LF, Wolff HG: Diseases of the neopallium. *Med Clin North Am* 42:677–689, 1958.
9. Luria AR: *The Working Brain*, London, Penguin Books, 1973.
10. Lipowski ZJ: *Delirium: Acute Brain Failure in Man*. Springfield, Ill, Charles C Thomas, 1980.
11. Goldstein K: *Aftereffects of Brain Injuries in War*. New York, Grune & Stratton, 1942.
12. Rice E: Organic brain syndromes and suicide. *Int J Psychoanal Psychother* 2:338–363, 1973.

Organic Brain Syndromes

New Classification, Concepts, and Prospects

13

Psychiatric manifestations of brain disorders are fast becoming a major area of research at the interface between psychiatry and the neurosciences. Neglected by investigators and clinicans alike for decades, the organic mental disorders (OMD) have attracted growing interest recently on account of their high prevalence and incidence among the elderly, whose numbers are increasing throughout the Western world and are expected to continue mounting in the coming years. Editorials in medical journals speak of an epidemic of dementia, for example, and call attention to its importance as a public health and social problem of staggering proportions. Clearly, organic psychiatric disorders can no longer be ignored by psychiatrists, who ought to play a leading role in efforts to advance knowledge and therapy in this area.

As a first step towards revitalization of this field it was necessary to revise the concept, terminology, and classification of the OMD, so as to facilitate case findings for epidemiologic and other studies, to improve communication, and to stimulate clinical investigations. As a result of the long neglect of the OMD, and in turn contributing to their conceptually underdeveloped state, the semantic and nosological aspects in this area of psychiatry had been marked by confusion and oversimplification. Undefined and overlapping terms had been used indiscriminately, and were compounded by an overly narrow conception of organicity and an oversimplified classification of the OMD. Preparation of the new official classification of the American Psychiatric Association, or DSM-III,[1] provided a timely opportunity to reassess and reformulate the whole category of OMD in the light of accrued clinical observations.

DSM-III represents a radical departure from the two previous American classifications, that is, DSM-I[2] and DSM-II.[3] Its main innovative features include the provision of explicit diagnostic criteria for every disorder, a multiaxial diagnostic system, and a predominantly descriptive approach to nosology. One of the most sweeping changes to be found in DSM-III concerns the classification and definitions of the OMD. As a member of the task force that developed DSM-III, I was closely involved with that effort and am familiar with the reasoning behind the changes. I propose to present in this chapter the salient features of the new definition and classification of the OMD and discuss their implications for research and practice.

Reprinted from *Canadian Journal of Psychiatry* 29:198–204, 1984. Copyright © 1984 by *Canadian Journal of Psychiatry*. Reprinted by permission. This work was supported in part by GP Special Training Grant MH-13172 from NIMH.

ORGANIC BRAIN SYNDROMES IN DSM-I AND DSM-II

To appreciate the extent of the changes introduced by DSM-III in its treatment of the OMD it is necessary to review briefly the core features of the approach to them in the two previous American classifications, that is, DSM-I[2] and DSM-II.[3] DSM-I, which came into force in 1952, included a category called "organic brain disorders," which were subdivided into acute or reversible and chronic or irreversible. DSM-II, adopted in 1968, substituted the word "syndromes" for "disorders" and subdivided them into psychotic and nonpsychotic, while the subdivision into acute and chronic syndromes was recommended as an option. The organic brain syndromes (OBS) were defined as a class of mental disorders caused by or associated with impaired brain tissue function. Their essential feature was stated to be "the basic organic brain syndrome," one characterized by impairment of orientation, all intellectual functions, memory, and judgment, and by lability or shallowness of affect. Thus, the OBS were defined almost exclusively in terms of a *global disorder of cognition*.

CRITIQUE OF DSM-I AND DSM-II

The above approach to and terminology of the OBS became firmly entrenched in North American psychiatry despite their serious flaws. The chief defect of the two previous classifications in the area of the OMD was their overly narrow and restricted definition. Presenting "the basic organic syndrome" as *the* essential criterion for their diagnosis, DSM-II restricted the class OMD to those that featured global cognitive impairment, and by implication excluded a whole range of noncognitive psychiatric correlates of brain disorders.

A search of the literature suggests[4] that the concept of the "basic organic syndrome" was derived from E. Bleuler's[5] "organic psycho-syndrome," which he introduced as a label for psychiatric manifestations of only the chronic, diffuse, cerebral cortical damage. E. Bleuler's son, Manfred, wrote of his father's concept that "forty years ago our clinic called this syndrome 'psycho-organic syndrome'; this was at a time when it was not known that *many other organically caused psychosyndromes existed*" (italics mine, ZJL).[6] In the same article, M. Bleuler described the chronic *focal* psychosyndrome, one associated with focal brain lesions and various endocrine disorders. The focal syndrome's essential features were to include altered emotionality, reduced or increased intensity of drives, defective impulse control, and relatively intact cognitive function.

M. Bleuler's landmark paper seems to have been overlooked by the compilers of DSM-I, which was published 1 year later and imposed E. Bleuler's explicitly delimited concept as the defining characteristic of the whole class of OMD. Thus, officially sanctioned, that restricted concept prevailed and likely helped slow down progress in the area of organic psychiatry for the next 30 years, until the introduction of DSM-III. Meanwhile, the rapid growth of general hospital psychiatry presented psychiatrists with an unprecedented opportunity to study psychopathological manifestations of a wide range of cerebral disorders, both acute and chronic, and both primary and secondary to systemic diseases and toxic agents. As a result, it became apparent that the basic organic syndrome failed to do justice to the true scope of psychiatric correlates of cerebral dysfunction.

Focal brain lesions, certain systemic diseases, and various exogenous chemicals tend to give rise to relatively circumscribed rather than across-the-board cognitive deficits or abnormalities, or to alteration of personality characteristics of the individual, or even to syndromes indistinguishable on a descriptive level from paranoid, schizophrenic, and affective disorders. All of these assorted psychopathological symptoms and syndromes logically belong to the "organic" category, in the sense that demonstrable or inferred cerebral dysfunction constitutes a necessary condition for their occurrence, yet they do not conform to the definition of the "basic organic syndrome." Consequently, there was no proper place for those psychiatric syndromes in the official classification. Clearly, the latter was flawed and had to be revised.

The subdivisions into psychotic versus nonpsychotic and acute (reversible) versus chronic (irreversible) OBS also had serious disadvantages.[7] The former subdivision was of little value in this area of psychiatry, as it conveyed little useful information, was ill defined and too arbitrary, and tended to stigmatize socially a patient labelled "psychotic." The acute versus chronic distinction created a spurious dichotomy, one based on a prognostic judgment that was often unwarranted for lack of reliable criteria for prediction. In many cases the clinician had to classify a patient on the basis of a cross-sectional clinical assessment which could be quite misleading with regard to prognosis. For example, a victim of a severe head injury or of cardiac arrest could display a marked degree of cognitive impairment which might over a period of months, or even years, remit partially or even completely. To ascertain the degree of restitution of cognitive function in such cases requires a prolonged follow-up and repeated careful evaluation of the patient. To diagnose the latter as suffering from a chronic, that is, irreversible, OBS in the absence of such a follow-up could be erroneous and have disastrous consequences for the patient so misdiagnosed. For example, it could result in a failure to detect and treat a cerebral disorder, such as normal pressure hydrocephalus, before permanent brain damage has occurred. Reversibility of cognitive dysfunction must not be viewed as an all-or-none attribute, but as a spectrum of degrees of functional recovery which could range from total, through partial, to none. The degree of reversibility of psychological deficits depends on current availability and timely application of treatment, on compensatory mechanisms deployed to make up for the functional losses, and on other pertinent factors.[7,8] It is remarkable in view of these serious flaws that the concepts of the acute and the chronic OBS have become so firmly entrenched in North American psychiatry. Perhaps the main reason for this is their appealing simplicity, which really amounted to oversimplification.

ORGANIC MENTAL DISORDERS IN DSM-III

THE KEY PREMISES

OMD are differentiated as a separate category in the classification of mental disorders on the assumption that demonstrable brain dysfunction constitutes a *necessary condition* for their occurrence. By contrast, the nonorganic (''functional'') mental disorders fail to meet this criterion at this time. Thus, the OMD are recognized as a separate class on the basis of an etiologic hypothesis. The etiology of the nonorganic disorders is either unknown or postulated to be multifactorial and to involve psychological, social, genetic, and other causative factors acting in various constellations. To set apart the ''organic'' disorders has practial consequences and advantages. It implies that the diagnosis and treatment of the putative underlying brain disorder should have an overriding priority.

The newly acknowledged heterogeneity of the OBS is postulated to reflect the nature and characteristics of the brain disorder causally related to the latter. Factors such as the rate of onset and progression as well as the nature of the pathological process, the degree of spread of the pathology, and the duration of cerebral dysfunction—all appear to influence which particular OBS will occur. For example, relatively widespread and either sudden or gradually progressive cerebral cortical damage is likely to give rise to the syndrome of dementia. By contrast, relatively widespread, acute, and transient derangement of cerebral metabolism and neurotransmission is considered to underlie delirium. The specific etiology of the brain damage and dementia or of the metabolic derangement and delirium can implicate one or more of many potential causative factors.[9]

To label a psychiatric disorder as ''organic'' does not at all imply that it is incurable or irreversible, or that it carries a more ominous prognosis than functional disorders. Furthermore, the term ''organic'' must not be misconstrued to imply that the only treatment to be applied is that which is targeted at the identified cerebral disorder. On the contrary, some combination of psychological, social, and psychopharmacological therapies should be used in every ''organic'' case, having been tailored to the given patient's specific needs. An OBS not only reflects brain pathology but also an individual's total psychosocial response to a cerebral insult. DSM-III stipulates that, apart from their defining essential clinical features, the OBS include a wide range of *associated features*, which represent individual patients' emotional, behavioral, and motivational disturbances induced by the brain disorder itself, or by the patient's appraisal of the personal consequences of the disorder for him, or by some other relevant factors. Thus, an ''organic'' patient may at times display practically any type of psychopathological symptoms, neurotic, psychotic, personality, or behavioral. Premorbid personality, age, education, intelligence, and the quality of interpersonal relationships (social supports) are all variables which influence the clinical picture displayed by a given patient.[7,9]

Finally, it must be stressed that the OMD may vary with regard to the *severity* of the symptoms and the *sequence* in which they appear in a given patient. For example, one delirious patient may be only mildly disoriented for time and may experience only a few visual illusions, while another one may be grossly disoriented in all three spheres and incessantly hallucinating. In an early stage of a progressive dementia, such as that due to Alzheimer's disease, the patient may display only inconsistent memory impairment and some personality change. It is most important for psychiatrists to be aware of the symptomatic *variability* of the OMD if they are to diagnose these conditions before they have progressed beyond recovery.

THE KEY CHANGES

Preparation of DSM-III offered a unique opportunity to update and reformulate the whole category of the OMD, and to weed out obsolete concepts and terms. The following major changes have been effected:

1. *Liberalization of the concept "organicity."* This concept refers to psychiatric correlates of cerebral dysfunction. As noted earlier, in the previous classifications organicity was narrowly defined in terms of the basic organic syndrome, that is, of global-cognitive impairment. In DSM-III, the concept of organicity has been markedly expanded and, as it were, liberalized, by allowing inclusion of a wide range of psychiatric syndromes into the organic category. The essential feature of the OMD has been reformulated to include any "psychological or behavioral abnormality associated with transient or permanent dysfunction of the brain."[1, p. 101] Note that the nature of the "abnormality" has not been spelled out so as to underscore its inherent *heterogeneity*. In other words, no single psychopathological symptom or syndrome may be regarded as a defining characteristic of the class of organic psychiatric disorders as a whole.

2. *Heterogeneity of the OBS.* Broadening the scope of the concept of organicity beyond the global cognitive impairment is clearly reflected in the dramatic increase in the number of the OBS in DSM-III. Previously, only *one* descriptive psychopathological syndrome, the so-called basic one, was regarded as organic. In DSM-III, by contrast, *ten* such syndromes are included, but only *seven* of them really represent discrete symptom clusters, while the remaining three are to be viewed as residual and are descriptively nonspecific. The new OBS span a broad range of psychopathology, are not confined to disorders of cognition, and overlap with "functional" psychiatric disorders.

3. *Overlap between OBS and "functional" disorders.* In DSM-III, the traditionally sharp distinction between the organic and the nonorganic ("functional") mental disorders has been drastically blurred. Patients displaying paranoid, schizophrenic, or affective (depressive or manic) disorders may now, in some cases, be classified as "organic," provided that the presence of a putative organic etiologic factor judged to be responsible for the given disorder has been demonstrated or reasonably inferred.

4. *Absence of subdivisions.* Previous subdivisions into psychotic versus nonpsychotic and acute versus chronic OBS have been eliminated. By implication, the concepts of reversibility and irreversibility of organically based psychopathology have been removed from the classification.

5. *Dual diagnostic criteria.* The diagnosis of an OMD according to DSM-III guidelines should involve two steps: (1) ascertainment of the presence of one of the recognized OBS; and (2) demonstration that "there is evidence, from the history, physical examination, or laboratory tests, of a specific organic factor that is judged to be etiologically related to the disturbance."[1, p. 101]

These two requirements imply that to diagnose an OMD one must satisfy two independent sets of criteria, namely, (1) to demonstrate the presence of a psychiatric disorder by means of mental status examination and psychiatric history; and (2) to show by means of nonpsychological methods (such as physical examination, radiology, electroencephalography) the presence of an organic factor judged to be responsible for the abnormal psychological state. The need for such dual diagnostic evidence is crucial in the case of those OBS whose presence does not constitute presumptive evidence that a brain disorder is present. For example, the presence of paranoid, schizophrenic, or affective symptoms in a given patient does not *by itself* allow the inference that a specific brain disorder is present. The presence of the latter has to be independently ascertained by recourse to medical data and must be judged to be causally related to the observed psychopathological symptoms. In the case of such OBS as dementia, delirium, and the amnesic syndrome, the positive correlation with brain pathology is well established, and thus the presence of one of these syndromes constitutes presumptive, if not conclusive, evidence that a specific cerebral disorder is present.

THE KEY TERMS AND DEFINITIONS

Terminology of organic psychiatric disorders has been notoriously muddled for decades.[7] Vaguely defined, overlapping, and inconsistently used terms have impeded meaningful communication and case finding. In DSM-III, an attempt has been made to overcome that semantic muddle by providing clear definitions for the terms used.

OMD designates the whole class of those psychiatric (mental) disorders which are associated with transient or permanent dysfunction of the brain. *DSM-III* distinguishes between OMD and OBS. An OBS constitutes a cluster of descriptive psychopathological symptoms and signs which tend to occur together and are either usually or more often than chance associated with cerebral disorders. So defined, the OBS lack any etiological specificity, that is to say, the presence of an OBS in a given patient gives no indication regarding the specific cause, say neoplasm or vascular disease, of the underlying brain dysfunction. Once the etiology of an OBS has been established or is presumed to be known, one speaks of an *organic mental disorder*. In other words, "organic mental disorder" is a designation for an OBS whose etiology is known or presumed. For example, when the clinician concludes that a given patient exhibits features of delirium whose cause is still unknown, he has diagnosed an OBS only. If, however, the delirium proves to be due to pneumonia, for instance, the clinician will have diagnosed an OMD, that is, delirium due to pneumonia. Each OBS is defined in terms of its purely descriptive, essential psychopathological features.

THE KEY ETIOLOGIC FACTORS

Any given OBS may be induced by one or more of a large number of potentially etiologic organic factors.[9] The latter comprise four major groups: (1) primary cerebral disorders; (2) cerebral disorders secondary to systemic diseases; (3) exogenous toxic agents affecting the brain; and (4) withdrawal from certain abused substances; such as alcohol or barbiturates.

THE KEY SYNDROMES

Ten OBs are listed and defined in DSM-III and have been grouped according to certain shared attributes as follows:

1. Delirium and dementia, distinguished by *global cognitive impairment.*
2. Amnesic syndrome and organic hallucinosis, which feature a relatively *selective (or circumscribed) cognitive abnormality.*
3. Organic delusional syndrome and organic affective syndrome, whose features resemble those of corresponding *"functional"* disorders.
4. Organic personality syndrome, in which the patient's *personality is altered* in some respects.
5. Intoxication and withdrawal, which are associated with ingestion or reduction in use of a *substance* and do not satisfy the criteria for any of the preceding OBS.
6. Atypical or mixed organic brain syndrome, a *residual category.*

It should be noted that only the first seven of the above OBS, that is, those in groups 1 to 4, are distinguished on the basis of their descriptive characteristics, while the remaining three OBS (groups 5 and 6) are diagnosed by their putative etiology or by exclusion, or by both. Strictly speaking, only those seven *descriptively specific* OBS constitute autonomous syndromes and hence one should really speak of *seven* rather than ten distinct OBS.[8] The discussion to follow will be confined to these seven syndromes.

The Seven Specific OBS

Limitations of space permit only a brief discussion of the essential features of the individual OBS. Readers are referred to more detailed accounts for additional information.[1,9-11]

1. *Delirium* is an OBS characterized by reduced clarity of awareness of the environment. Its essential features include: global cognitive impairment, that is, concurrent disturbances and abnormalities of memory, perception, and thinking; disordered attention, especially defective capacity to attend to stimuli selectively, to direct attention voluntarily, and to mobilize, sustain, and/or shift it at will; and disturbed sleep–wake cycle.[1,9,10] Furthermore, delirium has a characteristically acute onset and relatively brief duration (usually less than 1 month), while the severity of its symptoms tends to fluctuate over the course of a day and be highest at night. Delirium represents a transient disorder of cognition due to widespread derangement of cerebral metabolism and to imbalance of brain neurotransmission which may be brought about by one or more of a large number of organic factors, such as toxic agents, infections, and metabolic encephalopathies.[10] The usual outcome of delirium is full recovery, but the syndrome may end in death or be followed by dementia, or by some other OBS.

2. *Dementia* is an OBS characterized by loss of intellectual abilities of sufficient severity to impair the patient's occupational or social function, or both.[1] In a fully developed case, dementia features deficits of memory, abstract thinking, problem solving, reasoning, and judgment, which occur in a state of clear awareness and tend to be relatively stable from day to day. In addition, the patient often displays some type and degree of personality change, in that his habitual behavioral patterns become either markedly accentuated or truly altered. The degree of intellectual deterioration in

dementia may range from mild to very severe, depending on the extent of the under-lying brain pathology and on psychosocial factors, such as the level of anxiety and the availability of social supports and stimulation. A highly anxious or depressed, or a so-cially isolated, demented patient is likely to display more marked intellectual impair-ment than the individual free of these disadvantages. The course of dementia may be static, as after a single damaging insult to the brain; remitting, as in the case of chronic intoxication with an industrial poison; or progressive, as in the commonest type of de-mentia in the elderly, that associated with senile dementia of Alzheimer type. It should be noted that dementia as defined in DSM-III *no longer connotes irreversibility* of in-tellectual deficits, in contrast to its traditional meaning.

Like delirium, dementia is a cognitive disorder, one in which acquisition, process-ing, retrieval, and purposeful utilization of information are all defective to some ex-tent. Dementia differs from delirium in that its onset is often insidious and its course protracted or èven inexorably progressive; its manifestations do not fluctuate widely in severity over the course of a day; perceptual abnormalities and attentional distur-bances are often absent, or at least are less pronounced; and awareness of the environ-ment (consciousness) is as a rule undisturbed.[11,12] These distinctions are, however, relative rather than absolute, and the two syndromes do overlap. Dementia defined as a *syndrome* must be clearly distinguished from senile dementia, a degenerative brain *disease* which is a common, but not the only, cause of the syndrome. Indeed, the lat-ter can result from a large number of cerebral disorders.[9,11]

Delirium and dementia are generally recognized as the *most common and impor-tant* OBS. Both are highly prevalent among the elderly, that is, persons aged 65 and over. Continuing aging of the population ensures that the incidence and prevalence of these two OBS will predictably increase in the years to come.

3. *Amnestic syndrome* is an OBS whose essential feature is impairment in both short-term and long-term memory, occurring in a state of clear awareness (conscious-ness). The classical example of this syndrome is provided by the Wernicke–Korsakoff syndrome (in DSM-III it is labeled "alcohol amnestic disorder"). Memory pathology is the most conspicuous, or even the only, feature of this syndrome whose presence points to the involvement of diencephalic or medial temporal structures, or both. It may be caused by such factors as thiamine deficiency, trauma to the head, vascular or neoplastic brain lesions, encephalitis, or carbon monoxide poisoning.[9]

4. *Organic hallucinosis* is characterized by persistent or recurrent hallucinations, usually in the visual or auditory sphere, that occur in a state of normal awareness and may or may not be recognized by the patient as such. In other words, the patient may or may not hold the delusional belief that his hallucinations are true perceptions. A typical example of this syndrome is provided by alcohol hallucinosis, which usually consists of auditory hallucinations that are highly disturbing to the patient.[9] Other po-tential causes of this OBS include hallucinogens, brain tumor, certain medical drugs, and epilepsy.

5. *Organic delusional syndrome* features the presence of delusions that occur in a state of normal awareness and are due to an organic factor, such as amphetamine intoxication. The patient may display almost any symptom found in paranoid and schizophrenic disorders, but the presence of delusions is the only indispensable diag-

nostic characteristic and must be judged to be due to a demonstrable organic factor. Such a judgement is usually based on the knowledge that the given organic condition or the identified toxic substance is associated with delusions more often than chance. Delusional psychoses occurring in patients suffering from temporal lobe epilepsy or encephalitis fall into this category.

6. *Organic affective syndrome* is an OBS characterized by a disturbance of mood which resembles either a manic or a major depressive disorder, but is judged to be due to a specific organic factor such as a viral infection or Cushing's disease.

This OBS and the organic delusional syndrome exemplify the overlap between the organic and functional psychiatric disorders. Their respective psychopathological features do not indicate whether they are due to a cerebral disorder or to some other etiologic factors, and the appropriate diagnosis must be based on independent evidence, that is, on data obtained from history, physical examination, and various nonpsychological laboratory tests, that a specific organic factor is implicated and is believed to be responsible for the occurrence of the psychiatric syndrome. This is surely the most controversial feature of the new classification of the OMD, one whose validity will have to be confirmed or disconfirmed by future clinical observations and research. These syndromes have been included in DSM-III mainly to help resolve the issue of the etiology of the so-called symptomatic schizophrenic, paranoid, and affective psychoses, that is, those considered to be due to identifiable cerebral pathology.

7. *Organic personality syndrome* has as its essential diagnostic feature a marked alteration of personality due to a demonstrable organic factor. The relevant personality change typically involves emotional lability or apathy, increased or reduced intensity and expression of instinctual drives, defective control of impulses, and impaired social judgment.[10] A classical example of this OBS is provided by the so-called frontal lobe syndrome, which may result from head trauma, neurosyphilis, cerebral neoplasm, or vascular disease.

Organic Mental Disorders: The Prospects

As I stated earlier, the interest in the organic psychiatric disorders has been reawakened recently and is liable to grow. Three cogent reasons may be given for this development: (1) rising incidence and prevalence of the OMD related to the aging of the population; (2) reformulation of the "organic" section in DSM-III; and (3) availability of new technology for the study of brain function, exemplified by positron computed tomography, nuclear magnetic resonance imaging, and techniques to investigation neurotransmitter systems in the brain.

The convergence of the above three developments fully justifies the prediction that the study of the OMD will emerge as one of the fastest growing and challenging frontiers of psychiatric research in the 1980s and beyond. Epidemiology, pathogenesis, and treatment of the various OMD will increasingly attract researchers not only from psychiatry but also from other disciplines. Complexity of this area at the interface of psychiatry and the neurosciences necessitates collaborative, multidisciplinary investigations. Expected advances in this field should not only yield new knowledge of brain–behavior relationships, but also, and most important, result in effective therapies for such currently incurable conditions as Alzheimer's disease, which is estimated to affect about 25 per 1000 of the population over 65.[13]

On the clinical side, psychiatrists will be predictably called upon with growing frequency to assist in the diagnosis and treatment of the OBS, especially of dementia and delirium. General hospital and liaison psychiatrists are liable to be particularly so involved, given the fact that the elderly account for about 30% of the medical and surgical inpatients and of referrals for psychiatric consultation, and that the incidence and prevalence of delirium and dementia in this population are high.[14] Diagnostic problems in this area involve the often difficult distinction between dementia and pseudodementia[15] and delirium and pseudodelirium.[16] Furthermore, psychiatrists will need to be familiar with the treatable causes of dementia,[9,11] with the wide range of organic etiologic factors in delirium,[10,16] and with the proper use of psychotropic drugs in the physically ill, and especially the elderly patients suffering from an OBS.[17] All this clinical activity will require proper training of psychiatrists and the teaching of the whole subject of organic psychiatry will have to be properly emphasized in all training programs.[18] The time when psychiatrists can affort to ignore the OMD is over.

Conclusions

I have tried to present in this chapter the salient features of the revised concept, definitions, and classification of the OMD contained in DSM-III. I hope to have clarified the nature and extent of the effected changes, which are far-reaching and may appear overwhelming to someone used to the traditionally simplistic approach to this area of psychiatry. The relative complexity of the new classification is the inevitable result of expanding information about psychiatric correlates of cerebral disorders. To do justice to accruing empirical data some time-honored concepts had to be discarded or drastically modified. The traditional boundary between the organic and the functional psychiatric disorders has been blurred, and this may cause some confusion and controversy.

The main purpose of the revision outlined here is twofold: (1) to stimulate formulation of testable hypotheses about causal relationships and hence to encourage research; and (2) to raise the standard of psychiatric patient care by making medical evaluation an integral part of the diagnostic process in psychiatry. Etiologic hypotheses implied by the inclusion of a wider range of psychopathological phenomena in the organic category may not become validated in all cases. Research findings will have to settle this issue. There is reason to hope, however, that the new classification of the OMD will help revitalize this sorely neglected area of psychiatry and lead to badly needed theoretical and therapeutic advances in the coming years. Nobody could claim that DSM-III represents the last word on the subject of organic psychiatric disorders. On the contrary, the present classification reflects no more than our limited knowledge and working hypotheses, and will have to be revised in the future in the light of new data which will inevitably accrue as the hypotheses are tested.

REFERENCES

1. *Diagnostic and Statistical Manual of Mental Disorders*, ed 3. Washington, DC, American Psychiatric Association, 1980.
2. *Diagnostic and Statistical Manual of Mental Disorders*. Washington, DC, American Psychiatric Association, 1952.
3. *Diagnostic and Statistical Manual of Mental Disorders*, ed 2. Washington, DC, American Psychiatric Association, 1968.
4. Lipowski ZJ: Organic mental disorders: Their history and classification, with special reference to DSM-III, in Miller NE, Cohen GD (eds): *Clinical Aspects of Alzheimer's Disease and Senile Dementia*. New York, Raven Press, 1981, pp 37-45.
5. Bleuler E: *Textbook of Psychiatry*. New York, Macmillan Publishing Co. 1924.
6. Bleuler M: Psychiatry of cerebral diseases. *Br Med J* 2:1233-1238, 1951.
7. Lipowski ZJ: Organic brain syndromes: Overview and classification, in Benson DF, Blumer D (eds): *Psychiatric Aspects of Neurologic Disease*. New York, Grune & Stratton, 1975, pp 11-35.
8. Lipowski ZJ: A new look at organic brain syndromes. *AmJ Psychiatry* 137:674-678, 1980.
9. Lipowski ZJ: Organic mental disorders: Introduction and review of syndromes, in Kaplan HI, Freedman AM, Sadock BJ (eds): *Comprehensive Textbook of Psychiatry*, ed 3. Baltimore, Williams & Wilkins, 1980: pp 1359-1392.
10. Lipowski ZJ: *Delirium: Acute Brain Failure in Man*. Springfield Ill, Charles C Thomas, 1980.
11. Wells CE (ed): *Dementia*, ed. 2. Philadelphia, Davis, 1977.
12. Lipowski ZJ: Differentiating delirium from dementia in the elderly. *Clin Gerontol* 1:3-10, 1982.
13. Mortimer JA, Schuman LM (eds): *The Epidemiology of Dementia*. New York, Oxford University Press, 1981.
14. Lipowski ZJ: The need to integrate liaison psychiatry and geropsychiatry. *Am J Psychiatry* 140; 1003-1005, 1983.
15. Wells CE: Pseudodementia. *Am J Psychiatry* 136:895-900, 1979.
16. Lipowski ZJ: Transient cognitive disorders (delirium, acute confusional states) in the elderly. *Am J Psychiatry* 140:1426-1436, 1983.
17. Steinhart MJ: The use of haloperidol in geriatric patients with organic mental disorder. *Curr Ther Res* 33:132-143, 1983.
18. Lishman WA: *Organic Psychiatry*. Oxford, Blackwell, 1978.

Delirium, Clouding of Consciousness, and Confusion

14

Delirium has been for years the Cinderella of English-language psychiatry: taken for granted, ignored, and not considered worthy of study. Whatever the reasons for this neglect might be, several recent developments in psychiatry and psychology fully justify a reexamination of this syndrome and its conceptual framework. The growth of experimental psychopathology, and particularly the study of drug-induced model psychoses as well as of the psychological effects of variation of sensory input and of sleep deprivation, invite comparison with that "experiment of nature" which is delirium. The concept of consciousness has recovered its respectability in psychology and the class of disorders designated "disturbances of consciousness" has recently attracted the attention of scientists from various disciplines.[111] Progress in the understanding of the neural substrate of conscious experience has been spearheaded by neuroanatomists and neurophysiologists.[14, 36] The rapid development of general hospital psychiatry has given access and opportunity for the study of psychiatric complications of somatic disease to an extent unparalleled in the history of psychiatry. Psychiatrists working on the medical and surgical wards must deal with the diagnostic and therapeutic problems of delirium and related states as part of their liaison work.[86] There has been dissatisfaction with the current classification of the so-called organic brain syndromes and salutary recognition that their study "touches on the basic questions of the biological organization of drives, affects, and cognitive processes."[99] Current interest in cognition[60] should extend to delirium in which disorganization of cognitive processes is the chief feature.

Thus the climate of scientific interest in several areas, as well as the practical demands of psychiatric–medical liaison in general hospitals, calls for a reevaluation of delirium. The present writer has undertaken a review of this subject, in preparation for a planned long-term clinical study of it to be carried out on nonpsychiatric wards of a general and neurological hospital. It is also one of a series of papers designed to survey the psychiatric aspects of medical practice and thus expand the scope of psychosomatic medicine from a clinical viewpoint.[85,86]

Reprinted from *Journal of Nervous and Mental Disease* 145(3):227-255, 1967. Copyright © 1967 by The Williams & Wilkins Co. Reprinted by permission.

THE PROBLEMS OF DEFINITION

The area of psychopathology related to somatic illness in general, and cerebral disease in particular, presents a conceptual and semantic muddle. The meaning of the various terms found in the literature is unclear and often óverlapping. Unless some order is brought into the language of this area of psychiatry, little progress can be made in the elucidation of relevant etiological factors and physiological processes underlying the observed psychic phenomena. Before a set of definitions is offered it may be useful to review briefly the development and current meanings of the concept of delirium.

Viewed in historical perspective, the term "delirium" has undergone significant changes of meaning, although a core conception of it can be traced back to early medical writings. A striking example of it is offered by Thomas Willis who, in 1683, recorded some accurate observations of delirium.[131] He recognized that it was "a symptom" related to a variety of diseases, such as infections, intoxications, undernutrition, visceral disorders. He noted its reversibility and dominant cognitive defect, i.e., "incongruous conceptions, and·confused thoughts." According to Tuke's *Dictionary*,[119] the term was derived from Latin *deliro*, "I rave," and in a general sense designated disorder of the mind or insanity. In a narrower sense, however, it referred to a temporary psychic disturbance, occuring in connection with somatic diseases, particularly febrile ones. According to Tuke, descriptive characteristics of this disorder included incoherent speech, hallucinations, illusions, delusions, restlessness, watchfulness, and inability to fix attention. The main psychological impairment was in the sphere of intellect. Tuke's conception of delirium, which antedates Bonhoeffer's influential work, contains the core of the modern definition of this syndrome, as a reversible psychiatric disorder symptomatic of a wide range of cerebral disorders, primary or secondary. His stress on the impairment of the intellect is still valid but his description is too heavily weighted towards the more dramatic and inconstant clinical manifestations, such as perceptual distortions and increased psychomotor activity.

The conception of psychiatric disorders concomitant with somatic diseases has been greatly influenced by the work of Bonhoeffer.[11] This German investigator rejected the Kraepelinian view that each noxious agent affecting the brain evoked a specific psychiatric syndrome. Bonhoeffer postulated that any and all such pathogenic factors could cause one or more of the five "exogenous psychic reaction types": delirium, epileptiform excitement, twilight state, hallucinosis, and amentia. These descriptive syndromes were not sharply delimited, and could occur, in various combinations, in the same patient. Bonhoeffer's views have had a decisive influence on psychiatric thinking, especially in Germany, during the last 50 years. His classification has been modified (e.g., "amentia" has been excluded), but his general conception is still accepted.[7, 10] Russian workers have recently challenged the validity of Bonhoeffer's views. They claim that the type of pathogenic agent involved does influence the structure of the exogenous psychoses and that distinct syndromes are characteristic of infections such as malaria, tularemia, rheumatic fever.[110]

English-speaking psychiatrists responded favorably to Bonhoeffer's work.[58] One notes, however, a tendency to greater economy in classification, well illustrated by Adolf Meyer's work.[95] For him delirium was a prototype, and hallucinosis a variant, of dysergastic reaction, designating psychic disorders due to impaired "nutritive and circulatory support" of the brain.

Despite these efforts to define delirium clearly, there is still terminological chaos in the field of reversible organic psychiatric disorders. Terms such as "delirium," "confusional state," "toxic psychosis," "infective–exhaustive psychosis," "acute brain syndrome" are used indiscriminately, vitiating clear communication. The official American classification.[32] is not too helpful. It distinguishes the acute and chronic brain syndromes on the basis of reversibility of brain pathology and its accompanying psychic disorder. The acute syndrome is, by definition, reversible; the chronic syndrome, irreversible. Relevant clinical criteria involve a post hoc judgment, and distinction on clinical grounds between acute and chronic syndromes is not always possible. The diagnostic criteria (the so-called "basic syndrome") are also open to criticism, for they are too general and undefined. Moreover, they are based on the questionable assumption that *all* disorders caused by impairment of brain tissue function are characterized by them. Such a formulation leaves unclear the nosological position of hallucinosis, reversible amnesic syndrome, disorders due to amphetamines or cortisone, etc. These states can hardly be regarded as not related to cerebral dysfunction and yet do not present the "basic syndrome." Delirium is not defined in the classification and its position within the acute brain syndrome category is unclear. The term "acute brain syndrome" is little known or used by nonpsychiatrists,[43] while the term "delirium" is still widely employed. To list all shades of its meaning would be futile. Only two representative kinds of definition need be mentioned here as a basis for discussion.

Engel and Romano,[38] who have made original contributions to our understanding of delirium, call it a syndrome of cerebral insufficiency whose defining properties are (1) a reduction in the level of cognition and (2) a characteristic slowing of the EEG. In contrast to this broad definition, Victor and Adams[121] regard delirium as one of three syndromes belonging to the class of acute confusional states, characterized by one common feature: "Thinking with less than accustomed clarity and coherence." The other members of the class are primary mental confusion and beclouded dementia. Delirium in this classification is marked by increase in psychomotor and autonomic activity, vigilance, disorders of perception, and a relatively normal EEG. By contrast, the hallmarks of primary mental confusion are reduced alertness and responsiveness, psychomotor underactivity, little tendency to hallucinate, and an abnormal EEG.

It seems clear that delirium, as defined by Engel and Romano, embraces the whole group of acute confusional states. The main difference between the respective conceptions of these workers is this: for Victor and Adams delirium tremens is the model for the syndrome of delirium as a whole; for Engel and Romano, it is no more than an atypical variant of the more broadly conceived total syndrome. This distinction must be kept in mind as it is discernible in much of the published work on delirium and results in apparently contradictory statements about causes, clinical features, and EEG patterns. This reviewer endorses the definition of Engel and Romano as having the merits of greater logical consistency, inclusiveness, and clinical usefulness. Communication would be greatly improved if only one defition of delirium prevailed and superfluous groupings of symptoms were avoided.

CLOUDING OF CONSCIOUSNESS

The concept of delirium has been traditionally linked with that of disturbed or "clouded" consciousness.[15, 58, 102] A statement in a recent textbook of psychiatry expresses this relationship succinctly: "Disturbance of consciousness is the cardinal symptom of delirium."[99] Yet what does this statement really mean? To answer this question one has to consider the concept of consciousness, whose abnormality is postulated to characterize delirium. The epistemological aspects of this concept are a forbidding subject. Speculations about the nature of consciousness have been a pursuit of philosophers and the concept itself has been shunned by the behavioristically oriented psychologists. During the last decade, this situation has changed. The concept of consciousness has acquired scientific respectability. This change has paralleled a renewed interest in cognition and progress in the studies of the ascending reticular activating system. Representative of the changed climate in psychology is Hebb's[53] remark that consciousness is a useful construct, designating complex interaction of mediating processes in the intact, waking higher animal. Hebb proposes that consciousness is equivalent to complex thought processes, that it may diminish or increase responsiveness, and that it may lead to periods of sustained purposive behavior. Immediate memory, variability in degree of responsiveness to stimuli, insight, and purpose are all properties of consciousness.[52]

It would be beyond the scope of this article to attempt a review of the numerous definitions and views of consciousness. The reader is referred to relevant sources.[16,25,36,52,106] The psychiatric clinician is less concerned with the dispute about the nature of consciousness than with its usefulness as an explanatory concept, and the empirical criteria which justify its application.

Distinction has been made between consciousness as a state or process on the one hand, and its contents on the other. This concept can be approached in terms of introspective reports or of observable behavior, from which inferences can be drawn about subjective experience. The latter approach focusses on the observed transactions between an individual and his environment, or, more specifically, on his responses to sensory stimuli, verbal or nonverbal. The neurologist has traditionally relied on the stimulus–response model in his assessment of a patient's state of consciousness. The psychiatrist has tried to combine both the criterion of degree and type of responsiveness to environmental stimuli and that of reported subjective state. For the purpose of this discussion the writer offers the following definition: *Consciousness is that state of an organism which enables cognitive processes to occur.* Thus the evidence of occurrence of cognitive processes, based on introspective reports and observed behavior, is the empirical criterion of the theoretical concept "consciousness." Cognitive processes include perceiving, thinking, and remembering. Cognition deals with all aspects of symbolic behavior, but especially thinking.[60]

Consciousness is not an all-or-none concept. It is best viewed as a continuum, ranging from full awareness to unconsciousness. Hughlings Jackson[65] said, "There may be slight affections of consciousness, a slight confusion of thought, and from this there are all degrees down to deepest coma." This view leads us to the concept of clouding of consciousness. There are significant differences in the use of this term. Jaspers[66] distinguishes three types of disturbed consciousness: (1) reduced consciousness (torpor), i.e., those states that lie between consciousness and unconsciousness; (2) clouded consciousness, the hallmarks of which are fragmentation of psychic experience and appearance of fantasies and hallucinations; (3) altered consciousness, when the latter is restricted to certain areas, as in hysterical twilight states.

This classification seems to underlie the differentiation between "simple confusion"—in which consciousness is seen as quantitatively reduced, although this is not usually stated—and "delirium"—in which consciousness is perceived as "clouded," i.e., qualitatively changed, with often the appearance of hallucinations, delusions, etc. It is doubtful if this distinction is necessary. The writer suggests that "clouding of consciousness" be defined as a state characterized by a potentially reversible *global impairment of cognitive processes* of variable extent. Thus there should be evidence of some degree of simultaneous impairment of thinking, perceiving, and remembering, for the term "clouding" to be applicable. By "impairment" is meant decrement in functioning using the given individual as his own standard. It appears that a transient general impairment of cerebral cortical metabolism and/or a lesion of the ascending reticular activating system anywhere between the posterior hypothalamus and the tegmentum of the lower pons[97] are necessary conditions for the clouding of consciousness. This state designates the continuum of degrees of impaired cognition, ranging from its mildest blurring to coma.

There is some overlap between the consciousness–unconsciousness continuum and the wakefulness–sleep dichotomy.[71] Some writers[92] equate clouding of consciousness with a state of reduced wakefulness. Yet consciousness and wakefulness are not synonymous.[71] A high degree of alertness is usually concomitant with a high level of consciousness, but intermediate levels of the latter are compatible with either wakefulness or sleep. An individual behaviorally asleep but dreaming displays a degree of consciousness; in delirium the level of consciousness is low and yet the person is behaviorally awake, although he may be drowsy. The delirious patient's *awareness* of himself and his surroundings is always impaired, but his degree of *arousal* may vary from excitement to lethargy.

The attempt to define consciousness and its clouding is desirable, however inadequate and controversial it may be, in view of the current tendency to discuss "altered states of consciousness" as if they were a homogenenous group of phenomena.[88] Unless some differentiation is attempted in this vague field, it is unlikely that progress will be made in correlating psychological observations with neurophysiological mechanisms. There is need for descriptive delineation of relatively enduring clusters of cognitive–perceptual abnormalities, which can help define various altered states of consciousness. A recent attempt to do this for varying degrees of drowsiness[96] points in the right direction. Clouding of consciousness is seen as only one type of altered consciousness and one which is at present most closely correlated with a detectable neurophysiological change, i.e., change in the EEG pattern.

Clouding of consciousness is a psychological (or psychopathological) theoretical concept, whose defining property is reversible global impairment of cognition. Clinical syndromes of clouding include delirium, epileptic seizure, akinetic mutism, syncope, stupor, and coma. *Delirium* is a reversible psychiatric syndrome, defined by the following criteria:

1. The individual is awake and usually capable of responding verbally.
2. There is evidence of impairment of thinking, memory, perception, and attention. This impairment tends to fluctuate irregularly over time.
3. There is impaired ability to comprehend the environment and internal perceptions in accordance with the individual's past experience and knowledge (as a result of item 2), i.e., defective reality testing.
4. There is usually a concomitant change in the frequency of the EEG pattern, which tends to vary pari passu with the level of cognition.

All other psychological and physiological symptoms encountered in delirium may be regarded as inconstant and nonspecific; they will be described later. The syndrome has three possible outcomes: complete recovery: progression to irreversible amnestic syndrome or dementia; progression to irreversible coma and death. Delirium may last from minutes, as after a slight concussion, to months; its average duration does not exceed 1 week. A detailed analysis of its features follows.

DELIRIUM—A SYNDROME OF CLOUDED CONSCIOUSNESS

GENERAL REMARKS

In general, four mutually complementary ways of describing the phenomena of delirium may be distinguished:

1. Description of the patient's inner experience available from introspective reports and supplemented by empathic inferences from his communications and behavior.
2. Description in terms of observable verbal and nonverbal behavior of the patient in a given situation.
3. Description of the observed psychological events in terms of separate psychological functions or processes, such as perception or thinking.
4. Composite description in clinical terms, such as disorientation or defective grasp. This writer will try to combine the three latter approaches. The first one is well represented by Conrad.[26] Methodological problems of the introspective approach, as well as its advantages, are well illustrated by a comparative study of the LSD and delirium tremens experiences, respectively.[33]

Any critical survey of the literature on delirium encounters serious obstacles and pitfalls. These result from the problems of selection of the patient population studied, as well as from the vexing inconsistency and variability in the use of relevant terminology. Clinical reports of delirium differ, depending on whether the patients were studied in a psychiatric or a nonpsychiatric hospital setting. There is a tendency to transfer to psychiatric facilities those delirious patients who display grossly disturbed or "psychotic" behavior. Psychiatric consultants are generally asked to see delirious patients whose behavior *disturbs others*. The level of tolerance for such behavior varies markedly from one medical setting to another.

As a consultant to a general and neurological hospital, the writer is asked to see cases of delirium that attract the medical personnel's anxious or disapproving attention. For example a middle-aged lawyer, hospitalized for acute pancreatitus, wrote a note to his wife urging her to bring him his gun to the hospital. The wife passed the note to the attending physician and a psychiatric consultation was promptly requested. It turned out that the patient hallucinated Negroes entering his room through a hatch in the ceiling. They marched around his bed making threatening gestures. He wanted a gun to defend himself. A second patient, an elderly man, admitted for pulmonary insufficiency and treated with ephedrine, drew the attention of the staff by making repeated stereotyped movements as if he was throwing something. This was an "occupational delirium"; the man explained that he was a linesman on the docks. He was imitating his daily line-throwing.

Such examples of selective referrals could be multiplied. When the writer joined daily rounds on medical wards he encountered patients who smiled on approach and exchanged polite phrases with the doctors. When interviewed afterwards, many displayed marked disorientation and other cognitive defects. Such "good," i.e., quiet and compliant delirious patients, are practically never referred for consultation because they do not bother anybody. This suggests that published reports on delirium based on referred patients are likely to be significantly skewed towards the dramatic, obtrusive, and disturbing clinical features, such as restlessness, panic, threats, obvious hallucinations, and other "crazy" behavior. A balanced picture of the syndrome can hardly emerge from such selected clinical material. Engel and Romano[38,102,103] deserve special credit for repeatedly stressing these points.

The considerable confusion surrounding delirium has already been mentioned. In a recent paper dealing with the mental changes in acute pulmonary decompensation, it was stated that all patients had "obvious deterioration in mental acuity" but only 7 out of 50 had "transient psychotic reactions" with delusions, hallucinations, mania.[34] The word "delirium" was not mentioned. Some patients treated for chronic uremia were said to suffer from mental confusion, states like delirium tremens, or schizoid delusions.[120] These examples are typical. Sutton, who coined the term "delirium tremens" in 1813,[29] helped establish the enduring tendency to take his syndrome as a model for delirium as a whole. It has been suggested that the nondescript diagnostic term "acute brain syndrome" be abandoned and replaced by "acute confusional state."[43] Since delirium has the distinction of having been a familiar medical word for centuries, it is preferable to retain it but use it in a clearly defined and consistent manner.

There is a tendency to talk of delirium when the patient displays dramatic symptoms, such as overactivity and hallucinations, and use the word "confusion" when he shows cognitive impairment but is not manifestly disturbed. This tendency is deplorable. "Confusion" is a vague term devoid of clear diagnostic connotation. To say that a delirious patient is confused is superfluous; to say that a confused individual is delirious may be untrue. The term "confusion" has been applied by some writers[104, 108] to certain manifestations of schizophrenia and explained as a defense against the awareness of repressed affects.[107] It is proposed that unless "confusion" is clearly defined in a given communication its meaning is ambiguous and of no diagnostic or psychodynamic significance.

General Clinical Features

Clinical presentation of delirium may be variable. The onset may be rapid or gradual. In the early or prodromal stage, the patient may report mild and transient symptoms, difficuly in concentration and thinking coherently, anxiety, mild depression, or apathy. He may also show tendency to lose interest in activities and to become fatigued, restless, and irritable. His sleep may be disturbed by vivid dreams or nightmares. Such symptoms may be seen in ambulant patients.[123] and their recognition is vital, as they should alert the physician to the possibility of more serious disturbances developing later on. The writer recalls a young woman hospitalized for a viral infection who complained to the medical resident about anxiety and nightmares. These complaints were ignored and on the next night the patient wandered away from her bed, slipped into a laundry hatch on the ward, and fell several floors, sustaining multiple fractures of the spine and legs. At this point, an urgent psychiatric consultation was requested by her orthopedist, for patient was clearly disoriented and hallucinating.

A patient may not progress beyond early and mild symptoms. However, he may almost imperceptibly pass either into a manifestly turbulent phase of delirium or directly into coma.[38] At any stage of the syndrome, but especially in an early one, the patient may be aware of a degree of cognitive impairment and may develop dysphoric affects of depression, anxiety, anger, guilt, or shame. Ego mechanisms of defense may then be employed against the affects, and the patient will display denial, projection, conversion, withdrawal. The patient's usual personality style may be exaggerated or he may appear to be neurotic or psychotic. One may encounter depressive, paranoid, schizophrenic, phobic, or hysterical clinical pictures, reactive to the underlying cognitive impairment. Such secondary reactions may mask the delirium and give the false impression of a purely psychogenic illness. Many patients remain quiet, apathetic, and listless, and may not be recognized unless clinical examination of cognitive functions is repeatedly employed.

As the severity of the clouding of consciousness increases, the individual personality traits tend to give way to an increasingly undifferentiated disorganization. This development is analogous to that observed in individuals deprived of varying amounts of cerebral cortical tissue: the greater the amount of tissue loss, the greater the waning of individual characteristics, of differentiated affective response, and of defensive and compensatory psychological reactions.[22] The patient's perception of his environment becomes increasingly blurred and his inner experience impoverished; his capacity for purposive behavior decreases, and stupor and coma supervene. On emergence from coma, the patient invariable passes through a delirious phase, before regaining full awareness.

A single patient may show striking variability in his symptoms. A good recently described example of this sometimes protean character of delirium was given by a woman suffering from carcinoidosis.[75] Over a period of several weeks she showed excitement with a flight of ideas, anxiety, depression with guilt feelings, apathy merging into akinetic mutism, aggrssive outbursts, coma, catatonic and cataleptic symptoms. Unless it is recognized that all such symptoms are not inconsistent with an overall diagnosis of delirium, a number of possible irrelevant diagnostic labels may be applied to describe this single syndrome.

Not all delirious patients display such a wealth of psychopathology. Many remain apathetic and listless; others display excited, restless, and fearful or combative behavior; while still others remain depressed and withdrawn or euphoric or stoically unconcerned.

An important and frequent characteristic of delirium is the tendency for its manifestations to vary in severity over a 24-hr period. This is frequently described as fluctuations in the level of consciousness. So-called lucid intervals of varying duration, sometimes lasting only a few minutes, may appear unpredictably at any time. It has been asserted[38] that these fluctuations are related to psychological and environmental factors. In general, delirium tends to reach its peak at night—*nocturnal exacerbation*—when sensory cues, by which the patient may orient himself, are drastically reduced. As there is often associated insomnia, one may postulate that the effects of sleep deprivation have a contributory effect, and vivid dreams and hypnagogic phenomena may merge imperceptibly into waking hallucinations. There is progressive blurring of the boundaries between the inner psychic experience and the external environment. Thus a patient seen recently dreamed that she struck a skunk and was sprayed by its odorous secretion. She woke up and demanded a wash-basin so that she could wash off the foul-smelling fluid at once. Such manifestations can be observed only when one spends some hours at the patient's bedside. Daily rounds are not enough. This writer developed an interest in delirium after spending long periods with a patient who became delirious after surgery for cervical spondylosis, from which he emerged with quadriplegia and loss of sensation below the neck. This young man, a Negro minister, greeted the writer by shouting that he had lost his genitals in a car accident. A moment later he shouted that a dog was biting his penis; then he talked to himself about wonderful scents of some tropical flowers which he apparently hallucinated. After some minutes of such shifting psychotic experience, the patient suddenly looked at the writer attentively and said, "Am I sick? I seem to be hallucinating!" Told that this was so, the patient remained quiet for a few minutes, and then shouted, "Look, look, there's this dog again, biting me! Take this dog away!" The lucid interval was over.

In summary, no single description of delirium can do justice to the manifold character of its secondary symptoms. These are influenced by the individual's unique personality and past experiences, by his particular conflicts and preoccupations, and by his modes of reacting to cognitive disorganization. The quality and quantity of environmental stimuli also influence the clinical picture. In addition, the *intensity* of the psychological disturbance varies from case to case, and over a period of time in the same case. Only the *basic fact of global cognitive impairment is constant and diag-, nostic.* A detailed analysis of it follows.

COGNITIVE FUNCTIONS IN DELIRIUM

A search of the English psychiatric literature of the last half-century reveals a dearth of systematic studies of delirium. While clinical reports of this condition abound, their terminology, as well as their scientific rigor, vary greatly. Psychiatric textbooks seem to repeat uncritically a stereotyped set of descriptive features based on selected clinical material. The following attempt at a systematic presentation of delirium may highlight the gaps in our knowledge and thus stimulate research. It is based largely on the contributions of Romano and Engel,[38, 102, 103] whose studies have provided the groundwork for the modern conception of delirium.

There is relative agreement among clinicians that certain manifestations of delirium have special diagnostic importance. These characteristics are expressed in clinical terms and their relation to basic cognitive functions is unclear. They will be discussed first because of their diagnostic relevance.

Disorientation for time, place, and person, is often regarded as a *sine qua non* for the diagnosis of delirium.[77] Orientation for time, i.e., ability to correctly the date, day of the week, and time of day, is the first to be impaired and, as recovery progresses, the last to be regained.[77] Temporal disorientation may or may not be followed by impairment of orientation for place and person. In severe delirium, disorientation in all three spheres is the rule. There is a characteristic tendency for the delirious patient to mistake unfamiliar places and persons for familiar ones.[81] Thus the hospital may be mistaken for the patient's own home, or a familiar hotel, or a hospital which he knows best; doctors and nurses are misidentified as relatives or friends. A delirious patient walked into a hospital emergency clinic and was found fumbling in a refrigerator where drugs were kept; it turned out that he believed himself to be in his house and was looking for a bottle of beer! Weinstein and Kahn[126] studied patterns of disorientation in patients with cerebral disease. These authors felt that disorientation for place and time in their patients could not be attributed to defects in memory, calculation, or perception, but that the motivation to deny illness and leave the hospital was an important factor. Disorientation was further interpreted as a symbolic form of adaptation, used by the patient to avoid the "catastrophic reaction." Validity of this hypothesis is open to question.

In summary, disorientation is a diagnostically useful but not absolute indicator of delirium. In the early stage of delirium, orientation may be unimpaired.[11] The degree of disorientation tends to fluctuate pari passu with the fluctuations of consciousness, being usually most marked at night and immediately upon awakening. A patient suffering from dementia, severe anxiety, depression, or acute schizophrenia may show some degree of disorientation in the absence of delirium.

Grasp is another clinical term frequently noted in descriptions of delirium.[134] It designates ability to comprehend relationships among elements of one's environment, and relate them meaningfully to oneself and one's past experiences and knowledge. Grasp is a product of complex cognitive processes, and its impairment in delirium is an invariable sign of congitive disorganization.

Attention has been defined as selective central influence determining which aspect of the stimulus object will be responded to[52]; it is regarded by some writers as a criterion of the level of consciousness.[70] Hernandez-Peon[55] sees attention as the primary process underlying perception, memory, and thinking, and relates it to the vigilance system, i.e., arousing neurons in the brain stem, which can be activated by the specific sensory pathways and by descending projections from the cortex. Disturbances of attention observed in delirium include reduced span, fluctuation, difficulty in voluntary shifting, diffusion, contraction, and distractibility.[70]

DISTURBANCES OF THINKING

The only paper in English devoted specifically to the thought disorder in delirium is by Levin.[80] He found disturbances of association indistinguishable from those seen in schizophrenia and defects in reasoning of which the patients were unaware.

Thinking has been defined[56] as any behavior carried on in terms of ideas, i.e., in terms of representational or symbolic processes. For our purposes, two main varieties of thinking may be distinguished (1) associative, as in reverie, dreams and (2) directed, as in critical and creative thought.[56] Discussion of the pathology of thinking should include the following aspects of thought processes: (1) organization, i.e., selective ordering of symbols for the purpose of problem-solving and communication; (2) dynamics, i.e., evolution and pogression of thoughts over time sequences; (3) content; (4) concept-formation.

This general framework enables one to reivew thought disorder in delirium systematically. In general, one may postulate that thinking in delirium is impaired in the four aspects listed above. Thus, organization of thought is disrupted and fragmented to a varying extent, as implied in the term "incoherent." The patient has difficulty marshalling his thoughts logically and coherently.[38] Reasoning is defective, rules of logic disregarded. Unaccustomed bizarre thoughts, images, and fantasies intrude into awareness. There is a tendency for the primary process thinking to disrupt secondary process thinking. The ability to comprehend the environment and to solve problems is diminished, and capacity for purposive behavior reduced. The flow of thoughts may already be accelerated in the prodromal stage of delirium.[11] Or they may be slowed down, so that the patient responds to questions with difficulty and hesitation. In the area of concept-formation, there is a tendency towards predominance of the concrete over the abstract attitude. Regarding content, *delusions,* i.e., beliefs contrary to facts and resistant to correction, may appear. They are typically transient, unsystematized, and usually persecutory in character. The incidence of paranoid delusions in delirium differs in various reports, ranging from 39% to 100%.[39, 109, 134] These discrepancies may reflect differences in patient selection and in the definition of "delusion." It is likely that a random sample of delirious patients, taken from the medical wards, would show a lower frequency of delusions than a sample of patients referred to psychiatrists.

Weinstein and Kahn[126] found that among their brain-damaged patients those showing paranoid attitudes responded to their illness with fear and resentment, and showed marked concern with the overt attributes of masculinity and feminity.

Cameron's[19] remarks about behavioral disorganization in delirium are pertinent to the discussion of thought processes in this syndrome. He distinguishes four major manifestations of such disorganization: (1) incoordination, i.e., loss of the normal pace, direction, dependability, and predictability of thinking; (2) interpenetration, i.e., invasion into awareness of derivatives of unconscious primary processes; (3) fragmentation, i.e., repetition, perseveration, and stereotypy, as well as disruption of relatedness of thoughts; and (4) overinclusion, i.e., failure to limit the number and kind of thoughts to the most relevant ones. Cameron points out that, while these abnormalities are not confined to delirium, their association with disorientation, memory defect, delusions, and hallucinations is specific to this condition. The total effect of the cognitive disorganization in delirium is the patient's inability "to construct an intelligible whole out of his fragmented experience."

Perception has been defined as the mediating processes to which sensation gives rise directly.[52] Information about perception in delirium comes largely from descriptions by patients of their subjective experience. The writer has been unable to find any reports of systematic studies of perceptual processes in the syndrome. Nothing is known about quantitative aspects, such as intensity of the sensory components or sensory thresholds, in delirious patients. In the prodromal phase of delirium, the patient may complain of hypersensitivity to auditory and visual stimuli.[11] It has been suggested that a delirious patient is unable to maintain his habitual anticipatory and supporting attitudes in the presence of competing and discordant stimulation.

It is likely that perceptual processes are affected differently in delirium, depending on the degree of arousal. Thus some patients are drowsy and may show abnormalities described in different stages of drowsiness,[96] such as absence of expectancy and perceptual searching, coupled with difficulty in integrating meaningful percepts. Especially in cases of withdrawal from alcohol or sedatives, the level of arousal tends to be high and there is increased reactivity to sensory stimuli. In both cases, however, we may postulate that *perceptual discrimination is impaired.* It is of interest in this regard that perceptual discrimination was found to be poor with little stimulation of the reticular system, was more efficient with greater stimulation, and finally was poor again with further increases in stimulation.[41]

Some degree of impairment of perception is postulated to be one of the basic characteristics of delirium. This statement does not imply that more severe degrees of misperception, i.e., illusions and hallucinations, are also an invariable feature of this syndrome. They are not. If delirium is defined as an "hallucinosis with a clouded sensorium,"[100] then only hallucinating patients will be included in the sample, and the incidence of halluncinations will be reported as being 100%! If a broader definition, such as the one adopted in this paper, is accepted, hallucinations and illusions must be regarded as inconstant and diagnostically unessential components of delirium.

Illusions have been defined as premature or improper labeling of aspects of the perceptual field.[96] Their incidence in delirium is unknown, but they seem to be common.[134] Misinterpretations of visual, auditory, kinesthetic, and other sensory stimuli may occur. Visual illusions tend to predominate and may be relatively simple, as when the patient mistakes spots on the wall for insects, a fold in the bedcover for a snake, or the sound of a falling glass for a pistol shot. More complex illusions may also be experienced and seem to represent the projection of personally meaningful symbols and fantasies onto environmental objects. Thus a patient misperceived an ambulance as a hearse, and a stretcher as a coffin.[134] It has been suggested that these more complex (or fantasy) illusions represent intrusions of dream fragments within the perceptual field, resulting from a failure to separate inner images from outer percepts.[96] Illusions may precede or accompany hallucinations; the distinction between them may be difficult. Misinterpretations of stimuli may be incorporated in delusions, as in the case of a guilt-ridden barbiturate addict, who mistook her room for a prison cell from which she expected to be taken to be executed. She was caught opening a window (mistaken for a door) in an attempt to escape. In this case an urgent psychiatric consultation was requested not because the patient was delirious but because the staff interpreted her behavior as attempted suicide. A patient, delirious as a result of a temporal-lobe tumor, went to mow his lawn which he believed to be the Garden of Eden; he wanted to prepare it for the impending Day of Judgment. This patient was referred to the writer as a schizophrenic with religious delusions. Somatic and visceral sensations, such as paresthesias, may give rise to delusions of being poisoned or infested with lice. In delirium illusions, hallucinations, and delusions may intermingle and reinforce one another. Their affective concomitant is often anxiety which in turn enhances the susceptibility to perceptual and ideational distortions. The factors which predispose an individual to react with a paranoid attitude when consciousness is clouded need to be studied. This attitude may represent an archaic mode of response to the helplessness and adaptive incompetence resulting from cognitive disorganization—a state which for some individuals signifies the consequence or danger of malevolent interference. Whether this is the result of early experiences, inherited predisposition, and/or cultural factors is an open question.

Hallucinations, i.e., experiences having the character of perceptions but occurring without relevant or adequate sensory stimulation, have been reported in 39% to 73% of delirious patients.[10,39,109,134] These differences in observed incidence seem to reflect differences in the patient populations studied. The lowest incidence was reported in a study of patients aged 60 or older admitted to psychiatric wards of a general hospital.[109] Age may have been an important variable, since hallucinations are said to be less common in the older than in the younger delirious patients.[101] Inclusion of patients with delirium tremens in the sample studied may also influence the reported incidence of hallucinations, as these are usually regarded as one of the diagnostic criteria of this syndrome.[29] In one study of delirium, from which patients with delirium tremens were excluded (but which included 13% of alcoholic addicts), the incidence of hallucinations was only 54%.[30] It is of note that these were patients hospitalized in a psychiatric ward—an already selected group. When patients with clouding of consciousness due to metabolic disorder were studied on the medical wards the frequency of hallucinations was even lower—well under 50%.[34,116]

While hallucinations in *any* sensory modality may occur in delirium, *visual* hallucinations are most common.[10,134] In only one reported study was the incidence of auditory hallucinations higher than visual.[39] The content of visual hallucinations is highly variable and ranges from simple flashes of light, colored stars, etc., to formed and more or less complex visions of animals, inanimate objects, human figures, panoramic scenes, and even mythological figures.[15, 20, 26, 49, 134] In many cases these hallucinations are kaleidoscopic and fleeting; in some they resemble a continuous moviefilm. Visual distortions involving hallucinations, as well as true perceptions, such as polyopia, dysmegalopsia (micropsia or macropsia), metamorphopsia, and dysmorphopsia (alteration or distortion of shape) have been observed in delirium.[130] Darkness tends to increase the tendency to hallucinate, as observed by Hartley 200 years ago.[50] He noted that at the onset of delirium, patients hallucinate and "talk wildly," mostly when they are in the dark. When a candle is brought to them, they "recover themselves, and talk rationally, till the candle be removed again."

Visual hallucinations occurring in the course of the alcohol-withdrawal syndrome have attracted special attention.[12, 128] Animals of all kinds are a particularly common content of these hallucinations.[12] There is a tendency to hallucinate a variety of objects. Their reality is usually fully accepted by the patient and he reacts accordingly, i.e., with fear or amusement. The visions are often fantastic, e.g., a dragon with yellow eyes, a green head, and a red tongue.[128] There is a similarity between hallucinations in alcohol and other withdrawal syndromes on the one hand and those induced by LSD and mescaline on the other. Alcoholic addicts suffering from relapsing pancreatitis were found to hallucinate more often than those ill with pneumonia.[107]

Not only exteroceptors, i.e., vision and audition, but also proprioceptors and interoceptors may be involved in hallucinatory activity in delirium. Tactile and kinesthetic hallucinations are not uncommon.[134] Patients delirious in the course of typhus hallucinated sailing in ships, flying in planes, or falling into abysses.[49] Similar hallucinations have been described in poliomyelitis patients treated in a tank-type respirator.[94]

Disturbances of the body image, such as alteration in perception of the weight, size, shape, and position of the body or its parts, as well as their reduplication, including autoscopy, may occur in delirium.[89]

A number of questions may be raised regarding misperceptions in delirium. First what factors determine whether a delirious patient hallucinates or not? There is no conclusive answer to this at present. It has been suggested that the severity of clouding of consciousness is not the decisive factor; instead the *fluctuations* of consciousness provide a necessary condition for the appearance of hallucinations.[5] The theoretical model of informational underload (i.e., sensory deprivation) has been invoked to explain hallucinations.[13] It has been postulated that reduction of sensory input (both external and internal) can provide a necessary condition for the release of recorded percepts or memory traces. These can enter awareness and be experienced as hallucinations.[13, 128] Such an underload may possibly arise in delirium. Sensory input overload may have the same consequences and provide the mechanism for hallucinatory behavior in certain states of intoxication and conditions like delirium tremens. In the latter, the deprivation of the REM sleep and dreams has been hypothesized to result in hallucinations.[47]

While these hypotheses may help explain why hallucinations do occur, they throw no light on individual differences in susceptibility to hallucinations during states of clouded consciousness. Furthermore, conditions which result in delirium do so by virtue of a variety of biochemical and neurophysiological mechanisms which may have different potentials for releasing hallucinations. Genetic as well as acquired neurophysiological and personality characteristics may also be significant variables. Only future research can settle this.

Second, why do visual hallucinations predominate in delirium? It has been suggested that optic hallucinations are more concrete and environment-bound than the auditory ones and thus reflect the difference between the delirious and the autistic schizophrenic patient.[10] This hyopthesis would be stronger if it were shown that schizoid delirious patients tend to hallucinate in the auditory sphere. Some students of sensory deprivation have tried to account for the predominance of visual misperceptions in this state by hypothesizing that the amount of visual memory storage must be far greater than that of the other senses.[96] Thus the frequency of visual hallucinations would represent a proportionately high sampling of a rich storage of visual percepts. This hypothesis may be relevant to delirium as well. Another hypothesis proposes that in states of central disinhibition, entoptic images arising from anatomic structures of the eye, or in the retinal ganglionic network, may impinge on higher centers and there undergo secondary elaborations. The result could be the experience of visual illusions or hallucinations which follow the same psychodynamics as dream work.[61]

Third, to what extent is the *content* of hallucinations determined by the patient's conscious and unconscious wishes, conflicts and fears? A number of writers have postulated that such content does reflect the patient's remote and recent life-history as well as his needs and conflicts.[74, 94, 134] A postulated close relationship between delirious hallucinations and illusions on the one hand, and dreams on the other, has already been mentioned. These hypotheses are attractive but not yet validated by systematic studies. They are based on personal impressions, anecdotal material, and observations of individual patients. Klüver[72] draws attention to *formal* characteristics of hallucinations. He comments that to admit that distorted perceptions may have emotional significance is not the same as to assert that they are *created* by emotional factors. In addition to the formed and complex hallucinations one often finds elementary ones, such as bright spots, flashes of light, geometric figures, which seem to lack symbolic meaning.

To sum up, what has been said of the action of drugs may equally well apply to delirium; to what degree they create something new in the organism or only release that which is already present will remain an open question until physiological and psychological findings are more closely correlated.[59] One may add that what is released may be fragmented, chaotic, or randomly combined and therefore of limited signficance as a key to the patient's personality. There is no evidence yet that delirium is another "royal road" to the unconscious.

MEMORY

In delirium, there is disturbance of registration, retention, and recall of memories to a varying extent. Recent memory tends to be more severely impaired than memory for remote events. Retention and immediate recall are impaired. In some conditions such as Wernicke's encephalopathy certain types of encephalitis, and tuberculous meningitis, the defects of memory may stand out and persist longer than clouding of consciousness, or may even result in a permanent amnesic syndrome.[42, 129] Some patients confabulate. After recovery from delirium, there is usually partial or total amnesia for this period but clear memory for the hallucinatory episodes is not infrequent.[134] Some patients recall delirium as a "chaotic dream" or nightmare. The persistent amnesic gap after recovery provides an important retrospective diagnostic sign of a transient impairment of cerebral function.[129]

There are no published studies on the extent of amnesia following delirium. We do not know what effect, if any, the experience and persistent memory of delirium may have on subsequent psychic life of the individual. At least some delirious patients experience an invasion of unconscious, and presumably conflict-laden, material into awareness. One wonders how such experience is handled after recovery. In adults it has been found that delirium is only very rarely followed by schizophrenia.[10] It is not known whether the same is true of children, and if delirium experienced in childhood may predispose to later personality disorganization.

SECONDARY PSYCHOLOGICAL DISTURBANCES IN DELIRIUM

Clouding of consciousness and delirium have been defined in terms of disordered cognition, which represents the basic or primary psychological impairment in these states. Yet, as Chapman and Wolff[22] succinctly expressed it, delirium nay be viewed as a "more or less abrupt decline in high-level brain function featured by . . . a general mental cloudiness with fall-off in all functions." In their study of the effects of loss of varying amounts of cerebral cortical tissue these writers showed that such loss involves more than cognition. The whole adaptive capacity of the organism is affected, as shown by defects in (1) expression and control of drives (2) ability to tolerate frustration and anxiety, (3) maintenance of effective defense mechanisms, and (4) ability to initiate action. The same general considerations apply to delirium as well. In this syndrome, total adaptive behavior is temporarily affected to some degree. It is thus, in a full sense, an organismic reaction the cognitive aspects of which are only a partial, albeit invariable and diagnostically crucial, feature. For the sake of systematic presentation, the more important noncognitive disturbances will be discussed separately.

AFFECT

Affective change in delirium varies from patient to patient, and the same individual may exierience more than one affect concurrently or sequentially. Some writers stress *fear* as the most frequent affect in delirium,[134] while others stress *depression*.[38,39] There is little doubt that many delirious patients seen on the medical wards appear apathetic. The distinction between depression and apathy is not clear: the former implies some combination of sadness, hopelessness, and helplessness while the latter means absence of affect. Yet, in a recent study of the patterns of the depressive syndrome, apathetic behavior is considered to be a feature of one of the four clinical profiles of depression.[46] Apathy may be a symptom of the depressive syndrome, but it may also signify lack of affect in someone whose mental processes are impoverished and who is indifferent, lethargic, or somnolent. Such a distinction may be difficult to make in practice, and generalizations at this stage of our knowledge are not warranted. In the literature on delirium few authors distinguish between anxiety and fear. Anxiety can designate a syndrome, an affect, or a theoretical or explanatory concept.[84] As an affect, anxiety connotes anticipation of an imminent but intangible or improperly appraised danger. Therefore, while anxiety is a response to an unperceived or inadequate danger, fear is an affect evoked by a clearly perceived, objective threat. This difference is not a hard and fast one, for one can conceptualize continuum of affective response, with "pure" fear and anxiety representing opposite poles separated by intermediate or mixed affective states. Cognitive unclarity of danger in anxiety tends to intensify this affect and facilitate projection. The perception of physiological concomitants of anxiety also acts as a positive feedback and increases arousal. This semantic clarification of the descriptive terms for affects may serve as a background for a critical review of reported affective changes in delirium.

It appears that most writers on the subject are not concerned with a clear differentiation of the affects they observe or infer. This may partly account for variability in the reported incidence of the various affects. Some investigators note that "anxiety, apprehension, and fear" are present to some extent in all their patients, but also note that most patients are depressed.[134] In one study, depression was found to be the most common alteration of mood (40%) but "disturbance in affect" was noted in 44%, and a "shallow, constricted or flattened feeling tone" was present in 30% of all patients.[39]

One may state tentatively that the commonest affective disturbances in delirium are *anxiety, fear,* and *depression.* Less often one may see euphoria, rage, or apathy. Some patients do not show any disorder of affect. The abnormal affects may be assignable to the following variables:

1. *Personality structure.* Cognitive impairment, with the resulting loss of orientation, is stressful to many individuals. Some tend to react to cognitive blurring and instability with depression and shame, others with anxiety. Misperceptions as well as intrusion of primary process thinking may add further to the psychological stress and intensify the affects. The inner dangers are not infrequently projected on the environment and a paranoid attitude results.[134]

2. *The nature of the organic disease.* Certain conditions, such as delirium tremens, have a high potential for release of anxiety. Whether this is a result of the addict's personality or of a specific toxic effect in localized areas of the brain is unknown. By contrast, it has been observed that patients with hepatic encephalopathy tend to show euphoria or depression, while anxiety is uncommon.[30]

3. *Effect on the limbic system.* It may be postulated that a direct effect of the deranged metabolism in the anatomical substrate of emotions may release affects in a manner analogous to the ictal affects, or that affective change is the result of reduced cortical inhibition.

4. *Cultural factors.* It has been noted that members of different cultures respond differently to hallucinations. In Western cultures hallucinations often connote

insanity and its social consequences, while in some primitive cultures people tend to enjoy hallucinations, unless they have a threatening character.[124] Thus, in our culture, a delirious and hallucinating patient is likely to react to his experience with anxiety or depression or both. The content of and response to hallucinations in delirium may reflect cultural factors.

5. *Psychological stress of organic illness.* Delirium is often a complication of potentially life-threatening, or even terminal, illness. This fact may arouse fear and anxiety. The former is a realistic response to an actual danger, the latter is a result of activated intrapsychic conflicts related to the specific meaning of the illness for the patient. Depression may arise on the same basis.

A careful study of affective changes in delirium could add to our knowledge of the psychophysiology of affects. There is a need for precise descriptions and careful use of terms. It is probable that abnormal affects such as anxiety may intensify the clouding of consciousness and thus create a vicious cycle.

PSYCHOMOTOR BEHAVIOR

This may range from hyperactivity to lethargy and stupor. It is often stated that overactivity and restlessness are the rule.[134] but this seems to reflect the problem of patient selection, referred to earlier. Patients with delirium tremens are typically overactive.[29] It appears that certain agents, such as Artane,[113] tend to increase psychomotor activity, while conditions like hepatic encephalopathy[30] or Wernicke's encephalopathy[42] are usually characterized by underactivity. During the course of delirium the same patient may show a whole gamut of psychomotor behavior, as has been observed in many patients with uremia[6]: "The entire course of the illness may shift rapidly from states of overactivity with aggressiveness, crying, laughing, singing, dancing and swearing to states of lethargy...." Some patients may carry out complex movements imitating their usual work—occupational delirium. Others may try to get out of bed and wander away. Aggressive outbursts with attacks on others may occur. In more severe delirium one may observe purposeless overactivity, groping, picking at bedclothes, sudden choreiform movements, coarse tremor, etc. There is the possibility that the patient may accidentally hurt himself by falling out of bed or trying to escape his hallucinated or imagined dangers. Sometimes frantic efforts to escape may gived the appearance of a suicidal attempt, as when a patient tries to open a window and jump out of it. A true suicidal attempt may also be made. As often as overactivity, one observes *reduced activity,* and the patient appears lethargic, drowsy, slowed down, and even catatonic. Because they do not disturb anybody, such quiet patients often escape recognition by medical personnel. One finds that usually only overactive patients are referred for psychiatric consultation or admitted to psychiatric wards. This fact influences the standard descriptions of delirium given by psychiatric textbooks and papers.

Speech may be affected to a varying extent. It may be slow and slurred, or under pressure to the point of incoherence. Perseveration of psychomotor behavior, including speech, is common.[4, 79] There may be dysphasia or paraphasia. Incoherent muttering is usually a feature of severe delirium.

Autonomic Arousal

Physiological concomitants of anxiety and fear are encountered when these affects appear. Tachycardia, sweating, dilated pupils, mild pyrexia, flushing, tremor, etc. may be noted.[134]

Etiological Factors

A necessary condition for the development of delirium, as well as stupor and coma, is a disturbance in the production or utilization of energy involving cerebral cortex and those subcortical structures necessary for the maintenance of consciousness. Such disturbance can result from any interference with the supply of oxygen or substrate (mainly glucose) to, or with their uptake and utilization by, the neurons concerned. There may be interference with substrate or oxygen availability or enzymatic disturbances (lack of enzyme activators, inhibition of enzymatic activity, destruction of enzymes), or a combination of these factors.[40] If deprivation of energy reaches a critical degree of intensity or duration, irreversible cerebral damage and permanent psychiatric sequelae may result. Clearly the number of possible etiological factors and biochemical pathways must be large. Their full listing would go beyond the scope of this paper. More or less exhaustive lists of relevant factors are readily available in the literature.[23, 31] The following classes of organic conditions are more commonly associated with delirium:

Intoxication
1. Endogenous: hepatic encephalopathy, uremia, pulmonary insufficiency;
2. Exogenous: drugs, such as bromides, barbiturates, atropine, digitalis; alcohol; industrial poisons; addictive inhalants.

Drug withdrawal syndromes from alcohol (delirium tremens), barbiturates, meprobamate, chloral hydrate, paraldehyde, chlordiazepoxide, glutethimide, etc.

Infections.
1. Acute: intracranial; systemic.
2. Chronic: cerebrovascular syphilis.

Head trauma.

Epilepsy: postictal automatisms.

Metabolic disorders: endocrinopathies; excess or deficiency of minerals, electrolytes, water; avitaminosis (nicotinic acid, thiamine, B_{12}, folic acid); porphyria.

Intracranial space-occupying lesions.

Cerebrovascular and cardiovascular diseases.

Cerebral degenerative diseases: e.g., multiple sclerosis.

Collagen diseases, especially systemic lupus erythematosus.

Extracranial neoplasm, such as bronchogenic carcinoma.

Organic causative factors are more likely to result in delirium if more than one of them are present simultaneously. Thus, anoxia associated with electrolyte imbalance, blood pH changes, and the presence of endo- or exotoxins in the blood are more likely to cause delirium than any of these factors alone.

Absolute value of a given pathogenic factor, as well as the duration of its effect and the rate of change in the chemical milieu of the brain, seem to be significant variables, e.g., a fast-growing brain tumor and rapidly rising intracranial pressure favor the development of clouded consciousness.[9]

PREDISPOSING FACTORS

It is postulated that delirium may be the only psychiatric syndrome of universal susceptibility. There is no doubt however that there are *individual differences* in susceptibility to react with delirium to any given causative factor. Our knowledge of the predisposing conditions is surprisingly scanty. In this area there is more conjecture than established fact. A striking example of the differential susceptibility to delirium was given by Ebaugh *et al.*[35] These authors investigated delirious episodes in 200 patients undergoing courses of pyretotherapy, i.e., induction of fever in a hypertherm, heated to 130°–150°F. The patient's rectal temperature had to reach 104°–107°F in 1 hour. Of the 200 subjects so treated, 54% developed delirium at least once. Forty percent of those who became delirious had only one episode of delirium usually during the first treatment even though they had several exposures to the same conditions. It was hypothesized that initial anxiety increased the incidence of delirium during the first treatment session.

There is abundant clinical evidence that not every individual will develop delirium with equal ease, but our ability to predict such development in any given case is limited. The factors which have been established as increasing predisposition to delirium are

1. age fifty years or over;
2. addiction to alcohol or drugs;
3. cerebral damage due to any cause and sustained at any age.

There is no evidence for a hereditary predisposition to delirium.[10] No relationship could be found between predisposition to schizophrenia and delirium.[10] There is no excessive frequency of schizophrenia among relatives of patients who develop delirium, and no higher-than-average incidence of delirium in schizophrenics and their relatives.[10] This observation is important as there is a tendency to vaguely invoke inadequate ego strength as a predisposing factor to delirium. "Ego strength" is a weak explanatory concept, as it is too general to allow specific predictions to be based on it. No single psychological or personality variable has been established as imparting enduring predisposition to delirium. Abse[1] states that hysterics show proneness to it, but he does not substantiate this claim with supporting data. Bleuker *et al.*[10] conclude that knowledge of a person's personality does not allow one to predict whether he will be prone to delirium, or if he does develop it, what content it will show. One writer claims that patients who have had previous psychotic episodes, or those who have a history of postoperative or postpartum delirium, are more likely to become delirious when exposed to the stress of severe organic illness or operation.[118] It is not clear, however, if this statement is based on clinical impression or a systematic study. More research is needed to confirm or refute this and preceding claims.

PSYCHOLOGICAL STRESS AND DELIRIUM

There is growing evidence that certain conditions which affect the human organism primarily at the symbolic level of organization, and are best expressed in psychological terms, can precipitate, facilitate the onset of, or intensify delirium. The following is a tentative list of such factors:

VARIATION IN THE QUANTITY AND PATTERNING OF SENSORY INPUT

Experimental sensory deprivation has been found to have its principal effects on cognitive and perceptual processes. These effects include such changes as difficulty in directed (secondary process) thinking and concentration, "drifting" of thought with fantasies and daydreams (primary process), disorientation in time, illusions and hallucinations, paranoid delusions.[139] Ziskind *et al.*[136] postulate that a hypnoid syndrome, i.e., one of "reduced consciousness," is invariably present in sensory deprivation situations of sufficient intensity to cause symptoms. This syndrome includes (1) disturbances of perception (2) interference with goal-directed behavior, confusion, (3) somnolence, (4) anxiety, and (5) restlessness. The authors stress that this syndrome differs from the acute brain syndrome due to toxins in that confusion is fleeting and retrograde amnesia for the experience absent or reversible. These, however, seem to be quantitative rather than qualitative differences. The fact that slowing of the EEG has been found during various types of sensory deprivation of even brief duration[91, 138] further increases the probability that sensory deprivation results in mild clouding of consciousness and delirium.

A number of writers have pointed out the contributory role of reduced or destructured sensory input in delirium,[76] observed under various clinical conditions, such as eye surgery,[83, 127] placement in an intensive care unit[73, 93] and use of tank-type respirator in poliomyelitis patients.[94] It appears that patients 50 years old or older and those of any age who suffered brain damage are particularly likely to become delirous when sensory input is reduced. Inglis[62] hypothesizes that one of the ways in which sensory deprivation may affect cognitive functioning is by "depriving the acting, perceiving, problem-solving organism of the stimulus manifold against which his attempts at acting and problem-solving may continually be checked." He explains some clinical symptoms of deprivation as being due to interference with the normal feedback cycle in individuals handicapped in sensory storage capacity as a result of aging.

Closely related to sensory deprivation seem to be the factors of *social isolation*,[87, 135] *familiarity* of the environment,[78, 87] and *immobilization*.[82] It has often been observed that elderly patients admitted to hospital at first appear to be well compensated mentally, but they may rapidly develop manifest delirium. In these cases the loss of familiar sensory cues or separation from familiar people intensifies cerebral decompensation and results in manifestly disturbed behavior.

The effects of immobilization on behavior and EEG changes have been studied by Zubek and MacNeill.[137] They found that reducing the level of kinesthetic and proprioceptive stimulations by immobilizing the body can result in slowing of the EEG and impaired performance on intellectual tests as well as on two measures of perceptual–motor processes. In addition, some immobilized subjects reported hallucinatory experiences, complex and vivid dreams, temporal disorientation, anxiety, body-image disturbances, time distortions, and bizarre thoughts. Clinical relevance of these experimental findings has been postulated for patients with orthopedic, neurological, cardiac, and other disorders, necessitating prolonged periods of recumbency and immobilization.[82]

In summary, experimental and clinical observations converge to suggest that interference with the quantity and quality of sensory input is a significant variable in some cases of clinical delirium. This is an area of study with important theoretical and practical implications. Higher nervous activity may be affected by means other than direct physical or chemical assault on the brain. The mediating mechanisms of the effects described above are still unknown, although the ascending reticular activating system has been implicated. The practical consequences include provision of adequate sensory and social stimulation in hospital settings.

SLEEP DEPRIVATION

Experimental studies of sleep deprivation show a progressive disorder in cognition, visual perception, and time orientation, related to the duration of enforced sleeplessness.[96] Psychotic behavior tends to appear after about 120 hr of continuous sleep deprivation, although in one case studies it was absent during 264 hr of wakefulness.[48] It has been suggested that psychological changes during sleep deprivation closely resemble those found in altered consciousness brought about by sensory deprivation, bromide intoxication, and alcoholic hallucinosis.[96] The sleep-deprived subject experiences periods of drowsiness characterized by primary changes in attention, thinking, and interest.[96] Each level of drowsiness is accompanied by secondary changes in memory, perception, orientation, and affect, which are experienced by some but not all subjects.[96] One may tentatively suggest that sleep deprivation results in clouding of consciousness and delirium of varying degree of severity. It has been suggested that deprivation of sleep contributes to the onset of delirium following open-heart surgery, when the patients are tended in the recovery room and subjected to multiple awakenings.[73] Hinkle[57] states that symptoms of disordered brain function brought on by sensory and sleep deprivation, as well as by fatigue, differ little from those of the brain syndrome. He suggests that there is a wider range of individual susceptibility to the pathogenic effects of these factors than is the case with changes in body temperature, oxygen and glucose supply, etc. When one considers that insomnia is often a prodromal symptom of delirium, it is likely that it may contribute to the development and intensity of this syndrome.

PSYCHOLOGICAL REACTION TO ILLNESS

It has been suggested that threatening circumstances which engender conflict, or other excessive or prolonged stress, may impair high level brain function.[21] Physical illness may be regarded as one such form of psychological stress. If the affective response to illness is characterized by severe anxiety, the result may be an increased susceptibility to delirium. A similar result seems to follow massive denial of a threat and anxiety, as may happen in the case of impending surgery.

PSYCHOSOCIAL SITUATION IN WHICH SOMATIC ILLNESS DEVELOPS

When there is a setting of disturbed interpersonal relationships or heightened intrapsychic conflict, with resulting dysphoric affects, the individual may be more susceptible to cognitive disorganization. This can happen even when the physical illness is relatively mild.

THE QUALITY OF RELATIONSHIP BETWEEN THE PATIENT AND MEDICAL TEAM

It is postulated that the more trusting, conflict-free, and supporting such a relationship is, the less tendency will the patient show to gross cognitive disorganization.

The above variables are still largely hypothetical and their etiological importance is likely to vary from case to case. They deserve systematic study. We know little about the mediating physiological processes whereby various modes of psychological stress can result in impairment of brain function. This question offers a challenge to psychosomatic investigators and highlights the suitability of delirium for the study of the relationship between the mental and the physical. One may hypothesize that clouding of consciousness and delirium are the final common path for a variety of pathogenic factors, ranging on a continuum from organic to symbolic. This conception is strengthened by the common observation that psychological states, such as anxiety or depersonalization, can result from diverse causes, including focal cerebral disease, cerebral effects of systemic disease, as well as psychic conflict primarily involving the symbolic level of organization.

To conclude, delirium is seen as a truly psychosomatic condition, in the sense that both its determinants and manifestations encompass multiple biological and psychological variables. Whether psychological factors are a necessary condition for delirium to develop is an open question at present.

AN EXPLANATORY HYPOTHESIS

The most influential hypothesis attempting to explain the phenomena of delirium was advanced by Hughlings Jackson.[65] He proposed that this syndrome is an example of the dissolution of the highest nervous centers with retained control at the lower levels. The patient's condition is thus partly negative and partly positive. The negative mental state signifies loss of function of the "topmost layer" of the highest centers; the positive aspect represents activity at the lower level of the highest centers. Disorientation is an example of the negative aspect; misinterpretations of the environment represent a positive part of the syndrome and reflect activity at a lower level of organization. There is generally a reduction to a more automatic condition with the dominance of mentation devoid of its most differentiated, "highest," features. The highest and least organized and automatic centers are the physical basis of "most vivid consciousness." It is these centers that are affected in delirium.

The definition of clouding of consciousness proposed in this paper fits in with Hughlings Jackson's conception of dissolution. Directed or secondary process thinking is the evolutionarily highest, most complex, and specifically human attribute which is invariably impaired in delirium.

CLINICAL DIAGNOSIS OF DELIRIUM

The diagnosis rests on the recognition of descriptive features discussed earlier. Evidence of some degree of global cognitive impairment which tends to fluctuate in severity is diagnostically crucial. Presence of delirium can usually be established in the course of routine history-taking. Mental status examination which reveals no evidence of organic dysfunction is associated with a final diagnosis of functional mental illness with rare exceptions.[111] The following clinical tests are useful: serial subtraction, digit span, simple calculation, recitation of 6 mo forwards, orientation for time, orientation for place and person, ability to estimate passage of time, general information on current events, simple psychomotor tests eliciting perseveration.[4] All these procedures can be carried out at the bedside. Psychological tests, such as vocabulary and digit span subtests of the WAIS, Bender–Gestalt, Graham–Kendall, and Benton tests, may be employed.

The electroencephalogram is the most valuable laboratory tool aiding the diagnosis of delirium.[38, 103] Romano and Engel[103] carried out pioneering studies in this area. There is generally a tendency to progressive, diffuse slowing of the *basic* frequencies. In the complete absence of clouding of consciousness the EEG is seldom affected to any marked degree.[69] The degree of disturbance of consciousness is reflected with only rare exceptions in the degree of EEG changes.[17] Yet such exceptions do occur and some disturbed tracings are found where no change of consciousness exists and vice versa.[17, 69] At present these discrepancies are unexplained, but that does not alter the fact that in the majority of cases there is correspondence between psychological evidence of clouding of consciousness and EEG slowing. Delirium tremens provides an exception in that records showing low-to-moderate-voltage fast activity are more frequent than those with diffuse slow activity.[38] Of importance for resolving the problem of *fast* frequencies in the EEG of some delirious cases are recent studies by Itil and Fink.[64] These investigators experimentally induced delirium with Ditran and attempted to modify it with several antagonists. They found that anticholinergic hallucinogens led to a dissolution of the alpha rhythm with increases in delta and theta bands and superimposed fast beta activity. When this type of EEG disorganization was induced rapidly, behavior was characterized by clouding of consciousness and psychomotor hyperactivity. The alteration in the ratio of slow and fast frequencies was associated with the various aspects of the delirious state. With enhanced slow activity, there was predominance of stuporlike states. With relative increase in fast activity there was psychomotor hyperactivity and perceptual distortions. The writers postulate that these changes may be related to the effect on the medial ascending reticular activating system, which has cortical inhibitory function (slow waves in the EEG), as well as on the medial thalamic diffuse projection systems, which have a predominantly facilitatory influence upon the cortex (fast activity in the EEG). Increased activity of one or other of these systems may determine the type of delirium, i.e., whether psychomotor overactivity or underactivity predominates.

These findings and conclusions are significant in that they provide support for the *unitary* conception of delirium advocated in this review. They help encompass logically within one syndrome contrasting behavioral manifestations which may accompany clouding of consciousness.

DIFFERENTIAL DIAGNOSIS

This problem, discussed in some detail by Engel and Romano,[38] will only be touched upon here. It is acknowledged that many psychiatric disorders present cognitive–perceptual abnormalities. Schizophrenia, severe depression, or anxiety invariably impairs cognition to some extent. There is thus some overlap between these conditions and delirium, but this does not imply identity. Furthermore, a mixture of syndromes may be encountered clinically. A schizophrenic picture may accompany delirium. In this review delirium has been differentiated from other conditions by recognizing that is a reversible, global impairment of cognitive functions, with a tendency to fluctuations in the level of awareness, and usually a diffuse slowing of the EEG. The main practical importance of correctly diagnosing delirium is that such a diagnosis necessitates an inquiry into the underlying organic factor or factors and their prompt correction. An error of omission may result in irreversible cerebral damage with life-long psychological consequences.

Of particular diagnostic relevance are those states in which clouding of consciousness appears in the absence of detectable organic disease. There are reports in the literature of conditions named "acute confusion,"[114] "acute exhaustive psychoses,"[2] and "episodic confusions,"[68] which seem to be clinically indistinguishable from delirium and are regarded by the authors as psychogenic. No causative organic factors were found in these syndromes, even when death occurred and autopsy was performed. Clouding of consciousness has also been reported in a variety of states, such as the acute confusional type of schizophrenia, schizophreniform psychosis, oneirophrenia, and reactive psychosis.[8] The nosological status of these conditions is at present unclear and their relationship to delirium undefined. Combined clinical, electroencephalographical, and biochemical studies may clarify this in the future.

Certain drugs, such as amphetamines, cortisone, Atabrine, LSD, and mescaline, can cause psychoses which have to be distinguished from delirium. These conditions generally lack the features of clouding of consciousness as defined here.[63, 132] Their EEG characteristics also tend to be different. These states may be regarded as different modes of altered consciousness; their descriptive and neurophysiological characteristics await full elaboration.

Delirium also has to be distinguished from other reversible organic psychiatric syndromes, such as hallucinosis; transient amnesic syndrome; and the focal brain syndrome characterized primarily by a disturbance of affect and impulse expression and control.[9] All of these conditions should logically be included in the class of the "acute brain syndrome." The latter is clearly not coterminous with delirium, but a broader category including it.

Dementia, which is by definition irreversible, cannot always be readily distinguished from delirium. A prolonged observation and therapeutic trial may be necessary to settle the issue. On the whole, dementia does not display fluctuations of awareness, perceptual distortions, and reversible EEG changes. Reversible dementia, as recently described in folate deficiency,[115] is a contradiction in terms; it is clearly delirium.

MANAGEMENT OF DELIRIUM

Only the basic principles of therapy will be summarized. Other investigators have discussed them in detail[23,24,54]:

1. Treat the underlying cause (or causes) adequately.
2. Scrutinize all drugs which the patient is receiving and withdraw them if possible. Even therapeutic doses of a common drug, such as acetylsalicylic acid, may precipitate delirium on the basis of individual idiosyncrasy, or in the presence of cerebral, hepatic, or renal damage.
3. Insure electrolyte balance, adequate hydration, nutrition, and vitamin supply.
4. General care: adequate sensory stimulation to avoid sensory deprivation or overload effects, proper nursing care,[24] provision of familiar stimuli such as presence of close relatives, avoidance of physical restraints, the use of special attendants around the clock to avoid accidents and consequent medicolegal problems.
5. Psychiatric consultation: Psychiatrists working on the medical and surgical wards have more familiarity with delirium and its management than other physicians. An early psychiatric consultation may lead to prompt recognition and adequate treatment of the delirious patient.
6. Sedation: This is needed only when the patient is grossly overactive, violent, or anxious. Phenothiazines, chlordiazepoxide, and diazepam ar the most useful drugs for this purpose.
7. A small number of ECTs may on occasion be lifesaving.

EXPERIMENTAL DELIRIUM

An important recent development is the experimental production of delirium by pharmacological and other means. These methods provide a convenient way of studying psychological, neurophysiological, and biochemical aspects of this syndrome, under controlled conditions.

One of the earliest experiments was that by Cameron,[18] who showed that senile patients who tended to develop nocturnal delirium did so just as readily in daytime, if confined to a dark room. The delirium subsided in about 1 hr after the patient emerged from the darkness. This experiment illustrated the effect of reduction of visual cues on the development of delirium in those predisposed to it by brain damage.

In recent years drugs, mostly anticholinergic agents, such as Ditran,[44, 63, 64, 132] Sernyl,[44] benactyzine,[122] scopolamine,[28] amitryptyline,[5] have been used to produce delirium experimentally. The theoretically significant effects of Ditran, an anticholinergic drug, have already been mentioned. The psychotomimetic properties of benactyzine, a potent anticholinergic agent, have been explained on the basis of its interference with both acetylcholine and serotonin metabolism of the brain.[122] This group of drugs should be distinguished from other psychotomimetic agents, such as LSD and mescaline, as the former induce true delirium while the latter give rise to a syndrome which resembles more closely functional psychotic states.[132] A comparison of subjective effects of LSD and delirium tremens yielded significant differences although there was some overlap in the reported experiences, as well as considerable variation of individual response in both groups of subjects.[33] When LSD was administered to subjects with Ditran-induced delirium, there was an increase in alertness and psychomotor activity as well as more reports of perceptual distortions and thought disorder; the EEG showed increase in fast activity.[64] Ditran administered to alcoholic addicts who had experienced delirium tremens reproduced that syndrome.[44]

Other experimental methods of inducing clouding of consciousness include exposure to hyperbaric air[3] and to decreased barometric pressures in altitude chamber flights.[105]

CONTEMPORARY RELEVANCE OF DELIRIUM

Data on the frequency of delirium are rare. When one considers the confusion surrounding the subject discussed earlier, as well as the fact that the majority of the cases are found on the medical and surgical wards of general hospitals and likely remain undiagnosed, the statistical data available are not only questionable but misleading. A recent survey[45] of patients discharged with a psychiatric diagnosis from United States general hospitals over one year (1963-1964) shows that 70,854, i.e., 12% of the total, had the diagnosis of "brain syndrome" (no distinction was made between acute and chronic syndromes). The difficulties in determining the incidence of the acute brain syndrome as well as the importance of detection and proper management of this condition are emphasized in a recent study carried out in California.[43] Bleuler *et al.*[10] estimate that about 30% of the population between the ages of 20 and 70 years are likely to have suffered at least one episode of exogenous psychosis. The same writer estimates the incidence of such psychosis in the medical department of a general hospital at 5-10%. Some American authors report that as many as 40-50% of patients aged 60 years or over show evidence of delirium on admission to hospital.[101, 109] Anesthetists have observed delirium (referred to as "postanesthetic excitement" or "emergence delirium") in 5-6% of large samples of postoperative patients.[27, 37] The highest incidence of these postoperative deliria was in young patients who underwent operations associated with pain or emotional stress. Delirium developed in a relatively large proportion of children anesthetized with a barbiturate plus nitrous oxide-oxygen.[90] In a random sample of 200 surgical patients, delirium was found in 7.8%.[117] The investigators comment that delirium was often the first sign of a deterioration of the patients' medical condition and call for early recognition and prompt treatment.

Several writers[38, 77, 98] stress that delirium often goes unrecognized in the general hospitals and ascribe this fact partly to the neglect of organic aspects of psychiatry in the training of residents. It has been rightly suggested that the psychiatrist should be no less expert in the diagnosis and management of delirium as in the dynamic formulation of neuroses.[133]

A curious omission in the literature on delirium is the almost complete lack of reports on its incidence and consequences in childhood.[67] While it is often asserted that delirium is common in children, relevant statistics are missing. It is an important question whether delirium experienced in childhood has any effect on the psychological development of the individual and whether it predisposes him to psychiatric illness such as schizophrenia, anxiety, or dissociative states, in later life. An indication of the importance of this problem is found in an electroencephalographic study of children ill with apparently uncomplicated acute viral disease, such as measles, mumps, chickenpox, and rubella.[125] Nearly 30% of these children showed EEG changes identical with those found in manifest viral encephalitis. It was suggested that this indicated a mild encephalitis or metabolic encephalopathy and could explain persisting sequelae, such as mental retardation or behavior disorders.

Evidence that delirium is a common condition is accruing. Psychiatric consultants working on the medical and surgical wards find that organic brain syndromes constitute about 17% of referrals for consultation.[86] There is no doubt that this represents only a fraction of the true incidence. An increased awareness of the less dramatic and undisturbing modes of presentation of delirium is of practical importance, if permanent brain damage is to be avoided.

A number of factors contribute to the high, if not rising, incidence of delirium today. Increasing life-span of our population results in a growing number of elderly people, among whom delirium is particularly common and dangerous.[43, 109] The growing number of drugs, including tranquilizers, sedatives, and antidepressants, is a contributing factor to iatrogenic delirium and that resulting from withdrawal syndromes in people addicted to sedatives. Modern surgical procedures, such as heart surgery[51]; frequency of head trauma due to car accidents; industrial poisons; alcohol addiction—all these factors raise the incidence of delirium and make it a health hazard of major importance. Its theoretical interest rests in its being a condition in which cerebral pathophysiology and psychopathological manifestations occur in close temporal proximity, reinforce each other, and allow a study of brain–mind interaction. Both clinical and experimental studies of delirium now in progress should contribute to a clearer delineation of various altered states of consciousness, their psychological characteristics and neurophysiological correlates.

It is proposed that skill in diagnosing and treating delirium should be part of medical training. Systematic studies of it are needed to determine its incidence, causes, factors influencing its form and content, and the possible psychological sequelae in individuals recovering from it. Delirium highlights the dependence of man's unique attribute—his symbolic activity—on intact cerebral function and illustrates the manifold ways in which this activity can be impaired. This syndrome, which is likely as old as homo sapiens, is a major health problem today. It is psychosomatic condition par excellence and has been neglected too long.

REFERENCES

1. Abse WD: *Hysteria and Related Mental Disorders.* Bristol, Wright, 1966.
2. Adland ML. Review, case studies, therapy, and interpretation of the acute exhaustive psychoses. *Psychiatr Quart* 21:38-69, 1947.
3. Adolfson J: Deterioration of mental and motor functions in hyperbaric air. *Scand J Psychol* 6:26-32, 1965.
4. Allison, RS. Perseveration as a sign of diffuse and focal brain damage. *Br Med J* 2:1027-1032, 1966.
5. Arnold OH, Kryspin-Exner K: Das experimentelle Delir. *Wien Z Nervenheilk* 22:73-93, 1965.
6. Baker AB, Knutson J. Psychiatric aspects of uremia. *Am J Psychiat* 102:683-687, 1946.
7. Bash KW: Zur Psychopathologie akuter symptomatischer Psychosen. *Nervenarzt* 28:193-199, 1957.
8. Bellak, L, ed: *Schizophrenia: A Review of the Syndrome.* New York, Logos Press, 1958.
9. Bleuler M: Psychiatry of cerebral diseases. *Br Med J* 2:1233-1238, 1951.
10. Bleuler M, Willi J, Buehler HR: *Akute psychische Begleiterscheinungen koerperlicher Krankeiten.* Stuttgart, Thieme, 1966.
11. Bonhoeffer, K: Die Psychosen im Gefolge von akuten Infektionen, Allgemeinerkrankungen und inneren Erkrankungen, in Aschaffenburg GL (ed). *Handbuch der Psychiatrie,* Spez. Teil 3, Leipzig, Deuticke, 1912, pp. 1-60.
12. Boor W de: *Pharmakopsychologie und Psychopathologie.* Springer, Berlin, 1956.
13. Brawley P, Pos, R: The informational underload (sensory deprivation) model in contemporary psychiatry. *Can Psychiatr J* 12:105-124, 1967.
14. Brodal A: Anatomical points of view on the alleged morphological basis of consciousness. *Acta Neurochir (Wien)* 12:166-186, 1964.
15. Brown S: On the intervention of symptoms in the infective exhaustive psychoses. *J Nerv Ment Dis* 43:518-531, 1916.
16. Burt C: The concept of consciousness. *Br Psychol* 53:229-242, 1962.
17. Cadilhac J, Ribstein M. The EEG in metabolic disorders. *World Neurol* 2:296-308, 1961.
18. Cameron ED: Studies in senile nocturnal delirium. *Psychiatr quart* 15:47-53, 1941.
19. Cameron N: *Personality Development and Psychopathology.* Boston, Houghton Mifflin, 1963.
20. Cameron N, Magaret A: *Behavior Pathology.* Boston, Houghton Mifflin, 1951.
21. Chapman LF, Thetford WN, Berlin L, Guthrie TC, Wolff HG: Highest integrative functions in man during stress, in Solomon HC, Cobb S, Penfield W (eds): *The Brain and Human Behavior.* [Proc Ass Res Nerv Ment Dis] 36:491-534, 1958.
22. Chapman LF, Wolff HG: Disease of the neopallium and impairment of the highest integrative functions. *Med Clin North Am* 42:677-689, 1958.
23. Cohen S: The toxic psychoses and allied states. *Am J Med* 15:813-828, 1953.
24. Cohen S, Klein HK: The delirious patient. *Am J Nurs* 58:685-687, 1958.
25. Collier RM: A holistic-organismic theory of consciousness. *J Individ Psychol* 19:17-26, 1963.
26. Conrad K: Die symptomatischen Psychosen, in Gruhle HW, Jung R, Mayer-Gross W, Mueller M (eds): *Psychiatrie der Gegenwart,* Band 2, pp. 369-436. Berlin, Springer, 1960.
27. Coppolino GA: Incidence of post-anesthetic delirium in a community hospital: A statistical study. *Milit Med* 128:238-241, 1963.
28. Crowell EB Jr, Ketchum JS: The treatment of scopolamine-induced delirium with physostigmine. *Clin Pharmacol Ther* 8:409-414, 1967.

29. Cutshall BJ: The Saunders-Sutton syndrome: An analysis of delirium tremens. *Q J Stud Alcohol* 26:423–448, 1965.
30. Davidson EA, Solomon P: The differentiation of delirium tremens from impending hepatic coma. *J Ment Sci* 104:326–333, 1958.
31. Dewan JG, Spaulding WB: *The Organic Psychoses.* Toronto, Toronto University Press, 1958.
32. *Diagnostic and Statistical Manual of Mental Disorders.* Washington, DC, American Psychiatry Association, 1952.
33. Ditman KS, Whittlesey JRB: Comparison of the LSD-25 experience and delirium tremens. *Arch Gen Psychiatry (Chicago)* 1:47–57, 1959.
34. Dulfano MJ, Ishikawa S: Hypercapnia: Mental changes and extrapulmonary complications. *Ann Intern Med* 63:829–841, 1965.
35. Ebaugh FG, Barnacle CH, Ewalt JR: Delirious episodes associated with artificial fever: A study of 200 cases. *Am J Psychiatry* 23:191–217, 1936.
36. Eccles JC (ed): *Brain and Conscious Experience.* New York, Springer, 1966.
37. Eckenhoff JE, Kneale DH, Dripps RD: The incidence and etiology of post-anesthetic excitement. *Anesthesiology* 22:667–673, 1961.
38. Engel GL, Romano J: Delirium, a syndrome of cerebral insufficiency. *J Chron Dis* 9:260–277, 1959.
39. Farber IJ: Acute brain syndrome. *Dis Nerv Syst* 20:296–299, 1959.
40. Fazekas JF, Alman RW: *Coma: Biochemistry, Physiology and Therapeutic Principles.* Springfield, Il, Charles C Thomas, 1962.
41. Forgus RH: *Perception.* New York, McGraw-Hill, 1966.
42. Frantzen E: Wernicke's encephalopathy. *Acta Neurol Scand* 42:426–441, 1966.
43. Freedman DK, Troll L, MIlls AB, Baker P: *Acute Organic Disorder Accompanied by Mental Symptoms.* Sacramento, California Department of Mental Hygiene, 1965.
44. Gershon S, Olariu J: JB 329—A new psychotomimetic: Its antagonism by tetrahydroaminacrin and its comparison with LSD, mescaline and sernyl. *J Neuropsychiatry* 1:283–292, 1960.
45. Giesler R, Hurley PL, Person PH Jr: *Survey of General Hospitals Admitting Psychiatric Patients.* Washington, DC, US Dept. of Health, Education, and Welfare, 1966.
46. Grinker RR Sr, Miller J, Sabshin M, Nunn R, Nunnally JC: *The Phenomena of Depressions.* New York, Hoeber, 1961.
47. Gross MM, Goodenough D, Tobin M, Halpert E, Lepore D, Perlstein A, Sirota M, Dibianco J, Fuller R, Kishner I: Sleep disturbances and hallucinations in the acute alcoholic psychoses. *J Nerv Ment Dis* 142:493–514, 1966.
48. Gulevich G, Dement W, Johnson L: Psychiatric and EEG observations on a case of prolonged (264 hours) wakefulness. *Arch Gen Psychiatry (Chicago)* 15:29–35, 1966.
49. Guttman O: Psychic disturbances in typhus fever. *Psychiatr Quart* 26:478–491, 1952.
50. Hartley D: *Observations on Man, His Duty, and His Expectations.* London, Leake and Frederick, 1749.
51. Hazan SJ: Psychiatric complications following cardiac surgery: I. A review article. *J Thorac Cardiovasc Surg* 51:307–319, 1966.
52. Hebb DO: *A Textbook of Psychology.* Philadelphia, Saunders, 1958.
53. Hebb, DO: The American revolution. *Am Psychol* 15:735–745, 1960.
54. Henry DW, Mann AM: Diagnosis and treatment of delirium. *Cana Med Assoc J* 93:1156–1166, 1965.
55. Hernandez-Peon R: Physiological mechanisms in attention, in Russell RW (ed): *Frontiers in Physiological Psychology.* New York, Academic Press, 1966, pp 121–147.
56. Hilgard ER: *Introduction to Psychology,* ed 2. New York, Harcourt, Brace, 1957.
57. Hinkle LE Jr: The physiological state of the interrogation subject as it affects brain function, in Biderman AD, Zimmer H (eds): *The Manipulation of Human Behavior.* New York, Wiley, 1961, pp 19–50.
58. Hoch A: The problem of toxic-infectious psychoses. *NY State Hosp Bull* 5:384–392, 1912.
59. Hoch PH, Cattell JP, Pennes HH: Effects of drugs. *Am J Psychiatry* 108:585–589, 1952.
60. Holt RR: The emergence of cognitive psychology. *J Am Psychoanal Assoc* 12:650–665, 1964.
61. Horowitz MJ: The imagery of visual hallucinations. *J Nerv Ment Dis* 138:513–523, 1964.
62. Inglis J: Sensory deprivation and cognitive disorder. *Br J Psychiatry* 111:309–315, 1965.

63. Itil T: Quantitative EEG changes induced by anticholinergic drugs and their behavioral correlates in man. *Recent Adv Biol Psychiatry* 8:151-173, 1966.

64. Itil T, Fink M: Anticholinergic drug-induced delirium: Experimental modification, quantitative EEG and behavioral correlations. *J Nerv Ment Dis* 143:492-507, 1966.

65. Jackson JH: in Taylor J (ed): *Selected Writings*. New York, Basic Books, 1958, vols 1 and 2.

66. Jaspers K: *General Psychopathology*. Chicago, University of Chicago Press, 1963.

67. Kanner L: *Child Psychiatry*, ed 3. Springfield, Ill, Charles C Thomas, 1957.

68. Kasanin J: The syndrome of episodic confusions. *Am J Psychiat* 93:625-638, 1936.

69. Kiloh LG, Osselton JW: *Clinical Electroencephalography*. London, Butterworths, 1961.

70. Klein R, Mayer-Gross W: *The Clinical Examination of Patients with Organic Cerebral Disease*. London, Cassell, 1957.

71. Kleitman N: Sleep, Wakefulness, and consciousness. *Psychol Bull* 54:354-359, 1957.

72. Klüver H: Mechanisms of hallucinations, in McNemar Q, Merrill MA (eds): *Studies in Personality*. New York, McGraw-Hill, 1942, pp 175-207.

73. Kornfeld DS, Zimberg S, Malm JR: Psychiatric complications of open-heart surgery. *N Engl J Med* 273:287-292, 1965.

74. Kubie LS: The psychodynamic position on etiology, in Kruse HD (ed): *Integrating the Approaches to Mental Disease*, New York, Hoeber-Harper, 1957, p. 24.

75. Lehmann, J: Mental disturbances followed by stupor in a patient with carcinoidosis. *Acta Psychiatr Scand* 42:153-161, 1966.

76. Leiderman PH, Mendelson J, Wexler D, Solomon P: Sensory deprivation: Clinical aspects. *Arch Intern Med (Chicago)* 101:389-396, 1958.

77. Levin M: Delirium: A gap in psychiatric teaching. *Am J Psychiatry* 107: 689-694, 1951.

78. Levin M: Toxic delirium precipitated by admission to the hospital. *J Nerv Ment Dis* 116:210-214, 1952.

79. Levin M: Perseveration at various levels of complexity, with comments on delirium. *AMA Arch Neurol. Psychiatry* 73:439-444, 1955.

80. Levin M: Thinking disturbances in delirium. *AMA Arch Neurol Psychiatry* 75:62-66, 1956.

81. Levin M: Varieties of disorientation. *J Ment Sci* 102:619-623, 1956.

82. Levy R: The immobilized patient and his psychologic well-being. *Postgrad Med* 40:73-77, 1966.

83. Linn L, Kahn RL, Coles R, Cohen J, Marshall D, Weinstein EA: Patterns of behavior disturbance following cataract extraction. *Am J Psychiatry* 110:281-289, 1953.

84. Lipowski ZJ: Psychopathology as a science: Its scope and tasks. *Compr Psychiatry* 7:175-182, 1966.

85. Lipowski ZJ: Review of consultation psychiatry and psychosomatic medicine: I. General principles. *Psychosom Med* 29:153-171, 1967.

86. Lipowski ZJ: Review of consultation psychiatry and psychosomatic medicine: II. Clinical aspects. *Psychosom Med* 29:201-224, 1967.

87. Litin EM: Mental reaction to trauma and hospitalization in the aged. *JAMA* 162:1522-1524, 1956.

88. Ludwig AM: Altered states of consciousness. *Arch Gen Psychiatry (Chicago)* 15:225-234, 1966.

89. Lunn V: On body hallucinations. *Acta Psychiatr Scand* 41:387-399, 1965.

90. Malkin M, Hirsch AC: Postanesthetic delirium and its treatment. *Oral Surg* 21:738-742, 1966.

91. Marjerrison G, Keogh RP: Electroencephalographic changes during brief periods of perceptual deprivation. *Percept Mot Skills* 24:611-615, 1967.

92. Mayer-Gross W, Slater E, Roth M: *Clinical Psychiatry*. London, Cassell, 1954.

93. McKegney PF: The intensive care syndrome. *Conn Med* 30:633-636, 1966.

94. Mendelson J, Solomon P, Lindemann E: Hallucinations of poliomyelitis patients during treatment in a respirator. *J Nerv Ment Dis* 126:421-428, 1958.

95. Meyer A: in Winters EE (ed): *Collected Papers*, Baltimore, Johns Hopkins Press, 1951, vol 3, pp 304-305.

96. Morris GO, Singer MT: Sleep deprivation: The context of consciousness. *J Nerv Ment Dis* 143:291-304, 1966.

97. Plum F, Posner JB: *The Diagnosis of Stupor and Coma*. Philadelphia, Davis, 1966.

98. Reding GR, Daniels RS: Organic brain syndromes in a general hospital. *Am J Psychiatry* 120:800-801, 1964.

99. Redlich FC, Freedman DX: *The Theory and Practice of Psychiatry*. New York, Basic Books, 1966.

100. Robins AL, Schappell A, Wortis B: Psychiatric manifestations of organic disease of the brain. *Med Clin N Amer* 42:711-721, 1958.

101. Robinson WG Jr: the toxic delirious reactions of old age, in Kaplan OJ (ed): *Mental Disorders in Later Life*. Stanford, Stanford University Press, 1956, pp 332-351.

102. Romano J, Engel GL: Physiologic and psychologic considerations of delirium. *Med Clin North Am* 28:629-638, 1944.

103. Romano J, Engel GL: Studies of delirium: I. Electroencephalographic data. *AMA Arch Neurol Psychiatry* 51:356-377, 1944.

104. Rosenfeld HA: Note on the psycho-pathology of confusional states in chronic schizophrenias. *Int J Psychoanal* 31:132-137, 1950.

105. Sarnoff CA, Haberer CE: The technique of studying disturbances of consciousness at altitude. *J Aviat Med* 30:231-240, 1959.

106. Schiller F: Consciousness reconsidered. *AMA Arch Neurol Psychiatry* 67:199-227, 1952.

107. Schuster MM, Iber FL: Psychosis with pancreatitis. *Arch Intern Med (Chicago)* 116:228-233, 1965.

108. Searles HF: Concerning a psychodynamic function of perplexity, confusion, suspicion and related mental states. *Psychiatry* 15:351-376, 1952.

109. Simon A, Cahan RB: The acute brain syndrome in geriatric patients. *Psychiatr Res Rep* 16:8-21, 1963.

110. Simson TP: Infection psychoses. *Public Health Rep* 75:451-462, 1960.

111. Small IF, Small JG, Fjeld SP, Hayden MP: Organic cognates of acute psychiatric illness. *Am J Psychiatry* 122:790-797, 1966.

112. Staub H, Thoelen H (eds): *Bewusstseinsstoerungen*. Stuttgart, Thieme Verlag, 1961.

113. Stephens DA: Psychotoxic effects of benzhexol hydrochloride (Artane). *Br J Psychiatry* 113:213-218, 1967.

114. Stern ES: Acute confusional insanity and delirium. *J Ment Sci* 90:761-766, 1944.

115. Strachan RW, Henderson JG: Dementia and folate deficiency. *Q J Med* 59:189-204, 1967.

116. Summerskill WHJ, Davidson EA, Sherlock S, Steiner RE: The neuropsychiatric syndrome associated with hepatic cirrhosis and an extensive portal collateral circulation. *Q J Med* 25:245-266, 1956.

117. Titchener JL, Zwerling I, Gottschalk L, Levine M, Culbertson W, Cohen S, Silver H: Psychosis in surgical patients. *Surg Gynecol Obstet* 102:59-65, 1956.

118. Tucker WI: The prevention and management of toxic psychosis (post-operative psychosis). *Lahey Clin Bull* 13:268-271, 1964.

119. Tuke DH: *A Dictionary of Psychological Medicine*. Philadelphia, Blakiston, 1892.

120. Tyler RH: Neurological complications of dialysis, transplantation, and other forms of treatment in chronic uremia. *Neurology (Minneap)* 15:1081-1088, 1965.

121. Victor M, Adams RD. The acute confusional states, in Harrison TR, Adams RD, Bennett IL Jr, Resnik WH, Thorn GW, Wintrobe MM (eds): *Principles of Internal Medicine*. ed 4. New York, McGraw-Hill, 1962, pp 354-362.

122. Vojtechovsky M, Vitek V, Rysanek K: Experimentelle Psychose nach Verabreichung von Benactyzin. *Arzneimittel-forsch* 16:240-242, 1966.

123. Walker EF: The syndrome of delirium. *Dis Nerv Syst* 9:336-339, 1948.

124. Wallace AFC: Cultural determinants of response to hallucinatory experience. *Arch Gen Psychiatry (Chicago)* 1:58-69, 1959.

125. Weinmann HM: EEG changes in acute viral disease in infancy and childhood. *Electroenceph Clin Neurophysiol* 22:93, 1967.

126. Weinstein EA, Kahn RL: *Denial of Illness*. Springfield, Ill, Charles C Thomas, 1955.

127. Weisman AD, Hackett TP: Psychosis after eye surgery. *N Engl J Med* 258:1284-1289, 1958.

128. West LJ (ed): *Hallucinations*. New York, Grune & Stratton, 1962.

129. Whitty CWM, Zangwill OL (eds): *Amnesia*. London, Butterworths, 1966.

130. Willanger R, Klee A: Metamorphopsia and other visual disturbances with latency occurring in patients with diffuse cerebral lesions. *Acta Neurol Scand* 42:1-18, 1966.

131. Willis T: *Two Discourses Concerning the Soul of Brutes*. London, Bring, Harper and Leigh, 1683.

132. Wilson RE, Shagass C: Comparison of two drugs with psychotomimetic effects (LSD and Ditran). *J Nerv Ment Dis* 138:277-286, 1964.

133. Wohlrabe JC, Pitts FN Jr: Delirium and complex electrolyte disturbance. *Dis Nerv Syst* 25:44–47, 1965.

134. Wolff HG, Curran D: Nature of delirium and allied states. *AMA Arch Neurol Psychiatry* 33:1175–1215, 1935.

135. Ziskind E: Isolation stress in medical and mental illness. *JAMA* 168:1427–1431, 1958.

136. Ziskind E, graham RW, Kuninobu L, Ainsworth R: The hypnoid syndrome in sensory deprivation. *Recent Adv Biol Psychiatry* 5:331–346, 1963.

137. Zubek, JP, MacNeill M: Studies on immobilization: Behavioral and EEG effects. *Can J Psychol* 20:316–334, 1966.

138. Zubek JP, Welch G: Electroencephalographic changes after prolonged sensory and perceptual deprivation. *Science* 139:1209–1210, 1963.

139. Zuckerman M: Perceptual isolation as a stress situation. *Arch Gen Psychiatry (Chicago)* 11:255–276, 1964.

Delirium Updated

15

The new classification of organic mental disorders in *Diagnostic and Statistical Manual of Mental Disorders*. ed 3 (DSM-III)[1] features delirium as one of the seven organic brain syndromes. Acute failure of integrated cerebral functioning, due to a wide range of possible noxious factors, is manifested at the behavioral level by the syndrome of delirium.[2] Although well described by numerous writers since antiquity, delirium is still often misdiagnosed, and confusion about its essential features persists. For example, a recent report on lithium toxicity describes a patient as distractible, fully disoriented, and visually hallucinated, but curiously concludes that "despite the similarity of this illness to an acute delirium with occasional lucid intervals, the patient had no clouding of consciousness."[3] To counteract such diagnostic and related errors, an update of the diagnosis, pathogenesis, and management of delirium is presented, which supplements a previous extensive review.[4]

DEFINITION AND CLINICAL FEATURES

DEFINITION

Delirium may be defined as a transient mental disorder reflecting acute brain failure due to widespread derangement of cerebral metabolism. It is characterized by concurrent disorders of cognition, wakefulness, and psychomotor behavior.

DISORDER OF COGNITION

The first core feature of delirium is a relatively global impairment of cognitive functions. "Cognitive" refers to those mental functions that are involved in the acquisition, processing, storage, and retrieval of information about one's self, one's body, and one's environment. Thus, evidence of some degree of impairment of perception, memory, and thinking is essential for the diagnosis of delirium. As a result of such impairment, the patient's awareness of self and surroundings is reduced, and this is reflected in some degree of spatiotemporal disorientation, tendency to misidentify unfamiliar persons and surroundings for familiar ones, and difficulty in relating current perceptions to previously acquired knowledge. Patients and persons in attendance may

Reprinted from *Comprehensive Psychiatry* 21,(3):190–196, 1980. Copyright © 1980 by Grune & Stratton, Inc. Reprinted by permission.

use the term "confusion" to describe that state, but that word is devoid of precise meaning. It may refer to disorientation, muddled thinking, and/or difficulty in distinguishing perceptions from dreams and hallucinations. The latter occur in some 40–70% of cases and are not necessary for the diagnosis.[2] If hallucinations are present, they are most often visual or visual plus auditory.

Thinking is invariably disorganized to some extent. it may be slowed, labored, and impoverished, or on the contrary, speeded up and rich in personally meaningful and sometimes disturbing imagery. In either case, however, controlled and purposeful thinking, especially in the abstract mode, is impaired, and ability to reason and solve problems is reduced. The patient appears perplexed when asked simple questions and may not understand them, fails to appreciate logical connections and grasp similarities and differences between concepts, and has difficulty in grasping the current situation. Such thinking disorder seems to facilitate the common occurrence of transient delusions.

Memory is invariably impaired to some extent. Recall of memories formed before the onset of delirium is faulty, and ability to register and retain new information is reduced, resulting in partial amnesia for the duration of delirium after its resolution.

DISORDER OF WAKEFULNESS

The second core feature of delirium, one insufficiently stressed by most textbooks, is a disorder of wakefulness and sleep–waking cycle.[2] That disorder is manifested by disturbances of attention and by various combinations of drowsiness, insomnia, vivid dreams, nightmares, and oneiric or dreamlike mentation. The patient exhibits some difficulty in mobilizing, focusing, shifting, and sustaining attention. Alertness, that is, readiness to response to stimuli, may be increased or reduced. Some patients may be hyperalert and respond readily to stimuli but in an involuntary and indiscriminate manner. Vigilance, that is, sustained attention, is invariably reduced in delirium, regardless of whether the patient is hyperalert or hypoalert. A patient's capacity for selective and sustained attention tends to fluctuate during the course of a day. During the so-called lucid periods, alertness and vigilance may be relatively normal for minutes or even hours at a time, and the patient is then more accessible to questions. It is conceivable that disturbances of attention in delirium are primary and give rise to cognitive dysfunction.

Disturbances of the sleep–waking cycle have been observed in delirium since Hippocrates. Insomnia is the rule and may be total. Sleep–waking cycle may be reversed. Drowsiness and naps during daytime and insomnia at night are often combined. It appears that the normal sleep–waking cycle is disrupted and fragmented in delirium. Some patients describe the experience of delirium as an unpleasant twilight state between sleeping and waking.[2] The syndrome may be ushered in by insomnia and vivid dreams, and often becomes manifest first and is typically most pronounced at night. The patient wakes up and experiences confusion about his or her surroundings and often exhibits inability to distinguish dreams from hallucinations and true perceptions. A patient woke up to see his son at his bedside and said: "I recognize you from my dreams." It is likely that such subjective confusion between inner and outer reality, and the not uncommon sense of dreaming while awake, have encouraged hypotheses that delirium is a waking dream. Hunter[5] argued that delirium is "a diseased dream arising from what may be called diseased sleep." Such views were common in the 18th century and need to be reconsidered. The question whether hallucinations in delirium represent dreams remains open.[2] It is a fact, however, that many patients experience an oneiric state in which imagery, perceptions, hallucinations, and dreams merge and intertwine.

The ubiquity of disordered attention, alertness, vigilance, and sleep–waking cycle in delirium indicates that the syndrome represents in part a disorder of wakefulness.[2] That hypothesis offers advantages over the prevalent view of delirium as a disturbance of consciousness. The latter is an ambiguous term whose physiologic correlates have proven difficult to define. To propose that delirium is a disorder of wakefulness implies that the neurophysiologic and biochemical mechanisms subserving normal wakefulness are deranged. Since those mechanisms involve several neurotransmitters that are known to be imbalanced in many cases of delirium, my hypothesis has some empirical support. It will have heuristic value if it encourages studies on the relationship of delirium to disturbances of the sleep–waking cycle, to dreaming, and to their physiologic substrates.

A Disorder of Psychomotor Behavior

The third and last essential feature of delirium involves abnormal psychomotor behavior. The latter may extend over a whole spectrum, from ceaseless and purposeless hyperactivity, through sluggish inertia, to catatonic stupor. The patient's psychomotor behavior often shifts unpredictably from abnormally low to abnormally high. Some patients are predominantly underactive, others display hyperactivity. Purposefully modulated behavior is abolished in fully developed delirium. Speech may be slow and halting or fast but incoherent, and may very in volume from barely audible muttering to loud screaming, wailing, and other vocalizations. Various semipurposeful or involuntary movements may be present, such as tremor, grasping, picking at bedclothes, etc. Dysgraphia is the rule.[6] Differences in the level and form of psychomotor behavior between and within delirium patients contribute to the confusing variability of the clinical picture. Some authors include hyperactivity and excitement in their definition of delirium, contrary to clinical observations recorded since Hippocrates that it may feature a whole gamut of abnormal psychomotor activity.

Associated Features

Several associated, inconsistent features may be seen in delirium and add to its clinical variability. A whole range of emotions may be experienced and expressed by the patients. Fear, depression, apathy, rage, and euphoria may all be exhibited with their usual physiologic and expressive concomitants. No emotion is characteristic of delirium, however, even though some authors include fear in its definition. A fearful or angry patient may sustain injury while attempting to flee or fight. Fear in delirium is commonly a response to threatening hallucinations, persecutory delusions, or both.

Such psychotic symptoms are typically associated with hyperactive delirium and with increased autonomic, especially sympathetic, arousal, manifested by tachycardia, flushed face, sweating, dilated pupils, and elevated blood pressure.

Delirium is at times preceded for hours or even days by prodromal symptoms such as hypersensitivity to stimuli, difficulty in concentration and maintaining coherent train of thought, anxiety or lethargy, and vivid dreams and nocturnal visual hallucinations. In some cases coma and stupor precede delirium, as in concussion. Delirium usually lasts several days or a few weeks, rarely longer than a month. It is usually followed by recovery, but it may represent a terminal event or be succeeded by any other organic brain syndrome.

DIAGONOSIS OF DELIRIUM

Diagnosis of delirium should involve two aspects: clinical recognition of the syndrome and identification of the cause of brain failure. Diagnostic criteria for delirium in DSM-III[1] include

1. Clouding of consciousness (reduced clarity of awareness of environment) and disturbances of attention.
2. At least two of the following:
   Perceptual disturbance: misinterpretations, illusions, or hallucinations.
   Speech that is at times incoherent.
   Disturbances of sleep–wakefulness cycle with insomnia or daytime drowsiness.
   Increased or decreased psychomotor activity.
3. Disorientation and memory impairment.
4. Clinical features develop over a short period of time (usually hours to days) and tend to fluctuate over the course of a day.
5. Evidence, from the history, physical examination, or laboratory tests, of a specific organic factor judged to be etiologically related to the disturbance.

It is unfortune that DSM-III enshrines the vague and obsolete term ''clouding of consciousness,'' which itself begs to be defined. Abnormal thinking is left out and replaced by a vague reference to speech. Since evidence of a specific organic factor is occasionally lacking in practice, it would be prefereable to require laboratory evidence of disordered cerebral function instead. The EEG slowly was stressed by Engel and Romano[7] as a diagnostic criterion of delirium. Although slowing of the EEG background activity is not invariably present (being absent in delirium tremens,[8] for example), it remains a useful diagnostic aid, especially in cases where a specific organic factor cannot be found or the question of a focal lesion or a nonorganic mental disorder arises.[9,10]

PROBLEMS IN DIFFERENTIAL DIAGNOSIS

It is sometimes difficult to differentiate delirium from dementia, with which it may coexist. Since dementia no longer connotes irreversible and progressive intellectual deterioration, and a search for a treatable cause of it is the rule nowadays, such differentiation is less crucial than in the past. Dementia is a global cognitive disorder that is relatively stable and unaccompanied by fluctuating disturbance of wakefulness and attention.

It may be difficult to distinguish delirium from one of the disorders included in DSM-III under the terms schizophreniform disorder, brief reactive psychosis, and atypical psychosis. DSM-III states that in brief reactive psychosis there may be confusion with clouding of consciousness, disorientation, and impairment of recent memory. Such acute psychoses have been described in psychiatric literature for over 100 yr under a variety of names: acute delirium, Bell's mania, acute confusional insanity or state, psychogenic delirium, amentia, episodic confusion, exhaustion psychoses, psychogenic psychoses, bouffées délirantes, etc.[2] Those psychoses feature schizophrenic, affective, and delirious symptoms in various combinations and constitute a largely unexplored area of psychiatry at the boundary between delirium and functional psychoses. The EEG and sodium amytal interview are currently the main, if not entirely reliable, aids in the differential diagnosis between delirium and the psychoses under discussion.[7,9-11]

ETIOLOGY AND PATHOGENESIS

ETIOLOGY

Acute brain failure and delirium may result from a wide range of factors, acting singly or in various combinations, that bring about widespread derangement of cerebral metabolism.[2] Both intracranial diseases and systemic ones affecting the brain secondarily, as well as exogenous poisons and withdrawal from various substances of abuse, may cause delirium. In the absence of epidemiological data, one may only estimate that intoxication by medical drugs and substances of abuse, systemic metabolic disorders, and head trauma are the most common organic factors responsible for delirium today. Anticholinergic agents appear to be implicated particularly often.

The presence of one or more organic factors is a necessary condition for delirium to occur. Psychological stress, sleep and sensory deprivation, prolonged immobilization, and severe fatigue are likely to facilitate the onset of delirium and increase its severity.[2] Age of 60 yr and over, addiction to alcohol or drugs, and brain damage of any source predispose a person to delirium. Children are said to be particularly susceptible to it, but supporting data are lacking. Psychological predisposing factors have been postulated but never adequately demonstrated.[2]

PATHOGENESIS

Engel and Romano[7] postulated that a general derangement of brain metabolism underlies all cases of delirium and is reflected in reduced awareness and a slowing of the EEG background activity. A recent review[10] concludes that if delirium occurs in a severely ill medical patient and features reduced level of awareness and arousal, the EEG is liable to show some degree of diffuse slowing. If, however, delirium is of a predominantly hyperactive type, such as delirium tremens, the EEG slowing may be absent. This suggests that more than one pathogenetic mechanism may underlie delirium.

Direct studies of cerebral metabolism in delirium remain to be carried out. Positron emission tomography offers an intriguing possibility in this respect.[12] Recent studies of hypoxia and hypoglycemia show that even mild impairment of cerebral carbohydrate metabolism, insufficient to cause brain energy failure, results in reduced synthesis of acetylcholine and other neurotransmitters.[13] Blass and Gibson[13] have proposed that impairment of cholinergic function in the brain due to a variety of factors may play a key role in disorders of cognition. The reported efficacy of physostigmine, a cholinesterase inhibitor, in reversing delirium due not only to anticholinergics but also alcohol and cimetidine points to disordered cholinergic function in this syndrome.[2] Serotonergic and noradrenergic mechanisms in the brain may also be implicated in some cases. Serotonergic supersensitivity has been postulated to mediate delirium induced by prolonged levodopa therapy.[14] Central noradrenergic activity is reportedly increased in delirium tremens.[15]

Thus, recent studies support the view that widespread derangement of cerebral metabolism, coupled with imbalance of brain neurotransmitters, underlie delirium. Both cortical and subcortical structures are likely involved, as indicated by concurrent disorder of cognition and wakefulness. Future studies of regional cerebral metabolism and distribution of putative cerebral neurotransmitters in delirium of various etiologies should lead to identification of specific pathogenetic factors, and elucidate the origin of such clinical features as hypoactivity, hyperactivity, and hallucinations.

Management of Delirium

To identify the causative factor (or factors) and treat it, to offer supportive nursing care and maintain intake of fluids and nutrition, to sedate the restless and fearful patient, and to ensure sleep have been the key principles taught for centuries in the management of delirium.[2, 16] The only major recent addition has been a better selection of drugs. Haloperidol, with a few notable exceptions, has emerged as the drug of choice in delirium.[17, 18] It is effective in calming agitated, restless, and hallucinating patients and is remarkably safe in the presence of a wide range of physical illnesses and not likely to increase delirium. It is not recommended in several instances: in anticholinergic delirium, where physostigmine is the drug of choice[19]; in hepatic encephalopathy, in which benzodiazepines are preferable[20]; and in alcohol and drug withdrawal deliria, in which it offers no advantage over other commonly used drugs.[21]

Conclusion

Inclusion of delirium and formulation of its diagnostic criteria in DSM-III should improve its diagnosis and stimulate research that has been lagging for the past 30 yr. The high incidence of the syndrome in critical care medicine and in the aged, in whom it is one of the most common presenting features of physical illness and drug toxicity, underscores the need for its clinical recognition, management, and investigation. New research tools, such as positron emission tomography, are likely to help advance knowledge and diagnosis of delirium in the coming years.

REFERENCES

1. American Psychiatric Association: Diagnostic and Statistical Manual of Mental Disorders, ed 3. Washington DC, American Psychiatric Association, 1980.
2. Lipowski ZJ: *Delirium: Acute Brain Failure in Man.* Springfield Ill, Charles C Thomas, 1980.
3. Agulnik PL, Di Mascio A, Moore P: Acute brain syndrome associated with lithium therapy. *Am J Psychiatry* 129:621-623, 1972.
4. Lipowski ZJ: Delirium, clouding of consciousness and confusion. *J Nerv Ment Dis* 145:227-255, 1967.
5. Hunter J: *The Works of John Hunter, FRS* Palmer JF (ed). London, Longman, Rees, Orme, Brown, Green, and Longman, 1835, vol 1, p 333.
6. Chedru F, Geschwind N: Writing disturbances in acute confusional states. *Neuropsychologia* 10:343-353, 1972.
7. Engel GL, Romano J: Delirium, a syndrome of cerebral insufficiency. *J Chron Dis* 9:260-277, 1959.
8. Allahyari H, Deisenhammer E, Weiser G: EEG examination during delirium tremens. *Psychiatr Clin (Basel)* 9:21-31, 1976.
9. Obrecht R, Okhomina FOA, Scott DF: Value of EEG in acute confusional states. *J Neurol Neurosurg Psychiatry* 42:75-77, 1979.
10. Pro JD, Wells CE: The use of electroencephalogram in the diagnosis of delirium. *Dis Nerv Syst* 38:804-808, 1977.
11. Ward NG, Rowlett DB, Burke P: Sodium amylobarbitone in the differential diagnosis of confusion. *Am J Psychiatry* 135:75-78, 1978.
12. Editorial: Images of brain function. *Lancet* 2:725-726, 1979.
13. Blass JP, Gibson GE: Carbohydrates and acetylcholine synthesis: Implications for cognitive disorders, in Davis KL, Berger PA (eds): *Brain Acetylcholine and Neuropsychiatric Disease.* New York, Plenum, 1979, pp 215-236.
14. Nausieda PA, Kaplan LR, Weber S, et al: Sleep disruption and psychosis induced by chronic levodopa therapy. *Neurology (Minneap)* 29:553, 1979.
15. Athen D, Beckmann H, Ackenheil M, et al: Biochemical investigations into the alcoholic delirium: Alterations of biogenic amines. *Arch Psychiat Nervenkr* 224:129-140, 1977.
16. Lipowski ZJ: Organic mental disorders: Introduction and review of syndromes, in Freedman AM, Kaplan HI, Sadock BJ (eds): *Comprehensive Textbook of Psychiatry*, ed 3. Baltimore, Williams & Wilkins, 1980.
17. Ayd FJ: Haloperidol: Twenty years' clinical experience. *J Clin Psychiatry* 39:807-814, 1978.
18. Moore DP: Rapid treatment of delirium in critically ill patients. *Am J Psychiatry* 134:1431-1432, 1977.
19. Granacher RP, Baldessarini RJ: Physostigmine. *Arch Gen Psychiatry* 32:375-380, 1975.
20. Editorial: Sedation in liver disease. *Br Med J* 1:1241-1242, 1977.
21. Holzback E, Bühler KE: Die Behandlung des Delirium tremens mit Haldol. *Nervenarzt* 49:405-409, 1978.

Transient Cognitive Disorders (Delirium, Acute Confusional States) in the Elderly

16

> *Delirium and intoxication may be considered transient effects, from temporary causes, of that condition of sensorium which, more deeply fixed and longer continued, obtains the name and produces all the aspects of mental derangement.*
> HENRY HOLLAND, *Medical Notes and Reflections*, 1839

Cognitive disorders are on the rise. Their growing importance as a medical and psychiatric problem reflects the continued increase in the number of the elderly worldwide.[1, 2] In the United States, there are 25.5 million persons aged 65 years and older. Dementia and delirium, the main cognitive disorders, are most common among the elderly. Recent medical editorials speak of dementia as a "quiet epidemic" and "one of the greatest problems facing modern society."[3] [4] The elderly, and especially the demented, are uniquely prone to transient cognitive disorders, usually referred to in the literature as delirium or acute confusional states.[5] As the prevalence of dementia is expected to rise in the coming years because of the aging of the populaion, so the incidence of delirium is likely to follow suit. While dementia has attracted growing attention.[6, 7] delirium in the elderly continues to be neglected.[8, 9] A recent report of the Royal College of Physicians emphasizes that insufficient attention has been paid to this common and important mental disorder, one whose onset in an elderly patient usually heralds physical illness and hence calls for immediate medical evaluation.[8] Furthermore, delirium is still often mistaken for an irreversible dementia. The present overview may help prevent such grave diagnostic errors in the future and stimulate sorely needed research on transient cognitive disorders.

Reprinted from *American Journal of Psychiatry* 140(11):1426–1436, 1983. Copyright © 1983 by the American Psychiatric Association. Reprinted by permission.

EARLY STUDIES

In 1870, Hood[10] reported on several cases of "senile delirium" and concluded that it could develop in elderly persons free of prior "mental debility," required prompt treatment of the underlying cause, and was potentially reversible but could result in death from exhaustion. In 1904, Pickett[11] stressed the importance of distinguishing "confusion" and "delirium," two similar and curable mental disorders of the elderly, from senile dementia. Delirium, he believed, always had an organic cause, while confusion could result from bereavement, for example. This proposed distinction between delirium and confusion has remained an unexplored issue until today. By 1939 the concept of transient cognitive disorders in the elderly had been clearly formulated and the importance of differentiaing them from senile dementia fully recognized.[12] Unfortunately, progress in this area since then has been hampered by terminological chaos and lack of explicit diagnostic criteria. As a result, case identification, elucidation of causative factors and pathogenetic mechanisms, and clinical management have suffered. To facilitate communication, research, and teaching, the semantic muddle must be overcome.

DEFINITIONS: A WAY OUT OF THE SEMANTIC MUDDLE

Overlapping, inconsistently used, and poorly defined terms have bedeviled this area of psychiatry for decades. "Senile delirium," "acute confusional states," "acute brain syndrome," "acute brain failure," "pseudosenility," and "clouded states" are all terms that have been used to designate delirium in the elderly. Currently, "acute confusional states" and "delirium" are the most often used designations. The former term has been recommended by the World Health Organization and defined as a syndrome characterized by "features of delirium."[13] Derived from "confusion,"[14] an ambiguous quasimedical term that is widely used and all too loosely applied to the elderly,[15] "acute confusional states" is a designation favored by geriatricians and neurologists. It refers to some combination of spatiotemporal disorientation, difficulty in thinking coherently, memory impairment, and bewilderment.[15-17] In psychiatry, the terms "confusion" and "acute confusional states" have no established meaning, may be used in reference to a person of any age, and lack a clear etiological connotation of either organicity or psychogenicity.[16, 18] In DSM-III, "delirium" has replaced "acute confusional states" and is listed among organic brain syndromes. Ambiguity persists, however, as some writers include among acute confusional states both organic and presumably psychogenic transient cognitive disorders.[15, 16] while others use the word "delirium" in a narrow sense to denote a syndrome featuring hyperalertness, hyperactivity, frightening hallucinations, and high autonomic arousal.[19]

To clear up this semantic muddle I propose that (1) the term "delirium" be used exclusively for those transient global cognitive disorders that may occur at any age and that are judged to be of *organic* etiology, (2) the use of the ambiguous term "acute confusional states" be discouraged, and (3) the deliriumlike cognitive disorders judged to be functional be referred to as "pseudodelirium," by analogy with pseudodementia, until their nosological status has become clarified. (Such disorders cannot be called delirium, since DSM-III requires evidence of a "specific organic factor" for the latter.)

Delirium is defined as an organic brain syndrome characterized by global cognitive impairment of abrupt onset and relatively brief duration (usually less than 1 month) and by concurrent disturbances of attention, sleep–wake cycle, and psychomotor behavior (references 17, 20, 21, DSM-III). (For the sake of clarity, I will use the term "delirium" here even where the original source referred to used one of its synonyms.)

INCIDENCE AND IMPORTANCE OF DELIRIUM

Nearly every physical illness may give rise to delirium in an elderly person. As one geriatrician put it, "Acute confusion is a far more common herald of the onset of physical illness in an old person than are, for example, fever, pain or tachycardia."[22] "Confusion" is one of the most frequent reasons for referral of a patient to a geriatrician.[23] Failure to diagnose delirium and to identify and treat its underlying causes may have lethal consequences for the patient, since it may constitute the most prominent presenting feature of myocardial infarction, pneumonia, or some other life-threatening physical illness.

Few epidemiological studies have been done on delirium in the elderly. Its incidence is claimed to be four times higher in persons more than 40 years old[24] and is highest among those older than 70 years.[25] A geriatric multicenter British study found that 35% of patients aged 65 years and over had delirium on admission or developed it during the index hospitalization.[26] An even higher incidence, 80%, was found among 5000 patients 65 years and older admitted to the Oxford Geriatric Unit.[27] Of 534 patients aged 60 or older admitted to psychiatric wards of San Francisco General Hospital in 1959, 55% were diagnosed as having "acute organic brain syndrome" (i.e., delirium), which in about 80% of cases was associated with chronic brain disease.[28] Two studies of elderly patients admitted to general medical wards reported an identical incidence of delirium, 16%.[29, 30] Furthermore, other studies have shown that about 25% of those elderly patients who are judged to be cognitively intact on admission may be expected to develop delirium during the first month of hospitalization.[8, 26] Thus between one third and one half of the hospitalized elderly are likely to be delirious at some point during the index admission. If one considers that in 1980 the elderly occupied 38% of all beds in nonfederal short-stay hospitals,[31] it seems likely that the incidence and prevalence of delirium in these patients are higher than is often realized. Several investigators have reported that 10–15% of general surgical patients aged 65 or older become delirious after their operation.[32, 33] Clearly, the syndrome is sufficiently frequent among elderly medical and surgical patients to pose a formidable diagnostic and therapeutic challenge to all physicians, including general hospital psychiatrists.

Delirium is by definition transient, but this should not obscure the fact that in the elderly it is often a prelude to death or, probably less often, to dementia. Bedford[27] reported that fully 33% of 4000 patients exhibiting delirium on admission to a hospital died within a month. Of the survivors 80% recovered in less than a month and only 5% remained confused for more than 6 months. (By DSM-III criteria these patients would be likely to have a diagnosis of dementia.) In both the multicenter British study and the San Francisco study about one in four delirious elderly patients died within a month of admission.[26, 28] This mortality rate was about twice as high as that for comparable nondelirious patients.[26] In the two general hospital studies, 37% and 18%, respectively, of the delirious patients died.[29, 30] patients with the lowest mental test scores on admission, indicating most severe cognitive impairment, are likely to have a poor outcome.[30] The development of delirium in an elderly person must be regarded as a grave prognostic sign.

CLINICAL SYNDROME: PSYCHOPATHOLOGY AND COURSE

Studies of the phenomenology of delirium in old age are almost nonexistent, and the relevant literature is mostly anecdotal. The core features of the syndromes may be assumed to be the same in all age groups, however, and include disorders of cognition, attention, sleep–wake cycle, and psychomotor behavior.[5,12,17,20,32,34–38]

DISORDER OF COGNITION

Global disturbance of cogntion is one of the core features of delirum.[17] Perception, thinking, and memory—the three main aspects or phases of cognition—are all abnormal to some extent in delirium, as the adjective "global" implies. Cognitive processes whereby the individual acquires knowledge and guides his behavior are disorganized, rendering him helpless to some degree. Acquisition, processing, retention, retrieval, and utilization of information are all impaired, resulting in what both medical and lay observers often refer to as "confusion." This impairment may range from slight to profound; in the latter, organized cognitive activity practically ceases. As a result, the patient is less capable than normally of making sense of his environment and situation, of reasoning and solving problems, and of sustaining goal-directed behavior for any length of time.[17,20,34,35]

Disorganization and fluctuating efficiency of cognitive processes in delirium appear to facilitate the emergence of certain abnormal cognitive phenomena such as misidentifications, illusions, hallucinations, dreamlike (oneiric) thinking, delusions, and confabulations. The patient is always at least mildly disoriented in time and, in more severe delirium, also for place and person, but he practically never loses the sense of personal identity.[34] Typically, the disoriented delirious individual tends to misidentify unfamiliar places and persons as familiar ones.[39] The cognitive disorder characteristically fluctuates in severity over the course of a day, with so-called lucid intervals interspersed irregularly throughout, and is usually most pronounced during the night.

The elderly delarious patient often fails to show the more elaborate and flamboyant features such as hallucinations, oneiric thinking, and confabulations.[8, 32] Many of these patients suffer from concurrent dementia, which appears to limit their capacity to elaborate these symptoms.

Perception in delirium is marked by reduced ability to discriminate and integrate percepts and to distinguish them clearly from imagery, dreams, and hallucinations.[17] The patient may perceive objects as distorted, i.e., too big (macropsia), too small (micropsia), reduplicated (polyopsia), or misshapen (dysmorphopsia).[40] Stationary objects may be perceived as moving or flowing together. Illusions and hallucinations in any modality, but especially visual or mixed visual and auditory ones, are common but are neither invariably present in nor diagnostic of delirium. While some observers claim that only about 40% of the delirious elderly hallucinate,[28] others assert that most of these patients can be found to do so if one questions them systematically.[41] In about half of the patients hallucinations occur only at night.[42] They are typically experienced as real, three-dimensional, moving, bright, and colored images of people or nonhuman objects of natural size.[42] Most patients react to them with fear or anger and attempts at flight or fight, but some may actually enjoy them, especially the visions of cherished relatives or friends.

Thinking is disorganized and fragmented. Delirious patients of any age tend to experience uncontrolled and often disturbing dreamlike imagery or disjointed thoughts. The elderly delirious patient, however, is more likely to have only impoverished and incoherent thought processses. His ability to reason, use abstract concepts, judge, solve problems, and plan action is reduced. To think sequentially and logically, to grasp the meaning of words and define them, to see similarities and differences, and to direct thought at will are all abilities that have become difficult or impossible for the patient. A frankly paranoid attitude is common, and persecutory delusions, which tend to be poorly worked out, fleeting, changeable, and bound to the immediate stimuli, occur in 40% to 55% of the delirious elderly.[28]

Memory is impaired in all its aspects: registration, retention, and retrieval. Immediate recall is impaired, probably because of reduced attention span. Recent memory is more impaired than remote memory, and the ability to learn is reduced. Both retrograde and anterograde amnesia of some degree are present.[17] Unless the patient is also demented, he is likely to have relatively intact remote memory for both personal and public events.

DISORDER OF ATTENTION 'AND WAKEFULNESS

For about a century delirium has been linked with the concept of disordered or "clouded" consciousness, its alleged cardinal feature.[17] DSM-III includes clouding of consciousness among the diagnostic criteria for delirium and equates it with "reduced clarity of awareness of the environment," accompanied by "reawareness of the environment," accompanied by "reduced capacity to shift, focus, and sustain attention to environmental stimuli" (DSM-III, p. 107). For reasons discussed elsewhere,[17, 35] I shall use the more clearly defined and precise terms "attention" and "wakefulness," rather than "clouding of consciousness," a metaphorical concept that, in my view, is obsolete, vague, and redundant.

In delirium, attention is disordered in all of its main aspects: alertness (vigilance) or readiness to respond to stimuli, selectiveness, and directiveness. The patient shows diminished ability to respond to stimuli selectively, to mobilize, sustain, and shift attention at will, and to direct mental processes.[17] Alertness or vigilance may be abnormally increased or decreased, but capacity to deploy attention selectively and directively is invariably reduced.[17, 34, 35] Some writers regard abnormalities of attention as basic to and responsible for cognitive disorganization.[43] Basic or not, the characteristically fluctuating attentional disturbances in delirium enhance disruption of cognitive processes, impede communication with the patient, and render his behavior and performance erratic.

Disordered wakefulness and sleep–wake cycle are among the essential features of delirium (reference 17, DSM-III). Wakefulness is usually reduced during the day and abnormally increased at night. Night sleep is usually fragmented and reduced. For centuries many medical writers have viewed delirium as the "dreams of waking persons"[44] and as a manifestation of disordered sleep.[17] Kennedy[36] pointed out the similarities between delirium and dreaming, both of which are associated with EEG slowing and lessened attention. A typical elderly delirious patient is awake, restless, agitated, bewildered, and often hallucinating during the night and may oscillate between sleep and waking and betwen dreaming and hallucinating.[12, 17, 34, 45] In one study, about half of the patients were found to be "disturbing at night." The close association between fragmentation of the normal sleep–wake cycle and delirium is one of its most characteristic distinguishing features.[17]

DISORDER OF PSYCHOMOTOR BEHAVIOR

A delirious patient may be predominantly hyperactive or hypoactive or may repeatedly switch from one of these extremes to the other in the course of a day, as Soranus[46] had already observed in the second century A.D. His description of the patient's psychomotor behavior has not been surpassed:

> Quiet or loud laughter, singing or a state of sadness, silence, murmuring, crying, or a barely audible muttering to one's self; or such a state of anger that the patient jumps up in a rage and can scarcely be held back, is wrathful at everyone, shouts, beats himself. . .or seeks to hide in fear, or weeps, or fails to answer those who speak with him, while he speaks not only with those who are not present but with the dead.[46, p. 23]

Both speech and nonverbal behavior are disordered and may range from catatonia and lethargy to incessant aimless activity and vocalizations. About 10% of patients may display violence toward others.[28] Hypoactivity may predominate during the day, its opposite at night. Speech may be slurred, hesitating, disjointed, repetitious, circumlocutory, and paraphasic, and the patient's writing may show neographisms and spelling errors.[47, 48] Tremor, such as asterixis, and choreiform movements may occur, especially in metabolic encephalopathies and drug withdrawal delirium.

A variety of emotions, but most often fear, apathy, rage, or depression, may accompany delirium.[36, 38, 49] Autonomic, especially sympathetic, nervous system hyperarousal, manifested by flushed face, dilated pupils, tachycardia, and sweating, may occur in association with fear and hyperactivity.[17] Incontinence of urine and feces is not uncommon in the delirious elderly.

COURSE AND OUTCOME

Delirium comes on acutely over a few hours or days, often manifests itself first at night, and in the majority of cases clears up completely in 1–4 weeks. In the elderly, on the whole, it tends to last longer than in the younger patients.[12] About half of the survivors leave the hospital within a month.[26] For many patients delirium is a terminal event, as was mentioned earlier. The survivors have a good prognosis, as transition from delirium to dementia appears to be relatively uncommon. The favorable outcome is influenced by early detection and effective treatment of the syndrome. A demented delirious patient who is adequately treated is likely to return to his previous level of cognitive functioning, unless additional brain damage has occurred.

MULTIFACTORIAL ETIOLOGY

By definition, delirium is an organic brain syndrome, i.e., a mental disorder whose occurrence requires cerebral dysfunction due to one or more organic etiologic factors (references 8, 9, 17, DSM-III). The latter include systemic or cerebral disease, exogenous physical or chemical agents, and withdrawal from certain substances of abuse. The presence of one or more of these factors is a necessary, but not always sufficient, condition for delirium to occur. Some writers have emphasized the etiologic importance of psychosocial variables in delirium of the elderly.[15, 36, 37, 50] Kennedy,[36] for example, asserted that impaired brain function due to physical causes renders an elderly individual exquisitely vulnerable to a wide range of psychosocial stressors, such as bereavement, relocation to an unfamiliar environment, or destruction of the home, all of which may help precipitate delirium. Kral[37, 50] postulated that brain damage and lowered resistance to stress predispose many elderly persons to cognitive disorganization in response to both psychological stressors, such as loss of spouse or rejection, and physical ones, such as a hip fracture.

Etiologic organic factors could be identified in 80–95% of reported cases of clinically diagnosed delirium in the elderly.[26, 28, 51-53] The remaining 5–20% represent an unsolved puzzle. They could include patients with pseudodelirium as well as those in whom organic etiology escaped detection. Some investigators have reported relatively frequent concurrence of delirium and depression.[26,29,52,54-56] Elderly depressed patients are often malnourished and physically ill and are likely to be taking a variety of drugs, including tricyclic antidepressants. All of these factors are potentially deliriogenic.[26, 52, 54] A transient cognitive disorder has been reported to occur in 12% of elderly patients suffering from an acute affective psychosis,[56] and it may accompany other functional mental disorders as well.[57] It is not clear at this time what proportion of these cases represents psudodelirium rather than delirium.

Etiology of delirium in the elderly is typically multifactorial, in the sense that several causative organic factors are often implicated and their deliriogenic effect is frequently enhanced by such psychosocial stressors as bereavement, transfer to an unfamiliar environment, or excessive or deficient sensory inputs.[17] Sleep loss and fatigue may also play a contributory role. The elderly are highly vulnerable to the cognitively disorganizing effects of all of these factors because of certain ubiquitous predisposing conditions.[58]

PREDISPOSING FACTORS

Aging processes, brain damage or disease, and impairment of vision and hearing predispose the elderly to delirium.[8,17,26,32,34] Aging of the brain and of the special senses appears to facilitate cognitive disorganization in response to both physical and psychosocial stressors. Brain damage and disease, especially vascular and degenerative, increase predisposition to delirium even further. Capacity for homeostatic regulation and for resistance to stress is reduced in the elderly, possibly as a result of age-related changes in hypothalamic nuclei.[50, 59] Circadian rhythms undergo changes. Certain parts of the brain on whose integrity normal cognitive processes depend are susceptible to aging and show selective cell loss. There is loss of cells and reduction in the dendritic tree in the cerebral cortex.[59] Frontal cortex, hippocampus, and locus ceruleus are among the structures selectively involved.[60] Destruction of locus ceruleus or raphe nuclei or both has been blamed for the occurrence of nocturnal delirium in demented elderly patients.[61] The central cholinergic system is affected by aging, and even more so by degenerative brain disease, with resulting reduction in acetylcholine synthesis.[62] Since adequate functioning of this system is needed for normal memory, learning, attention, wakefulness, and sleep–wake cycle, its deficiency is likely to predispose to delirium. Some authors claim that rduced acetylcholine synthesis due to various systemic disorders is a common denominator in metabolic encephalopathies.[63] The normal elderly show reduction of cerebral blood flow and glucose metabolism, changes that are much greater in the presence of even mild and asymptomatic arteriosclerosis and are most pronounced in senile dementia.[64-66] The aging brain is highly vulnerable to hypoxia of any origin.

These changes related to aging, cerebral disease, or both are compounded by additional factors such as increased general susceptibility to, and a high frequency of, episodes of disease and high prevalence of chronic diseases. Furthermore, impaired mechanisms of drug metabolism render the elderly highly susceptible to drug-induced delirium.[17, 34]

ASSOCIATED PHYSICAL CONDITIONS

The most common physical illnesses associated with delirium in the elderly include congestive heart failure, pneumonia, urinary tract infection, cancer, uremia, malnutrition, hypokalemia, dehydration and/or sodium depletion, and cerebrovascular accidents.[26,28,30,51,52,56] Systemic diseases are much more often implicated than the primary cerebral ones. Intoxication with medical drugs is probably the most frequent single cause.[8,9,17,34]

The elderly are singularly prone to adverse drug reactions as a result of age-related changes in the metabolism and distribution of drugs in the body.[34,67] High drug consumption and frequent polypharmacy are notorious consequences of the current prescribing practices for elderly patients and no doubt increase the incidence of drug-related delirium.[34,67] Drugs with anticholinergic properties are among those most frequently prescribed for the elderly[68] and probably constitute the single most common cause of delirium in this age group. Delirium is especially likely to be induced when several anticholinergic drugs are administered concurrently.[68] Table 1 lists the more important organic causes of delirium in the elderly.[5,17,28,34,51,53,63,68,69]

PATHOGENETIC MECHANISMS

Almost 50 years ago, Hart wrote: "Of the precise processes by which delirium is mediated we know nothing. In discussing at the present time the possible pathogenesis of delirium we have therefore to leave the sphere of knowledge and enter that of hypothesis and speculation.[70, p. 747] This statement still holds. Several mechanisms are proposed to account for the occurrence of delirium in the elderly, and they may be classified as neurochemical, stress, information input, and sleep–wake cycle disturbance hypotheses.

Engel and Romano[71] postulated that a general reduction of cerebral metabolism underlies all cases of delirium and is reflected in concurrent cognitive impairment and a slowing of EEG background activity. Any factor reducing the supply, uptake, or utilization of substrates for oxidative metabolism could thus result in delirium. Blass and Plum[63] hypothesized that impairment of brain oxidative metabolism results in reduced

TABLE 1. Common Organic Causes of Delirium

Cause	Type
Drugs	Diuretics, sedative–hypnotics, analgesics, antihistaminics, antiparkinsonian agents, antidepressants, neuroleptics, cimetidine, digitalis glycosides
Alcohol intoxication or withdrawal Cardiovascular disorders	Congestive heart failure, myocardial infarction, cardiac arrhythmias, aortic stenosis, hypertensive encephalopathy, orthostatic hypotension, subacute bacterial endocarditis
Infections	Pneumonia, urinary tract infection, bacteremia, septicemia, cholecystitis, meningitis
Metabolic encephalopathies	Electrolyte and fluid imbalance; hepatic, renal, and pulmonary failure; diabetes and other endocrine diseases; nutritional deficiency (especially of vitamin B complex); hypothermia and heat stroke
Cerebrovascular disorders	Transient ischemic attacks, stroke, chronic subdural hematoma, vasculitis
Cerebral or extracranial neoplasm Trauma	Head injury, surgery, burns, hip fracture

synthesis of neurotransmitters, especially of acetylcholine, whose relative deficiency in the brain appears to provide a major, if not the only, pathogenetic mechanism in delirium. This hypothesis is supported by the ease with which delirium may be induced clinically or experimentally with anticholinergic drugs[17, 68, 72] and be reversed by physostigmine, a cholinesterase inhibitor.[17] Itil and Fink[72] have proposed that imbalance of central cholinergic and adrenergic mechanisms, affecting both the medial ascending reticular activating system and the medial thalamic diffuse projection system, underlies delirium. Increased central noradrenergic activity has been found in delirium tremens and probably accounts for its characteristic features, such as hyperalertness and hyperactivity,[73] as well as for the absence of EEG slowing.[74] Thus, imbalance of cerebral neurotranmitters, notably of acetylcholine and noradrenaline, appears to be implicated in many, possibly in most, cases of delirium.

Kral[37, 50] hypothesized that delirium in the elderly represents a reaction to acute stress, one mediated by abnormally high levels of circulating corticosteroids, or by increased vulnerability of the hypothalamus to their effects, or by concurrence of both of these conditions. In the elderly, secretion and plasma levels of cortisol are preserved while the rate of its degradation is reduced.[75] In response to stress, patients suffering from senile dementia show higher and more sustained increase in plasma cortisol levels than do the normal elderly.[50] Kral has speculated that excessive cortisol brings about delirium by virtue of its deleterious effect on the brainstem centrencephalic system. Cortisol does affect both cerebral and mental function and appears to interfere with selective attention and hence with processing of information,[76] but its role in delirium is still speculative. Adrenaline and noradrenaline levels tend to remain elevated for a longer time in stressed elderly people than in young individuals.[77] Since increased secretion of catecholamines leads to increased cerebral blood flow and oxygen consumption in experimental animals,[78] one may postulate that a stress-related increase of such secretion in the elderly, especially the demented, could accentuate cerebral metabolic demands and further reduce oxygen tension, thereby facilitating onset of delirium.

Levels of sensory stimulation needed for optimal cognitive activity decline with age, rendering the elderly susceptible to sensory overload and its disorganizing effects on cognition.[15, 79] Some authors believe that sensory deprivation contributes to delirium in the elderly. Recent work using positron computed tomography indicates that cerebral glucose metabolism in human beings decreases with reduced sensory inputs.[80] Cameron[81] observed that senile patients prone to nocturnal delirium could be made delirious by being put in a dark room in the daytime. He postulated that memory impairment rendered these patients dependent on uninterrupted input of visual cues, and abolition of such cues in the dark elicited spatial disorientation, anxiety, and delirium. Sensory deprivation has also been invoked to explain delirium in elderly patients undergoing cataract surgery.[17]

Nocturnal delirium, common in demented patients, has ben ascribed in part to sleep pathology. Feinberg and associates[82] observed that demented elderly patients tended to awaken abruptly from dream periods (REM sleep) and to display agitated delirium for up to 10 min. These researchers postulated that nocturnal delirium could in some cases be due to abrupt transition from dreaming sleep to wakefulness, with consequent intrusion of dreams into the waking state. More recently, Japanese researchers proposed that nocturnal delirium in dementia could be due to the occurrence of stage 1-REM (REM sleep without muscle atonia) caused by destruction of serotonergic neurons in raphe nuclei, or of noradrenergic neurons in locus ceruleus, or both[61] There is evidence of selective loss of noradrenergic neurons in locus ceruleus in senescence and especially in senile dementia.[83] Diurnal sleep–wake patterns in elderly subjects tend to be fragmented, with a high prevalence of sleep apnea, excessive daytime drowsiness, and microsleeps.[84] Disruptions of the sleep–wake cycle appear to be common in the elderly, especially in the presence of cerebral disease, and it is likely that they play an important part in the genesis of transient cognitive disorders. Psychosocial stress and sensory understimulation or overload, singly or in combination, may play a contributory role in some cases.

Diagnosis and Differential Diagnosis

Diagnosis of delirium involves two essential steps: (1) recognition of the syndrome and (2) identification of its cause (or causes).[17] The syndrome is recognized on the basis of its clinical features, described earlier, and by applying DSM-III diagnostic criteria. The patient's cognitive function and attention are tested as part of the psychiatric examination.[69] One of the clinical scales may be used for this purpose, such as the mental status questionnaire[85] or the minimental state.[86] Once delirium is diagnosed or suspected, the search for causative factors must start at once. All medical drugs that the patient is taking should be carefully scrutinized for their deliriogenic potential. Evidence of physical illness, either acute or chronic with acute exacerbation, must be looked for, as the patient's life may be at stake. *It must never be assumed a priori that a patient's transient cognitive disorder is due to a reported life change or psychosocial stress alone.* Such an assumption could result in failure to search for, diagnose, and treat an underlying physical illness, with possible fatal consequences for the patient. Physical, including neurological, examination and selected laboratory tests are called for in all cases. The choice of tests must depend on the clinician's judgment and may include some or all of the following: blood chemistries, hemogram, urinalysis, serology, ECG, chest X ray, blood culture, toxic drug screen, CSF examination, EEG, and CAT scan.

The EEG has been claimed to be the most sensitive and reliable indicator of cerebral metabolism generally and of its derangement in delirium in particular.[71] Bilateral diffuse slowing of EEG background activity has been shown to correlate positively with the degree of the delirious patient's cognitive impairment.[71] The EEG may help distinguish delirium from pseudodelirium and intracranial from systemic causes of the former.[87] In the elderly, however, the diagnostic value of the EEG is limited by the fact that generalized slowing is seen not only in delirium but also in primary degenerative dementia.[88] Repeated tracings may be needed to distinguish between these two conditions, since in delirium the EEG tends to normalize as the patient's cerebral disorder improves.

DIFFERENTIAL DIAGNOSIS

Delirium needs to be distinguished from dementia and pseudodelirium. Such differential diagnosis may at times be very difficult, because delirium in the elderly is often superimposed on dementia; i.e., there is an organic brain syndrome that also features global cognitive impairment. Furthermore, a demented patient may suffer from both depression and delirium or pseudodelirium at the same time. An adequate history may be unavailable for a patient who lives alone or with a demented spouse, and the patient is usually a poor historian. Because information about the mode of onset of the disorder (i.e., whether abrupt or insidious) and about the nature and duration of the symptoms is crucial for the clinical diagnosis, history must be sought from all available sources. As a general rule, a patient who by all accounts has functioned well intellectually and then suddenly develops a cognitive–attentional disorder that fluctuates in severity over the course of a day and becomes most marked at night is suffering from delirium unless proven otherwise.

DELIRIUM VERSUS DEMENTIA

It is important to distinguish delirium from dementia, as the two syndromes carry different prognostic implications.[89] It is a grave error to attach the label of senile dementia to a patient suffering only from delirium, yet such misdiagnosis is not uncommon and may cause disastrous consequences for the patient and his family.[90, 91] To avoid misdiagnosis one needs to consider the evolution of the patient's symptoms over time as well as his behavior and cognitive performance at the time of examination.[69,89] Table 2 may assist the reader in the diagnostic process.

Differential diagnosis is often complicated by the concurrence of delirium and dementia, since about one third of hospitalized demented patients are likely to suffer from superimposed delirium.[8] Moreover, the two syndromes, as they are currently defined in DSM-III, do overlap and are not sharply delimited. In an already demented patient the features of delirium tend to be modified. Complex hallucinations, dreamlike mentation, and confabulations are frequently lacking, and the patient exhibits mostly apathy interrupted by noisy restlessness, as well as more or less severe deficits of memory, general knowledge, and thinking ability. As a general rule, acute and fluctuating worsening of cognitive functioning in a patient known to suffer from dementia should suggest the onset of delirium and lead to appropriate medical management. It is not clear at this time how often pseudodelirium occurs in the course of dementia in response to stress.

DELIRIUM VERSUS PSEUDODELIRIUM

A transient cognitive disorder is not always delirium as this syndrome is defined in DSM-III. As noted earlier, in 5–20% of elderly patients with apparent delirium, no organic causative factor could be detected. The term "pseudodelirium" has been proposed to designate a deliriumlike transient cognitive disorder occurring in the absence of demonstrable organic causes.[92] Such disorders have been described in the

TABLE 2. Differential Diagnosis of Delirium and Dementia

Feature	Delirum	Dementia
Onset	Rapid, often at night	Usually insidious
Duration	Hours to weeks	Months to years
Course	Fluctuates over 24 hr; worse at night; lucid intervals	Relatively stable
Awareness	Always impaired	Usually normal
Alertness	Reduced or increased; tends to fluctuate	Usually normal
Orientation	Always impaired, at least for time; tendency to mistake unfamiliar for familiar place or person	May be intact; little tendency to confabulate
Memory	Recent and immediate impaired; fund of knowledge intact if dementia is absent	Recent and remote impaired; some loss of common knowledge
Thinking	Slow or accelerated; may be dreamlike	Poor in abstraction, impoverished
Perception	Often misperceptions, especially visual	Misperceptions often absent
Sleep–wake cycle	Always disrupted; often drowsiness during the day, insomnia at night	Fragmented sleep
Physical illness or drug toxicity	Usually present	Often absent, especially in primary degenerative dementia

literature for over a century and have been called "acute confusional insanity or state," "acute delirious mania," and "psychogenic delirium."[17, 70] The elderly, particularly those with some degree of chronic cognitive impairment, are especially prone to exhibit pseudodelirium as a feature of an affective, schizophrenic, brief reactive, paranoid, or atypical psychosis.[56, 57] Disorientation, bewilderment, incoherence, and perceptual and psychomotor disturbances of rapid onset appear to characterize pseudodelirium. In contrast to delirium, however, laboratory evidence of diffuse cerebral dysfunction is absent. The incidence of pseudodelirium is unknown. Its clinical features have not been systematically studied and contrasted with those of delirium. This is an unexplored area of geropsychiatry, one clamoring for research.

To differentiate pseudodelirium from delirium on clinical grounds alone may be impossible at times, because the two syndromes resemble each other too much. Signs of physical illness, such as fever or asterixis, should suggest delirium. In the latter, the patient's level of awareness tends to fluctuate irregularly in the daytime and is usually lowest during sleepless nights. Pseudodelirium, like pseudodementia, may be suggested by inconsistencies in cognitive performance, as when a patient claims to be unaware of his whereabouts yet is oriented for time and has no trouble finding his way around.[93] The probability of pseudodelirium being present is increased if the patient has a past history of psychiatric illness, displays marked depressive or manic features, is grossly and consistently delusional, or appears to be unmotivated to perform on bedside cognitive tests rather than truly impaired. Persistent questioning may reveal that the patient is cognitively more or less intact but is too preoccupied with his own thoughts, too agitated, or too withdrawn to perform on request.

If doubt persists about whether delirium is present, additional tests, such as the amobarbital interview, the EEG, and the dexamethasone suppression test (DST) may help.[93, 94] In pseudodelirium cognitive performance tends to normalize under amobarbital, the EEG is normal (unless dementia is also present), and DST results are likely to be abnormal if a major depressive disorder underlies the transient cognitive disorder in the absence of advanced primary dementia or inanition.[94]

TREATMENT

Therapy of delirium is two-pronged. First and foremost, one must look for the putative organic factors and treat or remove them. Drugs that the patient has taken may have to be withheld or their dosage reduced. Concurrently, symptomatic and supportive treatment must proceed.[9,15,17,30,34,58,69,95] Fluid and electrolyte balance and nutrition must be maintained. A proper sensory environment for the patient needs to be secured, one that guards against both extremes of sensory input. A quiet, well-lighted room, a clock and a calendar, and a few familiar objects or photographs may help reduce anxiety and cognitive disorganization. Good nursing—consistent, supportive, and orienting—is essential.[15] Sleep may be aided by a hynotic such as temazepam, 15–30 mg at bedtime. It must be kept in mind that practically all hypnotics may at times increase confusion. Finally, sedation may be necessary for an agitated patient who could sustain a fracture or some other serious injury, or even be killed, as a result of an attempt to run away or fight, especially at night when confusion tends to peak. Haloperidol is the drug of choice in this situation.[17] It is effective and relatively safe and has only mild anticholinergic activity. Its main side effects in the elderly are extrapyramidal. It may be given orally or intramuscularly in doses of 0.5–5 mg twice daily, depending on the degree of the patient's agitation.

COMMENT

Fifteen years ago I called delirium the Cinderella of American psychiatry: taken for granted, ignored, and seldom studied.[20] The situation has changed little since then, and the syndrome, despite its high frequency among the elderly, remains almost totally neglected by researchers. Much still needs to be learned about its incidence, phenomenology, pathogenesis, and prevention. The current upsurge of interest in geropsychiatry, occasioned by the continued aging of the population as a whole, may at last include delirium and the conditions that mimic it and stimulate badly needed clinical research. The relation of delirium to psychological stress, disordered biorhythms, sleep pathology, dreaming, dementia, and acute functional psychoses has never been properly explored, yet its nature touches on basis issues of the mind–body problem.

Application to this syndrome of the newest techniques for studying the brain–behavior relationship, such as positron emission tomography, may help clarify its pathogenesis in the future. Such methods may finally allow us to establish the theoretically and practically important relation of delirium to pseudodelirium. Can psychological stress alone give rise to acute cerebral dysfunction manifested behaviorally as delirium? Is the DSM-III definition of this syndrome too restrictive by requiring presence of a "specific organic factor" as a necessary diagnostic criterion? Hart[70] raised the former question 50 years ago and thought that such a possibility was logically tenable, but this issue has never been satisfactorily resolved. Meanwhile, however, epidemiological and clinical studies should be undertaken. A recent study by a group of nurses, though flawed, points in the right direction.[96] Liaison psychiatrists are strategically placed to carry out such research in collaboration with geropsychiatrists and neuroscientists.[97]

In clinical practice, the often difficult task of differentiating delirium from pseudodelirium and dementia will occur with growing frequency, as the number of very old persons will predictably increase in the coming years. The importance of this task is underscored by the authors of a recent study: "Psychiatrists and other mental health professionals must be able to differentiate organic brain syndrome from functional psychiatric illness in order to avoid increased mortality and morbidity in elderly patients."[98] Such differentiation presupposes knowledge of the distinguishing clinical features of the syndromes involved and highlights the need for appropriate research and teaching. To differentiate delirium and conditions that mimic it from dementia is a matter vitally important for the elderly patient's welfare and even survival, and should be a required skill for mental health workers and all other health workers. Since liaison psychiatrists and geropsychiatrists are, on the whole, the physicians most familiar with transient cognitive disorder, they should play a key and active role in the requisite teaching.[97]

Finally, there is need to attempt prevention of delirium whenever possible. Liaison psychiatrists have demonstrated that this can be achieved, with resulting reduction of the length of hospitalization and hence its cost.[99] Considering that the elderly, on the average, stay in the hospital for treatment of acute disorders 30% longer than younger patients do[31] and that the development of delirium tends to prolong their stay, preventing its onset could result in substantial savings and in avoidance of protracted disability due to cognitive impairment.[97, 99, 100] The patient would also avoid the risk of being branded as demented, with all the undesirable consequences of such a label. Efforts to prevent delirium must involve a revision and reform of current uninhibited prescribing practices for elderly patients, as the syndrome is so reaily induced by medical and psychotropic drugs.[69]

References

1. Siegel JS: Demogrpahic background for international gerontological studies. *J Gerontol* 36:93–102, 1981.
2. McFarland DD: The aged in the 21st century: A demographer's view, in Jarvik LF (ed): *Aging into the 21st Century*. New York, Gardner Press, 1978.

3. Dementia: The quiet epidemic (edtl). *Br Med J* 1:1-2, 1978.

4. Alzheimer's disease (edtl). *Br Med J* 2:1374-1375, 1980.

5. Jolley D: Acute confusional states in the elderly, in Coakley D (ed): *Acute Geriatric Medicine* London, Croon Helm, 1981.

6. Schneck MK, Reisberg B, Ferris SH: An overview of current concepts of Alzheimer's disease. *Am J Psychiatry* 139:165-173, 1982.

7. Wells CE: Chronic brain disease: an overview. *Am J Psychiatry* 135:1-12, 1978.

8. Organic mental impairment in the elderly. *J R Coll Physicians Lond* 15:141-167, 1981.

9. Senility reconsidered. *JAMA* 244:259-264, 1980.

10. Hood P: On senile delirium. *Practitioner* 5:279-289, 1870.

11. Picket W: Senile dementia: a clinical study of two hundred cases with particular regard to types of the disease. *J Nerv Ment Dis* 31:81-88, 1904.

12. Robinson GW: Acute confusional states of old age. *South Med J* 32:479-485, 1939.

13. *Psychogeriatrics.* World Health Organization Technical Report 507. Geneva, WHO, 1972.

14. Berrios GE: Delirium and confusion in the 19th century: A conceptual history. *Br J Psychiatry* 139:439-449, 1981.

15. Wolanin MO, Philips LRF: *Confusion.* St. Louis, CV Mosby Co, 1981.

16. Lishman WA: *Organic Psychiatry.* Oxford, England, Blackwell, 1978.

17. Lipowski ZJ: *Delirium: Acute Brain Failure in Man.* Springfield, Ill, Charles C Thomas, 1980.

18. Campbell RJ: *Psychiatric Dictionary*, ed. 5 New York, Oxford University Press, 1981.

19. Adams RD, Victor M: *Principles of Neurology*, ed. 2 New York, McGraw-Hill, 1981.

20. Lipowski ZJ: Delirium, clouding of consciousness and confusion. *J Nerv Ment Dis* 145:227-255, 1967.

21. Lipowski ZJ: A new look at organic brain syndromes. *Am J Psychiatry* 137:674-678, 1980.

22. Hodkinson HM: *Common Symptoms of Disease in the Elderly.* Oxford, England, Blackwell, 1976.

23. Brocklehurst JC: Psychogeriatric care as a specialized discipline in medicine. *Bull NY Acad Med* 53:702-709, 1977.

24. Doty EJ: The incidence and treatment of delirious reactions in later life. *Geriatrics* 1:21-26, 1946.

25. Willi J: Delir, daemmerzustand und verwirrtheit bei koerperlich kranken, in Bleuler M, Willi J, Buehler HR (eds): *Akute Psychische Begleiterscheinungen Koerperlicher Krankheiten,* Stuttgart, Thieme Verlag, 1966.

26. Hodkinson HM: Mental impairment in the elderly. *J R Coll Physicians Lond* 7:305-317, 1973.

27. Bedford PD: General medical aspects of confusional states in elderly people. *Br Med J* 2:185-188, 1959.

28. Simon A, Cahan RB: The acute brain syndrome in geriatric patients. *Psychiatr Res Rep* 16:8-21, 1963.

29. Bergmann K, Eastham EJ: Psychogeriatric ascertainment and assessment for treatment in an acute medical ward setting. *Age Ageing* 3:174-188, 1974.

30. Seymour DG, Henschke PJ, Cape RDT, et al: Acute confusional states and dementia in the elderly: the role of dehydration/volume depletion, physical illness and age. *Age Ageing* 9:137-146, 1980.

31. National Center for Health Statistics: *Vital and Health Statistics*, series 13, number 64: Utilization of Short Stay Hospitals, Washington, DC, NCHS, 1982.

32. Seymour DG, Pringle R: Post-operative complications in the elderly surgical patient. *Gerontology* 29:262-270, 1983.

33. Millar HR: Psychiatric morbidity in elderly surgical patients. *BR J Psychiatry* 138:17-20, 1981.

34. Lipowski ZJ: Delirium (acute confusional states), in Albert ML (ed:): *The Clinical Neurology of Aging.* New York, Oxford University Press, 1984.

35. Lipowski ZJ: Delirium updated. *Compr Psychiatry* 21:190-196, 1980.

36. Kennedy A: Psychological factors in confusional states in the elderly: *Gerontol Clin* 1:71-82, 1959.

37. Kral VA: Confusional states: description and management, in Howells JG (ed): *Modern Perspectives in the Psychiatry of Old Age.* New York, Brunner/Mazel, 1975.

38. Roth M: Some diagnostic and aetiological aspects of confusional states in the elderly. *Gerontol Clin* 1:83-95, 1959.

39. Levin M: Delirious disorientation: the law of the unfamiliar mistaken for the familiar. *J Ment Sci* 91:447-450, 1945.

40. Willanger R, Klee A: Metamorphopsia and other visual disturbances with latency occurring in patients with diffuse cerebral lesions. *Acta Neurol Scand* 42:1-18, 1966.

41. Aggernaes A, Myschetzky A: Experienced reality in somatic patients more than 65 years old. *Acta Psychiatr Scand* 54:225–237, 1976.

42. Frieske DA, Wilson WP, Formal qualities of hallucinations: a comparative study of the visual hallucinations in patients with schizophrenic, organic and affective psychoses, in Hoch PH, Zubin J (eds): *Psychopathology of Schizophrenia*. New York, Grune & Stratton, 1966.

43. Hernandez-Peon R: Physiological mechanisms in attention, in Russell RW *Frontiers of Physiological Psychology*. New York, Academic Press, 1966.

44. Quincy J: *Lexicon Physicomedicum*. London, Bell, Taylor, Osborn, 1719, p 103.

45. Strejilevitch SM: La turbulence nocturne du viellard psychotique. *Encephale* 51:238–262, 1962.

46. Aurelianus C: *On Acute Diseases and on Chronic Diseases*. Edited by Drabkin IE. Chicago, University of Chicago Press, 1950.

47. Chedru F, Geschwind N: Disorders of higher cortical functions in acute confusional states. *Cortex* 8:395–411, 1972.

48. Chedru F, Geschwind N: Writing disturbances in acute confusional states. *Neuropsychologia* 10:343–353, 1972.

49. Simon A, Lowenthal MF, Epstein LJ: *Crisis and Intervention*. San Francisco, Jossey-Bass, 1970.

50. Kral VA: Stress and mental disorders of the senium. *Med Serv J Can* 18:363–370, 1962.

51. Flint FJ, Richards SM: Organic basis of confusional states in the elderly. *Br Med J* 2:1537–1539, 1956.

52. Kay DWK, Roth M: Physical accompaniments of mental disorder in old age. *Lancet* 2:740–745, 1955.

53. Purdie FR, Honigman TB, Rosen P: Acute organic brain syndrome: a review of 100 cases. *Ann Emerg Med* 10:455–461, 1981.

54. Fish F, Williamson J: A delirium unit in an acute geriatric hospital. *Gerontol Clin* 6:71–80, 1964.

55. Roth M: The psychiatric disorders of later life. *Psychiatr Ann* 6:417–445, 1976.

56. Roth M: The natural history of mental disorder in old age. *J Ment Sci* 101:281–301, 1955.

57. Whitehead T: Confusing the causes of confusion. *Nurs Mirror* 151:38–39, 1980.

58. Dunn T, Arie T: Mental disturbance in the ill old person. *Br Med J* 2:413–416, 1973.

59. Samorajski T, Hartford J: Brain physiology of aging, in Busse EW, Blazer DG (eds): *Handbook of Geriatric Psychiatry*. New York, Van Nostrand Reinhold Co, 1980.

60. Brady H: Neuroanatomy and neuropathology of aging, in Busse EW, Blazer DG (eds): *Handbook of Geriatric Psychiatry*. New York, Van Nostrand Reinhold Co, 1980.

61. Hishikawa Y, Lijima J, Shimizu T, et al: A dissociated sleep state "stage 1-REM" and its relation to delirium in Baldy-Moulinier M (ed): *Actualités en Médecine Expérimentale*.

62. Gibson GE, Peterson C, Jenden DJ: Brain acetylcholine synthesis declines with senescence. *Science* 213:674–676, 1981.

63. Blass JP, Plum F: Metabolic encephalopathies, in Katzman R, Terry RD (eds): *The Neurology of Aging*. Philadelphia, FA Davis, 1983.

64. Obrist WD: Cerebral circulatory changes in normal aging and dementia, in Hoffmeister F, Müller C (eds): *Brain Function in Old Age*. Berlin, Springer-Verlag, 1979.

65. Farkas T, Ferris SH, Wolf AP, et al: ^{18}F-2-Deoxy-2-fluoro-D-glucose as a tracer in the positron emission tomographic study of senile dementia. *Am J Psychiatry* 139:352–353, 1982.

66. Sokoloff L: Effects of normal aging on cerebral circulation and energy metabolism, in Brain Function in Hoffmeister F, Müller C. (eds): *Brain Function in Old Age*. Berlin, Springer-Verlag, 1979.

67. Vestal RE: Drug use in the elderly: A review of problems and special considerations. *Drugs* 16:358, 1978.

68. Blazer DG, Federspeil CF, Ray WA, et al: The risk of anticholinergic toxicity in the elderly: a study of prescribing practices in two populations. *J Gerontol* 38:31–35, 1983.

69. Liston EH: Delirium in the aged. *Psychiatr Clin North Am* 5:49–66, 1982.

70. Hart B: Delirious states. *Br Med J* 2:745–749, 1936.

71. Engel GL, Romano J: Delirium, a syndrome of cerebral insufficiency. *J Chron Dis* 9:260–277, 1959.

72. Itil T, Fink M: Anticholinergic drug-induced delirium: Experimental modification, quantitiative EEG and behavioral correlations. *J Nerv Ment Dis* 143:492–507, 1966.

73. Hawley RJ, Major LF, Schulman EA, et al: CSF levels of norepinephrine during alcohol withdrawal. *Arch Neurol* 38:289–292, 1981.

74. Allahyari H, Deisenhammer E, Weiser G: EEG examination during delirium tremens. *Psychiatr Clin (Basel)* 9:21-31, 1976.

75. Vernadakis A, Timiras PS (eds): *Hormones in Development and Aging.* New York, SP Medical & Scientific Books, 1982.

76. Carpenter WT, Gruen PH: Cortisol's effects on human mental functioning. *J Clin Psychopharmacol* 2:91-101, 1982.

77. Faucheux BA, Bourliere F, Baulon A, et al: The effects of psychosocial stress on urinary excretion of adrenaline and noradrenaline in 51- to 55- and 71- to 74-year-old men. *Gerontology* 27:313-325, 1981.

78. Carlsson C, Hagerdal M, Kaasi AE, et al: A catecholamine-mediated increase in cerebral oxygen uptake during immobilisation stress in rats. *Brain Res* 119:223-231, 1977.

79. Lipowski ZJ: Sensory and information inputs overload: behavioral effects. *Compr Psychiatry* 16:199-221, 1975.

80. Mazziotta JC, Phelps ME, Carson RE, et al: Tomographic mapping of human cerebral metabolism: sensory deprivation. *Ann Neurol* 12:435-444, 1982.

81. Cameron DE: Studies in senile nocturnal delirium. *Psychiatr Q* 15:47-53, 1941.

82. Feinberg I, Koresko RL, Schaffner IR: Sleep electroencephalographic and eye-movement patterns in patients with chronic brain syndrome. *J Psychiatr Res* 3:11-26, 1965.

83. Bondareff W, Mountjoy CQ, Roth M: Loss of neurons of origin of the adrenergic projection to cerebral cortex (nucleus locus ceruleus) in senile dementia. *Neurology (NY)* 32:164-168, 1982.

84. Dement WC, Miles LE, Carskadon MA: "White paper" on sleep and aging. *J Am Geriatr Soc* 30:25-50, 1982.

85. Kahn RL, Miller NE: Assessment of altered brain function in the aged, in Storandt M, Siegler HC, Elias MF (eds): *The Clinical Psychology of Aging.* New York, Plenum, 1978.

86. Anthony JC, La Resche L, Niaz U, et al: Limits of the "Mini-Mental State" as a screening test for dementia and delirium among hospital patients. *Psychol Med* 12:397-408, 1982.

87. Obrecht R, Okhomina FOA, Scott DR: Value of EEG in acute confusional states. *J Neurol Neurosurg Psychiatry* 42:75-77, 1979.

88. Obrist WD: Electroencephalographic changes in normal aging and dementia, in Hoffmeister F, Müller C (eds): *Brain Function in Old Age.* Berlin, Springer-Verlag, 1979.

89. Lipowski ZJ: Differentiating delirium from dementia in the elderly. *Clin Gerontologist* 1:3-10, 1982.

90. Libow LS: Pseudosenility: acute and reversible organic brain syndrome. *J Am Geriatr Soc* 21:112-120, 1973.

91. Glassman M: Misdiagnosis of senile dementia: Denial of care to the elderly. *Social Work* 25:288-292, 1980.

92. Goldney R: Pseudodelirium. *Med J Aust* 1:630, 1979.

93. Wells CE: Pseudodementia. *Am J Psychiatry* 136:895-900, 1979.

94. McAllister TW, Ferrel RB, Price TRP, et al: The dexamethasone suppression test in two patients with severe depressive psudodementia. *Am J Psychiatry* 139:479-481, 1982.

95. Bayne JRD: Management of confusion in elderly persons. *Can Med Assoc J* 118:139-141, 1978.

96. Chisholm SE, Deniston OL, Igvisan RM, et al: Prevalence of confusion in elderly hospitalized patients *J Gerontol Nurs* 8:87-96, 1982.

97. Lipowski ZJ: The need to integrate liaison psychiatry and geropsychiatry. *Am J Psychiatry* 140:1003-1005, 1983.

98. Waxman HM, Carner EA, Dubin W, et al: Geriatric psychiatry in the emergency department: Characteristics of geriatric and non-geriatric admissions. *J Am Geriatr Soc* 30:427-432, 1982.

99. Levitan SJ, Kornfeld DS: Clinical and cost benefits of liaison psychiatry. *Am J Psychiatry* 138:790-793, 1981.

100. Warshaw GA, Moore JT, Friedman SW, et al: Functional disability in the hospitalized elderly. *JAMA* 248:847-850, 1982.

The Concept and
Psychopathology of Dementia

17

A Historical Note

The term "dementia" stems from the Latin word *demens*, which implies being out of one's mind or crazy. The term was probably used for the first time in the medical literature by Celsus in the 1st century A.D.[1] In his description of delirium, or phrenesis, he noted that it could sometimes be followed by "dementia continua." Aretaeus of Cappadocia, active in the 2nd century A.D., classified diseases into acute and chronic and included among the chronic ones senile dementia, which had its onset in old age and featured deterioration of the intellect.[1] Juvenal,[2] the Roman poet and satirist of the 2nd century A.D., gave a vivid vignette of senile dementia in one of his satires: "Worse by far than all bodily hurt is dementia: for he who has it no longer knows the names of his slaves or recognizes the friend with whom he has dined the night before, or those whom he has begotten and brought up" (p. 718). This brief description suggests that the word "dementia" was used by the Romans in a manner similar to the contemporary one and encompassed one of the core features of the syndrome, namely, failing memory. In the English-language medical literature, however, the term had been used until the 19th century as a general designation for insanity or as a synonym to delirium.[1]

At the end of the 18th century, the French psychiatrist Pinel[3] introduced the term "demence," or dementia, which he included among five main classes of mental derangement and defined as the "abolition of the thinking faculty." Its features were to include a rapid succession of unconnected ideas, volatile emotions, and wild eccentricity. This description suggests that Pinel may have used the word "dementia" to refer to schizophrenic and manic psychoses. More important, however, Pinel stated explicity that mental disorders differed in regard to their etiology: "Derangement of the understanding is generally considered as an effect of an organic lesion of the brain, consequently as incurable; a supposition that is, in a great number of instances, contrary to anatomical fact" (p. 3).

Pinel's student Esquirol[4] developed the concept of dementia further. He defined it as a cerebral affection featuring weakened sensibility, understanding, and will, as well as impaired memory, reasoning, and attention. Moreover, he distinguished three varieties of dementia: acute, chronic, and senile, and differentiated it explicitly from amentia, or mental retardation. Acute dementia could be caused by fever or hemorrhage and was curable; chronic dementia could be caused by masturbation, drunkenness, or excessive study or follow mania or epilepsy, and it was rarely cured. Senile

dementia resulted from advanced age and was heralded by general excitement and irritability, followed by deficits of recent memory and other intellectual functions. It
could not be cured, but its progress could be slowed down by exposure to country air
and by moderate exercise. In general, dementia could be due to either organic disease
or moral causes.

The influence of the writings of Pinel and Esquirol spread outside France. In 1837,
an English psychiatrist, Prichard,[5] developed the concept of dementia still further. He
delineated two classes: primary and secondary to disorders of the brain such as mania, apoplexy, or paralysis. He described four stages of dementia and thus outlined
its natural history. The first stage featured impairment of recent memory; the second,
loss of reason; the third, loss of comprehension; and the fourth, loss of instinctive action. All these stages could be found in the gradual progression of senile dementia,
which was not to be viewed as due to old age alone but rather to harmful conditions
such as excessive striving for success, intense pursuit of studies, and abuse of alcohol. Prichard asserted that in its later stages dementia was characterized by change of
the patient's personality, by abolition of his capacity to reason, and by total disorganization of the mind.

Several students of Esquirol observed that dementia could be a feature of the
general paralysis of the insane and thus result from demonstrable brain pathology. This
discovery, in the 1820s, stimulated an intense search for cerebral causes of other forms
of mental derangement and let to the belief that insanity was a manifestation of brain
disease. At the end of the 19th century, Kraepelin purified, as it were, Esquirol's concept of chronic dementia by detaching from it several clinical subtypes of what he designated "dementia praecox."[1] He used the term "organic dementias" for psychoses
caused by diseases of the central nervous system such as neurosyphilis. In 1924,
Bleuler[6] described the clinical features of dementia due to chronic diffuse cerebral
cortical damage or disease and called it the "organic psychosyndrome." It was characterized by impairment of memory, judgment, critical faculty, perceptual discrimination, attention, and orientation as well as by labile emotionality and defective impulse
control. Bleuler's formulation of this syndrome constituted a landmark in the history
of the development of the concept of dementia and of the organic mental disorders
generally. His organic psychosyndrome, however, became adopted uncritically by the
compilers of the first American official classification of mental disorders, DSM-I, as
the hallmark of the whole class of organic mental disorders.[7] This erroneous and misleading conception had persisted until the appearance of DSM-III in 1980 and, in my
opinion, helped to hamper research in the field of organic psychiatry. Bleuler was
hardly responsible for this undesirable development, since he made it very clear that
his psychosyndrome was a feature of only chronic and diffuse cerebral damage, and
not of acute or focal brain disease. The term "dementia" had come to signify an *irreversible* syndrome, or what the DSM-I and DSM-II referred to as the "chronic brain
syndrome."[7]

In the 1960s, writers in England and Germany began to call for a revision of the
concept of dementia and pointed out that the syndrome could be partly or even fully
reversible.[7] Neurologists started to speak of "reversible dementia," an obvious contradiction in terms in view of dementia's traditional connotation of irreversibility. The

current American classification, DSM-III, reflects the evolution of the concept of dementia in the course of this century.[8] It states explicitly that the syndrome may be progressive, static, or remitting. Its mode of onset and subsequent course depend on the underlying pathology and, in some cases, on the application of appropriate and timely treatment. It is essential to distinguish clearly dementia as a *syndrome* due to many possible causes from *senile dementia of Alzheimer type (SDAT)*, a brain disease and the most common cause of the syndrome in the Western world.

INCIDENCE AND PREVALENCE

Recent editorials speak of the coming epidemic of dementia, one that casts a shadow over the future of society.[9,10] There is general agreement that the prevalence of dementia is increasing as a direct result of the growing numbers of the elderly, those aged 65 years and older, and especially of the very old.[11] Studies carried out in the last 30 years show the prevalence of severe dementia to be between 1.3% and 6.2% of persons over the age of 65, and of milder intellectual deterioration, between 2.6% and 15.4%.[11] These marked differences in the reported prevalence of dementia reflect different diagnostic criteria and methods of case finding. The median prevalence of severe dementia in the elderly is probably about 4%.[11] Considering that in the United States 25.5 million persons are 65 years old or older, the estimate of the number of those with severe dementia is about 1.2 million. The prevalence of SDAT is estimated to be about 25 per 1000 of the population over 65, i.e., approximately 750,000 persons, or 60% of all cases of dementia in that population.[11] Multiinfarct dementia is believed to account for about 9 cases per 1000, i.e., approximately 270,000 persons. There are virtually no data on the prevalence of dementia in persons under 65 years of age.

The incidence of dementia is difficult to establish, as the syndrome is typically insidious and may not be detected until it is advanced. Estimates of its annual incidence in the elderly vary from 1% to 2.3%.[11]

PSYCHOPATHOLOGY

The essential feature of dementia is a *loss of intellectual abilities that is sufficiently severe to interfere with the individual's social or occupational functioning, or both.*[8] Dementia may be regarded as a global disorder of cognition, in the sense that several cognitive functions are impaired concurrently. They include memory, judgment, and abstract thinking. The work "impairment" in this context implies a decrement or deterioration of these functions in comparison with the given individual's premorbid level of performance. In addition to the cognitive disorder, dementia usually features personality change, that is, either accentuation or alteration of some of the person's characteristic traits.

One should keep in mind that dementia is not an all-or-none concept but rather a descriptive term for a clinical syndrome whose essential features may occur in various degrees of severity, time sequences, and constellations. For example, the syndrome may initially feature no more than annoying forgetfulness and difficulty in dealing with novel tasks or situations. At this early stage, the patient is likely to dismiss such symptoms as universal accompaniments of old age. At the other end of the spectrum, the clinical picture is dramatically different, with the patient impressing one as being a shell of his previous self: totally disoriented, incoherent, incontinent, and helpless. Between these two extremes lies a wide spectrum of degrees of the cognitive and behavioral disorder and of personality change. In some patients the latter may actually dominate the clinical picture from the beginning, whereas in others the personality remains intact until intellectual deterioration becomes profound. Such variability of the clinical picture of dementia is further accentuated by fluctuations in its severity in response to several possible factors. The degree of cognitive impairment may increase temporarily under the influence of such variables as personally stressful life change, intense emotions, physical ill health, and excessive or deficient environmental stimulation. A classical example of this is provided by a mildly demented man who becomes depressed after the death of his wife and displays rapid and profound, though potentially reversible, intellectual deterioration.

Clearly, no single definition of dementia or description of its essential and diagnostic features can do justice to the remarkable variability of its clinical picture displayed by the patients over time. In addition to the variables touched on previously, such factors as the nature of the underlying brain disease, the patient's level of education and intelligence, and the availability of social supports are all likely to influence the course and clinical manifestations of dementia in a given case. For all its variability, however, the syndrome features a set of psychopathological characteristics that can be discerned in a fully developed case. These characteristics include the following:

1. *Deterioration of overall intellectual function.* Dementia involves some degree of loss of intellectual abilities that the individual possessed prior to the illness, as attested by the level of his scholastic and occupational achievement as well as by the formal intelligence quotient (IQ). In dementia, the patient's IQ declines and formal testing discloses greater deterioration of the performance IQ than of the verbal IQ.[12] In everyday situations this intellectual impairment is likely to be most conspicuous when the patient is faced with novel and complex tasks, or those that demand shifts in problem-solving strategy. Time pressure tends to impair the patient's performance even further. On the contrary, he may still be able to perform efficiently when given a familiar and well-practiced task. (A patient of mine, for example, an outstanding lawyer who developed Alzheimer's disease, showed severe intellectual deterioration on psychologic testing, yet was still able to offer apparently sound legal advice to his clients, provided that his son was present during such consultations and interrupted them tactfully when his father began to repeat himself too often. The patient's clients seemed to be unaware of his dementia.) On the whole, the demented patient's performance is less efficient than before, and he tends to exhibit unaccustomed early fatigue and to become frustrated and flustered or angry while trying to perform.

2. *Impairment of memory.* Research on memory indicates that both short-term and long-term memory are impaired in the demented patient.[12] These patients are slow to

learn and, according to some investigators, have defective acquisition of new information.[12] Disturbed attention might be responsible for these deficits, but this issue is still unresolved. It has also been suggested that new information that enters long-term memory may be inefficiently coded in dementia and hence result in defective recall.

Clinically, memory impairment is an early and prominent feature in dementia. The patient tends to forget not only names but also actual events that have taken place hours or days before. Kral[13] has described what he called "malignant type of senescent memory dysfunction," which characterizes patients with primary degenerative dementia. The malignant type is marked by the inability of the patient to recall events of the recent past, so that whole experiences and not just bits of experiences cannot be recalled. Such loss of recent memories leads, in Kral's view, to disorientation for time and place and to retroactive loss of remote memories. Events that have special emotional significance for the patient may still be recalled. The patient displaying malignant forgetfulness is typically unaware of this defect.

Recent work has shown that long-term (remote) memory is indeed impaired in dementia, even though patients often assert that their recent memory is more affected than the remote.[14] Some authors have postulated that in dementia the retrograde amnesia extends over many decades and is equally distributed over time.[15]

A demented patient tends to understate or deny his memory deficits and may or may not confabulate to fill the memory gaps. If he is also depressed, however, he is likely not just to complain of being forgetful but actually to exaggerate his memory deficits.

3. *Impairment of abstraction.* The ability to display the abstract mode of cognitive functioning is one of the essential features of dementia. It was Goldstein[16] who postulated that the normal individual exhibits two basic types of attitudes toward the world: the concrete and the abstract, respectively. The former attitude is characterized by a response to an object or situation that is conditioned and bound by its immediate and unique features. In contrast, one displays the abstract attitude when one transcends the immediate stimulus object or situation and views it in a broader, conceptual context. To employ the abstract attitude is to compare, generalize, analyze or synthesize, apply general principles, discern essential features, and form concepts. On the basis of his extensive studies of brain-damaged patients, Goldstein proposed that impairment of abstraction is a core psychopathologic consequence and feature of brain damage.

Goldstein's conceptions have not gone unchallenged. Reitan,[17] for example, asserted already 25 years ago that a clear-cut dichotomy between "concrete" and "abstract" attitude or behavior had not been supported by research findings. The concept of abstraction ability, however, and the postulate that the latter is impaired in the brain-damaged individual remain heuristically valuable. More recently, Reitan[18] has proposed that *loss of abstraction*, of *reasoning ability*, and of the *capacity to understand the essential nature of a problem* together constitute the fundamental cognitive deficit in dementia. As a consequence of this impairment, the demented patient performs less efficiently than before in his accustomed occupational, social, and recreational activities. Such performance is likely to be even more strikingly affected if the task at hand is unfamiliar to the patient or is complex, or both, and if in addition it requires a prompt response and problem solving. The degree of this impairment may range from mild to severe and tends to fluctuate in such a way that it is likely to be most pronounced when the patient is anxious, depressed, physically ill, or tired.[19]

4. *Language impairment.* Disorder of language due to brain dysfunction is included among the diagnostic criteria of dementia in the official classification of mental disorders, although it is acknowledged that not all cerebral diseases that give rise to dementia feature it.[8] Language impairment is associated with diffuse degenerative diseases of the brain that account for the majority of cases of dementia in the elderly.[20,21] In the initial phase of the syndrome language disorder, although present, may not be readily detectable. In conversation the patient may impress a listener as being vague, but his speech is still relatively fluent as well as syntactically and phonologically correct, yet semantic paraphasias may be observed.[20] In the more advanced stage of dementia language impairment becomes manifest. Patients display impoverished vocabulary in narrative speech and dysphasic phenomena, both receptive and expressive. Verbal perseveration, that is, repetition of words or ideas, is common. The patient may have difficulty naming objects but, in contrast to subjects suffering from aphasia due to focal lesions, he appears to misidentify the object rather than to be unable to produce the correct word.[12] In severe dementia, when the patient is fully disoriented and has marked memory impairment, he may speak jargon, or utter meaningless sentences, or be mute.[20] Language disorder in the demented individual tends to progress proportionately to the deterioration of cognitive functions.

5. *Other disturbances of higher cortical function.* Apraxia, agnosia, and "constructional difficulty" are included in this group of diagnostic criteria for dementia.[8] These deficits have been observed mostly in Alzheimer's disease, and it is not known to what extent, if any, they occur in dementia due to other cerebral diseases. Moreover, impairment of memory and language makes it difficult to interpret agnostic and dyspraxic phenomena in these patients. Visual agnosia has been held responsible for defective naming of objects observed in some demented individuals.[12] Both ideational and ideomotor apraxia occur in many patients with Alzheimer's disease. The former connotes a failure to use objects correctly despite intact sensory and motor functions, whereas the latter refers to an inability to carry out on demand an action that the patient is able to perform spontaneously.

6. *Personality change.* Alteration of the individual's characteristic ways of reacting and acting, that is, of his personality style, is a common feature of dementia, one that may dominate the clinical picture from the onset of the disorder. Such alteration may involve either a conspicuous accentuation of the individual's personality characteristics or a true change of personality. In the latter case, the patient shows behavior that differs from his habitual conduct. Thus a meticulous person may start to show unaccustomed sloppiness, or a usually polite and tactful individual may begin to display coarse manners and use obscene or insulting language. In contrast, a patient may strike one as a caricature of his usual self, in the sense of being more than ever impulsive or compulsive or irascible or suspicious. Some patients attract attention because of their frankly antisocial or even criminal conduct, which they had never manifested before. Sexual molesting of minors, promiscuity, assaultive behavior, and shoplifting are examples of misdemeanors that may be a conspicuous feature of personality change and result in conflict with the law.

Bleuler[6] summed up succinctly the more common features of personality altera-tion: "Tenderness, consideration, tact, piety, esthetic sensibility, sense of duty, sense of right, feeling of sexual shame—all these may fail at any moment, even when they are present."

Personality alteration appears to reflect a combination of several contributing fac-tors. The patient's ability to control and modulate the expression of emotions and im-pulses is reduced. His social judgment, that is, capacity to anticipate other people's reaction to his behavior and to be concerned about it, is frequently diminished. Finer emotions and sensibility are often blunted, as is appreciation of ethical and aesthetic values and norms. At the same time, the affected individual tends to be unaware of his personality change and other people's reaction to it. The pathogenesis of person-ality change is not well understood. Damage to the frontal lobes may play a part in some cases, but the type of change and behavior described here may occur with focal lesions of the brain other than the frontal ones. It is equally plausible to hypothesize that the personality alteration represents a behavioral response to the distressing aware-ness of one's failing memory and intellectual performance and waning sense of con-trol over one's surroundings. Despite his denial, the patient is often aware, especially in the early stages of dementia, of a pervasive threat to his survival as a person, and this appears to be a major determinant of personality change. The latter may actually represent the patient's attempts to ward off the sense of failure and to maintain a meas-ure of mastery. Regardless of what explanations one may advance to account for the alteration of the personality in dementia, it represents a frequent and clinically and so-cially important aspect of the syndrome.

7. *Associated features*. Emotional, cognitive, and behavioral responses that a de-mented patient evolves as a reaction to his subjective awareness of intellectual deteri-oration and memory deficits fall under this heading. Some patients become more or less severely depressed, anxious, or both, especially in the early stages of dementia. Symptoms of a depressive or anxiety disorder may actually overshadow initially those related to intellectual and memory impairment as well as serve to accentuate them. Some patients become hypochondriacal and seek medical consultation for assorted so-matic symptoms for which no organic basis can be found. Others may develop a frank paranoid psychosis, with delusions of persecution or jealousy or of having things sto-len from them. Such a paranoid demented patient may threaten, assault, and even kill a falsely accused other person. For example, a patient who develops a delusion that his wife is unfaithful may murder her in a fit of rage. Demented individuals tend to tolerate alcohol poorly and may become grossly disinhibited while drinking.

Faced with a difficult problem-solving task, a demented patient is likely to become flustered, irritable, and anxious and may actually experience a full-blown anxiety at-tack. Goldstein[16] called such emotional responses to a difficult task a "catastrophic reaction" and argued that a considerable part of a brain-damaged individual's behavior can be explained by his attempts to avoid experiencing the highly distressing sense of failure and to ward off the catastrophic reaction.

The above *reactive*, *protective*, and *compensatory* emotional and behavioral responses frequently exhibited by demented individuals cannot be neatly separated from the so-called personality change discussed earlier. Indeed, they may constitute components of such a change. The whole issue of separating the essential from the accessory or associated features of dementia represents our efforts to identify the more or less invariable, and hence diagnostic, characteristics of this syndrome and to distinguish them from the relatively more inconstant and variable ones. In clinical practice, however, such boundaries are by no means clear-cut, as one is dealing with a totality of a patient's behavior.[22,23]

COURSE AND PROGNOSIS

The course and outcome of dementia are determined by the nature of the underlying brain disorder, by the timely application of proper treatment, and by psychosocial factors. Since the definition of the syndrome in DSM-III does not include the criterion of gradual and inexorable progression of intellectual deterioration, one can no longer speak of a more or less uniform natural history of dementia. Rather, it is more cogent to discuss the course and prognosis of the syndrome in relation to its specific etiology.

The onset of dementia may be *acute*, as when its cause is head injury, severe hypoxia or hypoglycemia, acute poisoning that results in brain damage, or encephalitis. In some cases, the onset is *subacute*, as in chronic intoxication with drugs or industrial poisons or in an endocrinopathy or metabolic encephalopathy. In the majority of cases, however, especially of older individuals, the onset of dementia is characteristically *insidious*, as is the case in Alzheimer's disease.

Similarly, the course of dementia may be static, remitting, or more or less steadily progressive. A patient who sustains a severe head injury, or some other cerebral insult resulting in widespread brain damage, may show improving intellectual function for months or even several years and then tends to reach a static level of impaired intellectual performance. In constrast, a victim of cardiac arrest or a metabolic encephalopathy may recovery completely over a period of months or a few years. Patients with cerebrovascular disease and multiinfarct dementia typically display an irregularly progressive course in that each new infarction is likely to be followed by an increment in intellectual deterioration. Patients with Alzheimer's disease usually show progressive intellectual deficits, but the rate of the cognitive deterioration tends to vary considerably from patient to patient.

An issue that has attracted much attention in recent years is *reversibility* of dementia. Larson et al.[23] have rightly argued that the notion of a clear-cut dichotomy (reversible–irreversible) may have been overemphasized and is of little clinical value. The majority of their series of patients with reversible dementia showed improvement with appropriate treatment but failed to reverse to normal. Finally, attempts are underway to develop diagnostic criteria for *mild dementia*, a problem of considerable clinical importance.[24]

SUMMARY AND CONCLUSIONS

The concept of dementia, in the current meaning of this term, has developed gradually over the past 1700 years. For much of the present century the term "dementia" carried a connotation of an irreversible and usually progressive intellectual deterioration from a premorbid state of cognitive functioning. As currently defined, however, dementia refers to cognitive impairment that may be static, remitting, or steadily or irregularly progressive. Considerable confusion has resulted from a common tendency to equate the term "dementia," a descriptive *syndrome*, with the senile dementia of Alzheimer type, a *disease* of the brain that is the most common cause of the syndrome of dementia in the elderly population. This semantic confusion has led to unwarranted conclusions about the natural history and outcome of dementia conceived as a syndrome. The issue of reversibility of this syndrome has been overemphasized and has resulted in an unduly sharp dichotomy of reversibility versus irreversibility. It seems more appropriate to speak of *degrees* of potential or actual restitution to the premorbid mental capacity of the patient, which may range from full to none.

Dementia is currently the subject of unprecedented interest and research on many fronts. One may predict that this situation will lead to a gradual refinement of the concept and perhaps its complete abandonment in favor of a more differentiated taxonomy and nosology of the states of cognitive impairment in man.

REFERENCES

1. Lipowski ZJ: Organic mental disorders: Their history and classification with special reference to DSM-III, in Miller NE, Cohen GD (eds): *Clinical Aspects of Alzheimer's Disease and Senile Dementia.* New York, Raven Press, 1981, pp 37–45.
2. Juvenal: Quoted in Brothwell D. Scandison AT (eds): *Diseases of Antiquity.* Springfield, Ill, Charles C Thomas, 1967, p 718.
3. Pinel P: *A Treatise on Insanity.* New York, Harper, 1962.
4. Esquirol JED: *Mental Maladies.* New York, Harper, 1965.
5. Prichard JC: *A Treatise on Insanity.* Philadelphia, Haswell, Barrington, and Haswell, 1837.
6. Bleuler E: *Textbook of Psychiatry.* New York, Macmillan, 1924.
7. Lipowski ZJ: Organic mental disorders: Introduction and review of syndromes, in Kaplan HI, Freedman AM, Sadock BJ (eds): *Comprehensive Textbook of Psychiatry,* ed 3. Baltimore, Williams & Wilkins, 1980. pp 1359–1392.
8. *DSM-III. Diagnostic and Statistical Manual of mental Disorders,* ed 3. Washington, DC, American Psychiatric Association, 1980.
9. Editorial: Dementia: The quiet epidemic. *Br Med J* 1:1–2, 1978.
10. Plum F: Dementia: An approaching epidemic. *Nature* 279:372–373, 1979.
11. Mortimer JA, Schuman LM (eds): *The Epidemiology of Dementia.* New York, Oxford University Press, 1981.
12. Miller E: The nature of cognitive deficit in senile dementia, in Miller NE, Cohen GD (eds): *Clinical Aspects of Alzheimer's Disease and Senile Dementia.* New York, Raven Press, 1981.
13. Kral VA: Senescent forgetfulness: Benign and malignant. *Can Med Assoc J* 86:257–260, 1962.
14. Kahn RL. Zarit SH, Hilbert NM, Niederehe G: Memory complaint and impairment in the aged. *Arch Gen Psychiatry* 32:1569–1573, 1975.
15. Albert MS, Butters N, Brandt J: Patterns of remote memory in amnestic and demented patients. *Arch Neurol* 38:495–500, 1981.
16. Goldstein K: Functional disturbances in brain damage, in Ariet: S, Reiser MF (eds): *American Handbook of Psychiatry,* edition 2. New York, Basic Books, 1975, vol 4, pp 182–207.
17. Reitan RM: Impairment of abstraction ability in brain damage: Quantitative versus qualitative changes. *J Psychol* 48:97–102, 1959.
18. Reitan RM: Neuropsychological concepts and psychiatric diagnosis, in Radoff VM, Stancer HC, Kedward HB (eds): *Psychiatric Diagnosis.* New York, Brunner/, 1977, pp 42–68.

19. Reisberg B (ed): *Alzheimer's Disease.* New York, The Free Press, 1983.
20. Bayles KA, Boone DR,, Kaszniak AW, Stern LZ: Language impairment in dementia. *Arizona Med* 39:308–311, 1982.
21. Obler LK: Language and brain dysfunction in dementia, in Segalowitz S (ed): *Language Function and Brain Organization.* New York, Academic Press, 1977.
22. Hemsi L: Living with dementia. *Postgrad Med J* 58:610–617, 1982.
23. Larson EB, Reifler BV, Featherstone HJ, English DR: Dementia in elderly outpatients. *Ann Intern Med* 100:417–423, 1984.
24. Henderson AS, Hupper FA: The problem of mild dementia. *Psychol Med* 14:5–11, 1984.

Consultation–Liaison Psychiatry IV

The articles in this section comprise a comprehensive overview of all the major aspects of the work of consultation–liaison psychiatrists. A reader looking for a general introduction to this subspecialty of psychiatry would be well advised to start with Chapters 18, 19, 21, and 27. Chapter 24 focuses on the currently controversial relations among liaison psychiatrists and nurses and the practitioners of behavioral medicine. Chapter 25 provides data on the types of patients referred for psychiatric consultation from medical and surgical discussions of general hospitals, and Chapter 26 focuses on the growing importance of psychopathology exhibited by elderly medical and surgical patients.

Review of Consultation Psychiatry and Psychosomatic Medicine

18

I. General Principles

One of the most significant developments in American psychiatry since World War II has been the growth of general-hospital psychiatric units. Several excellent books[39,46,80] have been devoted to this subject, but they do not attempt to evaluate specifically the importance of this development for psychosomatic medicine. Most relevant to the latter is consultation or liaison work carried out by psychiatrists in the nonpsychiatric departments of a general hospital. This consultative activity is one of the chief functions, as well as an outgrowth, of the psychiatric units. Kaufman, one of the pioneers in this field, calls liaison psychiatry "the most significant division for the role of psychiatrists in a general hospital."[38] There is a growing number of publications dealing with different facets of consultation psychiatry[11,24,27,31,32,40,42,48,59,60,71] and several general reviews are among them.[5,41,53,64,76] Each of these contributions, however, tends to stress one or more aspects of this field to the relative exclusion of others, and thus a comprehensive outline of this area of psychiatric activity is worth attempting. It may serve as a guide to the relevant literature for the increasing numbers of young psychiatrists wishing to spend some part of their training on a consultation service and perhaps choose it as their main area of psychiatric work. Another purpose of this paper is to point out the relevance and implications of consultation psychiatry for the wider field of psychosomatic medicine, and thereby supplement a review, by Wittkower and the author,[78] of recent trends in psychosomatic research.

The ill-defined area of psychosomatic medicine can be seen as developing most vigorously in two directions: that of psychophysiological research, which attempts to correlate events at the psychosocial and biological levels of abstraction, respectively; and that of consultation or liaison psychiatry, which is primarily a clinical and teaching activity applying and propagating the psychosomatic approach. Psychophysiological research becomes increasingly laboratory-based and dependent on experimental replication of presumed analogs of naturally occurring psychological stress. Consultation psychiatry has a hospital and medical practice as its base of operation and offers unique opportunities for the study of the interplay of biological and psychosocial variables in a clinical setting. It is the main goal of this review to outline the scope, tasks,

Reprinted from *Psychosomatic Medicine* 29(2):153–171, 1967. Copyright © 1967 by The American Psychosomatic Society, Inc. Reprinted by permission of Elsevier Science Publishing Co., Inc.

and fascinating possibilities for advancing the knowledge of man of this relatively new "area of special interest" in psychiatry.

THE SCOPE OF CONSULTATION (LIAISON) PSYCHIATRY

Consultation psychiatry may be defined as that area of clinical psychiatry which includes all diagnostic, therapeutic, teaching, and research activities of psychiatrists in the nonpsychiatric parts of a general hospital. Such a broad operational definition is felt to delimit the field with reasonable clarity by stressing the actual physical and social setting in which these activities take place. There is little doubt, however, that there is no conceptual boundary between consultation psychiatry as here defined and the consultative services which psychiatrists render to other physicians, such as general practitioners, in other types of setting. Indeed these two areas of psychiatric activity have much in common in that their primary concern is the sick person. Furthermore, the respective patient populations share almost universally one important characteristic: They communicate their distress, regardless of its origin, in somatic terms—i.e., in the form of bodily discomfort or symptoms. The diagnostic and theoretical implications of this fact are of crucial importance to the psychiatric consultant and will be discussed in later sections of this review.

The designation "consultation psychiatry" does not convey adequately the true scope of the activities and theoretical concerns of psychiatrists working in this field. While there is no doubt that consultation is the focus and practical raison d'être of this area of psychiatry, the actual extent of the latter is considerably wider. The consultants consult, but they usually teach and often do clinical research as well. Their area of work, interests, teaching, and investigation is that of psychosocial and psychopathological aspects of medical practice in general and of hospital practice in particular. It appears that the term "consultation psychiatry" has gained popularity because it stresses the service aspect of the work and thus its usefulness to the other physicians. The tendency to avoid the word "psychosomatic" in this context is striking and no doubt related to its ambiguous meaning. A consultant in "psychosomatic medicine" would likely become a victim of misinterpretation of his function and be considered an expert in the limited area of the so-called psychosomatic disorders, with resulting limitation of his scope of work and usefulness.

Another source of ambiguity in calling our area of interest "consultation psychiatry" is the fact that psychiatrists serve in consulting capacity in courts, community agencies, etc., where the problems and techniques are different from those under consideration here. In some centers, the terms "liaison psychiatry" and "liaison service" are used in an apparent attempt at clearer communication, but these terms are rather nondescript and offer little advantage. In the end, of course, what matters is not which designation is used, but the clear definition of its meaning and the actual activities of the people who use it. In this paper the terms "liaison" and "consultation" psychiatry will be used synonymously.

The scope of consultation psychiatry as defined in this paper is a wide one: It comprises both the activities listed above and the body of observation and theory on which these activities depend. In general, consultation psychiatry is concerned with psychological aspects of illness and of medical practice in a general hospital. Its special focus is the consultation proper. This review can do no more than offer an outline of the various facets of this whole field. The relevant literature is vast and clearly cannot be adequately covered here. Several books[6,33,34,45,62,75,77] give a more general presentation of the psychological aspects of medicine, and even though their respective scopes and emphases differ rather widely, they are valuable as basic references for the consultant. In addition, there are available books and papers which deal with the psychological aspects of various medical specialties, such as neurology,[72] obstetrics and gynecology,[43] ophthalmology,[61] pediatrics,[51] surgery,[14,73] dermatology,[55] and otolaryngology.[3] These publications are indispensable for the psychiatric consultants working in those respective departments. Two problems of medical practice in all specialities which are of particular importance to the consultant must be singled out: the management of the dying patient[23] and the psychological aspects of neoplastic diseases.[65,68] Both have adequate literature and will not be discussed here.

PSYCHIATRIC CONSULTATION SERVICE IN A GENERAL HOSPITAL

ORGANIZATION

The organizational basis for the practice of consultation psychiatry in a general hospital is the consultation or liaison service. As Richmond[57] rightly emphasizes, it is through this service that the impact of a psychiatric unit on the hospital as a whole can be effected. The same author states that in the United States such services range from large units, which provide consultants to each medical specialty, to a one-man unit in which one psychiatrist serves as a consultant to all departments. Exact information on the number of liaison services in the North American community hospitals is, however, lacking, and a detailed survey which would include facts about staffing, procedures, number of patients seen annually, etc. is overdue. Kaufman[37] reports that at the Mount Sinai Hospital in New York every service has a psychiatrist or a team of psychiatrists assigned to it. A similar organizational model seems to be at work at Michael Reese Hospital in Chicago[5] and the Beth Israel Hospital in Boston.[80] Our own unit at the Royal Victoria Hospital in Montreal consists of three part-time staff psychiatrists and three senior psychiatric residents—a number which we feel is unequal to the task. While the size of the service is inevitably dictated by the size of the hospital, its readiness to accept psychiatrists as members of a medical team, and the availability of consultants, it is proposed as a goal that at least in a teaching hospital psychiatrists should be assigned to each specialty as well as to the medical outpatient clinics and the emergency department. Some of these assignments can be filled by senior residents or clinical fellows with special interest in this type of work. These junior members of the service could rotate through the various departments to gain experience of the specific problems presented by each of them. The writer had such varied training at the Massachusetts General Hospital and found it most rewarding.

Whatever the number of the members of the consultation service, they should function as a team and share their experiences in a formal weekly case conference. Other aspects of their cooperation are discussed under *Teaching*. It is generally desirable that each consultant should become a member of the professional team in the department to which he is assigned.[32] This involves participation in daily or at least weekly clinical rounds, even if that is time-consuming and at times appears to be unrewarding. The consultant should be prepared to tolerate fluctuations of his colleagues' interest in his role and contribution. He may be ignored, especially at the beginning, or asked questions on purely medical matters. If he can hold his ground in these testing situations and display sound knowledge of general medicine, his services as a psychiatrist may then be sought with increasing frequency and sense of purpose. As Beigler *et al.*[5] remark, liaison psychiatry is a phasic process in the sense that the degree of acceptance of a consultant, the types of problems he is asked to deal with, and the related effectiveness and value of his contribution all go through a series of stages before reaching an optimum state.

The present writer recalls vividly his first experience as a consultant to a medical ward in a famous American hospital. He attended daily rounds on the ward and for the first 2 weeks was totally ignored by all members of the medical team who had been informed about the nature of his assignment. At the end of this "quarantine," during which he remained a silent witness, he was asked jokingly by the attending physician whether his role was to watch the chief or the residents. Having explained that his role was not that of a spy but of a consultant who would try to be of some use in dealing with problem patients, the author began to be noticed with a less wary eye. He was at first drawn into purely medical discussions and later asked to try to rehabilitate a few chronic alcoholics with advanced cirrhosis and Korsakoff's syndrome. It would be nice, he was told, if these unhappy men could be persuaded to stop drinking and take up gainful occupation. In the next phase of his work, he was called upon to suggest a sedative for a loudly abusive, delirious woman and here came his first modest success, received with polite thanks. Having proved his practical usefulness to the team, the author was asked for assistance with some diagnostic problems and his expert advice was acknowledged. It was only after a few months that his help with management problems began to be sought—e.g., in the case of a coronary patient who refused to stay in bed or a woman who angrily complained that too much blood was being taken from her for tests. In this way, the consultant's relationship with the team progressed through fairly distinct phases, from isolation to meaningful cooperation. While this is surely not a universal model, it does illustrate fairly typical vicissitudes of a consultant's liaison with his medical colleagues.

The role of a psychiatric consultant was succinctly stated by Kaufman[38]: he should be "of practical assistance in the total evaluation and furtherance of treatment of any given patient." The emphasis must be put on "practical assistance." To be useful, the consultant has to be readily available; waiting for a consultation slip in a room distant from the ward is not good enough. Furthermore, unless the psychiatrist is thoroughly familiar with the personnel of the wards to which he is assigned, he can hardly be of help with the problems involving conflicts between the patient and the people who take care of him. These matters are obvious to experienced consultants, but have to be brought home to the psychiatrists beginning to work in this area. The author feels strongly that at least some of the members of the consultation service should have full-time assignments and devote themselves entirely to liaison work. While this may not often be possible in the case of the senior members for whom adequate salaries are seldom available, one may make use of full-time clinical fellows or residents with at least 2 but preferably 3 years' experience of psychiatry. These junior consultants should be largely free from other duties. It is seldom appreciated by those not working in this field that consulting on medical wards is a time-consuming job. Success depends on the degree to which the consultant proves his usefulness to the medical team, and this means that he is available when needed, communicates adequately with all concerned, and follows up at least some of the patients he sees throughout their hospitalization. A good deal of the teaching that the consultant does takes place during informal contacts with the medical residents and others. All this makes for a full day's work if the job is to be done right.

An important aspect of the organization of the service is that of recording what is being done.[18] A standardized form containing basic data about the patients seen should be filled out as soon as the consultation is over. This procedure is necessary if any information is to be retrieved later for statistical and research purposes. It may be of value for the full-time consultant to record daily his contacts, exchanges, and observations pertaining to his work on the wards. Such records may yield interesting data about social interaction in the milieu in which problems with patients arise. This type of record was usefully employed by Myer and Mendelson.[53] These workers made detailed reports of their daily activities as well as of the circumstances and manner of presentation of the requests for consultation. They also recorded their own responses to the situations in which they were involved. The results of their data-gathering threw important light on what they call the natural history of the consultation process, and will be referred to later. Such extensive recording could hardly be recommended as a routine procedure and really falls into the category of clinical research.

In summary, a consultation service should be a close-knit, organized unit consisting of at least some full-time psychiatrists who at the same time are members of the medical team in close daily contact with it and with the medical wards. Only in this way can the service fulfill its main function as a psychiatric–medical liaison endeavor.

THE CONSULTANT AND HIS ENVIRONMENT

To list the qualities of an ideal consultant would be an exercise in futility. Yet there is little doubt that certain qualities impede while others facilitate work in this area. It follows that, if the service is to work smoothly, a careful selection of the candidates for it is of utmost importance. Smith,[69] a sociologist, calls the psychiatrist a marginal man of the medical profession. He remarks that this marginality of the psychiatrist "may also be experienced in general hospitals where he is likely, as a widely ranging consultant, to be an outsider on another physician's or service's ward." Smith also observes that psychiatrists are accused of the "imperialistic intention of making medicine its adjunct" and through their missionary zeal to educate other men, provoke their medical colleagues to try to push them back.

These remarks are pertinent and highlight the sensitivity of the position of the psychiatric consultant whose personal conduct and attitude may spell the difference between success of the service and its death of disuse atrophy. It is not enough for the consultant to be a competent expert in the fields of psychodynamics and psychopathology. He has to have sound knowledge of and some continued interest in general medicine, as well as in the speciality to which he is assigned. Yet, as Kaufman[38] emphasizes, the psychiatrist's contribution to medicine must be made mainly as a psychiatrist and not under the guise of pretended medical expertness. This view does not seem to be shared by all, since Engel et al.[21] report that at the University of Rochester Medical Center the liaison service is staffed by men who were first trained as internists and then as psychiatrists and can thus be expected to be experts in both fields. Apart from medical knowledge, the consultant should possess personal qualities which enable him to be an acceptable member of a medical team. This position requires tact, ability to communicate clearly and without psychiatric jargon, flexibility, and genuine respect for the other man's job. Striking peculiarities of manner, condescending attitude, professional fanaticism, and salesmanship are definitely out of place here. The psychiatrist can make a valuable contribution to the running of a medical service, and he can learn perhaps more than he is able to teach, but his usefulness has limitations inherent in the state of psychiatric knowledge and therapeutic efficacy. To deny this latter fact, implicitly or explicitly, would amount to fanaticism or bluff.

A problem which a young consultant will have to work through is that of his own professional identity: Is he primarily a psychiatrist, with his bias psychosocial rather than biological and thus a "marginal man," or is he a biologically oriented physician? Should he wear a white coat on rounds, carry a stethoscope, stand out, or merge into the background? These questions and related ambiguity of role may be stressful. With time, however, the young man is likely to accept that he is what he is—a psychiatrist with a holistic bias—and leave it at that.

An account of the consultant's job would be incomplete without mentioning some of its strains and frustrations. The author's remarks are based on 7 years' experience of consulting with varying periods spent in three hospitals widely known for their contribution to medical progress. His general impression is that, despite all the talk about comprehensive medicine and pious incantations about the holistic approach to patients, many physicians have little interest in and appreciation of the psychosocial factors in illness and even less conviction that psychiatry has something useful to contribute to the practice of medicine.[12,19] The most desirable attitude to this problem which one's colleagues may display is that of benevolent skepticism. What one often encounters, however, is indifference, prejudice, derogatory stereotypes, and outright hostility. It is not without good reason that an editorial in a medical journal[20] comments on the "calumniatory denigration" with which some of his professional colleagues regard the psychiatrist. The latter is often represented as a scientifically unsophisticated, medically ignorant, and impractical man, given to sweeping statements about other people's motives based on abstruse theories of questionable validity. It is up to the consultant to live down some of these stereotypical notions.

Mendelson and Meyer[52] review some of the countertransference reactions of the psychiatric consultant related to the inconveniences, dilemmas, and frustrations of his work. Their remarks can be endorsed by this writer from his own experience. There are, however, important satisfactions in this type of work. One applies one's knowledge and skill to situations where effects of such intervention tend to be prompt and sometimes dramatic, in contrast to the slow gains in some other areas of psychiatric work. In addition, there is cognitive and aesthetic satisfaction in working with a class of existential crises equally interesting to the biologist and the humanist.

THE CONSULTATION

OBJECTIVES AND STRATEGIES

Consultation is the main focus of a psychiatrist's work on a medical service. Kahana[35] rightly stresses that psychiatric consultation concerned with the management of patients on the medical and surgical wards is "an immediate exercise in the integration of psychological thought in medical practice." Caplan[15] has done much to clarify the meaning, modes, and procedures of mental health consultation. He defines the latter as "the process of interaction between two professional persons—the consultant, who is a specialist, and the consultee, who invokes his help in regard to a current work problem with which the latter is having some difficulty, and which he has decided is within the former's area of special competence." Caplan distinguishes four types of mental health consultation, two of which are applicable to the work with patients: client-centered case consultation, the immediate goal of which is to assist the consultee in finding proper treatment for his client (patient); and consultee-centered case consultation, which focuses upon the consultee and his particular difficulty with the given client. The former type of consultation is equivalent to the diagnostic evaluation and consequent therapeutic recommendations and thus conforms to the traditional model of medical consultation, while the latter type represents a significant shift from the tradition in its concern with the consultee. Bartemeier[4] stresses that a psychiatric consultant, unlike other medical specialists, needs to concern himself not only with the patient referred to him but also with the specific problems of the referring physician insofar as they influence his professional relationship with the patient. In general, one notes three trends among writers who deal with psychiatric consultations in a general hospital: (1) the patient is the primary focus of the consultant's interest (a patient-oriented approach), as in Weisman and Hackett's[76] conception of therapeutic consultation; (2) the referring physician's motives for requesting a consultation and his related difficulties and expectations are the center of the consultant's inquiry and advice (a consultee-oriented approach);[60] (3) interpersonal transactions of all the members of the clinical team involved in the care of the patient for whom consultation had been requested are taken into account to understand the patient's behavior and the consultee's concern about it (situation-oriented approach).[42,53]

There can be little doubt that the three approaches described above are not mutually exclusive and that an experienced consultant will shift his interest according to the demands of the situation. What needs special emphasis, however, is the increased scope of the consultation process and its growing complexity and psychosocial sophistication. It is enough to compare Campbell's[13] witty account of medical consultations, as practiced both in the past and now, with a recent discussion of psychiatric consultations by Meyer and Mendelson,[53] to appreciate how fundamentally the latter differ from the former. The crucial difference lies in the psychiatric consultant's awareness that a consultation is incomplete if the patient is considered apart from the social field is which he finds himself. The operational group,[53] of which the patient is the center and which includes the physicians, nurses, and social worker concerned with his care, is viewed as a social field within which transactions take place between the participants. These transactions exert decisive effect on the patient's adaptation of his illness, hospitalization and therapeutic procedures, and thus significantly influence his behavior. The psychiatric consultant enters the group as a participant observer and from his relatively detached position applies his knowledge of dynamics in an attempt to identify sources of strain in the group and to offer practical measures for their removal or attenuation. Conceptualized in this way, the consultant's activity combines all three approaches to consultation listed above: its focus is the disturbed patient; the crisis which his disturbed behavior creates in his relationship with his doctor and members of the clinical team, as well as the effect of the latter on the patient.

This discussion of the general objectives and strategies of a psychiatrist's consultative activity in the medical wards should not obscure the fundamental goal of this activity, which is *the promotion of improved patient care*. Regardless of whether the immediate strategy is patient-or consultee-centered, the ultimate target must always be the patient. It is not the consultant's task to offer covert "psychotherapy" to the referring doctor. While the latter's increased self-awareness, which Bibring[8] stresses may result from his contact with the psychiatrist, this acquired insight is relevant to the consultant's job only insofar as it improves his medical colleague's professional functioning. This formulation of the consultant's primary objective puts the emphasis squarely on his *medical* role and responsibility. His unique contribution is his knowledge of individual psychodynamics (and psychopathology), as well as his work methodology based on this knowledge. His professional goals, however, are shared with other members of the clinical team.

CONSULTATION AS A PROCESS

In a recent paper, Wolfe[79] distinguishes three interdependent operational aspects of consultation: role, function, and process. Consultant role is what the consultant thinks he is and what others think he is; function is what he does; and process, how he does it. The role aspect was discussed above; the elements of the process and the functions of psychiatric consultation in a general hospital remain to be examined.

Viewed as a process, consultation consists of a sequence of events which can be conceptualized in different ways. Such a sequential analysis has the advantage of clarifying for the consultant his general mode of operating. Meyer and Mendelson[53] offer the most thorough and sophisticated analysis available of what they call the natural history of the consultation process. They distinguish three main elements of the process: the request for consultation, the psychiatrist's redefinition of the patient situation, and the psychiatrist and the operational group. While this conceptual model can be usefully applied to a considerable part of consultative activity, it is not valid for all of it. The authors themselves remark wisely that one must "beware of premature stereotypes.'' A different conceptual model is proposed by Sandt and Leifer.[59] Theirs is a "sociocommunicational analytic model in which the consultation is seen as a communication which may be divided into three components: the sender, the message and the receiver.'' This scheme, as elaborated by the authors, does clarify an important aspect of consultative activity by stressing the influence of language on the transactions between the consultee, the patient, and the consultant.

The present writer prefers to offer a scheme which in his opinion has more general validity and practical usefulness by being less abstract and more descriptive. He views the consultation process as consisting essentially of three phases: reception of a request for consultation, gathering of information, and communication of the consultant's findings, opinions, and advice. It is the writer's contention that these three elements are most basic to the consultation process and are never absent, regardless of whether the consultant redefines the situation he encounters, attempts therapeutic intervention, uses consultation as a teaching medium, becomes a participant of the operational group— or does none of these things. The only exception to the proposed sequence of events occurs when the consultant who is a member of a medical team himself initiates a consultation, in which case no request is received. The latter, however, is an atypical situation.

REQUEST FOR CONSULTATION

The usual custom is for the consultee, who is the physician in charge of the patient, to make the request by sending a standard slip, or directly, verbally. In either case, it is important for the consultant to note how the message is worded as they may offer clues as to how the consultee perceives his problem. It has been pointed out[60] that the request may bear little relevance to the real nature of the problem and that the more diffuse and unclear the message, the more likely is the consultee helpless and in need of the consultant's assistance. It is the latter's task in such a case to redefine the problem to achieve semantic clarity which in itself may help the consultee find a correct solution. It may be stated as a general rule that the request for consultation is not in the full sense received until the consultant has *clarified its meaning*. To do so he has to discuss with the consultee the reasons for the request. At this point, the first phase of the process merges with the second—viz., gathering of information. What is the consultee's problem? That is the first question which the consultant attempts to answer.

The meaning and the genesis of the request for consultation are thus the first steps of the consultant's inquiry. The request may originate with the patient, but in practice this is not common. The initiative usually comes from the physician—attending or resident—in charge of the patient, or much less often, from one of the nurses or the social worker. In any case, it is customarily the physician who communicates the request to the consultant. Before a request is made, there must be acknowledgment that a problem exists which necessitates expert advice. What types of problems can lead to this? Meyer and Mendelson[53] suggest that two conditions are required for a physician to request psychiatric consultation: uncertainty about the nature of the patient's behavior and responsibility for doing something about it. The former implies a cognitive stalemate; the latter, frustrated readiness for action. In more concrete terms, the following are the commonest reasons for request for a psychiatric consultation: diagnostic uncertainty; recognition of a gross psychiatric disorder; patient's deviant behavior with regard to medical procedures and therapies, ward routine, etc., which disturbs smooth functioning of the medical team; crisis in the doctor–patient relationship; patient's admission of serious psychosocial difficulties. In all these instances, the consultee, and to a lesser degree other members of the medical team, are of decisive importance. The consultee's own value system which determines what he regards as "deviant" or "abnormal," his tolerance of an ability to deal with such "abnormality" and with conflict, and his ideas about what his psychiatric consultant can do, all influence the decision to request a consultation and its timing.

GATHERING OF INFORMATION

Information-gathering starts with the inquiry into the nature of the problem which leads to the request for consultation. The consultant speaks to the referring doctor and the head nurse, and examines the patient's chart. In the latter, the nurses' notes are usually most informative and may, for example, suggest the diagnosis of delirium even before the patient is seen. It is important to inquire if the patient knows that a psychiatrist was asked to see him, and to insist that he be told about the consultation in advance.[56] The patient is interviewed, if at all possible, in a private place. To fail to observe this need for privacy may vitiate the interview, as a colleague's experience illustrates: He started to interview a female patient on a public ward when he heard the penetrating whisper of an old lady lying in another bed: "Listen, listen, he is bugging her, he is the bug man!" Such interferences do not promote rapport.

The interview proper cannot be schematized. Ruesch et al.[58] point out that the initial psychiatric evaluation is focal in nature, and answers to clearly formulated questions should be sought. This is an important point. The consultant is often faced with emergency situations, as when an acutely ill patient refuses consent to an operation, in which the problem on hand must be the overriding focus of the inquiry. Such situations test the consultant's skill in eliciting relevant information in the shortest possible time and call for high flexibility and improvisation in the conduct of the interview. Careful testing of the cognitive functions (sensorium) is a must in all cases. In some complicated diagnostic problems, the consultant may have to take a truly comprehensive case history, including a careful functional inquiry, to discern the nature of the different symptoms. These diagnostic problems will be taken up in detail in a later section of this review. To repeat, the focus, direction, and technique of the interview will be dictated by the presenting problem and no rigid schematization is possible. A psychiatrist accustomed to the more leisurely tempo of office practice may find the exigencies of medical ward consultations too much to bear; this kind of work certainly does not suit every temperament.

In some cases, the phase of information-gathering is not completed without further inquiry which may involve the nurses, social worker, and members of the patient's family. Meyer and Mendelson[53] call this the expanded psychiatric interview. It may yield data of crucial importance without which the consultation would fail to be of use.

COMMUNICATION OF RESULTS

In the final phase of the consultation, the consultant is faced with the task of communicating his findings, opinions, and recommendations to the consultee and frequently to other members of the clinical team, such as interns, nurses, and the social worker. Customarily this communication is verbal, as well as by means of a written report to be included in the patient's chart. It is mostly at this stage that the consultant can exert some influence on the situation of the patient. Thus, what he communicates, how he does it, and to whom are of decisive importance for the success of the consultation. In general, such a communication should satisfy the following four criteria: *relevance, explanatory value, intelligibility,* and *practicability.* The need for relevance cannot be stressed too strongly. It implies that what is communicated must have a direct bearing on the problem at hand. An inexperienced consultant asked to see a patient for a preoperative evaluation may come up with a lengthy life history and a neat, dynamic formulation of the patient's personality, conflicts, and defenses, but fail completely to select that material which is relevant to the problem and of predictive value in the given situation. Apart from being selective and relevant, the communication should help the consultee understand why the patient behaves (and this includes complains) as he does. The consultant's opinions and advice are of little or no value if communicated in a language and in a referential frame which the consultee cannot understand. As Proctor[56] points out, the referring doctor wants "concrete suggestions as to therapy, not a lot of psychiatric jargon that he cannot understand or comprehend." Finally, consultation is incomplete unless it leads to a course of action, and this must be clearly stated and follow logically from the findings and opinion of the consultant.

The problem of writing psychiatric reports has been well dealt with in a paper by Dean.[17] His main postulates are worth restating here because of their relevance. He recommends that such written reports should be conceived as a guide to action, free from professional jargon and verbiage, factual rather than speculative, clear in respect of what is speculation or opinion and what is thought to be fact, and organized—i.e., in orderly form, stating the problem, its elucidation, and proposed action for its solution.

Apart from the formal written report, it is essential for the consultant to talk the matter over the the consultee in a more extended and informal manner. It is often difficult to convey all nuances of the case in a concise written note and there may be aspects of the doctor–patient relationship, conflict within the operational group, etc., which do not belong in the official record. It is in these direct personal contacts with people concerned with the patient's care that the consultant fulfills his clarifying, conflict-reducing, teaching, and constructively manipulative role. These functions of the consultation can now be discussed in more detail.

FUNCTIONS OF A CONSULTATION

The various uses to which psychiatric consultations in a general hospital may be put are by no means mutually exclusive. The emphasis in any given case will depend on the situation and to some extent on the consultant's predominant interest and conception of his role. He may see himself primarily as a diagnostician, therapist, teacher, or medicosocial reformer manipulating interpersonal transactions to reduce strain, conflict, etc. In practice, the main functions of consultation are as follows: *diagnosing, advising on management of patients, therapy, resolving conflicts within the operational group (patient and clinical team)*, and *teaching*. These functions will now be discussed in some detail.

Diagnostic Evaluation

To diagnose means "to recognize the presence of a disease by examination and assessment of the symptoms and signs."[9] In a wider sense, it means "to identify by careful observation."[66] In this discussion, we will assume that the diagnosing function of the consultant includes both the strictly medical connotation of searching for the disease or disorder underlying the presenting symptoms, and the broader connotation of identifying the patient's chief personality features, his characteristic conflicts and defenses, and his current psychosocial situation. The actual diagnostic problems which commonly confront the psychiatric consultant in medicine will be considered in Part II of this review (Chapter 19, this volume) and only some general remarks will be made at this stage.

Kaufman[37] observes that the spectrum of diagnostic categories into which the patients seen by the psychiatric consultant fall is "an index of the psychiatrist's role in modern medicine." In his study of over 2000 consultations over a 2-year period, Kaugman found that in 61.4% the problem was one of differential diagnosis. This figure highlights the frequency with which psychiatric consultants are called upon to contribute to the diagnostic process in its more narrowly medical sense. Faucett,[22] discussing the application of psychiatric interview to medical diagnosis, points out that the psychiatrist who is asked for a diagnostic consultation on a patient with somatic symptoms should pay particular attention to the rationale on which his opinion is based. He should satisfy himself that the clinical and psychodynamic picture of the patient and his psychogenetic history support one another and provide adequate explanation for the timing of the onset of illness and for the choice of the given symptoms as an expression of psychic conflict. If these criteria cannot be satisfied, the consultant should suspend his judgment and encourage further investigation. Faucett's postulates are certainly good policy for a responsible consultant but in practice one often has to be satisfied with degrees of probability rather than with certainty. This writer believes that there is a pressing need for an analysis of the psychiatric diagnostic process in general, and as it is applied to somatic symptoms in particular, comparable to Ledley and Lustig's analysis[44] of the reasoning foundations of medical diagnosis. While psychiatrists are usually expert at eliciting data in the course of a diagnostic interview, they generally pay little attention to the formal logical aspects of drawing inferences from their data. This neglect results in the frequent impression of fanciful improvisation which psychiatric conclusions convey to other physicians and consequent distrust in practical recommendations based on such conclusions.

Magraw[49,50] contributes two useful papers on the process of comprehensive diagnosis for medical patients. He suggests that the narrow concept of diagnosis centered about disease entities is an inadequate theoretical model which hinders the application of comprehensive medical care. He postulates that the more correct approach to diagnosis is one in which the goal is understanding of the patient's complaints in terms of the various mechanisms which produce them. The psychiatric consultant in a general hospital is one of the few physicians who nowadays apply the principles of comprehensive or psychosomatic diagnosis in this sense. If he were to confine himself to a purely psychiatric diagnostic evaluation or to sketching of psychodynamic personality profiles with little regard to the patient's somatic and social reality, he would fail in his task as diagnostician and teacher.

An important and practically useful facet of the diagnosis is identification of the patient's basic personality style. The perfection of this area of inquiry is a special contribution of a group of psychiatrists under the leadership of Bibring at the Beth Israel Hospital in Boston. In a series of papers[7,8,36] these workers develop a psychoanalytically oriented medical psychology to serve as a guide to the management of medical patients. This approach is based on the assumption that if "the main structure and probable etiology of the presenting symptom, in this case the leading personality trait, has been understood, the therapeutic intervention follows logically and simply as in any clinical science."[8] Thus the diagnosis of personality structure becomes an indispensable part of the evaluation of the management problem patient. To facilitate such diagnosis, Kahana and Bibring[36] describe seven basic classes of personality type and attitudes: (1) the dependent, overdemanding (oral); (2) the orderly, controlled (compulsive); (3) the dramatizing, emotionally involved, capitulating (hysterical); (4) the long-suffering, self-sacrificing (masochistic); (5) the guarded, querulous (paranoid); (6) the superior-feeling (narcissistic); and (7) the uninvolved and aloof (schizoid) personality. The authors postulate that each of these normal personality types, as well as its psychopathological counterpart (included above in parentheses), will react to the stress of illness, hospitalization, etc., and consequent anxiety, with *increased intensity* of his basic characterological defenses. These in turn will result in certain predictable attitudes and behaviors which may interfere with, but can be utilized to secure, the patient's cooperation with the medical management. The meaning of illness is different to each of these personality types and the physician's awareness of this greatly increases his understanding of the patient's behavior and improves his therapeutic effectiveness.

Advising on Management

The function of consultation merges imperceptibly with the preceding discussion of comprehensive, and especially personality, diagnosis. A survey of specific management problems confronting the psychiatric consultant will follow in Part II of this review (chapter 19, this volume) and only general principles will be discussed at this stage.

The above-mentioned Beth Israel Hospital group has developed a most useful theoretical framework to serve as a practical guide to solving management problems of psychological origin on the medical wards. They call their approach "therapeutic manipulation" or "adaptive intervention."[35] The Bibrings, as quoted by Zinberg,[80] define the word "manipulation" as the "employment of various emotional systems existing in the patient for the purpose of achieving therapeutic and adjustive change." This technique can be utilized directly by the consultant in his contacts with the patient or offered to the consultee to increase his effectiveness in dealing with the patient and help the latter "utilize the strength of his personality in cooperatively combatting illness."[35] Bibring[8] presents fascinating clinical vignettes illustrating this approach in its practical operation with problem patients. This is application of psychodynamics to concrete medical problems at its best.

Therapy

The therapeutic function of consultation can hardly be clearly differentiated from the foregoing. Its focus, however, is directly on the patient rather than on the consultee. Kahana,[35] following the Bibrings' formulations, stresses the value of suggestion and clarification as psychotherapeutic agents. Suggestion involves the "induction by the physician of ideas, impulses, and actions of the patient" while clarification is achieved by the physician's explanations to the patient of the meaning of his symptoms and attitudes, as well as of the reasons for the various medical tests, procedures, and recommendations. For many patients, some degree of cognitive clarity regarding what is happening and being done to them results in reduction of anxiety and related disturbing behavior.

Weisman and Hackett[76] develop their own conception of "therapeutic consultation," which is formulated as a crisis intervention. They describe four elements of such consultation: rapid evaluation; psychodynamic formulation of the major conflict, ego functions, and object relationships; rational programming of a therapeutic intervention; and active implementation by the consultant himself. The focus of this approach is the crisis or conflict with which the patient is confronted as a result of his illness, hospitalization, therapeutic procedures, vicissitudes of the doctor–patient relationship, etc. The consultant tries to establish himself as an understanding and supportive ally of the patient—a role deliberately modeled after some "good" figure in the patient's past life—and attempts to help him utilize those ego assets which helped him cope with life crises in the past. In two other papers,[29,30] Hackett and Weisman illustrate their approach as applied to the management of operative syndromes. This technique adds a valuable and practically useful tool to the consultant's clincial armamentarium and thus increases his overall usefulness.

Resolving Conflicts

This function of consultation is the liaison function proper. The consultant fulfills the role of go-between and interpreter between the patient and one or more members of the medical team. The moment a patient is admitted to a medical ward, he becomes a member of a specific subculture in which the chief roles are played by members of the medical and ancillary professions.[63] A person's customary freedom of action becomes curtailed by virtue of his becoming a hospital patient. He is subjected to routines which are foreign to him and his privacy is largely disregarded. Other people—

members of the clinical team—become authorities, deciding what is wrong with him, what investigative and therapeutic procedures he is to undergo, what restrictions to observe, and which behavior is permissible and which not. The patient enters this environment bringing to it his characteristic modes of coping with stress, his attitudes towards dependence, passivity, authority figures, and uncertainty—aspects of his status as a hospital patient. Most people seem to adjust to this situation in a manner which does not draw disapproving attention of the medical team. But the situation creates favorable conditions for conflict between the patient and those taking care of him. Such conflict may grow to the point of crisis, which implies that the threshold of tolerance in one or more participants has been exceeded and disruptive affects of anxiety, anger, resentment, guilt, and shame appear, resulting in behaviors which interfere with adequate medical care.

A brief clinical vignette from our recent experience can illustrate this. The patient, a young woman, was admitted to a medical ward for treatment of acute pyelonephritis. Within a day or two, she was up and about and immediately took it upon herself to visit all patients on the ward to inquire if they were satisfied with the nursing care and had any special requests. She then took all complaints and wishes to the head nurse, urging appropriate action. After a few days of this activity, which was at once resented by the nurses as interference with their prerogatives, the head nurse complained to the resident with an intensity which prompted him to request an emergency psychiatric consultation.

We have here a typical situation of ward conflict which the psychiatric consultant may be asked to resolve by influencing somehow the disturbing patient. It is clear, however, that the consultant's intervention in this crisis has to go beyond the patient and reach the "offended" members of the team if the conflict is to subside and proper therapeutic situation be restored.

Several authors[5,27,42,53] deal specifically with this aspect of the consultant's job. Meyer and Mendelson[53] introduce their useful concept of the operational group, referred to earlier, for which the consultant functions as enabler of interpersonal communication, interpreter of the patient's behavior, and reducer of disruptive conflict. They note that the patients may display unsuspected adaptive responses which are the result of the reduction of strain in the operational group and consequent reduction of the patient's isolation from the members of the medical team on whom he is dependent. Such strain is, according to these authors, the result of mutual distrust, inhibited communication, and distorted mutual perceptions among members of the operational group.

An important aspect of the conflict-reducing function is the help offered by the consultant to the members of the medical team in understanding their own responses to the various patients. Bibring[8] discusses this aspect in some detail and points out that "the doctor's intuitive functioning, his diagnostic ability, is at its best when unhampered by inhibitions, resistances, apprehensions and prejudices." This is surely an ideal state to which the psychiatric consultant can make only a modest contribution by taking care to discuss tactfully and in the framework of a good personal relationship some of the implications of the consultee's own attitudes to the behavior of his patients. Some physicians habitually provoke in some of their patients unduly dependent, hostile, anxious, seductive, or withdrawing responses, and a friendly discussion of these recurrent patterns with the consultant may improve the consultee's professional functioning as a result of a measure of insight gained. The same applies to the nurses[10] or the social workers.[5]

Teaching

This function of consultation has attracted more attention in the literature than any other and would require a separate review for comprehensive coverage. There is room here for only some general remarks, and the reader is referred to the relevant sources.[1,2,16,21,25,26,28,35,54,67,70]

At the 1962 Conference on Graduate Psychiatric Education[74] a good deal of attention was devoted to manpower shortage in psychiatry and the related need to disseminate psychiatric knowledge among nonpsychiatric physicians. There is little doubt that members of a psychiatric consultation team are, by virtue of their close contact with physicians and special interest in the psychological aspects of medical practice, in a particularly advantageous position to play a key role in such teaching. The present writer acted for 6 years as the senior instructor in charge of teaching psychiatry to third-year medical students at the Allan Memorial Institute of Psychiatry and, as the chief of the Consultation Service, had an opportunity to meet his students again when they became interns and residents on the medical wards of the Royal Victoria Hospital. He was consistently struck by these young doctors' inability to apply their knowledge of psychiatry after 4 years of an unusually comprehensive undergraduate training in psychiatry offered by McGill University. He believes that such training should be reoriented in such a way as to impress the student with its relevance to his day-to-day medical practice; this can be done best by those psychiatrists who have extensive knowledge of the psychological aspects of medicine. Psychiatric consultations on the medical and surgical wards provide a unique opportunity for imparting such knowledge to the medical students. Techniques of interviewing and history-taking, comprehensive diagnosing, psychosocial factors in illness, importance of the doctor–patient relationship, assessment of the patient's personality as an aid to his management— these are only some of the crucial skills and conceptions which the psychiatric consultant can effectively demonstrate to the students in the course of his liaison work. Engel *et al.*[21] give a particularly comprehensive account of such teaching of the medical students by members of the Liaison Service at Rochester. While their program can be regarded as unusual in its scope and degree of involvement of the consultants in the undergraduate teaching of medicine, more modest endeavors are reported by many other centers and suggest an increasing trend in medical education. The recent emphasis on comprehensive medicine[45,70] makes this trend inevitable.

The teaching function of consultation is not confined to medical students. It applies to the medical residents,[21,28,35,54,67] attending physicians,[57] and nurses.[10] With these groups, the teaching tends to be less formal and regular than with medical students and the response varies.[28] Last but not least, consultation work provides invaluable experience for the psychiatric residents,[2,26] and a period of time spent on the consultation service should be made a required part of psychiatric training programs.

Perhaps the most important advantage to the psychiatric residents lies in an opportunity to learn to communicate effectively with nonpsychiatric health professions, which with the present emphasis on community psychiatry becomes an essential skill. In addition, the psychiatrist in training learns how to apply his knowledge of psychopathology in its comprehensive sense[47] to patients found in a setting in which psychological, social, and biological components of behavior demand equal attention.

SUMMARY AND CONCLUSIONS

Consultation psychiatry in general hospitals has showed considerable development in the last two decades. Its growth has paralleled the growth of general-hospital psychiatric units. It is important to distinguish between such units and consultation service which provides liaison with all nonpsychiatric facilities of a general hospital.[41] The principal function of such a service is to bring the unique knowledge and skills of psychiatrists to bear on the comprehensive diagnosis and management of medical patients and on the social interaction on the medical wards in the interests of better patient care. In addition, the consultants are increasingly in the forefront of teaching psychosocial aspects of medicine to nonpsychiatric physicians, nurses, etc., an activity which assumes strategic importance in view of the growing gap between the demand for psychiatric services and available manpower. As the training of psychiatrists becomes geared to meeting current social needs, apprenticeship with a consultation service will be one of the indispensable clinical experiences for psychiatric residents.

Consultation psychiatry can be conceptualized according to two prevalent models: as a branch of *preventive psychiatry* by virtue of its intervention in individual and interpersonal crisis situations to forestall personality and social disorganization; and as the practice and teaching of *psychosomatic medicine* as a science of and approach to human life phenomena which attempts to bring together the organismic and the psychosocial modes of abstraction.

Part II of this review (Chapter 19, this volume) will survey common diagnostic and management problems encountered by psychiatrists on the medical wards. Also, an attempt will be made to evaluate the implications of this special interest area in psychiatry for psychosomatic medicine.

REFERENCES

1. Aldrich CK: Psychiatric teaching on an inpatient medical service. *J Med Educ* 28:36, 1953.
2. Barnes RH, *et al:* The training of psychiatric residents in consultative skills. *J Med Educ* 32:124, 1957.
3. Barry MJ: Psychiatric aspects of the eye, ear, nose and throat. *Int Rec Med* 10:170, 1957.
4. Bartemeier LH: Psychiatric consultations. *Am J Psychiatry* 111:364, 1954.
5. Beigler JS *et al:* Report on liaison psychiatry at Michael Reese Hospital, 1950–1958. *AMA Arch Neurol* 81: 733, 1959.
6. Bellak L (ed): *Psychology of Physical Illness.* New York, Grune & Stratton, 1952.
7. Bibring GL: Preventive psychiatry in a general hospital. *Bull World Fed Ment Health* 3:224, 1951.
8. Bibring GL: Psychiatry and medical practice in a general hospital. *N Engl J Med* 254:366, 1956.

9. *The British Medical Dictionary*. Philadelphia, JB Lippincott Co, 1961.

10. Bursten B: The psychiatric consultation and the nurse. *Nurs Forum* 2:7, 1963.

11. Butler RN, Perlin S: Psychiatric consultations in a research setting. *Med Ann DC* 27:503, 1958.

12. Bynder H: Physicians choose psychiatrists: Medical social structure and patterns of choice. *J Health Hum Behav* 6:83, 1965.

13. Campbell AD: Consultations then and now. *Can Med Assoc J* 89:1030, 1963.

14. Cantor AJ, Bailey CP, (eds): *Psychosomatic Aspects of Surgery.* New York, Grune & Stratton, 1956.

15. Caplan G: Types of mental health consultation. *Am J Orthopsychiatry* 33: 470, 1963.

16. Clyne MB: Undergraduate teaching in psychological medicine as applicable to general practice. *J Med Educ* 38:961, 1963.

17. Dean ES: Writing psychiatric reports. *Am J Psychiatry* 119:759, 1963.

18. Denney D: A record keeping system for a psychiatric consultation service. *J Nerv Ment Dis* 141:474, 1965.

19. Eaton JW *et al:* Resistance to psychiatry in a general hospital. *Ment Hosp* 16:156, 1965.

20. Editorial: Science and psychiatry. *Can Med Assoc J* 89:902, 1963.

21. Engel GL, *et al:* A graduate and undergraduate teaching program on the psychological aspects of medicine. *J Med Educ* 32:859, 1957.

22. Faucett RL: Psychiatric interview as tool of medical diagnosis. *JAMA* 162:537, 1956.

23. Feifel H (ed): *The Meaning of Death.* New York, McGraw-Hill Book Co, 1959.

24. Fischer KH: The hospital bedside interview. *Psychosomatics* 2:445, 1961.

25. Fox HM: Psychiatric consultation in general medical clinics, an experiment in postgraduate education. *JAMA* 185:999, 1963.

26. Fox HM: Psychiatric residency on a medical service. *AMA Arch Gen Psychiatry* 11:19, 1964.

27. Greenberg IM: Approaches to psychiatric consultation in a research hospital setting. *AMA Arch Gen Psychiatry* 3:691, 1960.

28. Greenhill MH, Kilgore SR: Principles of methodology in teaching the psychiatric approach to medical house officers. *Psychosom Med* 12:38, 1950.

29. Hackett TP, Weisman AD: Psychiatric management of operative syndromes: I. The therapeutic consultation and the effect of noninterpretive intervention. *Psychosom Med* 22:267, 1960.

30. Hackett TP, Weisman AD: Psychiatric management of operative syndromes: II. Psychodynamic factors in formulation and management. *Psychosom Med* 22:356, 1960.

31. Heron MJ: Functions and problems of psychiatric units in general hospitals, *Br Med J* 2:1529, 1962.

32. Hockaday WJ: Experiences of a psychiatrist as a member of a surgical faculty. *Am J Psychiatry* 117:706, 1961.

33. Hollender MH: *The Psychology of Medical Practice.* Philadelphia, WB Saunders Co, 1958.

34. Jaco EG (ed): *Patients, Physicians, and Illness.* Glencoe, Ill, Free Press, 1958.

35. Kahana RJ: Teaching medical psychology through psychiatric consultation. *J Med Educ* 34:1003, 1959.

36. Kahana RJ, Bibring GL: Personality types in medical management, in Zinberg EN (ed): *Psychiatry and Medical Practice in a General Hospital.* New York, International Universities Press, 1964.

37. Kaufman RM: A psychiatric unit in a general hospital. *J Mount Sinai Hosp* 24:572, 1957.

38. Kaufman RM: The role of the psychiatrist in a general hospital. *Psychiatr Quart* 27:367, 1953.

39. Kaufman RM (ed): *The Psychiatric Unit in a General Hospital.* New York, International Universities Press, 1965.

40. Kenyon FE, Rutter ML: The psychiatrist and the general hospital. *Comp Psychiatry* 4:80, 1963.

41. Kornfeld DS, Feldman M: The psychiatric service in the general hospital. *NY State J Med* 65:1332, 1965.

42. Koumans AJR: Psychiatric consultation in an intensive care unit. *JAMA* 194:163, 1965.

43. Kroger WS (ed): *Psychosomatic Obstetrics, Gynecology and Endocrinology.* Springfield, Ill, Charles C Thomas, 1962.

44. Ledley RS, Lustig LB: Reasoning foundations of medical diagnosis. *Science* 130:9, 1959.

45. Lidz T, Fleck S: Integration of medical and psychiatric methods and objectives on a medical service. *Psychosom Med* 12:103, 1950.

46. Linn L (ed): *Frontiers in General Hospital Psychiatry.* New York International Universities Press, 1961.

47. Lipowski ZJ: Psychopathology as a science: Its scope and tasks. *Comp Psychiatry* 7:175-182, 1966.

48. Litin EM: Preoperative psychiatric consultation. *JAMA* 170:1369, 1959.

49. Magraw RM: Psychosomatic medicine and the diagnostic process. *Post-grad Med* 25:639, 1959.

50. Magraw RM: The patient's presenting complaint—signpost or goal. *Univ Minn Med Bull* 29:329, 1958.

51. MacKeith R, Sandler J (eds): *Psychosomatic Aspects of Pediatrics*. New York, Pergamon Press, 1961.

52. Mendelson M, Meyer E: Countertransference problems of the liaison psychiatrist. *Psychosom Med* 23:115, 1961.

53. Meyer E, Mendelson M: Psychiatric consultations with patients on medical and surgical wards: Patterns and processes. *Psychiatry* 24:197, 1961.

54. Meyer E, Mendelson M: The psychiatric consultation in postgraduate medical teaching. *J Nerv Ment Dis* 130:78, 1960.

55. Obermayer ME: *Psychocutaneous Medicine*. Springfield, Ill, Charles C Thomas, 1955.

56. Proctor RC: Consultative psychiatry. *Med Times* 86:1043, 1958.

57. Richmond JB: Relationship of the psychiatric unit to other departments of the hospital, in Kaufman RM (ed): *The Psychiatric Unit in a General Hospital*. New York, International Universities Press, 1965.

58. Ruesch J, et al: *Psychiatric Care*. New York, Grune & Stratton, 1964.

59. Sandt JJ, Leifer R: The psychiatric consultation. *Comp Psychiatry* 5:409, 1964.

60. Schiff KS, Pilot ML: An approach to psychiatric consultation in the general hospital. *AM Arch Gen Psychiatry* 1:349, 1959.

61. Schlaegel TF: *Psychosomatic Ophthalmology*. Baltimore, Williams & Wilkins Co, 1957.

62. Schottstaedt WW: *Psychophysiologic Approach in Medical Practice*. Chicago, Year Book Publishers, 1960.

63. Schottstaedt WW, et al: Sociologic, psychologic, and metabolic observations on patients in the community of a metabolic ward. *Am J Med* 25:248, 1958.

64. Schwartz LA: Application of psychosomatic concepts by a liaison psychiatrist on a medical service. *J Mich Med Soc* 57:1547, 1958.

65. Senescu RA: The development of emotional complications in the patient with cancer. J Chron Dis 16:813, 1963.

66. *The Shorter Oxford English Dictionary*. Oxford, Clavendon press, 1955.

67. Silverman S: Teaching psychoanalytic psychiatry to medical residents. *J Med Educ* 31:436, 1956.

68. Simmons HE: *The Psychosomatic Aspects of Cancer*. Washington, DC, Peabody Press, 1956.

69. Smith HL: Psychiatry in medicine: Intra- or interprofessional relationships? *Am J Sociol* 63:285, 1957.

70. Steiger WA, et al: Experiences in the teaching of comprehensive medicine. *J Med Educ* 31:241, 1956.

71. Stewart MA, et al: A study of psychiatric consultations in a general hospital. *J Chron Dis* 15:331, 1962.

72. Teitelbaum, HA: *Psychosomatic Neurology*. New York, Grune & Stratton, 1964.

73. Titchener JL, Levine M: *Surgery as a Human Experience*. New York, Oxford, University Press, 1960.

74. *Training the Psychiatrist to Meet Changing Needs*. Washington, DC, American Psychiatric Association, 1963.

75. Wahl CW (ed): *New Dimensions in Psychosomatic Medicine*. Boston, Little, Brown & Co, 1964.

76. Weisman AD, Hackett TP: Organization and function of a psychiatric consultation service. *Int Rec Med* 173:306, 1960.

77. Weiss E, English SO: *Psychosomatic Medicine*. Philadelphia, WB Saunders Co, 1957.

78. Wittkower ED, Lipowski ZJ: Recent developments in psychosomatic medicine. *Psychosom Med* 28:722–737, 1966.

79. Wolfe HE: Consultation: Role, function, and process. *Ment Hyg* 50:132, 1966.

80. Zinberg EN (ed): *Psychiatry and Medical Practice in a General Hospital*. New York, International Universities Press, 1964.

Review of Consultation Psychiatry and Psychosomatic Medicine

19

II. Clinical Aspects

In Part I of this review[73] an attempt was made to outline the scope, organization, and functions of consultation psychiatry in general hospitals. Part II surveys the types of diagnostic and management problems encountered by psychiatric consultants in the medical and surgical divisions of a general hospital. For clarity of presentation, the writer will first review some studies of the prevalence of psychiatric illness in this type of hospital and the frequency of and trends in referrals for psychiatric consultation. While such a survey may give some information about the *quantitiative* aspects of the problem, it can tell little about the manifold *quality* of psychopathological and social phenomena which psychiatrists can observe in a medical setting. To do justice to this broader and theoretically far more important aspect, a synopsis of psychiatric aspects of medical practice in a general hospital will be presented. It is expected that such treatment of the subjects will make the review more useful for a wider circle of readers and offer clearer implications for teaching, therapeutic needs, research possibilities, and use of psychiatric manpower.

The writer is aware of the vagueness of the phrase "psychiatric aspects of medical practice" but can offer no better substitute at present. His selection of clinical material is based both on the problems which psychiatric consultants are actually asked to help with and on his judgment that a given class of facts can be more adequately observed, understood, and managed if a psychiatrist's special knowledge and techniques are brought into play. This does not, of course, mean that everything that falls into this category is necessarily "abnormal" and in need of psychiatric therapeutic intervention. To describe what psychiatric consultants see and what they are called upon to deal with would be of only limited interest. More important are the varieties of human behavior and experience that can be observed in a medical setting, which are usually ignored by nonpsychiatric observers and are yet of importance both for overall medical care and for their theoretical interest to the students of human behavior.

Reprinted from *Psychosomatic Medicine* 29(3):201–224, 1967. Copyright © 1967 by The American Psychosomatic Society, Inc. Reprinted by permission of Elsevier Science Publishing Co., Inc.

Quantitative Aspects

Psychiatric Morbidity in Hospitals' Nonpsychiatric Areas

Prevalence studies are intended to estimate the number of patients with a mental disorder of recognized severity in a population at one point in time.[96] For practical purposes, however, this means the number counted not at one instant but at any time during the period of survey. Such studies are of value for estimating the need for psychiatric care. Data about the prevalence of psychiatric illness in various nonpsychiatric divisions of general hospitals are still limited and inconclusive. It appears that the most frequently studied population have been the patients attending medical outpatient clinics.[17,42,53,66,68,98,125-127] Culpan and Davis[17] tabulated findings from some previous reports on the number of patients with psychiatric illness in various "medical" populations and arrived at a mean percentage of 27.3 This is a low estimate compared with their own study in which they found that 51% of 100 consecutive new referrals to a medical outpatient clinic and 21% of corresponding referrals to a surgical clinic had psychiatric illness. Stoeckle et al.[127] have recently reviewed surveys of psychiatric illness in medical practice (not confined to general hospitals) and comment that criteria of case selection and definitions used by the various studies make comparisons between them practically impossible. The writer concurs with this opinion. Stoeckle et al. studied the incidence of "psychological distress" in 101 new patients attending the medical clinic at the Massachusetts General Hospital and found it to be 84%. They emphasize the importance of such distress for the timing of the patient's decision to attend the doctor.

Kaufman and Bernstein[53] studied the records of 1000 consecutive patients referred to the outpatient diagnostic clinic at the Mount Sinai Hospital in New York and found that 81.4% had psychological factors as the basis for their complaints. Thus only 16.6% of the 1000 patients had organic illness without a psychological component. It appears that in 69% of the patients no organic disease was present.

The similar findings of Stoeckle and Kaufman and of others suggest that the prevalence of psychiatric morbidity in outpatient clinic populations is indeed high and may actually be higher than the occurrence of organic disease. The implications of this finding for the organization and staffing of such clinics are apparent. There is clearly a need for the availability of psychiatric consultants in medical outpatient departments and for the provision of community mental health clinics.

Studies of the prevalence of psychiatric morbidity among medical and surgical impatients are relatively few.[19,40,55,85,89,93,97,109,140] Table I shows the total number of patients studied by each investigator and the percentage of those showing psychiatric disease or distress. The wide range of the reported frequency of psychiatric illness is notable. How meaningful and practically useful are these figures? The only generalizations that can be made at this stage are methodological ones. The following variables appear to be directly relevant to the evaluation of these studies:

1. Type of setting studied—general or private hospital, ward or outpatient clinic, medical or surgical, etc.
2. Demographic characteristics of the patient population (e.g., Denney et al.[19]

TABLE 1. Prevalence of Psychiatric Morbidity in "Medical" Populations

	Patients in study	
Investigator	No.	Percent with psychiatric disease
Denney et al.[19]	39	72
Denney et al.[19]	54	32
Helsborg[40]	500	41
Kaufman et al.[55]	253	66.8
Mittelman et al.[85]	450	30
Payson et al.[89]	109	72.5
Querido[93]	1630	46.6
Richman et al.[97]	184	36
Schwab et al.[109]	100	15
Zwerling et al.[140]	200	86

found twice as much psychiatric morbidity among the medically indigent as in private patients).

3. Case-finding methods—psychiatric interview, self-administered questionnaires, personality scales, or the judgment of a nonpsychiatrist.

4. Presence or absence of a psychiatric unit in the hospital studied. (One could expect that if such a unit were present, some patients would be steered to it directly, thus reducing the incidence of purely psychiatric illness on the medical wards.)

5. Definition of psychiatric disorder or distress. This seems to be the most difficult variable to control, and unless such definitions are operational and rigorously adhered to, the meaning of the survey is doubtful.

The crucial question is: How relevant is the finding of a certain prevalence of psychiatric illness to the needs for psychiatric treatment and, as a result, manpower? For example, one finds in Zwerling's[140] study that as many as 86% of his 172 surgical patients had "psychiatric disorder," but that this included 108 (54%) with character and behavior disorders such as passive–aggressive and emotionally unstable personalities. (These two types accounted for almost 100% of this diagnostic subgroup.) One wonders what the value is of such an overinclusive diagnostic dragnet for any prevalence study and especially for rational planning of psychiatric services. (Perhaps the most urgent and promising task is to focus research endeavors on that *rara avis*–a medical patient defying psychiatric diagnosis.) More realistic and practically useful is the type of survey reported by Querido[93] from Amsterdam. He tried to assess the prevalence of distress—defined as social and/or psychic tensions too heavy for the patient to bear—in a sample of medical patients and predict the chances of each patient's recovery from somatic illness. He found distress in 46.6% of his patients and states that a follow-up investigation showed a significant difference in frequency of recovery between distressed patients and those without distress. A conclusion was reached that distress is a highly significant variable which adversely influences the effectiveness of medical treatment. Predictive studies of this type are likely to offer a realistic basis for planning preventive measures.

In summary, the frequency of psychiatric morbidity in nonpsychiatric divisions of general hospitals is not known with certainty, but there is some evidence that 30–60% of inpatients and 50–80% of outpatients suffer from psychic distress or psychiatric illness of sufficient severity to create a problem for the health professions. Carefully designed (particularly predictive and longitudinal) studies are needed to establish not only the quantity of but also the type, severity, and duration of such illness as a basis for rationing planning of services and action.

REFERRALS FOR PSYCHIATRIC CONSULTATION

What percentage of medical and surgical inpatients are referred for psychiatric consultations? How does the frequency of such referrals compare with the prevalence of psychiatric morbidity? What are the characteristics of the referred patient populations? What seems to influence the decision for and timing of requests for psychiatric consultations? There is some published information which can help answer, however tentatively, these questions. [12,19,24,31,52,58,64,83,89,97,102,107-112,115,119,123,135,136]

Frequency

Published data giving the total number of patients admitted to the medical and surgical wards over a period of time and the percentage of patients referred for psychiatric consultation are still too few. The several American publications available[12,19,64,83,89,107,123,135] show the range as being 4 to 13%, with an average of 9%. A striking exception is the low figure of 2.2% reported by Eilenberg[24] from the Mayo Clinic. However, since the time periods under consideration vary from 3 months[24,89] to 8 years,[64] it is difficult to talk about general trends. A national survey of all general hospitals is clearly indicated. The two British studies[31,115] give the percentage of referrals as 0.7 and 1.34, respectively, and these figures contast strikingly with the American ones. The Norwegian study by Rud[102] gives the figure of 4.9% of patients referred to a psychiatrist over a $3^1/_2$-year period. It seems clear that such figures are likely to differ from country to country and from hospital to hospital, and to reflect a variety of factors. It is likely that American teaching hospitals, especially those possessing a well-established consultation service, will generally show the highest frequencies of psychiatric referrals.

Comparison with Actual Prevalence of Psychiatric Morbidity. Studies such as those by Richman *et al.*[97] and Denney *et al.*[19] suggest a discrepancy between estimated psychiatric morbidity and the frequency of referrals. While these studies may reflect no more than purely local conditions, a comparison of the estimates quoted above of psychiatric morbidity among medical and surgical inpatients with the reported frequency of psychiatric referrals strongly suggests that there is a wide disparity between the number of referrals and patients who could presumably benefit from a consultation. Does this mean that the prevalence figures are unrealistically high and thus of little value for the planning of psychiatric services in general hospitals; that nonpsychiatric physicians are woefully unaware of what their patients need; or that they deal with the psychiatric problems without our assistance? There are no ready answers to these questions at the present time. What is also involved here is the wider issue of medical philosophy, namely: Where does a physician's professional responsibility end? Is he expected to take into account and *somehow* deal with psychosocial distress and classifiable personality disorder in all his patients, or call upon his psychiatric consultant to do it for him even if this applies to 60, 70, or 86% of the patients at any given time? Surely a line has to be drawn somewhere if we are not to advocate a medicosocial utopia.

Diagnostic Characteristics

The number of published studies giving pertinent data is still small[12,31,64,109,119,123,135] and comparison among them is made difficult by diverse and/or undefined diagnostic terminology used by the authors. Until there is greater uniformity and consistency in the usage of psychiatric classification such surveys will be of limited value. In addition, the samples tend to be small, which limits their usefulness even more. The six American studies which this writer succeeded in finding and which give diagnostic breakdown of the patient populations[12,64,109,119,123,135] show that the relative frequency of psychiatric diagnoses differed from study to study, making general conclusions difficult.

The study by Wilson and Meyer[135] calls for special comment as it illustrates the value of consistency in the use of psychiatric diagnostic terms. These authors compared two groups of patients referred to a psychiatric liaison service in each of 2 successive years and found "a high degree of concordance in the diagnoses assigned by the service." One notes that the organic brain syndromes accounted for 21% and 28% of the diagnoses made in the 2 years, respectively, and were thus the commonest condition referred, followed by personality disorder, psychoneurosis (excluding depression), and depression (neurotic and psychotic). Schizophrenia was found in only 9% of the entire group. In another comparable study,[64] depression and personality disorders were each found in 21% of the referred patients and were thus most frequent. In a third study,[12] psychoneurosis topped the list, but the authors note that the symptom of depressive mood prompted the referral in 30% of the patients. Poe *et al.*[91] encountered depression in 52% of 192 patients referred for psychiatric consultation. Thus the overall impression from the studies quoted is that the group of depressions is probably the commonest class of psychiatric syndromes referred to psychiatric consultants.

One striking finding is that of the 808 consultation referrals reported in the American studies only 46 (6%) were given that vague but officially approved diagnosis of psychophysiologic reaction. The so-called psychosomatic disorders are mentioned in three sutdies,[12,24,64] and accounted for only 2, 6.1, and 7% respectively, of all the consultation requests. The writer's impression from his own consultation service confirms this very low frequency of referrals of "psychosomatic" patients. These findings highlight our medical colleagues' lack of faith in our ability to contribute to the management of this class of patients. It appears that years of psychiatrists' preoccupation with these conditions and the massive volume of published studies have had little impact on medical practice beyond the spread of vague specificity stereotypes. There is little doubt that the bulk of a psychiatric consultant's work on medical and surgical wards consists of clinical problems unrelated to the psychosomatic disorders in the strict sense of the term. This fact can be expected to further divert research interests away from these disorders and consequently influence psychosomatic theory.

One general conclusion that can be drawn from a review of the studies referred to above is that the standard of reporting is generally low and more factual information is badly needed. It should be possible to organize a national survey of data possessed at present by all the psychiatric consultation services in the general hospitals on this continent. Such pooled information would surely encompass thousands of patients referred for consultation over a number of years, and provide meaningful data which are lacking at present. One has to consider that the six American studies quoted here pertain to a total of only a little over 800 referrals—a sample which any psychiatric consultation service in a large hospital could collect in 1–2 years. This writer and his group do 350–400 public consultations and about 200 private consultations a year and will publish their findings when these are analyzed.

The three British studies[31, 58, 115] are difficult to compare with the American ones because of different diagnostic terminology. One notes, however, that the British authors also found depression to be the commonest psychiatric syndrome referred to psychiatrists, although Shepherd et al.[115] report a slightly higher percentage of toxic and organic reaction.

Patterns

The reasons for the requests for psychiatric consultation are specified in a number of studies.[12,24,31,52,58,64,123] Here again the lack of homogeneous terminology thwarts any attempts at meaningful comparison. There is a need for an agreement to record and report such data in a standardized fashion; otherwise the published reports will largely remain of limited value, if any, with no general trends discernible. Some writers give "psychiatric problem" or "psychiatric symptoms" as a reason for referral and do not specify whether the request was primarily for diagnosis, management, or disposition. Thus one study[52] reports that 61.4% of referrals were for differential diagnosis, while another[12] does not mention diagnosis at all but gives percentage of referrals for "psychiatric symptoms," "drugs and procedures," and "no organic explanation for symptoms." If any generalization can be drawn from these reports it is that diagnostic uncertainty on the part of ten physicians and a need for advice on management of patients are the main reasons for consultation.

There is also little information regarding the type of patient referred irrespective of psychiatric diagnosis. Payson[89] noted that patients from higher social classes, the middle-aged, women with little education, and highly educated men who had low occupational status were all favored in referrals. Wilson and Meyer[136] found that residents selected for psychiatric consultation younger (i.e., those less than 49 years of age) patients with less serious medical illnesses. These authors emphasize what others have already noticed, that "the quietly depressed patient whose behavior is unremarkable" is the one usually unrecognized by both physicians and nurses as he does not disturb them in their work. Patients with organically impaired brain function are often not referred since, as has been suggested,[19] there is pessimism regarding our therapeutic efficacy when the patient's cerebral function is impaired. Schwab *et al.*[107,109-112] discuss in a series of papers the characteristics of 100 hospitalized medical patients referred for psychiatric consultation and draw some conclusions regarding referral patterns. They found that their referred patients were characterized by "long-standing illnesses, intractable in quality, and unchanging in symptomatology." It is of note that less than half of these patients had positive physical findings related to their symptoms. These writers suggest that when a patient gives a history of increase in a chronic illness, combined with a high number of adverse events in the past and unsatisfactory home life, there is increased probability that he will be referred. Regarding timing of the referral for consultation, Schwab *et al.* found that when physical diagnosis on admission is negative, the patient is likely to be referred early; but if he has serious organic disease and abnormal physical findings and laboratory results, referral is late. These investigators make a strong plea for referrals to the psychiatric consultants early in the period of hospitalization if the physician finds evidence of significant psychopathology on admission.

In a separate paper Schwab *et al.*[108] report that despite common fear among physicians that patients may react adversely to a psychiatric referral, the majority of the patients whom they studied and who had been referred reacted favorably to their physician's decision to arrange for a psychiatric assessement. A more general and theoretical discussion of the factors which influence a physician's decision whether and when to refer a patient for psychiatric consultation can be found in Meyer's articles[81,82] and in Part I of this review (Chapter 18, this volume).

PSYCHIATRIC DIAGNOSTIC PROBLEMS ON MEDICAL WARDS

A psychiatric consultant on the medical and surgical wards is often called to assist in the diagnostic process. Apart from relatively few cases of gross psychiatric disorder, the two questions he is asked most frequently are (1) is this particular bodily complaint (or set of complaints) explicable as an expression of psychological ill-health i.e., is it partly or wholly psychogenic? (2) Is the inner experience of psychic change reported by the patient or his observable behavior explicable as the direct results of, or a psychological reaction to, organic disease? The only method by which the consultant can attempt to answer these questions is the psychiatric interview, possibly supplemented by interviews with other observers. All this is common knowledge, but its theoretical implications are seldom analyzed and discussed. Psychiatrists in training and physicians in general are urged to avoid diagnosis by exclusion, and high value is set on "positive" diagnosis of psychopathology—a salutary goal, but what does it really imply and can it always be achieved in practice? Studies of the prevalence of psychiatric morbidity indicate that it is relatively easy to attach an acceptable "positive" psychiatric diagnosis to as many as seven or eight out of every ten "medical" patients. In the case of somatic symptoms we have at our disposal the unfailing wastebasket called the psychophysiologic reaction. Yet what is the practical value of this labeling and is relevance to the given diagnostic problem? Faced with the question about the determinants of a given somatic symptom (e.g., pain), the consultant can (1) affirm that is is psychogenic, e.g., a symbolic expression of conflict; (2) discuss the diagnosis in descriptive psychiatric and/or psychodynamic terms while evading the question about the symptom itself or stating his inability to explain its nature; (3) attempt to show that the symptom is meaningful and fully accounted for by consideration of the patient's personality dynamics, past history, and current life situation—even though no symbolic meaning has been discerned; (4) express the opinion that further medical investigations are needed to rule out organic basis. The crucial question is: How reliable is the psychiatric interview as a diagnostic tool when applied to the elucidation of somatic symptoms? Sandt and Leifer[104] give a clear answer to this question as it relates to pain, the commonest presenting complaint. According to them psychiatric consultation which depends upon psychological or psychodynamic investigation can only add to the diagnosis but not differentiate psychogenic from physical illness. The writer agrees with this viewpoint but with some reservations. The consultant has the choice of either confining himself to a psychodynamic exploration or expanding it to include a functional inquiry and critical evaluation of the symptom from the medical viewpoint. A psychiatrist's interviewing skills and his ability to secure the cooperation of the patient may allow him to obtain vital information which has eluded the patient's physician and which may help in establishing an organic diagnosis. Should the psychiatrist shirk this opportunity because of a rigid conception of his role as an expert in psychodynamics only? The writer does not believe so. A psychiatric consultant to medicine must surely be more than a peripatetic sketcher of psychodynamic profiles.

The problem of diagnosis could be easier to solve if we had a better understanding of the determinants and psychophysiological mechanisms of somatic symptoms not directly due to organic disease. Szasz,[129] Kepecs,[59] Seitz,[113] Malmo et al.,[77] and others have made important contributions to this problem—an area of clinical research to which psychiatrists working on the medical wards could usefully contribute. An example of such an endeavor can be found in Lipin's paper.[72] This author presents some psychiatric methods of determining the nature of somatic symptoms. He postulates that pain and other somatic sensations may be a manifestation not only of organic or hysterical illness but also of memories of bodily symptoms experienced during a forgotten childhood illness, brought into awareness through association with current experiences. This hypothesis is worth attempting to validate. What we need is a theory of somatic symptoms and practical guides to differential diagnosis based on it.

From the psychological viewpoint, each somatic symptom can be regarded as a perception and/or communication. Thus a person can report a somatic perception, just communicate psychological distress in bodily metaphors, or do both. Pain, weakness, and tingling are all sensations which immediately give rise to cognitive and emotional responses. How the patient feels about his symptom will depend on its *meaning* to him, conscious and unconscious. The meaning in turn depends on the patient's past experience, level of knowledge, personality organization, conflicts and modes of coping with them, and current psychosocial situation. What results may be an extremely complex network of variables which change the quality and intensity of the original sensation and may result in secondary, tertiary, etc., symptoms. These symptoms can be partly physiological concomitants or equivalents of affective arousal (e.g., anxiety), and partly an expression of the symbolic meanings of the original and derivative symptoms and their inclusion in the intrapsychic conflict. These processes are further complicated by the perceived responses of others to the communication of the symptom, by cultural norms, etc. It is clear that what the patient experiences and how he communicates it to his physician is the resultant of mulstiple psychic processes as well as the doctor–patient relationship. We have yet to learn how to identify and evaluate the relative contribution of these multiple variables to the patient's presenting complaints.

A common pitfall for the beginning and even the experienced consultant is to include the presenting somatic symptoms into a plausible psychodynamic formulation. The symptom is then presented as a bodily expression of an ideational content. The writer recalls reading a senior psychiatric resident's consultation note on a patient presenting with paraplegia:

"This patient shows severe castration anxiety which he displaced from his penis to his legs and hence the paralysis. The diagnosis is conversion hysteria. Psychotherapy is recommended." This was a truly positive diagnosis but, as it turned out, equally positive was the patient's Wassermann reaction. While the resident's remarks about the castration anxiety may have been correct, the causal chain including the patient's paralysis was an artifact, however plausible it appeared. This raises the crucial problem of degrees of relevance in the psychological interpretation of somatic symptoms. The symptom may seem to fit a dynamic formulation, but in fact the latter can be partly or totally irrelevant to it. How can such compromising mistakes be avoided? The reviewer believes that psychiatric residents should be taught to exercise appropriate caution in drawing inference and to temper their interpretative zeal with careful observation and logical reasoning.

Guze[37] offers a schema for comprehensive diagnosis which is worth keeping in mind. He proposes that every patient should be examined in terms of four points of reference: (1) factors in the environment (or life situation); (2) heredity and past experience; (3) changes in the function and structure of organs and tissues; and (4) contribution of these changes to subsequent behavioral responses and nature of the latter.

Such schemes are useful as general guidelines, but they do not facilitate a consultant's task when faced with a concrete diagnostic problem. Directly relevant to the consultant's work is the growing literature on the psychiatric aspects of pain,[10,25,61,80,94,122,129,132] some of which will be dealt with in detail below.

In summary, an attempt to integrate the various theoretical and experimental approaches to the understanding of somatic symptoms is overdue. Such a study might provide practical guidelines for differential diagnosis which are lacking at present. Woolly generalities about comprehensive or positive diagnosis should not conceal our ignorance in this area.

CLASSIFICATION

Psychiatric diagnostic problems encountered on the medical wards may be grouped as follows:

1. Psychological presentation of organic disease
2. Psychological complications of organic disease

3. Psychological reactions to organic disease
4. Somatic presentation of psychiatric disorders
5. "Psychosomatic" disorders

It is clearly impossible to review all the relevant material on this subject—a book would be required for adequate coverage. This review only attempts to outline and organize the facts, viewpoints, and procedures which constitute the field of consultation psychiatry in general hospitals. The above grouping is an empirical one and reflects the actual modes of presentation of diagnostic problems to the consultant. There is obvious overlapping of the different groups, but a more rigidly defined classification would artifically delimit what in nature is intertwining, fluid, and shifting.

Psychological Presentation of Organic Disease

A person suffering from an organic disease can present with complaints expressed in psychological terms; i.e., in terms of disordered cognition, perception, and/or affect. Or the patient may not complain of anything but people around him notice changes in his behavior which physicians sometimes refer to as "personality change." Such change may be either an accentuation of the patient's characteristic personality style (i.e., he appears to be more obsessional, hysterical, or psychopathic), or a display of behavior which is unusual and atypical for the patient. Thus a cautious and pedantic businessman may become reckless or a normally outgoing housewife morose and withdrawn, etc. Such personality change occurring in patients who are over the age of 40 raises the suspicion of cerebral disease, primary or secondary. Chapman and Wolff[13] give a particularly useful account of psychological changes brought about by disease of the neopallium. It is not only cerebral disease that can present with psychological manifestations; e.g., carcinoma of the body and tail of the pancreas is well known for its tendency to simulate psychiatric illness.[90] The writer saw three patients on the same ward within a few months who had been referred to him as sufferers of pure depression but actually suffered from unsuspected pancreatic cancer. In all three he postulated the presence of organic disease on the basis of a careful history and evaluation of the presenting symptom of pain, even though the patient did suffer from varying degrees of depression.

Some patients unconsciously deny or consciously conceal significant somatic symptoms and may even present the consultant with their own diagnosis of a psychological illness. The writer is always on guard when a patient tells him from the start: "It's all psychosomatic, doctor." Such introduction calls for particular care in evaluation of the symptoms. Anxiety or depression aroused by subjective awareness of physical ill health and its possible ominous implications may mask the underlying disease. This has been repeatedly observed in the case of brain tumor.[39] Conditions such as epilepsy[16, 46, 76] or pheochromocytoma[21] may give rise to anxiety attacks indistinguishable clinically from those accompanying psychogenic illness. Stengel[122] suggests that it was one of Paul Schilder's main contributions to psychopathology to recognize that the same symptoms, such as depersonalization or body–image disturbances, can be produced by both organic and psychogenic causes. The theoretical implications of this fact should be brought into focus again.

In general, any organic disease may give rise to any type of neurotic or psychotic symptoms, depending on the patient's personality structure; and these symptoms overshadow those of the basic disease. The practical implications of this fact are clear: The psychiatric consultant in a general hospital must have the knowledge of and be constantly aware of the psychological presentation of organic disease which may *mask* the latter and be easily overlooked by physicians.[101]

Psychological Complications of Organic Disease

Psychiatric disorders which fall roughly into the category of acute and chronic brain syndromes can be regarded as a direct result of organic disease on the highest integrative functions of the brain. Their hallmark is the impairment of cognitive functions, either global or relatively selective. The acute syndrome is by definition reversible; the chronic one, irreversible. the two syndromes may, of course, coexist in the same patient. Prolonged observation may be necessary before the extent of apparent irreversibility can be reasonably established. Etiological factors are many[20,41] since any factor which interferes with the supply, uptake, and/or utilization of oxygen or glucose by the cerebral neurons may bring about an organic brain syndrome. Predisposing factors are inadequately known, particularly the psychological ones.

These syndromes are a strangely neglected subject in the English-language literature. Their terminology, psychopathology, and diagnostic criteria are in need of revision. Various authors use terms such as "delirium," "acute confusional states," "exogenous reaction type," "toxic psychosis," "infective–exhaustive psychosis," etc., to denote the reversible syndrome. Clear definitions and classification are needed before progress can be made in this important area. A few authors[27,67] have called attention to the general lack of interest in delirium and the frequent failure of both physicians and psychiatrists to recognize it clinically.[95] Psychosomatic investigators have shown hardly any interest in the reversible syndrome. This is surprising since it is a condition in which both organic and psychological changes occur in close temporal proximity, and their interaction would deserve study. Perhaps in the future delirium will come to be regarded as a model of a psychosomatic disorder. Engel and Romano[27] offer one of the best available reviews of delirium in English and point out that many seriously ill hospitalized patients display some degree of it. This claim is borne out by incidence studies carried out in the nonpsychiatric hospitals.[95,99,116] It has been found that as many as 50% of patients over 60 years of age may show evidence of delirium on admission to hospital.[99,116] Bleuler,[9] using a different terminology, estimates that 5–10% of medical patients in his Swiss hospital suffer from the acute exogenous reaction type. If this estimate is a generally valid one, it follows that only a fraction of such patients are referred to psychiatric consultants. A survey of ten publications giving relevant figures[12,24,31,38,58,64,95,115,123,135] shows that the two brain syndromes constitute about 17% of all referrals.

A psychiatric consultant can make several contributions in this area: first, diagnosis[27,41,118]; second, help with the management[41]; third, clinical research.[38,79] The consultant is often the only physician sufficiently familiar with delirium and allied states to make a correct diagnosis. This is not an academic matter since medical progress brings with it a new crop of potential causes of organic psychoses. It is enough to mention steroids,[92] open-heart surgery,[65] and psychotropic drugs[28,50] as representative examples. Withdrawal states from alcohol,[18] barbiturates,[7] and opiates[6] are often treated on the medical wards, and the psychiatric consultant may be called upon to play a key role in their diagnosis and therapy. He can draw attention to some psychological aspects of the care of delirious patients, such as the need for adequate sensory stimulation, human contact, etc. An outstanding example of a consultant's imaginative contribution to such problems is the management of delirium after eye surgery.[134]

With regard to research, psychiatric consultants have a unique opportunity to study all degrees and varieties of delirium. Mendelson *et al.*[79] illustrate this potential in their study of the psychiatric theory of psychopathological disturbances in poliomyelitis patients confined in a respirator. Suggested problems in need of organized inquiry are (1) classification of the reversible syndrome which, in the writer's opinion, is at present too crude and muddled; (2) investigation of psychopathological features from the viewpoint of modern psychology, e.g., the concepts of "confusion" and "clouding of consciousness"; (3) psychological predisposing factors in delirium, e.g., degree of ego strength, personality structure, etc.; (4) psychodynamic meaning of delirious productions (generally taken for granted but seldom investigated); and (5) the possible effect of delirium experienced in childhood on psychological development and predisposition to psychiatric disorders.

One can consider delirium and allied states from the theoretical viewpoint as a class of disorders of consciousness. As such they invite comparison with and delineation in psychological and physiological terms from model psychoses, disturbances attending alterations of sensory input, effects of sleep and dream deprivation, psychogenic confusional states, and dissociative reactions. This is surely an intriguing area of comparative psychopathology almost untouched by psychosomatic research. Much of the relevant clinical material can be found on the medical and surgical wards.

In contrast to the English school, German psychiatry has a long tradition of interest in psychiatric disorders complicating organic diseases. Since Bonhoeffer delineated the acute exogenous reaction type more than half a century ago, there has been a massive output of relevant literature recently reviewed by several authors.[9,15,30] Bleuler[8] distinguishes three different subtypes of this reaction type: (1) reduction of consciousness, (2) alteration (clouding) of consciousness with confusion, and (3) dysmnesic or Korsakoff's syndrome. He claims that each of these forms has its own psychopathology and pathophysiology This seems to be a more adequate classification than lumping together diverse states under the heading "acute brain syndrome." The latter offers no room for such disorders as toxic psychosis due to amphetamine or cortisone where "clouding of consciousness" does not usually occur.

In summary, psychiatric complications of organic disease are an area on the borderlands between psychiatry and medicine which has been untapped by psychosomatic research. Accruing evidence indicates the relatively high incidence of these complications in general hospitals and their high priority in a psychiatric consultant's work. They offer wide scope for cooperative investigation likely to be appreciated by our medical colleagues and to open new vistas for psychosomatic research and theory.

Psychological Reactions to Organic Disease

The distinction between psychological "reactions" and "complications" is an arbitrary one and no clear-cut line can be drawn between them. The organic brain syndromes have been traditionally distinguished on the basis of impairment of cognitive functions (i.e., remembering and thinking); but it is generally known that affective disturbances, such as lability of affect, are often present, too.[118] On the other hand, impaired intellectual functioning and judgment as well as confusion may be present in acute schizophrenia.[118] Yet as a general rule lack of evidence of organic dysfunction is usually associated with a final diagnosis of functional mental illness, and vice versa.[118] While allowing for a continuum and intermingling of the "organic" and "psychogenic" consequences of organic disease, there is still heuristic merit in separating the predominantly affective and symbolic effects of such disease from those due to demonstrable cerebral insufficiency.[27]

Psychological reactions to physical illness have been variously conceptualized in terms of psychological stress,[26,45] psychological trauma,[4] crisis,[126] change in body image,[3,106] or shift in libido economy.[29] Each of these approaches tends to emphasize different facets of the total human response. The writer finds Engel's[26] conception of psychological stress a particularly comprehensive and useful conceptual framework. Engel regards broadly conceived injury or threat of injury to the body as a special category of psychological stress. Thus his general outline of responses to such stress can be applied logically to physical illness. These responses can be summarized as follows:

1. Formation of an unpleasant affect, or sequence of affects (anxiety, guilt, hopelessness, helplessness, shame, disgust).

2. Pathological affective states, i.e., long-lasting and/or excessively intense affects associated with manifest bodily changes.

3. Employment of ego mechanisms of defense against the unpleasant affect. (This results in development of neurotic or psychotic symptoms and character disorders.)

4. Inadequate evaluation and avoidance of external stresses as possible consequence of developments under Item 3.

5. Harmful somatic effecs of the physiological concomitants of dysphoric affects (e.g., precipitation of anginal pain).

6. Influence of secondary somatic effects (Items 4 and 5) on the psychic functions; this could be called "positive feedback" effect on the original psychological stress.

Bellak[3] proposes a different scheme of psychological reactions to physical illness: (1) "normal" reaction, (2) avoidance reaction, (3) reactive depression, (4) channeling of premorbid pathological anxiety into preoccupation with the physical disease, and (5) psychological invalidism.

Particularly useful clinically is the list of possible psychological responses to serious physical disease, such as cancer, suggested by Senescu[114]: (1) the dependency response or revival of dependent patterns of behavior, (2) the feeling of damage and reduction of self-esteem (3) the anger response, (4) the guilt response, (5) the loss of gratification or pleasure, and (6) the responses to the physician's attitude and behavior.

Other important contributions to the subject include Kahana's and Bibring's[49] discussion of the meaning of illness and its implications for the patient's behavior and management in terms of different personality types. A valuable sociological concept is that of illness behavior[78] which refers to ways in which different patients perceive, evaluate, and act (or not act) upon their symptoms. This concept stresses the individual differences in the reaction to disease.

This writer believes that a set of variables influences any patient's psychological response to disease to a varying extent. These include such factors as

1. Personality structure and unconscious conflicts[4,49]
2. The meaning and importance for the patients of the affected organ, lesion, actual bodily change, changed proprioceptive sensations, and body image
3. The degree and nature of the inclusion of Item 2 into unconscious conflicts
4. Psychodynamic effect of the beliefs about the cause of disease[2]
5. Cultural[105] and educational[75] factors
6. The state of the patient's current interpersonal relationships
7. The actual extent of mutilation and loss of function and their socioeconomic consequences for the patient
8. Previous experience with disease
9. The patient's state of awareness and cognitive functioning
10. Degree of acceptance by him of the "sick role"[78]
11. The doctor–patient relationship

All these variables have to be evaluated when the consultant wants to obtain an overall picture of a patient's psychological response to his illness as a basis for therapeutic action. Senescu[114] suggests some practical behavioral criteria for the assessment of pathological reactions to illness.

From the nosological viewpoint, psychological reactions to organic disease spread over the whole spectrum of neuroses, psychoses, and personality disorders. The incidence of more extreme degrees of personality disorganization in response to illness is virtually unknown. Kaufman et al.[55] found the prevalence of psychiatric illness on a medical service to be as high as 66.8%, but one half of these patients suffered from "benign psychiatric disorder." Functional psychosis was found in only 7.5% of the patients; it is not clear what proportion of them suffered from it prior to the onset of organic disease. Some studies[22,124] indicate that a considerable proportion of patients became depressed as a result of severe illness. More data are clearly needed.

Up to this point the psychological reactions have been dealt with in general terms, and a premature impression might be gained that such reactions are totally independent of the type of organic disease present. There is actually some evidence that certain diseases are more likely than others to precipitate disorders having the features of functional rather than organic psychiatric illness. As examples one may mention viral infections,[36] such as hepatitis,[74] which are often followed by a depression; systemic lupus erythematosus;[87] multiple sclerosis;[35] porphyria;[1] and Cushing's syndrome [120] The relative importance of the disease in question as an etiological factor in psychiatric illness is difficult to evaluate.[23] Quarton et al.[92] offer a brilliant paradigm for the evaluation of the variables and hypotheses relevant to psychiatric disorders due to ACTH and cortisone. Their schema could well be applied by consultants to other drugs and diseases.

Somatic Presentation of Psychiatric Disorders

The inclusion of the whole gamut of functional psychiatric disorders would be of little practical value. Only those disorders which give rise to diagnostic difficulties in medical settings are described below.

Depression. The depression syndrome is the most common and versatile imitator of organic disease. The range of somatic symptoms accompanying the various types of depression is wide.[14] Fatigue, insomnia, localized and diffuse pain, impotence, paresthesias, and palpitations are some of the commonest complaints noted.[5,10,47,91,125] As many as 25% of patients suffering from a psychotic depression may present with physical symptoms.[47] Depressed patients seem to form the bulk of those at medical clinics who present with somatic complaints not supported by positive signs of organic disease.[125] The diagnosis rests on characteristic psychological symptoms.[91,125] The language of emotions is foreign to some patients while others unconsciously or consciously deny any awareness of depressed mood, making diagnosis difficult. The term "depressive equivalent" has been used to describe such depressions.[5] In a doubtful case with negative physical signs a therapeutic trial with antidepressants may be used.

Conversion Reaction and Hysteria. Nearly 30 years ago Lindemann[71] discussed hysteria as a problem in a general hospital, and his observations are still pertinent. He noted that in conversion symptoms we are dealing with functional physiological alterations, but that knowledge of how "psychogenic factors operate to cause physiologic change is not available yet." There is little that we can add to his remarks today. The whole concept of hysteria has disintegrated in the last two or three decades, prompting a historian of this disease[131] to ask if it has really disappeared in modern life. Psychiatric consultants in the general hospital can reassure the historian that it has not. A typical comment is:"...men, women, and children continue to suffer illnesses diagnosed as conversion hysteria, in numbers similar to illnesses considered far from uncommon."[70] Other consultants also confirm that they see "substantial numbers" of conversion reactions on the medical wards.[137] The same observers discuss operational diagnostic criteria and a conceptual model of conversion reaction.[137-139] They point out that the diagnosis of this reaction cannot be established by either psychiatric or physiological considerations alone but requires assessment of both these aspects. In this writer's experience it is indeed rare that a convincing symbolic meaning of a symptom can be established during a single psychiatric consultation—a degree of probability is usually all one can achieve. A discovery of a symbolic meaning for a symptom does not settle the issue of diagnosis since any organically derived symptom may acquire secondary symbolic elaboration.

While the concept of hysteria has been officially replaced by conversion and dissociative reactions, some authors still claim[34] that hysteria is a syndrome with characteristic clinical features of which conversion symptoms are not an essential part.

The frequency of the different conversion symptoms is not known but it appears at present that pain is the commonest of them.[137] Engel[25] observes that the largest number of patients with "psychogenic" pain belongs to the conversion reaction category. Merskey[80] reports that persistent pain shows common association with hysteria. Yet Slater[117] issues a chilling warning: "The diagonsis of 'hysteria' is a disguise for ignorance and a fertile source of clinical error." In a similar vein, Walters[132] suggests that the term "hysterical pain" be abandoned in favor of "psychogenic regional pain." Thus the controversy continues.

Whether pain and other more circumscribed symptoms are the commonest form of conversion reaction is still an open issue. The more dramatic manifestations believed by some to be extinct are still with us.[62] Lipin[72] describes gross mental disturbances with depersonalization, amnesia, and emotional outbursts occurring during the early weeks following the onset of a major conversion symptom. He emphasizes that when there is no major psychic decompensation at that stage, the symptoms are not likely to be conversion. It is notable that Lipin's interesting observations on the natural history of conversion were made in a neurological hospital. This writer has been struck by the relative frequency with which various types of conversion symptoms can be found on the wards of the neurological hospital where he is consultant. The wards of the general and neurological hospitals are some of the best settings in which to study conversion reactions, affording consultants another opportunity to contribute to psychopathology.

In summary, conversion reaction and hysteria are concepts currently in a state of revision and flux. The relevant phenomena, however they may be named, do exist and pose common and sometimes difficult diagnostic problems for consultants. Conversion symptoms may coexist with and mask organic disease, severe depression, or schizophrenia. Diagnostic criteria could be improved; the definition of conversion reaction in psychodynamic terms tends to impede diagnosis. Physiological mechanisms are still unknown.

Anxiety Reaction. Anxiety is a much used and abused term. Three related meanings of it may be distinguished: it is an affect, a clinical syndrome, and a theoretical concept. These three meanings are seldom explicitly distinguished and this causes confusion. The clinical syndrome can occur in association with any disease, psychiatric or organic, and it is only when anxiety dominates the clinical picture in the absence of psychosis that the term "anxiety reaction" applies. The syndrome consists of a cognitive aspect, feeling tone, observable behavior, and physiological concomitants. At times only the latter are in evidence—an anxiety equivalent. Somatic complaints are always part of the syndrome and may be the presenting complaint. One of the best descriptions of the syndrome is still that by Freud.[32] Current psychiatric textbooks tend to devote more space to psychodynamic generalizations about anxiety than to description of its clinical features. Kolb[63] gives a useful presentation of diagnostic criteria.

Particularly difficult for the diagnostician are isolated symptoms, such as headache or hyperhidrosis. Hyperventilation is a common concomitant of chronic and acute anxiety and gives rise to a variety of symptoms which may imitate organic disease, from coronary thrombosis to epilepsy.[69] Such symptoms may be unilateral and suggest neurologic disease.[130] The predominantly cardiovascular symptoms in the so-called neurocirculatory asthennia is another diagnostic pitfall.[60] Many patients presenting with painful somatic symptoms, such as headache, suffer from an anxiety reaction.[61]

In conclusion, psychiatric consultants to medicine have an opportunity to see varied symptomatic presentation of anxiety reaction. They encounter anxiety states precipitated by organic disease or resulting from focal epilepsy[16,46,76] or pheochromocytoma.[21] They could contribute to the building of a truly psychosomatic theory of anxiety which would integrate descriptive, psychodynamic, and biological approaches. The tendency of anxiety to have primarily autonomic, and that of conversion reaction to have largely nonautonomic, physiological concomitants suggests two different biological modes of response to danger—internal or external.

Schizophrenia. This syndrome is often accompanied by somatic symptoms. Of special practical importance for psychiatric consultants as well as medical practitioners is the fact that many schizophrenic patients go from one medical clinic to another presenting their somatic complaints for diagnostic considerations. The true diagnosis is probably often missed,[88] especially in early and in so-called ambulatory schizophrenia.[43,84] These patients seem to have a predilection for neuromuscular symptoms, such as backache,[61] as well as gastrointestinal and EENT[84] complaints and those referred to the genitourinary tract.[86] The ambulatory or borderline schizophrenic patients often suffer from such somatic symptoms, regard themselves as physically ill, and resent referrals to psychiatrist.[43] Many of them suffer from psychogenic pain and fail to be correctly diagnosed.[25] Engel[25] regards such pain as a delusion and claims that correct diagnosis can be made if the patient is allowed to give his own explanation for the pain. It seems that many of these patients are labeled in medical clinics as hypochondriacs or psychophysiologic reactions. Miller[84] provides some useful diagnostic clues, such as the highly personalized and excessive character of the complaints, their bizarreness, etc. Another writer[133] offers a practical set of suggestive clinical features that permit the diagnosis of early schizophrenia. One should mention especially the disturbances of the body image which may bring such a patient to a plastic surgeon with the request for surgical correction of the shape of his nose or penis. The reviewer recalls a young man, circumcised in infancy, who went from surgeon to surgeon demanding that his prepuce be "replaced" by a new one to allow him to have an erection. Not all these patients are easy to spot early since many come with ordinary somatic complaints, such as headache. Unless a thorough discussion of the presenting complaint is attempted on the first interview, the patient may end up with a full diagnostic workup and be told that he is really quite well. A psychiatric consultant should be called in early in such cases.

Hypochondriasis. This term has been dropped from the official American classification but it is still used as evidenced by a spate of recent papers devoted to it.[44,56,57,61,121] The revived interest no doubt stems from the fact that every medical clinic has its hard core of chronic complainers showing relatively fixed somatic complaints in the absence, or as overlay, of organic disease. Some of these patients are frankly delusional and, in any case, give the impression of being persecuted by their symptoms, such as pain.[25] They tend to describe their complaints with an intensity, persistence, and urgency which is in striking contrast to the typically indifferent hysteria.[25] Some of these patients are prepsychotic, and it is of interest that hypochondriasis shows rather common association with frank schizophrenia.[121] It appears, however, that many of these patients never fully decompensate into psychosis; those who do are likely to develop paranoid schizophrenia.

It would seem that the group of patients just described is a fairly homogeneous one, but this is denied by others. Kreitman[66] found that about one fifth of them were suffering from depression. Kenyon[56,57] discusses the meaning, history, and current state of hypochondriasis as a clinical entity. He lists 18 different usages of the term and suggests that hypochondriasis is always part of another syndrome, especially an affective one, and that there is no such entity as "primary hypochondriasis."

This writer believes that there may be some merit in retaining the term hypochondriasis to designate a group of chronic complainers with a paranoid personality structure. The writer repeatedly saw such patients as a consultant. He recalls a man who for some 30 years complained of rectal pain which he described "like a big stick trying to push through a small hole" and ascribed it to a rectal examination before an appendectomy. This man was a single and lonely individual with marked but not conscious homosexual interests who decompensated into a schizoaffective psychosis on several occasions. When psychotic, he claimed that his rectal pain was unbearable. This type of chronic patient should be distinguished from one who has transient hypochondriacal complaints as part of a depressive or anxiety reaction. It is well known that medical students suffer from fears of disease and various feelings of ill health; but as Hunter *et al.*[44] point out, these should be seen as a largely occupationally based nosophobia while hypochondriasis is rare and has serious significance.

Psychiatric consultants to the medical clinics are strategically placed to study this whole problem and to come up with a definitive statement on the issue of hypochondriasis.

"Psychosomatic" Disorders

Little needs to be said about these conditions here. As noted earlier they constitute but a fraction of the cases referred to psychiatric consultants. The focus of medical–psychiatric cooperation has largely shifted away from these disorders. The vast quantity of research carried out on them has left us with a body of valuable observation and such outstanding works as Engel's study of ulcerative colitis or Mirsky's formulation of the necessary conditions for the development of peptic ulcer. The value of our contribution to the therapy of these disorders has fallen far short of the promise of the "great-leap-forward" phase of psychosomatic medicine. We are also perhaps less sanguine in our search for psychogenicity which, as Schilder[106] remarked, is not very likely to solve the problem of organic disease.

What is a "psychosomatic disorder?" In this reviewer's opinion it is a misnomer with a vague meaning. It haunts the consultant like a bad ghost from the past. The consultant has to repeatedly correct the impression that all there is to psychosomatic medicine begins and ends with dependence, repressed anger, and the internalized bad mother symbolically nibbling at the gastric mucosa. Stereotypes die hard! It is an open question if it is methodologically sound to retain the concept of the psychosomatic disorders at all. In any case, those disorders are of importance to psychiatric consultants only insofar as they are presented by patients who have significant psychiatric difficulties, whether or not they antedated and/or followed the onset of the given disorder.

MANAGEMENT PROBLEMS ON MEDICAL WARDS

PSYCHIATRIC ASPECTS

As noted above, up to one half of requests for psychiatric consultation concern problems of management of patients. A general discussion of this aspect of the consultant's role as well as the more important techniques of dealing with the problems can be found in Part I[73] of this review. What remains is to list and briefly discuss some of the commoner problems to which the consultant may usefully contribute solutions. Such a list can hardly be complete, but it gives substance to the vague term "management problems" and conveys some idea of the scope of psychiatric consultants' work.

1. *Suicidal attempt or threat.* The consultant is called in to evaluate every patient admitted as a consequence of a suicidal attempt or attempting or threatening suicide during his hospitalization. (Some 10–20%[12,31,58] of referrals to consultation may stem from this cause.) Brown and Pisetsky[11] found the suicide rate in a general hospital to be 1.55 per 10,000 admissions. All the general ward patients in their series were chronically or terminally ill and suffered pain, dyspnea, or severe disability. Jumping from windows was the commonest method of suicide. The authors conclude that while suicide cannot be infallibly predicted, good rapport between doctor and patient offers the best possibility of assessing suicidal hazard.

Stoller and Estess[128] report on 33 patients who committed suicide in the medical and surgical wards. All had severe physical illness and were older men with few relatives. The authors stress the importance of training medical personnel in recognition of depression and adequate reporting by the nurses of their behavioral observations. Early and adequate psychiatric consultation is recommended. A report on a series of patients admitted to a general hospital after a suicidal attempt notes that none made another attempt during the hospitalization.[33]

2. *Grossly disturbed behavior.* Delirium, functional psychosis, agitated dementia, panic state, nondiagnosable outbursts of rage, etc., are examples of this problem. In these cases, thorough familiarity with psychotropic drugs is necessary if the consultant is to be helpful. A well-sedated patient may remain on the ward with minimum interruption of investigations and treatment, avoiding an emegency transfer to a psychiatric facility.

3. *Excessive emotional reactions.* This problem is characterized by fear, anger, depression, or suspicion related to hospitalization,[81] diagnostic procedures,[51] ward

routine (such as rounds),[54] therapy and its effects,[45] and disclosure of the diagnosis.[54]

4. *Refusal to cooperate.* This includes such problems as refusal to undergo recommended surgery or other medical or surgical procedure or therapy, and signing out from the hospital against medical advice.[48] This type of problem is usually related to Item 3 above, but may also be an expression of conflict between the patient and his doctor. In that case, refusal to cooperate is only a symptom of a crisis in relationship.

5. *Delayed convalescence.* Every physician knows the type of patient who displays disability incompatible with obejctive findings of pathology, or who shows an apparent relapse or new symptoms when discharge is mentioned. These responses may be related to the patient's separation anxiety at the prospect of leaving the hospital on whose personnel he has become dependent; or to his fear, rational or irrational, regarding his state of health; or to his enthusiastic acceptance of the "sick role" for socioeconomic reasons. A psychiatrist is often called in to elucidate the problem and offer practical advice on how to speed up the patient's recovery. Such patients are often resented by the medical staff as weaklings and parasites—which only serves to complicate matters. The consultant may help overcome the stalemate.

6. *Conflict between patient and personnel.* Apart from refusal to cooperate with major aspects of the medical management, a patient may fall into a conflict with any member of the medical or nursing staff with resulting disruption of the therapeutic relationship.[82] Any patient who is demanding, complaining, openly critical of the hospital, unduly flirtatious, or hostile may draw disapproving attention of a doctor or nurse; the result is usually some form of rejection and possibly avoidance of the patient. When this happens, tension affects the entire ward; the patient may demand immediate discharge or try to pick a quarrel with his doctor. In this event, a psychiatrist usually receives an urgent call. The writer was asked to see a man who insisted on smoking at times when it was not allowed, which quickly led to a major crisis on the ward. It turned out that the patient could not tolerate authority, particularly if exercised by women (nurses). He had to assert his masculine and masterful position at any cost. The case was dealt with by explaining the situation to the staff and patiently pointing out to the patient why certain rules had to be observed on the wards for his own and others' comfort and safety. It worked and the conflict was settled.

7. *Patient with psychiatric history.* Many physicians work on the unspoken assumption that "once a crock, always a crock." If a patient gives history of previous psychiatric hospitalization, especially for schizophrenia, he is likely to be watched with suspicion and fear. Such a patient may be discharged earlier than thorough diagnostic workup and adequate therapy would justify. All his symptoms tend to be taken with skepticism, and serious organic disease may be overlooked. If such patient has difficulty in communicating, his fate is sealed. The same applies to previous diagnosis of hysteria. Such labels do stick! It is often up to the psychiatric consultant to take a careful history from such patients and point out to the referring physician that psychiatric and organic disorders are not incompatible—a truism often forgotten.

This writer recalls being asked, prior to the patient's hysterectomy, to see a woman because her old chart showed diagnosis of hysteria. During a lengthy and difficult interview, it transpired that the patient had recently developed spells in which she noticed a bad smell. "I am a clean woman!" she protested. A tentative diagnosis of uncinate fits due to an expanding lesion was made by the reviewer. A series of specialist consultations and tests followed and resulted in a conclusion that the patient was "just a hysteric." A few days after the operation she developed tentorial pressure cone and died. A large aneurysm of the tip of a temporal lobe was found at autopsy. The case was instructive for the many people concerned, but the patient was dead!

8. *Psychiatric side effects of drugs.* This management problem is encountered with drugs such as steroids and cannot be elaborated here.

9. *Selection and/or preparation of patients.* Elective surgery, and other therapeutic procedures, such as hemodialysis,[103] sometimes evoke reactions like those described in Items 3 and 4 above. When there are reasons to expect such undesirable responses, a predictive psychiatric assessment and preparation of the patient are called for.[45,100]

10. *Disposition.* Ideally, this problem, which includes transfer of patients to the psychiatric ward and commitment, should occupy a fraction of a consultant's time if his work is efficient.

SUMMARY AND CONCLUSIONS

In this review an attempt has been made to present the scope of consultation psychiatry in the general hospitals. The evaluation of the importance of this whole area of work for psychiatric practice, teaching, and theory is left to the readers. The widening of the scope of psychosomatic medicine resulting from the diversification of the consultants' work and experience seems to be beyond doubt. A survey of the diagnostic and management problems confronting us in the various parts of the general hospitals has been presented here. The writer has aimed at comprehensiveness rather than intensive treatment of specific areas, each of which would deserve a separate paper. This approach was chosen deliberately with a view to illustrating the manifold quality of the psychosocial and psychopathological phenomena encountered in the medical settings. The writer considered it worthwhile to try and encompass this diversity in one review. He hopes to counteract the current malaise and uncertainty regarding the nature, scope, and goals of psychosomatic medicine. There is no need for defeatism. Fascinating vistas for clinical psychosomatic research are opening up. They should be welcome to all those disillusioned with the meager practical and theoretical results of the decades of search for psychogenic etiological factors in relatively few and elusive diseases. We are now closer to the truly comprehensive conceptions of that great, if too-little-recognized, pioneer of psychosomatic medicine Paul Schilder. In the preface to his most significant book[106] he wrote: "It would be erroneous to suppose that phenomenology and psycho-analysis should or could be separated from brain pathology. It seems to me that the theory of organism could and should be incorporated in a psychological doctrine which sees life and personality as a unit. . . .I have always believed that there is no gap between the organic and the functional."

Consultation psychiatry, despite its modest designation, has practical value for teaching and for collaboration with the rest of medicine. But beyond that it deals with the facets of the human condition which are of importance for the science of man, and such science must be *psychosomatic* in the full sense of the word.

REFERENCES

1. Ackner B, *et al:* Acute porphyria: A neuropsychiatric and biochemical study. *J Psychosom Res* 6:1, 1962.
2. Bard M, Dyk RB: Psychodynamic significance of beliefs regarding the cause of serious illness. *Psychoanal Rev* 43:146, 1956.
3. Bellak L: *Psychology of Physical Illness.* New York, Grune & Stratton, 1952.
4. Beres D, Brenner C: Mental reactions in patients with neurological disease. *Psychoanal Quart* 19:170, 1950.
5. Biloon S, Karliner W: The clinical picture of manic-depressive equivalents. *N Engl J Med* 259:684, 1958.
6. Blachly PH: Management of the opiate abstinence syndrome. *Am J Psychiat* 122:742, 1966.
7. Blachly PH: Procedure for withdrawal of barbiturates. *Am J Psychiatry* 120:894, 1964.
8. Bleuler M: Akute psychische Veraenderungen bei akuten Koerpererkrankungen. *Schweiz Med Wschr* 92:1521, 1962.
9. Bleuler M, *et al: Akute psychische Begleiterscheinungen K¼orperlicher Krankheiten.* Stuttgart, Thieme, 1966.
10. Bradley JJ: Severe localized pain associated with the depressive syndrome. *Br J Psychiatry* 109:741, 1963.
11. Brown W, Pisetsky JE: Suicidal behavior in a general hospital. *Am J Med* 29:307, 1960.
12. Butler RN, Perlin S: Psychiatric consultations in a research setting. *Med Ann DC* 27:503, 1958.
13. Chapman LF, Wolff HG: Disease of the neopallium. *Med Clin North Am,* 42:677, 1958.
14. Cleghorn RA, Curtis GC: Psychosomatic accompaniments of latent and manifest depressive affect. *Can Psychiatr Assoc* J4 (suppl):13, 1959.
15. Conrad K: Die symptomatischen Psychosen, in Gruhle HW ed: *Psychiatrie der Gegenwart* (Bd 2). Berlin, Springer, 1960.
16. Court JH: Anxiety among acute schizophrenics and temporal lobe patients. *Br J Soc Clin Psychol* 4:254, 1965.
17. Culpan R, Davis B: Psychiatric illness at medical and surgical outpatient clinic. *Compr Psychiatry* 1: 228, 1960.
18. Cutshall BJ: The Saunders-Sutton syndrome: An analysis of delirium tremens. *Q J Stud Alcohol* 26: 423, 1965.
19. Denney D, *et al:* Psychiatric patients on medical wards. *Arch Gen Psychiatry (Chicago)* 14:530, 1966.
20. Dewan JG, Spaulding WB: *Thee Organic Psychoses.* Toronto, University Press, 1958.
21. Doust BC: Anxiety as a manifestation of pheochromocytoma. *Arch Intern Med (Chicago)* 102:811, 1958.
22. Dovenmuehle RH and Verwoerdt A. Physical illness and depressive symptomatology. 1. Incidence of depressive symptoms in hospitalized cardiac patients. *J Am Geriatr Soc* 10:932, 1962.
23. Eilenberg MD: Psychiatric illness and pernicious anemia. A clinical reevaluation. *J Ment Sci* 106:1539, 1960.
24. Eilenberg MD: Survey of inpatient referrals to an American psychiatric department. *Br J Psychiatry* 111:1211, 1965.
25. Engel GL: "Psychogenic" pain and the pain-prone patient. *Am J Med* 26:899, 1959.
26. Engel GL: *Psychological Development in Health and Disease.* Philadelphia, WB Saunders Co, 1962.
27. Engel GL, Romano J: Delirium, a syndrome of cerebral insufficiency. *J Chron Dis* 9:260, 1959.
28. Essig CF: Newer sedative drugs that can cause intoxication and dependence of barbiturate type. *JAMA* 196:714, 1966.
29. Ferenczi S: Disease- or pathoneuroses, in *Further Contributions to the Theory and Technique of Psycho-Analysis.* London, Hogarth Press, 1926.
30. Fleck U: Symptomatische Psychosen (1941-1957). *Fortschr Neurol Psychiatr* 28. Heft 1, 1960.
31. Fleminger JJ, Mallett BL: Psychiatric referrals from medical and surgical wards. *J Ment Sci* 108:183, 1962.
32. Freud S: The justification for detaching from neurasthemia a particular syndrome: The anxiety-neurosis, in *Collected Papers.* New York, Basic, 1959, vol 1, p 76.

33. Friedman JH, Cancellieri R. Suicidal risk in a municipal general hospital. *Dis Nerv Syst* 19:556, 1958.
34. Gatfield PD, Guze SB: Prognosis and differential diagnosis of conversion reactions. *Dis Nerv Syst* 23:623, 1962.
35. Geocaris K: Psychotic episodes heralding the diagnosis of multiple sclerosis. *Bull Menninger Clin* 21:107, 1957.
36. Gould J. Virus disease and psychiatric ill-health. *Br J Clin Pract* 11:1, 1957.
37. Guze SB: A formulation of principles of comprehensive medicine with special reference to learning theory. *J Clin Psychol* 9:127, 1953.
38. Guze, SB, Cantwell DP: The prognosis in "organic brain" syndromes. *Am J Psychiatry* 120:878, 1964.
39. Haberland C: Psychiatric manifestations in brain tumors. *Akt Fragen Psychiatr Neurol* 2:65, 1965.
40. Helsborg HC: Psychiatric investigations of patients in a medical department. *Acta Psychiatr Neurol Scand* 33:303, 1958.
41. Henry DW, Mann AM: Diagnosis and treatment of delirium. *Can Med Assoc J* 93:1156, 1965.
42. Hilkevitch A. Psychiatric disturbances in outpatients of a general medical outpatient clinic. *Int J Neuropsychiatry* 1:371, 1965.
43. Hollender M: Ambulatory schizophrenia. *J Chron Dis* 9:249, 1959.
44. Hunter RCA, *et al:* Nosophobia and hypochondriasis in medical students. *J Nerv Ment Dis* 139:147, 1964.
45. Janis IL: *Psychological Stress.* New York, John Wiley & Sons, 1958.
46. Jonas AD: *Ictal and Subictal Neurosis.* Springfield, Ill, Charles C Thomas, 1965.
47. Jones D, Hall SB: Significance of somatic complaints in patients suffering from psychotic depression. *Acta Psychother (Basel)* 11:193, 1963.
48. Kahana RJ: Teaching medical psychology through psychiatric consultation. *J Med Educ* 34:1003, 1959.
49. Kahana RJ, Bibring GL. Personality types in medical management, In Zinberg EN (ed): *Psychiatry and Medical Practice in a General Hospital.* International Universities Press, 1964, New York.
50. Kane FJ Jr, Ewing JA: Iatrogenic brain syndrome. *South Med J* 58:875, 1965.
51. Kaplan SM: Laboratory procedures as an emotional stress. *JAMA* 161:677, 1956.
52. Kaufman RM: A psychiatric unit in a general hospital. *J Mount Sinai Hosp NY* 24:572, 1957.
53. Kaufman RM, Bernstein S: A psychiatric evaluation of the problem patient. *JAMA* 163:108, 1957.
54. Kaufman RM, *et al:* The emotional impact of ward rounds. *J Mount Sinai Hosp NY* 23:782, 1956.
55. Kaufman RM, *et al:* Psychiatric findings in admissions to a medical service in a general hospital. *J Mount Sinai Hosp NY* 26:160, 1959.
56. Kenyon FE: Hypochondriasis: A clinical study. *Br J Psychiatry* 110:467, 1964.
57. Kenyon FE: Hypochondriasis: a survey of some historical, clinical and social aspects. *Br J Med Psychol* 38:117, 1965.
58. Kenyon FE, Rutter ML: The psychiatrist and the general hospital. *Compr Psychiatry* 4:80, 1963.
59. Kepecs JG: Some patterns of somatic displacement. *Psychosom Med* 15:425, 1953.
60. Keyes JW: Iatrogenic heart disease. *JAMA* 192:951, 1965.
61. Klee GD, *et al:* Pain and other somatic complaints in a psychiatric clinic. *Maryland Med J* 8:188, 1959.
62. Knight JA: Epidemic hysteria: A field study. *Am J Public Health* 55:858, 1965.
63. Kolb LC: Anxiety and the anxiety states. *J Chron Dis* 9:199, 1959.
64. Kornfeld, DS, Feldman M: The psychiatric service in the general hospital. *NY State J Med* 65:1332, 1965.
65. Kornfeld DS, *et al:* Psychiatric complications of open-heart surgery *N Engl J Med* 273:287, 1965.
66. Kreitman N: Hypochondriasis and depression in out-patients at a general hospital. *Br J Psychiatry* 111:476, 1965.
67. Levin M: Delirium: A gap in psychiatric teaching. *Am J Psychiatry* 107:689, 1951.
68. Lewis BI: A psycho-medical survey of a private out-patient clinic in a university hospital. *Am J Med* 14:586, 1953.
69. Lewis BI: The hyperventilation syndrome. *Ann Intern Med* 38:918, 1953.
70. Lewis WC, Berman M: Studies of conversion hysteria. *Arch Gen Psychiatry (Chicago)* 13:275, 1965.
71. Lindemann E: Hysteria as a problem in a general hospital. *Med Clin North Am*, 22:591, 1938.
72. Lipin T: Psychic functioning in patients with undiagnosed somatic symptoms. *Arch Neurol Psychiatry* 73:239, 1955.

73. Lipowski ZJ: Review of consultation psychiatry and psychosomatic medicine. I. General principles. *Psychosom Med* 29:153, 1967.

75. Mabry JH: Lay concepts of etiology. *J Chron Dis* 17:371, 1964.

76. Macrae D: Isolated fear. A temporal lobe aura. *Neurology (Minneap)* 4:497, 1954.

77. Malmo RB, *et al:* Specificity of bodily reactions under stress, in Wolff HG (ed): *Life Stress and Bodily Disease. Assoc. Research Nervous Mental Disease.* Baltimore, Williams & Wilkins, 1950.

78. Mechanic D: The concept of illness behavior. *J Chron Dis* 15:189, 1962.

79. Mendelson J, *et al:* Hallucinations of poliomyelitis patients during treatment in a respirator. *J Nerv Ment Dis* 126:421, 1958.

80. Merskey H: The characteristics of persistent pain in psychological illness. *J Psychosom Res* 9:291, 1965.

81. Meyer E: Disturbed behavior on medical and surgical wards: A training and research opportunity, in Masserman JH (ed): *Science and Psychoanalysis: Psychoanalytic Education.* New York, Grune & Stratton, 1962, vol 5.

82. Meyer E, Mendelson M: Psychiatric consultations with patients on medical and surgical wards: Patterns and processes. *Psychiatry* 24:197, 1961.

83. Meyer E, Mendelson M: The psychiatric consultation in postgraduate medical teaching. *J Nerv Ment Dis* 130:78, 1960.

84. Miller MH: The borderline psychotic patient: The importance of diagnosis in medical and surgical practice. *Ann Intern Med* 46:736, 1957.

85. Mittelman B, *et al:* Personality and psychosomatic disturbances in patients on medical and surgical wards: a survey of 450 admissions. *Psychosom Med* 7:220, 1945.

86. Nussbaum K: Somatic complaints and homeostasis in psychiatric patients. *Psychiatr Quart* 34:311, 1960.

87. O'Connor JF, Musher DM: Central nervous system involvement in systemic lupus erythematosus. *Arch Neurol (Chicago)* 14:157, 1966.

88. Offenkrantz W: Multiple somatic complaints as a precursor of schizophrenia. *Am J Psychiatry* 119:258, 1962.

89. Payson HE, *et al:* Recognition and referral of psychiatric illness on a university medical inpatient service. Scientific Proceedings of the 117th Annual Meeting of the American Psychiatric Association, Washington, 1961.

90. Perlas AP, Faillace LA: Psychiatric manifestations of carcinoma of the pancreas. *Am J Psychiatry* 121:182, 1964.

91. Poe RO, *et al:* Depression *JAMA* 195:345, 1966.

92. Quarton GC, *et al:* Mental disturbances associated with ACTH and cortisone: A review of explanatory hypotheses. *Medicine (Baltimore)* 34:13, 1955.

93. Querido A: Forecast and follow-up: an investigation into the clinical, social and mental factors determining the results of hospital treatment. *Br J Prev Soc Med* 13:33, 1959.

94. Rangell L: Psychiatric aspects of pain. *Psychosom Med* 15:22, 1953.

95. Reding GR, Daniels RS: Organic brain syndromes in a general hospital. *Am J Psychiatry* 120:800, 1964.

96. Reid DD: *Epidemiological Methods in the Study of Mental Disorders.* Geneva, World Health Organization, 1960.

97. Richman A, *et al:* Symptom questionnaire validity in assessing the need for psychiatrists' care. *Br J Psychiatry* 112:549, 1966.

98. Roberts BH, Norton NM: The prevalence of psychiatric illness in a medical out-patient clinic. *N Engl J Med* 246:82, 1952.

99. Robinson WG Jr: The toxic delirious reactions of old age, in Kaplan OJ (ed): *Mental Disorders in Later Life.* Stanford, Stanford University Press, 1956.

100. Rosenbaum M, Cohen YA: Psychological preparation of the individual for medical and surgical care, in Liebman S (ed): *Understanding Your Patient.* Philadelphia, JB Lippincott Co, 1957.

101. Rossman PL: Organic diseases simulating functional disorders. *GP* 28:78, 1963.

102. Rud F: Psychiatric activities and instruction at a general hospital. *J Clin Exp Psychopathol* 14:139, 1953.

103. Sand P, *et al:* Psychological assessment of candidates for a hemodialysis program. *Ann Intern Med* 64:602, 1966.

104. Sandt JJ, Leifer R: The psychiatric consultation. *Compr Psychiatry* 5:409, 1964.

105. Saunders L: *Cultural Differences and Medical Care.* New York, Russell Sage Foundation, 1954.

106. Schilder P: *The Image and Appearance of the Human Body.* New York, International Universities Press, 1950.

107. Schwab JJ, *et al:* Differential characteristics of medical in-patients referred for psychiatric consultation: A controlled study. *Psychosom Med* 27:112, 1965.

108. Schwab JJ, *et al:* Medical patients' reactions to referring physicians after psychiatric consultation. *JAMA* 195:1120, 1966.

109. Schwab JJ, *et al:* Problems in psychosomatic diagnosis: I. A controlled study of medical inpatients. *Psychosomatics* 6:369, 1964.

110. Schwab JJ, *et al.* Problems in psychosomatic diagnosis: II. Severity of medical illness and psychiatric consultations. *Psychosomatics* 6:69, 1965.

111. Schwab JJ, *et al.* Problems in psychosomatic diagnosis: III. Physical examinations, laboratory procedures, and psychiatric consultations. *Psychosomatics* 6:147, 1965.

112. Schwab JJ *et al:* Problems in psychosomatic diagnosis: IV. A challenge to all physicians. *Psychosomatics* 6:198, 1965.

113. Seitz PFD: Symbolism and organ choice in conversion reactions. *Psychosom Med* 13:254, 1951.

114. Senescu RA: The development of emotional complications in the patient with cancer. *J Chron Dis* 16:813, 1963.

115. Shepherd M *et al:* Psychiatric illness in the general hospital. *Acta Psychiatr Neurol Scand* 35:518, 1960.

116. Simon A, Cahan RB: The acute brain syndrome in geriatric patients. *Psychiatr Res Rep Am Psychiatr Assoc,* May 16, 1963.

117. Slater E: Diagnosis of "hysteria." *Br Med J* 1:1395, 1965.

118. Small IF *et al:* Organic cognates of acute psychiatric illness. *Am J Psychiatry* 122:790, 1966.

119. Spencer RF: Medical patients: Consultation and psychotherapy. *Arch Gen Psychiatry (Chicago)* 10:270, 1964.

120. Starr AM: Personality changes in Cushing's syndrome. *J Clin Endocrinol.* 12:502, 1952.

121. Stenbäck A, Rimon R: Hypochondria and paranoia. *Acta Psychiatr Scand* 49:379, 1964.

122. Stengel E: Pain and the psychiatrist. *Br J Psychiatry* 111:795, 1965.

123. Stewart MA *et al:* A study of psychiatric consultations in a general hospital. *J Chron Dis* 15:331, 1962.

124. Stewart MA *et al:* Depression among medically ill patients. *Dis Nerv Syst* 26:479, 1965.

125. Stoeckle JD, Davidson GE: Bodily complaints and the other symptoms of a depressive reaction, its diagnosis and significance in a medical clinic. *JAMA* 180:134, 1962.

126. Stoeckle JD, Davidson GE: The use of "crisis" as an orientation for the study of patients in a medical clinic. *J Med Educ* 37:604, 1962.

127. Stoeckle JD *et al:* The quantity and significance of psychological distress in medical patients. *J Chron Dis* 17:959, 1964.

128. Stoller RJ, Estess FM: Suicides in medical and surgical wards of general hospitals. *J Chron Dis* 12:592, 1960.

129. Szasz TS; *Pain and Pleasure,* New York, Basic, 1957.

130. Tavel ME: Hyperventilation syndrome with unilateral somatic symptoms. *JAMA* 187:301, 1964.

131. Veith I: *Hysteria. The History of a Disease.* Chicago, University of Chicago Press, 1965.

132. Walters A: Psychogenic regional pain alias hysterical pain. *Brain* 84:1, 1961.

133. Weinstock HI: Discussion of schizophrenia in: Early recognition and management of psychiatric disorders in general practice. *J Mount Sinai Hosp NY* 25:137, 1958.

134. Weisman AD, Hackett TP: Psychosis after eye surgery. *N Engl J Med* 258:1284, 1958.

135. Wilson MS, Meyer E: Diagnostic consistency in a psychiatric liaison service. *Am J Psychiatry* 119:207, 1962.

136. Wilson M, Meyer E: The doctors vs. the nurses' view of emotional disturbances. *Can Psychiatr Assoc J* 10:212, 1965.

137. Ziegler E J *et al:* Contemporary conversion reactions: A clinical study, *Am J Psychiatry* 116:901, 1960.

138. Ziegler FJ, Imboden JB: Contemporary conversion reactions. II. A conceptual model. *Arch Gen Psychiatry (Chicago)* 6:279, 1962.

139. Ziegler FJ et al: Contemporary conversion reactions. III. Diagnostic considerations. *JAMA* 186:307, 1963.

140. Zwerling I *et al:* Personality disorder and the relationship of emotion to surgical illness in 200 surgical patients. *Am J Psychiatry* 112:270, 1955.

Psychiatric Liaison with Neurology and Neurosurgery

20

There is a growing realization that psychiatry and neurology have drifted apart to the detriment of both. One notes recent appeals for their closer collaboration, particularly in the area of residency training.[1,2] Rose, in his presidential address to the American Neurological Association in 1969, stated: "To meet the future, neurology should join with those similarly disposed in psychiatry to make clinical training a more relevant experience."[3] Such "similarly disposed" psychiatrists are logically those engaged in consultation–liaison work with the nonpsychiatric physicians. This area of clinical psychiatry has developed rapidly in the past two decades, and its practitioners are experienced in collaborative teaching.[4,5]

In this paper I will describe a joint teaching conference I conducted at the Montreal Neurological Institute from January 1, 1968, to July 31, 1971. This venture represented the teaching aspect of the liaison with the institute undertaken by the Psychiatric Consultation Service to the Royal Victoria Hospital in Montreal. Our consulting activities at the institute as well as the characteristics of patients referred to us and the problems they presented are reported in detail elsewhere.[6] That report, based on nearly 1000 patients seen, offers a comprehensive survey of the borderlands between psychiatry and neurology.

THE SETTING

Neurology and neurosurgery, like every other specialty, present psychiatric consultants with diagnostic and management problems that are in some respects unique. This uniqueness is enhanced by the characteristics of the setting. The latter include the personalities of the professionals involved, their standing, and their attitudes toward psychiatry, as well as the physical aspects of the hospital milieu. Hence a brief description of the setting and its patient population is in order.

The Montreal Neurological Institute, founded in 1934, has 135 beds for neurological and neurosurgical patients. There are about 1000 annual admissions to the three neurology services and as many to neurosurgery. The institute conducts research in most neurosciences, has pioneered in the field of neurosurgery, and provides under-

Reprinted from *American Journal of Psychiatry* 129(2):136–140, 1972. Copyright © 1972 the American Psychiatric Association. Reprinted by permission.

graduate and postgraduate teaching. Some 250 fellows studied there between 1960 and 1970. Its standing as a clinical, research, and teaching facility is well known. Its reputation, particularly that of Dr. Wilder Penfield, attracts patients from many countries. This is important, since such patients often have very complex and obscure symptoms of long standing; at the same time they have very high expectations that they will be correctly diagnosed and cured. This makes formidable demands on the staff, including the psychiatric consultants, who see about 7% of all admissions.[6]

The patients present several salient features from the psychiatric viewpoint. First, a large proportion of them suffer from disorders of the central nervous system and thus show varying degrees and patterns of impairment of the highest integrative functions of the brain. Second, many are admitted for intracranial surgery, which arouses anxiety at least equal to that provoked by cardiac operations. It is indeed striking that most of them cope with this experience without psychological breakdown. Third, there is a high proportion of patients who have sustained a dramatic interruption of their psychic processes as a result of head injury, stroke, epilepsy, or other causes. Fourth, many patients suffer from chronic diseases of the nervous system with attendant problems of disability in crucial areas of living: locomotion, speech, use of hands, control of elimination, sexual function, etc. Such defects are likely to have deep personal meaning in terms of threat, loss, and disrupted interpersonal relationships.[7,8] Some of these chronic disorders, such as multiple sclerosis or myasthenia gravis, are marked by high uncertainty; others, such as epilepsy, carry social stigma; others, such as trigeminal neuralgia, involve pain; still others, such as facial paralysis, involve disfigurement. Fifth, diseases of the nervous system are particularly likely to be used for unconsciously motivated simulation as a mode of expression and communication. The number and variety of conversion symptoms, alone or in conjunction with organic disease, is exceptionally high. They constitute about 16% of all psychiatric referrals.

This then is the setting for our teaching conference, which will now be described. It must be clear that it provided unusually rich and varied clinical material for collaborative teaching.

THE CONFERENCE

Our joint teaching exercise was initiated by the senior neurologists, who became convinced that their residency training needed more emphasis on psychosocial aspects of illness. Having been closely involved in consulting at the institute for some 8 years, I was invited to conduct it. It was agreed that the conference would be patient centered and not a formal seminar on psychiatric topics. My stated objective was to demonstrate that every patient presents both unique and common psychological and social facets to his illness and these must be considered in diagnosis and management.

The conference was held for 1 hr every Friday. A patient from the institute was selected by its staff for discussion of a diagnostic and/or management problem for which psychiatric advice was sought. It was stipulated that we were not looking for pure "psychiatric" problems. The patient's history and examination results were briefly summarized by his resident. I then interviewed the patient for 15–20 min in front of the group, which consisted of physicians, medical students, social workers, nurses, and other interested professionals. There followed a short discussion and my summing up. The latter focused on what had transpired during the interview and attempted to highlight one or two general principles based on the case. I invariably ended by suggesting concrete recommendations for therapeutic action. This could involve suggestions for specific psychological management, use of psychotropic drugs, follow-up, etc. This needs emphasis. A liaison conference confined only to a discussion of fine points of diagnosis or psychodynamics is of little value. Information elicited during the interview, and subsequent explanations, must lead to *practical conclusions* for it to be truly educational.

Some participants tended to induce me to speculate about the patient's unconscious life. Such temptations had to be resisted. The surest way to discredit the conference would have been to indulge in freewheeling psychodynamic interpretations that, however plausible, could hardly be convincing to untrained observers watching a brief interview. Another pitfall set up by some residents was to bring a mute, aphasic, or grossly demented patient. In the first case, an ad hoc sodium amytal interview revealed a florid schizophrenic psychosis and provided an occasion for a discussion of catatonia and differential diagnosis of stupor. In the other two cases the interview was short but gave rise to a discussion of the problems of an aphasic patient, and various causes and management of dementia, respectively. No patient was deemed unsuitable or uninteresting; each offered a learning experience.

THE PATIENTS

Each patient was asked to consent to appear at the conference. Of about 120 patients selected over the three and one-half years, only one or two refused. There was nothing to suggest that a tactfully conducted interview was traumatic to any of them. Care was taken to avoid public disclosure of personal matters that the patient was clearly reluctant to discuss.

To illustrate the conduct of the conference a few brief vignettes are given.

Case 1. Miss B. S., aged 23 was admitted with a history of frequent seizures that turned out to be hysterical fits. She also suffered from well-documented epilepsy but neglected to take anticonvulsants. Her fits came on in a setting of conflict over a love affair and separation from her parents. My comment: Frequently in our experience true epilepsy and hysterical fits are associated. The patient used her cerebral seizures as a model for communicating conflict and adopting the sick role, with its primary and secondary gains. Physical and emotional illness often do coexist and reinforce each other. The social setting and its meaning to the patient must be understood. A transfer to the pyschiatric unit was recommended.

Case 2. Mrs. B. C., aged 58, was diagnosed as suffering from Guillain–Barré syndrome; she was quadriplegic. She made incessant demands on the nurses, especially at night, and was increasingly resented by them. She complained about nursing care, food, etc. In the interview she described the sudden onset of her illness: "I couldn't believe this was happening to me—I was always so healthy and active." She described herself as always hardworking and independent, as one who helped everybody and needed nobody to help her. My comment: This patient's illness threatened her self-image and deprived her of her chief coping strategies by making her immobile and utterly dependent. Her angry demands and complaints reflected her anxiety and her desperate attempts to regain some control and keep dependent needs in check. The nurses were asked to refrain from retaliating for her criticisms. (They told me afterwards that it was revealing for them to see this patient as frightened rather than simply obnoxious.)

Case 3. Mr. A. B., aged 37, had just undergone a unilateral thalamotomy for severe paralysis agitans. The day after the operation he announced that the surgeon found an oily substance in his skull that indicated the presence of syphilis. He said the doctors then decided to kill him "humanely" and that he had actually heard his own obituary on the radio. There was no doubt in his mind, he said, that he was doomed and all he could do was to resign himself to his fate. He spoke calmly; affect was blunt. He reported having been in a mental hospital a few years previously because of his fear that he would be assassinated. He had not thought it important to mention this to his surgeons before the operation. My comment: The patient suffered from paranoid schizophrenia, exacerbated by fear of cranial surgery. His mental state and psychiatric history should have been known preoperatively, but his calm manner misled the surgeon. Thioridazine (Mellaril) was recommended as well as psychiatric consultation prior to an anticipated second thalamotomy later on. (This patient responded rapidly to thioridazine, was seen 6 months later before his second operation, and had an uneventful course while on that drug.)

Case 4. Miss N. L., aged 19, was admitted for quadriplegia of sudden onset, thought to be Guillain-Barre syndrome. She recovered power in her arms after 1 month but remained paraplegic, with sensory loss below T_4 and no bowel or bladder control. She had been told initially she would recover fully, but the lack of progress led to a change of diagnosis to transverse myelitis, with almost certain permanent paraplegia. The neurologists disagreed among themselves about how much she should be told about her changed prognosis. She was an attractive, compliant girl engaged to be married a few months later. She evoked sympathy in everyone. I was told that she was euphoric and unaware of the seriousness of her illness. She was presented for advice on how to handle the disclosure of the truth to her and how she would probably react. In the interview she expressed awareness that her future was bleak and said she thought the doctors had reassured her out of kindness. Her fiancé and family would not discuss her illness with her, she said. She was calm but not euphoric.

My comment: She knew more about her predicament than was believed and suffered from the lack of frank communication. My recommendations were, first, to tell her that her diagnosis and prognosis had to be revised and she would most likely remain paralyzed; second, to stress her recovering use of her upper limbs and the consequent opportunities for rehabilitation and manual work; third, to hold a joint session with her, her parents, and her fiancé to discuss her condition and future prospects and thus remove blocks to communication and decisions; fourth, to start occupational therapy and offer emotional support for the expected depressive reaction.

This last intervention illustrates important points. The conference helped resolve conflict among the staff members and allowed them to express feelings of guilt and doubt. It opened communication with the patient and corrected the mistaken impression that she was denying her illness. Finally, it prepared the way for realistic planning for her and her family. Thus the objectives of psychiatric liaison and teaching could be achieved in an hour. Clearly, not every conference was equally productive; the focus may have been on diagnosis, for example. But the emphasis on the need to view the patient as an individual interacting with a given social milieu and attempting to cope with it and/or his illness or disability was never absent.

THE TOPICS

The above vignettes are a sample of the histories of some 120 patients seen. Over the years we had a chance to see and talk about almost every major type of psychosocial and psychiatric problem encountered in neurology and neurosurgery. Since these topics offer an overview of the interface between neurology and psychiatry, they are summarized in Table 1.

DISCUSSION

The conference may serve as a model for the teaching of psychosocial aspects of medical and surgical specialities anywhere. Specific topics may vary, but certain general principles are common to all. Such a conference provides the most effective medium for teaching the psychosomatic approach in its broad sense.[4,5]

What has the conference accomplished? There are no definitive answers to this, just a few suggestive observations. We noted that referrals for psychiatric consultation increased by 170% in 1968 (the year the conference started) as compared to 1967 and this higher rate has persisted. In fact, in the first 6 months of 1971 more patients were referred than in any previous entire year.[6] Whatever success has been achieved must be due in large part to the unfailing warm support that successive chief neurologists gave the conference Their presence added a certain authority to it in the eyes of residents. Further, we noticed two significant developments: a definite improvement in the quality of medical records from the psychosocial viewpoint; and the friendly and helpful reception extended to members of our service in all wards of the institute. A bridge evidently has been built where none had existed before.

Our colleagues seemed to agree. In his annual report for 1968, the neurologist-in-chief wrote: "Perhaps the most important teaching development of the year in the M.N.I. has been the establishment of a weekly Psychiatric Conference.... This is our first joint teaching conference and it fills an important gap in the residency training program.... The late Dr. Stanley Cobb once wrote that 'Progress is achieved by ignoring the boundaries of academic disciplines.' "

Such a conference offered the following advantages for neurologists and psychiatrists, respectively. First, it gave the former a perspective on their work that some of them, especially the residents, may have overlooked. Second, some concrete ad-

TABLE 1. Topics Discussed at the Neuropsychiatric Conference

Diagnostic and/or therapeutic problems

1. Psychogenic versus organic symptoms: their similarities and differences; criteria for their
   differentiation; their common coexistence, e.g.,
       Epilepsy versus hysterical fits (pseudoseizures)
       Psychogenic versus organic pain
       Multiple sclerosis and conversion symptoms
       Organic and psychogenic depersonalization
       Hysterical versus organic tremor
       Epileptic versus hysterical fugue
2. Personality change and/or psychiatric syndrome as initial or most prominent presenting symptom
   of neurological disease, e.g.
       Change or accentuation of the patient's personality style as manifestation of early cerebral
           disease, such as tumor or Huntington's disease (chorea)
       Severe depression, anxiety, etc., "masking" coexistent organic symptoms
       Denial of illness and resulting diagnostic pitfalls
3. Psychological reactions to illness, surgery, etc., and their determinants, e.g.,
       Personal meaning of specific disability, such as paralysis, aphasia, tremor, and resultant emo-
           tional reactions and behavior
       Individual modes of communication of symptoms and resultant misunderstandings
       Individual coping styles and strategies, and enhancement of adaptive ones[9]
4. Organic brain syndromes: delirium, dementia, amnestic syndrome
5. Syndromes with marked psychological component, e.g.,
       Tension headache, migraine, narcolepsy
6. Psychosocial aspects of epilepsy[10]

Ward management problems

1. Personality-derived, e.g.,
       Paranoid or dependent attitudes[11]
2. Illness-derived, e.g.,
       Psychosis, panic, withdrawal, regression, giving up
3. Family-derived: the importance of interaction with significant others for illness behavior and
   outcome
4. Hospital-milieu-derived, e.g.,
       Conflicts with physicians or nurses and ways of resolving them
       Emotional responses to: the hospital environment; strict ward rules: sight of psychotic be-
           havior of postoperative patients, seizures, etc.

vice was given on management of patients. Third, neurology residents got some exposure to interviewing techniques, psychiatric diagnostic formulations, and the proper
use of psychotropic drugs. All these facets could hardly fail to be of use in their
practice.

For the psychiatrists involved it was a demanding teaching exercise, calling for
maximum clarity in thinking and communication. There is hardly a better teaching experience than one with a skeptical group. Further, we gained access to clinical material that reflected an unusually wide range of human experience and psychosomatic
relationships.[6,12,13] This aspect makes a conference like this a valuable learning experience for psychiatric residents before they retire to their narrow professional niche.

We have demonstrated that liaison with neurology is possible and mutually rewarding. We hope others may be encouraged to follow suit.

REFERENCES

1. Rose AS: The integration of neurology into psychiatric education. *Am J Psychiatry,* 123:592–594, 1966.
2. Wilson WP, Wells CE, Irigaray PJ: Should psychiatry and neurology integrate? *Am J Psychiatry* 128:617–622, 1971.
3. Rose AS: The current status of education for neurology. *Trans Am Neurol Assoc* 94:1–10, 1969.
4. Lipowski ZJ: New Perspectives in psychosomatic medicine. *Can Psychiatr Assoc J* 15:515–525, 1970.
5. Lipowski ZJ: Consultation–liaison psychiatry in general hospital. *Compr Psychiatry* 12:461–465, 1971.
6. Lipowski ZJ, Kiriakos RZ: Borderlands between neurology and psychiatry: observations in a neurological hospital. *Psychiatry Med* 3:131–147, 1972.
7. Beres D, Brenner C: Mental reactions in patients with neurological disease. *Psychoanal Quart* 19:170–191, 1950.
8. Lipowski ZJ: Psychosocial aspects of disease. *Ann Intern Med* 71:1197–1206, 1969.
9. Lipowski ZJ: Physical illness, the individual and the coping processes. *Psychiatry Med* 1:91–102, 1970.
10. Horowitz MJ: *Psychosocial Function in Epilepsy.* Springfield, Ill, Charles C Thomas, 1970.
11. Kahana RJ: Teaching medical psychology through psychiatric consultation. *J Med Educ* 34:1003–1009, 1959.
12. Lipowski ZJ (ed): *Psychosocial Aspects of Physical Illness.* Basel, Karger, 1972.
13. Teitelbaum HA: *Psychosomatic Neurology.* New York, Grune & Stratton, 1964.

Consultation–Liaison Psychiatry

An Overview

21

An overview of consultation–liaison psychiatry from the perspective of 15 years of personal work in this area provides an opportunity to highlight some current trends in psychiatry. Liaison psychiatrists have kept in touch with seminal developments in clinical practice, education, research, and modes of health care delivery in both general medicine and psychiatry. The last 15 years have brought far-reaching changes in all of these areas. Consultation–liaison psychiatry provides a fit vantage point for watching the changes that permit prediction of future directions in psychiatry as a *medical discipline*. The kind of psychiatry that the consultants practice and the type of training, skills, and professional attitudes that their work requires represent a model that is likely to prevail in psychiatry in the coming years. This contention is based on the observable trends in health care delivery and the scientific, social, and economic factors that influence them. These issues will be discussed here in the framework of a survey of the scope, assumptions, organization, and functions of consultation–liaison psychiatry.

A Historical Perspective

Consultation–liaison psychiatry has developed over the past 40 years as an outgrowth of general hospital psychiatric units.[1-5] Their development represents a landmark in the history of psychiatry that has led to fundamental changes in the management of psychiatric patients. The continued growth of general hospital psychiatry has done much to overcome their isolation from the community and from general health care and to open psychiatry to the advances in the medical and behavioral sciences with the resulting diversification of therapies, research, and theory. In turn, the entry of psychiatry into the mainstream of medicine has fostered changes in medical education and in the management of the physically ill in the direction of comprehensive medicine.[6]

The first viable general hospital psychiatric unit in this country was opened in the Albany Hospital in 1902.[7] At the last count there were about 770 such units in the country, and 22.4% of all psychiatrists worked there (C. Kanno, personal communication, March 21, 1971). The provision of psychiatric consultations to the medical was given additional impetus by the emergence in the 1920s of psychosomatic medicine. In 1929 appeared Henry's classical paper on "Some Modern Aspects of Psychiatry in General Hospital Practice."[8] It marks the beginning of consultation–liaison psychiatry as it is practiced today. Henry's article has not lost its relevance. His emphasis on careful observation rather than inspired guessing, on jargon-free communication, and on flexibility in the choice of therapy is still valid. His observation that physicians tend to dismiss as irrelevant patients' complaints that are not directly pertinent to physical illness is still largely true today.

In 1934 the Rockefeller Foundation funded the establishment of five psychiatric liaison departments in university hospitals. One of them was organized at the Colorado General Hospital in Denver.[9] Another, at the Columbia University Medical Center, was led by Flanders Dunbar, one of the pioneers of psychosomatic medicine. She and her collaborators helped expand the theoretical basis on which consultation–liaison work rests.[10] Dunbar forecast optimistically that "the time should not be too long delayed when psychiatrists are required on all our medical and surgical wards, and in all our general and special clinics."[10] That prediction, made in 1936, is still unfullfilled, and its realization is nowhere in sight. Yet progress has been made, particularly since the end of World War II. M. R. Kaufman and his collaborators deserve much credit for this. They organized model psychiatric services, with particular stress on close liaison with the medical and surgical wards and clinics, at the Mount Sinai Hospital in New York in 1945.[11-13] Liaison psychiatrists were to play a key role in building a bridge between psychiatry and medicine by virtue of their clinical and teaching activities. Kaufman and Margolin spelled out the goals of this teaching in 1948.[13] They emphasized indoctrination of physicians in psychoanalyic psychology and psychosomatic medicine. These teaching objectives have been modified and expanded since then and will be discussed later.

The past 30 years have brought a gradual growth of consultation–liaison psychiatry in all of its aspects. A 1966 survey showed that 76% of all psychiatric training centers in the United States offered instruction in consultation work.[14] Although more recent figures are unavailable, informal inquiries indicate that most postgraduate training programs in psychiatry demand that the residents spend some time consulting on the medical and surgical floors. A recent worldwide survey shows that the growth of consultation–liaison psychiatry has occurred in most of the developed countries.[15] There is extensive literature on it that includes a general review,[1-3] a handbook,[16] a reference guide,[17] and a critical review of consultation research.[18] Some of this literature deals with mental health consultation in settings other than the medical ones that are the focus of this paper. Despite certain shared assumptions and techniques, medical–psychiatric consultation work differs from that in nonmedical settings such as schools, social and correctional agencies, and industry. The chief differences are (1) operation in the context of health care delivery both administratively and conceptually; (2) adherence to the psychosomatic approach, one that proposes that human health and disease result from an *interaction* of biological, psychological, and social factors; and (3) focus on people whose psychiatric problems are related to physical illness and disability and those who communicate their distress in terms of somatic symptoms.

Much of the literature on consultation–liaison psychiatry is descriptive, but several notable works stand out as attempts to conceptualize the consultant's mode of operation, assumptions, and aims.[19-23] Particularly important is Miller's application of the general systems approach to psychiatric consultation.[21,22] These articles should become recommended reading for psychiatric trainees.

The current role of consultation–liaison psychiatry has been succinctly, if incompletely, summed up by the American Hospital Association:

> The development of liaison psychiatric services is based on the acknowledged fact that psychiatry applied in general or specialty medicine contributes to the quality of care provided, affects hospital utilization, and results in a savings of the physician's time.... The liaison psychiatrist often serves the unserved, by helping to ensure the identification and appropriate management of mental and emotional aspects of illness throughout the hospital.[24, pp. 26-27]

This statement acknowledges the contribution of consultation–liaison psychiatry to improved patient care and to preventive medicine and psychiatry.

THE SCOPE OF CONSULTATION–LIAISON PSYCHIATRY

Consultation–liaison psychiatry has been defined as the area of clinical psychiatry that encompasses clinical, teaching, and research activities of psychiatrists and allied mental health professionals in the nonpsychiatric divisions of a general hospital.[4] This definition is already too narrow. While it is true that the medical and surgical wards, outpatient clinics, and emergency departments of general hospitals provide the main operational base for liaison psychiatrists, their activities are gradually spreading beyond the hospital walls. The scope of consultation–liaison psychiatry has expanded to include collaboration with all categories of health professionals in all types of health care facilities, be they community health clinics, rehabilitation centers, convalescent hospitals, nursing homes, or doctor's private offices.

The designation "consultation–liaison" reflects two interrelated roles of the consultants. "Consultation" refers to the provision of expert diagnostic opinion and advice on management regarding a patient's mental state and behavior at the request of another health professional. "Liaison" connotes a linking up of groups for the purpose of effective collaboration. In the present context, liaison involves *interpretation and mediation*. The consultant mediates between mental health and other health professionals, respectively. In clinical settings he interprets the attitudes and behavior of patients and of those taking care of them in an attempt to maintain communication and cooperation and to allay conflicts among them. Mutual distrust and misunderstandings between patients and staff interfere with optimal care and functioning of a hospital ward or clinic as a therapeutic setting.[20,25] Patients who are markedly demanding, hostile, dependent, or uncooperative readily evoke negative feelings and retaliatory behavior on the part of the staff. As a result, communication breaks down and quality of care deteriorates. The liaison psychiatrist applies his knowledge of motivation of behavior and his skills in gathering pertinent information to identify sources of conflict, explain contentious attitudes, and thus help restore communication and cooperation. This mediating role is facilitated if the consultant is an accepted member of the medical team, maintains regular contact with it, and knows the staff well. A weekly conference of the health team of a ward or clinic provides a good forum for him to discuss problem patients, the staff's ways of coping wtih them and with their own countertransference reactions, and the strains within the team.

At another level, the liaison psychiatrist acts as a mediator and bridge builder between two professional groups: the medical–biological and the psychiatric–behavioral, respectively. Members of each of these groups tend to ignore, misunderstand, and disparage the viewpoints and modes of operation of the other group. This state of affairs fosters the spread of derogatory stereotypes and mutual suspicion. As a result, collaboration in patient care, teaching, and research is poor. Liaison psychiatrists and their few allies in other specialties help keep an interprofessional dialogue and cooperation alive.

Consultation and liaison are mutually complementary. A consultation should encompass three interlocked foci: the patient, the consultee, and the therapeutic team.[1] This implies that consultation is most effective if the consultant has personal contact with both the patient and those taking care of him. In addition, communication with and knowledge about the patient's family and other significant people in his social milieu are indispensable for the evaluation of the psychosocial consequences of his illness.[26] One also has to take into account the influence of his disability and illness behavior on his family. People tend to become ill and seek medical help and hospitalization at times of psychosocial stress, which, magnified by that of illness, may lead to emotional disorder and deviant illness behavior, such as psychogenic invalidism, noncompliance with physician's advice, and overutilization of health and social welfare facilities.[27] The attitudes and behavior of the patient's family members play a key role in bringing about these undesirable behavior patterns. In turn, a patient's illness and behavior are often a source of distress and psychiatric disorder for his spouse and other family members.[28]

Since the most prevalent forms of serious illness today are of the chronic type, the importance of the psychosocial factors in medicine is increasingly recognized. At the same time, medical training, with its emphasis on narrow specialization and the purely biological aspects of disease, does not prepare physicians to recognize and deal with the influence of these factors on their patients. By default, this role is often relegated to the liaison service. It is in this area that psychiatrist can discharge their responsibility to medicine.[29]

No organized form of human activity can survive in an ideological vacuum. Ideology is implied here as a set of beliefs, assumptions, definitions, and stated goals that furnish a professional activity with a raison d'etre that justifies its continuation in the eyes of its practitioners, their clients, and concerned observers. If an ideology becomes diffuse and ambiguous, the whole purpose and legitimacy of the activity based on it is liable to be challenged. As a result, the practitioner's sense of meaningful commitment is undermined; they experience an identity crisis. This condition is the lot of many psychiatrists today, as highlighted by the recent formation of a task force that is to define the terms "psychiatrist" and "mental illness."[30] The liaison psychiatrist is potentially vulnerable to confusion about his professional identity too. Working as he does at the boundary between two professions and two distinct conceptual approaches to illness he is liable to be viewed with a critical eye by colleagues on either side. They may question his role, allegiance, credentials, and goals. To formulate his ideological base has relevance for the specialty as a whole.

Consultation–liaison psychiatry has derived conceptually from an old tradition in human thought, one that advocates a view of man as a body–mind complex in ceaseless dynamic interaction with the social and nonhuman environments. This holistic, antireductionist conception of man has achieved wide currency in the last 50 years. It has been applied to the theory and practice of medicine and psychiatry under the term "psychosomatic medicine."[3,31,32] The latter encompasses a body of assumptions, a research strategy, and a mode of approach to clinical practice. Unfortunately, psychosomatic medicine is often erroneously identified with a search for psychogenesis of ever more somatic disorders. This distorted view of the field has historical reasons. Psychosomatic medicine's first phase of development, roughly between 1930 and 1950, was dominated by psychoanalytic investigators and their attempts to explain the occurrence of certain somatic diseases, misnamed "psychosomatic," by invoking unconscious psychic processes and mechanisms. This reductionist tendency was most prominently and vocally represented by Alexander and his specificity hypotheses.[33] The foundering of his methodological approach nearly brought down with it psychosomatic medicine as a whole. It is necessary, therefore, to reaffirm a broad perspective of the field.

Psychosomatic medicine has recovered and grown in the past 20 years. It has a scientific and a clinical dimension. The former is represented by systematic research (experimental, clinical, and epidemiological) on the psychophysiological responses of the effects of these responses on health and disease. Related lines of research focus on the contribution of these social and psychophysiological factors to the predisposition to, precipitation, and time of onset, as well as course and outcome of, all diseases. Concurrently, other studies have explored the influence of physiological and biophysical variables on human behavior and subjective experience, normal and abnormal. The clinical dimension of psychosomatic medicine encompasses guidelines for a comprehensive approach to the diagnosis, management, and prevention of illness, and clinical and teaching activities applying psychosomatic postulates to the care of patients.[3,31]

Alexander, despite his methodological errors, deserves credit for formulating the principles of the psychosomatic approach.[33] His prediction of the course that psychiatry would follow is as timely as it is unfulfilled: "A growing integration of the biologic, psychodynamic and sociologic approaches, and the emergence of comprehensive psychiatry which no longer attempts to solve the great mystery of human behavior form one single restricted point of view."[34]

Consultation–liaison psychiatry represents application of the psychosomatic approach to clinical work. Its hallmark is the gathering and applying of information from several levels of abstraction relevant to patient care. Its basic assumption is that an integrated approach results in optimal health care, one sensitive to people's needs, mindful of prevention, and economically sound. Liaison psychiatrists can only modestly contribute to such care. Their major function is to demonstrate that it can be done and how. In the present fragmented state of medical practice resulting from overspecialization of physicians, the liaison psychiatrist is one of the few health professionals with a broad enough perspective to achieve a measure of integration of diverse data relevant to comprehensive evaluation and management of patients. To do so, the consultant needs training and experience of unique breadth as well as conceptual tools to integrate complex information and draw practical conclusions from it expeditiously.[21,22] He must think and communicate clearly and welcome complexity as an intellectual challenge. As our health delivery system becomes increasingly integrated and attuned to social demands, the need for broadly trained mediators will grow. Psychiatrists should aim deliberately at assuming the role of integrating health care and mediating between the overspecialized physicians on the one hand and the psychosocially oriented but medically naïve behavioral scientists on the other.

ORGANIZATION AND FUNDING

To be optimally effective and ensure continuity of service the consultants should work as a team. A consultation–liaison service should be an administrative unit treated as an integral and indispensable component of every psychiatric department of a general hospital or a community health clinic. Lack of organizational structure is liable to make the provision of consultations haphazard and vulnerable to the changing attitudes toward them of the heads of the departments of psychiatry, medicine, and other specialities. Only a firmly established service can function effectively, maintain liaison with other departments, and do justice to its clinical, teaching. and research commitments. A critic recently wrote that in the future, consultation services should be supplanted by the involvement of all full-time members of a psychiatric faculty in the work on the medical and surgical floors.[35] Yet to expect that all psychiatrists would be able and willing to act as consultants in unrealistic. This work requires special training and interest. Many competent psychiatrists choose to stay away from the often trying conditions of liaison work and contact with the physically ill. Neither competence nor interest in this work can be decreed. The practice of consultation–liaison psychiatry has always relied on a core group of people who freely chose to do it. The number of such individuals is liable to grow in response to changing emphases and incentives in health care delivery.

A consultation–liaison service should be staffed by full-time and part-time psychiatrists, liaison nurses,[36] social workers, and psychologists. They should form the operational core and be free to call upon willing colleagues to contribute to clinical work and teaching. The number of people involved will obviously depend upon the size of the hospital and the availability of staff and funds. The person in charge should be a senior psychiatrist who is experienced in this type of work, able to coordinate the activities of the service, and able to negotiate with other physicians on an equal footing.

It is generally desirable for a consultant to develop a special interest in and liaison with a particular department, ward, or clinic. Close liaison facilities continuity of service, development of a good relationship with staff, intimate knowledge of psychosocial problems characteristic of the given specialty, and collaborative research. There are valuable reports on liaison work with a wide range of specialties and clinical settings, such as internal medicine,[37] surgery,[38] pediatrics,[39] neurology and neurosurgery,[40] intensive care units,[41] oncology,[42] hemodialysis units,[43] emergency departments,[44] outpatient clinics,[45] and rehabilitation.[46]

One notes with concern that relatively few psychiatrists remain in liaison work for more than a few years. Reasons for this undesirable mobility need to be examined and overcome. Economic factors seem to play a major part. Under the prevailing conditions, no psychiatrist can earn an average income by confining himself to consultation–liaison work. Much of what he does, if he does it right, is highly time-consuming and not remunerated. Insurance plans pay for a consultation but not for time spent in liaison work. The best solution is a salary for a block of time, which could be spent consulting, supervising residents, teaching, etc. A properly functioning liaison service cannot be financially self-sufficent if it relies on fees for consultations. Funds have to come from the department of psychiatry, from the departments that avail themselves of the consultant's liaison services, and from insurance plans.

Conditions of work discourage some consultants. Relationships with consultees may be frustrating.[47,48] A consultant encounters much indifference, ambivalence, and overt and covert hostility from his medical and surgical colleagues. Their negative attitudes are often expressed subtly and jovially and are sometimes disguised with effusive cordiality. The enmity of a department head may thwart liaison work. The consultant's advice may be acknowledged but not acted upon, patients may be referred to him without adequate preparation,[49] or they may be abruptly discharged before he has completed his evaluation. It may take years of close liaison with a particular department before a consultant becomes accepted and can work effectively. Much depends on his own attitude and ability to demonstrate his usefulness. If he is able to communicate clearly, displays sound clinical judgment, offers useful advice on the management of patients, and teaches well, he stands a good chance of becoming a valued member of the team.[40]

To endure, the consultant needs reasonable economic security, the support of his colleagues, time for continued study, and interest in his work. He needs ties with his department of psychiatry, where he can contribute his special expertise and psychosomatic viewpoint. His professional satisfaction derives from viewing his work as useful and rich in intellectual challenge provided by ever new and often highly complex clinical problems.

FUNCTIONS OF CONSULTANTS

These functions fall into three categories: clinical work, teaching, and research. They deserve separate discussion.

CLINICAL WORK

In addition to liaison work, diagnostic and therapeutic activities constitute a consultant's clinical function. The diagnostic problems that he encounters fall into several types. First, the patient may present with somatic complaints for which no convincing organic explanation can be found.[50] They may indicate the presence of a psychiatric disorder or psychosocial stress or both. Depression of all degrees of severity is the commonest disorder encountered and may mimic, accompany, or mask many somatic diseases.[2] Hysterical, anxiety, and hypochondriacal neuroses are common; schizophrenia is less so.[2] Second, a patient may display a change in his habitual behavior, i.e., either accentuation or alteration of his characteristic personality. This may signify cerebral disease, functional psychiatric disorder, or an unclassifiable behavioral response to physical illness or interpersonal stress or both.[2,26] To evaluate such change demands familiarity with psychological manifestations of cerebral disorders and of many systemic diseases: endocrine, neoplastic, etc.[51] Third, the patient may suffer from an obvious psychiatric disorder that the consultee has recognized and for which he wants advice on management. And fourth, the patient may display deviant illness behavior, such as self-destructive noncompliance with medical advice, excessive dependence, gross denial of illness, a given-up attitude, factitial illness, or suicide threats or attempts.[3]

Such a broad range of diagnostic problems is not usually encountered in other areas of psychiatry. They call for a comprehensive evaluation that may require several interviews and a thorough knowledge of medicine and psychiatry. In many cases no definitive diagnosis can be reached due to lack of reliable techniques to discern the underlying pathogenic mechanisms of many complaints, both psychological and somatic. To label a symptom as "conversion," "psychosomatic," or "psychophysiological" is often an admission of ignorance. To fit a patient's unexplained somatic symptoms into a plausible cause-and-effect sequence involving his intrapsychic dynamics may be deceptively easy but misleading. To establish such a relationship may be impossible in the short time available. There is a pressing need for more research aimed at development of diagnostic techniques in the area of "mysterious medical complaints,"[50] which are found in more than 50% of medical outpatients and in at least 30% of all inpatients, regardless of whether a physical illness is known to be present. Investigations and medical treatment of such symptoms cost vast sums of money.[52] The initial psychosocial evaluation every patient could help reduce the rising costs of health care related to redundant laboratory tests and treatment of psychosocial problems by medical and surgical techniques.

A consultation is useless unless it results in practical recommendations. Additional investigations may be suggested, concrete advice on the psychological approach to the patient or his family given, and specific therapy or disposition recommended. The consultant may have to follow up the patient in the hospital and after discharge and carry out therapeutic procedures himself. It is misleading to view a consultation as consisting of but a brief, single diagnostic interview. We average two visits for every referred inpatient; many are seen daily for a week or more. Medical wards and clinics are a valuable setting for time-limited psychotherapy (individual, group, marital couple, and family).[53] Group therapy is useful for special groups, such as survivors of myocardial infarction.[54] Behavior modification, biofeedback, and hypnosis are used for selected medical problems. A thorough familiarity with psychotropic drugs, their deleterious side effects in various somatic disorders, and their application for psychiatric emergencies common in medicine, such as delirium, is essential.

Thus a consultant is invariably a therapist. His intervention is guided by the following principles: clear and prompt definition of therapeutic goals, both immediate and long-term, based on comprehensive assessment; choice of therapy tailored to a given patient's individual needs and coping capacity; flexibility in the conduct of therapy; and incisive intervention by the therapist in order to achieve his goals expeditiously. It is erroneous to assert that the results of such intervention are at best symptomatic and that its goals are confined to treating the immediate crisis. Whenever possible, an attempt is made to facilitate self-understanding, prevent maladaptive coping, and enhance personal growth. Emerging trends in health care delivery will increasingly favor this type of approach, i.e., selective, time-limited, and preventive.[55]

TEACHING

Every liaison psychiatrist acts as a teacher. The teaching need not be formal: He can teach by providing a conceptual model and example. His role in teaching psychiatry, especially as it pertains to medical practice, has expanded steadily.[56] This teaching is extended to medical students and residents, physicians, nurses, social workers, and physicians' assistants. Medical students are the prime concern of the liaison teacher. He can demonstrate at the bedside and in clinical conferences, seminars, and informal discussion groups such crucial skills as interviewing techniques, approach to comprehensive diagnosis and management, personality assessment, proper use of drugs and brief psychotherapy, etc.[56] At our hospital every senior medical student is expected to act as a consultee, that is, to initiate a referral for psychiatic consultation, follow its progress, and discuss the findings and recommendations with the consultant. In this way the students learn what to expect from a psychiatric consultation, how to prepare a patient for it, and how to act on the advice received.

Psychiatric residents should spend at least 3 months in full-time liaison work in their second or third year of training. In this way they learn to view patients comprehensively, that is, to take into account psychodynamic, somatic, social, and economic factors as elements of an integrated approach to diagnosis, treatment, and prevention of any illness.[57] In addition, experience on a liaison service helps them learn to communicate clearly, collaborate with other health professionals, and apply psychiatric knowledge and therapy under time pressure. Use of woolly jargon, fanatical adherence to a single psychiatric theory or technique, and free-floating psychodynamic speculation based on sparse information are discouraged. Such training helps develop skills that the residents will find useful in future practice.

CLINICAL RESEARCH

Liaison psychiatrists have made numerous and varied research contributions. They have access to vast clinical material and excellent laboratory facilities. There are many opportunities for collaborative clinical research at the interface of the medical and behavioral sciences.[5] Some of the most exciting research today lies in the borderlands between the various scientific disciplines concerned with man.[27,29,31,32,58]

Liaison psychiatrists have investigated such diverse topics as delirium, fainting, and hyperventilation; clinical psychophysiology of all body systems; attitudes toward death and experience of fatal illness and dying; psychosocial antecedents of illness on-set; psychological reactions to and coping with all types of illness and disability; psychiatric aspects of new medical technologies; psychological impact of hospital environ-ments; and the process of consultation and its outcome.[10,18,20,27,31,59] These are merely representative examples to illustrate the fact that closer liaison with medicine has opened up an area of research relevant to both medicine and the science of behavior.

CONSULTATION-LIAISON: A MODEL FOR FUTURE PSYCHIATRY

Comprehensive health care is medicine's overriding social objective today. In order to achieve it, we will need professionals skilled at integration. Their integrative skills should include referral, consultation, liaison, and interprofessional communication necessitated by increasing differentiation of roles in the health care field.[60] Basic to these skills are cognitive foundations enabling a holistic approach to individual patients. As health professionals become increasingly specialized, their ability and willingness to perceive and deal with more than a circumscribed segment of a patient's problems decrease. For some patients a focal approach suffices, but for the majority it does not. Someone will have to evaluate and integrate the medical and psychosocial data per-taining to diagnosis, management, and prevention of illness. Communication and liaison between the medically and the psychosocially trained members of a health team, with their distinct conceptual approaches, techniques, and languages, will have to be main-tained. *It is in the area of integration of comprehensive health care that the psy-chiatrist's future role will lie.* He will function mostly as consultant, integrator, and liaison man.[35] Consultation–liaison psychiatry provides a relevant role model, evolved over the past 40 years, that the specialty should adopt in order to secure a distinct place in tomorrow's health system and avoid disintegration. This postulate has obvious im-plications for psychiatrist's training, attitudes, and skills. It is germane to spell them out.

Training of unique breadth and complexity is indispensable. Its two basic com-ponents are thorough medical training and acquisition of expert knowledge about man as a body–mind complex in social interaction. This implies that psychiatrists must be both physicians and broadly trained experts in the sciences of individual and group be-havior. Only such psychosomatic and humanistic cognitive preparation can enable the psychiatrist to function as an integrator within a highly differentiated health team. We cannot afford opportunistic shortcuts in training for the sake of expediency. The psy-chiatrist as a half-baked doctor with an ill-defined psychosocial orientation and nar-row therapeutic skills would become an extinct professional. Attempts to restrict psy-chiatric training to a single school of psychiatric thought or therapeutic technique must be resisted.

The core training should include exposure to all behavioral sciences and ground-ing in the broad range of therapeutic techniques available today. It should foster clear communication, diagnostic reasoning, and an open-minded scientific attitude. Com-plexity, uncertainty, and diversity inherent in our field should be presented to the trainees as an intellectual challege that makes this profession uniquely exciting. Those who cannot tolerate complexity and the lack of immutable, easily assimilable verities and guidelines should be discouraged from continuing psychiatric training. The future psychiatrist will need familiarity with all treatment modalities that offer some relief of suffering of individuals and help them attain what growth, as persons, they are capable of. He can be proficient in only one or a few of them. There is no therapy that only a psychiatrist can perform. Much of the treatment he now performs will be taken over by other specialized professionals. His therapeutic work will but complement his liaison and consulting functions, which *together* will comprise his specific role within a health team.

The professions of psychiatry and medicine can best discharge their social and mutual responsibilities by collaborating closely in teaching, disease prevention, research, and health care delivery. Liaison psychiatrists have contributed toward this goal. Their work provides a viable model for the psychiatry of tomorrow.

REFERENCES

1. Lipowski ZJ: Review of consultation psychiatry and psychosomatic medicine: General principles. *Psychosom Med* 29:153–171, 1967.
2. Lipowski ZJ: Review of consultation psychiatry and psychosomatic medicine, II: Clinical aspects. *Psychosom Med* 29:201–224, 1967.
3. Lipowski ZJ: Reivew of consultation psychiatry and psychosomatic medicine, III: Theoretical issues. *Pschosom Med* 30:395–422, 1968.
4. Lipowski ZJ: Consultation-liaison psychiatry in a general hospital. *Compr Psychiatry* 12:461–465, 1971.
5. Kaufman MR (ed): *The Psychiatric Unit in a General Hospital.* New York, International Universities Press, 1965.
6. Guze SB, Matarazzo JD, Saslow G: A formulation of principles of comprehensive medicine with speical reference to learning theory. *J Clin Psychol* 9:127–136, 1953.
7. Sweeney GH: Pioneering general hospital psychiatry. *Psychiatr Q* 36(suppl, part 2):209–268, 1962.
8. Henry GW: Some modern aspects of psychiatry in general hospital practice. *Am J Psychiatry* 86:481–499, 1929.
9. Billings EG: The psychiatric liaison department of the University of Colorado Medical School and Hospitals. *Am J Psychiatry* 122 (June suppl): 28–33, 1966.
10. Dunbar FH, Wolfe TP, Rioch JM: Psychiatric aspects of medical problems. *Am J Psychiatry* 93:649–679, 1936.
11. Kaufman MR: A psychiatric unit in a general hospital. *J Mount Sinai Hosp, NY* 24:572–579, 1957.
12. Bernstein S, Kaufman MR: The psychiatrist in a general hospital. *J Mount Sinai Hosp, NY* 29:385–394, 1962.
13. Kaufman MR, Margolin SG: Theory and practice of psychosomatic medicine in a general hospital. *Med Clin North Am* 32:611–616, 1948.
14. Mendel WM: Psychiatric consultation education—1966. *Am J Psychiatry* 123:150–155, 1966.
15. Krakowski AJ: Consultation psychiatry: present global status—a survey. *Psychother Psychosom* 23:78–86, 1974.
16. Schwab JJ: *Handbook of Psychiatric Consultation.* New York, Appleton-Century-Crofts, 1968.
17. Mannino FV: *Consultation in Mental Health and Related Fields.* Chevy Chase, Md, National Institute of Mental health, 1969.
18. Mannino FV, Shore MF: *Consultation Research in Mental Health and Related Fields.* Public Health Monograph No 79. Washington, DC, US Department of Health, Education, and Welfare, 1971.
19. Bibring GL: Psychiatry and medical practice in a general hospital. *N Engl J Med* 154:366–372, 1956.
20. Meyer E, Mendelson M: Psychiatric consultations with patients on medical and surgical wards: patterns and processes. *Psychiatry* 24:197–220, 1961.

21. Miller WB: Psychiatric consultation, part I: A general systems approach. *Psychiatry Med* 4:135-145, 1973.
22. Miller WB: Psychiatric consultation, part II: conceptual and pragmatic issues of formulation. *Psychiatry Med* 4:251-271, 1973.
23. Sandt JJ, Leifer R: The psychiatric consultation. *Compr Psychiatry* 5:409-418, 1964.
24. American Hospital Association: *Mental Health Services and the General Hospital.* Chicago, AHA, 1970.
25. Issacharoff A, Redinger R, Schneider D: The psychiatric consultation as an experience in group process. *Contemp Psychoanaly* 8:260-275, 1972.
26. Brodsky CM: A social view of the psychiatric consultation. *Psychosomatics* 8:61-68, 1967.
27. Lipowski ZJ: The patient, his illness and environment: psychosocial foundations of medicine, in Ariet: S (ed): *American Handbook of Psychiatry*, ed. 2, New York, Basic Books vol 4, 1975, pp. 3-42.
28. Livsey CG: Physical illness and family dynamics, in Lipowski ZJ (ed): *Psychosocial Aspects of Physical Illness.* Basel, Karger, 1972, pp 237-251.
29. Engel GL: Is psychiatry failing in its responsibility to medicine? *Am J Psychiatry* 128:1561-1563, 1972.
30. What is a psychiatrist? *Psychiatr News*, Nov 21, 1973, p 13.
31. Lipowski ZJ: New perspectives in psychosomatic medicine. *Can Psychiatr Assoc J* 15:515-525, 1970.
32. Lipowski ZJ: Psychosomatic medicine in a changing society: some current trends in theory and research. *Compr Psychiatry* 14:203-215, 1973.
33. Alexander F: *Psychosomatic Medicine.* New York, WW Norton & Co, 1950.
34. Alexander F: The next ten years in psychiatry. *Am J Psychother* 12:438-442, 1958.
35. West LJ: The future of psychiatric education. *Am J Psychiatry* 130:521-528, 1973.
36. Barton D, Kelso MT: The nurse as a psychiatric consultation team member. *Psychiatry Med* 2:108-115, 1971.
37. Abrahams D, Golden JS: Psychiatric consultations on a medical ward. *Arch Intern Med* 112:766-774, 1963.
38. Baudry F, Wiener A: Initiation of a psychiatric teaching program for surgeons. *Am J Psychiatry* 125:1192, 1969.
39. Rothenberg MB: Child psychiatry-pediatrics liaison. A history and commentary. *J Am Acad Child Psychiatry* 7:492-509, 1968.
40. Lipowski ZJ: Psychiatric liaison with neurology and neurosurgery. *Am J Psychiatry* 129:136-140, 1972.
41. Cassem NH, Hackett TP: Psychiatric consultation in a coronary care unit. *Ann Intern Med* 75:9-14, 1971.
42. Janes RG, Weisz AE: Psychiatric liaison with a cancer research center. *Compr Psychiatry* 11:336-345, 1970.
43. Kaplan De-Nour A: Role and reactions of psychiatrists in chronic hemodialysis programs. *Psychiatry Med* 4:63-76, 1973.
44. Bartolucci G, Drayer CS: An overview of crisis intervention in the emergency rooms of general hospitals. *Am J Psychiatry* 130:953-960, 1973.
45. Lipowski ZJ, Ramsay RA, Villard HP: Psychiatric consultations in medical and surgical outpatient clinics. *Can Psychiatr Assoc J* 14:239-245, 1969.
46. Gunther MS: Psychiatric consultation in a rehabilitation hospital. *Compr Psychiatry* 12:572-585, 1971.
47. Mendelson M, Meyer E: Countertransference problems of the liaison psychiatrist. *Psychosom Med* 23:115-122, 1961.
48. Abram HS: Interpersonal aspects of psychiatric consultations in a general hospital. *Psychiatry Med* 2:321-326, 1971.
49. Hale ML, Abram HS: Patients' attitudes toward psychiatric consultations in the general hospital. *Va Med Mon* 94:342-347, 1967.
50. Goodwin DW: Psychiatry and the mysterious medical complaint. *JAMA* 209:1884-1888, 1969.
51. Peterson HW, Martin MJ: Organic disease presenting as a psychiatric syndrome. *Postgrad Med* 54:78-83, 1973.
52. Goshen CE: Functional versus organic diagnostic problems. *NY State J Med* 69:2332-2338, 1969.
53. Stein EH, Murdaugh J, Macleod JA: Brief psychotherapy of psychiatric reactions to physical illness. *Am J Psychiatry* 125:1040-1047, 1969.
54. Rahe RH, Tuffli CF, Suchor RJ, *et al:* Group therapy in the out-patient management of post-myocardial infarction patients. *Psychiatry Med* 4:77-88, 1973.

55. Paris J: Psychiatric practice in Canada pre- and post-medicare. *Can Med Assoc J* 109:469–470, 1973.
56. McKegney PF: Consultation-liaison teaching of psychosomatic medicine: opportunities and obstacles. *J Nerv Ment Dis* 154:198–205, 1972.
57. Small IF, Foster LG, Small JG, et al: Teaching the art and skill of psychiatric consultation. *Dis Nerv Syst* 29:817–822, 1968.
58. Lipowski ZJ, Lipsitt DR, Whybrow PC (eds): *Psychosomatic Medicine: Current Trends, and Clinical Applications.* New York, Oxford University Press, 1977.
59. Lipowski ZJ (ed): *Psychosocial Aspects of Physical Illness.* Basel, Karger, 1972.
60. Harper AC: Towards a job description for comprehensive health care–A framework for education and management. *Soc Sci Med* 7:291–301, 1973.

Psychiatric Consultation

Concepts and Controversies

22

Consultation is one of the main professional activities of psychiatrists. Nearly 70% of the respondents to a 1970 nationwide survey of American psychiatrists stated that they engaged in it.[1] Consultation accounted for about 10% of their working time and was practiced in 18 different settings. Consultation was not explicitly defined in the survey, but it was distinguished from direct patient contact. Thus, by implication, the authors of the survey and the respondents considered consultation to be an indirect service, one not involving contact with patients. This view of psychiatric consultation is not shared by all of its practitioners. There is no general agreement on what the term implies. Such ambiguity leads to misunderstandings. Clarification is worth attempting if we are to talk intelligibly about the role of the psychiatrist as a consultant. I will focus my discussion on current concepts and controversies in this important area of psychiatry.

DEFINITIONS OF TWO LEADING MODELS

One may distinguish two major models of consultation in the mental health field today. I shall refer to them as the *psychiatric–therapeutic* and the social–reformist or *community mental health* models, respectively. The former may be defined as rendering a professional opinion on a patient's mental state or psychiatric problem, as well as its management, at the request of another health professional. This type of consultation usually involves explicit consent (if not an actual request) by the patient, is focused on him, and may be regarded as an integral aspect of health care delivery. The consultee acts as an agent for the patient and is given information on the patient by the consultant for the purpose of adequate diagnosis and proper management. The purpose of this type of consultation is diagnostic and therapeutic.[2]

Community mental health consultation refers to provision of advice on problems related to mental health to clients who wish to improve their ability to identify, prevent, and help solve such problems in other people. The ultimate purpose of such consultation is improvement of a society's level of mental health according to preconceived norms and standards. In this sense one can refer to this consultation model as social–

reformist. Its practitioners strive to prevent the occurrence of what they regard as undesirable attitudes, feelings, and behaviors and to promote desirable ones in as many people as possible. They do so primarily by offering guidance to willing helpers, who need not be health professionals.

These two models will be further described and contrasted with reference to their basic dimensions.

BASIC DIMENSIONS OF CONSULTATION

Every consultation, psychiatric or otherwise, may be viewed as having the following six basic aspects or demensions: goal, participants, setting, process, methods, and outcome.[3] These dimensions must be specified for the given type of consultation for the purpose of meaningful comparison, study, and evaluation. I shall first define these dimensions for the class of consultations that I have termed "psychiatric-therapeutic," hereafter referred to as "psychiatric."

PSYCHIATRIC–THERAPEUTIC CONSULTATION

Psychiatric consultation may be viewed as a modified form of the traditional medical consultation. It continues an ancient custom of providing professional advice on the diagnosis and management of a patient to a colleague who requests it. Such advice presupposes special expertise on the part of the consultant. It is usually based on a direct contact with the patient. Psychiatric consultation follows this model with some important modifications.[2] Its primary focus is the patient's psychological state and well-being. In contrast to the traditional medical consultation, however, the inquiry and recommendations often encompass the patient's interpersonal relationships, especially those with his family, the doctor, and other members of the medical team. Conflicts and inadequate communication between the patient and these relevant others constitute an extended focus of psychiatric consultation in health care settings. Furthermore, the consultant often attempts direct therapy even within the scope of a single diagnostic interview. This fact justifies calling this type of consultation "psychiatric–therapeutic."

The goal of psychiatric consultation is the provision of optimal health care for the individual patient. This implies accurate diagnosis, effective management and rehabilitation, and prevention or amelioration of psychiatric morbidity. The participants include a consultant who is a trained mental health professional, one or more consultees who are health professionals concerned with patient care, and a patient. The term "patient" designates any person who believes himself, or has been found by a health professional, to be ill and is thus a candidate for the sick role. One of the functions of psychiatric consultation is to help decide whether a given patient's assumption of the sick role should be legitimized and encouraged or discouraged.

The consultant may be a psychiatrist or a psychiatrically trained nonmedical expert, such as a clinical psychologist, a psychiatric social worker, or a liaison nurse. The degree and specific area of a consultant's expertise will vary depending on the scope of his training and professional experience. A consultee is, by definition, a trained provider of some aspects of health care. The setting for psychiatric consultation is any health care facility, be it hospital, community clinic, or a consultant's office. The process and method of psychiatric consultation vary according to the kind of participants and setting involved. Typically, the process is composed of several stages that include receipt of a request for consultation, formulation of the problem to be explored, gathering of information relevant to it, drawing and communicating conclusions from the received information, and making practical recommendations. The principal method of the consultation is the interview.

The above are the basic elements of psychiatric consultation. It is an activity that involves definable knowledge, method, and skills. It has a clear-cut focus and therapeutic as well as teaching and preventive functions. Its objectives are pragmatic and attuned to the needs of a large but operationally delimited constituency of people, namely, those who seek medical attention. Before further discussing the role of the psychiatrist as a consultant in this context, I will examine the second conception of consultation.

COMMUNITY MENTAL HEALTH CONSULTATION

The National Institute of Mental Health (NIMH) has published a monograph titled *The Practice of Mental Health Consultation*.[4] Its authors defined mental health consultation as "the provision of technical assistance by an expert to individual and agency caregivers related to the mental health dimensions of their work" (pp. 4–5). This definition seems to be inspired by Caplan's view of mental health consultation as an activity aimed at the promotion of mental health.[5] It was also he who proposed that the consultees should include a broad spectrum of people called the "caregiving professionals," ranging from physicians and nurses to clergymen, lawyers, and policemen. This conception of consultation differs in several crucial aspects from psychiatric consultation as here defined. These differences will be made explicit for the purpose of comparison.

The promotion of mental health as a goal of consultation contrasts with provision of optimal patient care. It is a much broader aim, one that must predicate a point of view about the criteria of mental health. There is no universally accepted set of such criteria, as Jahoda argued in her monograph on the concepts of positive mental health.[6] She remarked perceptively that mental health workers display almost religious fervor and see in positive mental health "a panacea for all evil and all social problems or for the whole improvement of mankind." This penetrating comment was written before the peak flowering of the community mental health movement. To label this conception of consultation as "social–reformist" captures its thrust. It is clearly distinct from the psychiatric–therapeutic conception. The participants include a wide range of potential consultees, the caregiving professionals. As the authors of the NIMH-sponsored monograph stated, "There is a mental health and human relations dimension to all human activities; consequently, almost anyone in the community may seek consultation from a community mental health center."[4, p. 11] The crucial point is that a consultation in this context is sought and provided for the promotion of *somebody else's* mental health. The patient is not a participant in the process. In fact, the very word "patient" is irrelevant in this context.

The settings, process, and methods of mental health consultation also differ from those of psychiatric consultation. The direct therapeutic aspect is absent. The number of possible settings is infinite, and they are certainly not confined to health care facilities. Thus the two conceptions of consultation differ from each other on most of the basic elements. This observation does not imply that either conception should be viewed as the only valid one. There is room for the practice of both types of consultation. However, controversies arise when one addresses the issues of priorities in the deployment of consultants and of their role and the boundaries of their expertise. One's position on these issues tends to reflect personal bias and convictions since factual data are notoriously scarce. My bias is that of a psychiatric consultant working in a general hospital. I believe that the consultant's role should be defined and restricted by his training, professional experience, and skills. I propose that in view of the actual needs for service and the limited manpower, the consultants should function primarily in the framework of the health care delivery system.

The main criticisms of the community mental health consultation may be summarized as follows: Its objectives are unduly vague. It purports to promote mental health, a concept that is laden with value judgments and lends itself to exploitation by political and other special interest groups concerned with power and manipulation of people rather than with health. The role of the consultant in this context is unclear and can be readily misconstrued. He may be viewed as an infallible judge, prophet, and fixer of human attitudes and behavior. If he gives in to the temptation to play such a role, he will run the risk of being called an impostor. Psychiatrists would be rightly discredited if they assumed the roles of social reformers and engineers, roles for which they neither are trained nor possess the requisite knowledge and skills.

The above criticisms must not be misunderstood to imply that psychiatrists should not practice preventive psychiatry when this is soundly based. It is surely desirable to offer mental health consultation to schools, industry, courts of law, and other institutions and organizations, provided that the consultants are trained for the type of work and setting in which they operate and that they confine their advice to problems of bona fide *mental health*.

NEED TO RESTRICT SCOPE OF CONSULTATIONS

The consultant's role ought to be restricted to avoid the pitfalls of unrealistic promises inherent in the overly broad and vague definition of consultation. No individual can claim to be an expert in all facets of a human behavior and thus a potential consultant to all and sundry. This obvious stricture needs to be stressed in view of the current tendency to propagate the role of the mental health consultant as an ominiscient fixer of faulty psychosocial functioning of any kind and in every setting. For example, the sociodynamic model of consultation, promulgated by some writers, is said to focus on "mental health input to the wide range of agents and agencies comprising the socialization community."[7] The hollow ring of this statement reflects the conceptual muddle that pervades much of the writing on mental health consultation. The concept of the "caregiving professional" is so diffuse that it perilously overextends the consultant's role and scope of operation. The latter should be restricted to the mental health concerns of a particular institution or organization, be it school, court, or factory, with whose specific problems the consultant is familiar and where he can consult as an expert.

PSYCHIATRIC CONSULTATION IN HEALTH CARE CONTEXTS

I wish to propose that psychiatric consultation should be an integral aspect of mental health services offered in the context of comprehensive health care systems. As Coleman and Patrick[8] have argued, the medical facilities are the only social resource that can provide adequate and generally accessible primary health care; psychiatric services should be part of this care. Thus medical facilities of all types should be the setting in which most psychiatric consultants operate. There is a vast unmet need for psychiatric services, including consultation–liaison activities, in medical settings, in which psychiatrists can use their uniquely broad training to the best advantage and most effectively.

PREVALENCE OF PSYCHIATRIC MORBIDITY IN MEDICAL SETTINGS

Epidemiological studies carried out during the last 20 years have documented the high incidence of emotional disorders in all major segments of medical practice.[9-13] A recent British survey revealed that 109 patients of every 1000 who went to general practitioners suffered from a mental disorder.[12] In the United States it has been reported that 12% to 15% of adult patients who went to family physicians had symptoms of an emotional disorder[9]; These patients account for an estimated 30% of all office visits during any one year.[9] A recent report from the Columbia Point Health Center in Boston, Massachusetts, revealed that during a typical year 109 of every 1000 people who went to the health center received at least one psychiatric diagnosis[14]; this figure is identical to that found in the British morbidity survey cited by Shepherd.[12] Canadian family physicians have reported that 8% of their patients had psychiatric disorders; depression and anxiety neurosis headed the list of psychiatric diagnoses and ranked ahead of diabetes, hypertension, and ischemic heart disease.[13]

The incidence of psychiatric morbidity has been reported to be even higher in medical outpatient clinics than in family practice. A study of 4000 consecutive new patients admitted to the medical clinic of a large Canadian teaching hospital revealed that 30% had a psychiatric disorder believed to be relevant to the presenting symptoms.[13] The most common symptoms were abdominal and chest pain; these were attributed to a psychiatric disorder in 28% and 26% of the cases, respectively. These percentages were underestimates; they did not include patients who received no diagnosis at all. A review of the literature showed that 30% to 60% of medical inpatients and 50% to 80% of medical outpatients had a psychiatric disorder.[15] Studies of prevalence of depression alone among medical inpatients revealed that 20% to 25% were significantly depressed.[10,16] The incidence of depression among hospitalized cardiac patients has been reported to be about 65%.[10] Furthermore, a number of studies have documented a positive association between psychiatric and physical illness.[10]

Studies of referrals for psychiatric consultation in general hospitals have shown that only 5% to 10% of the medical and surgical patients were referred.[15] Depression was the most common disorder diagnosed by liaison consultants and accounted for at least 50% of all referrals.[17] A study by my associates and me of 1000 referrals for psychiatric consultation showed that 23% of the referred inpatients had no evidence of a physical illness and 68% had both a medical and a psychiatric disorder.[17] These findings highlight the existence of two major patient populations in need of psychiatric consultation and liaison in the medical setting: those who present somatic symptoms in the absence of organic pathology and those who suffer from concurrent physical and psychiatric illness.

The so-called worried–well patients, who perceive themselves as sick in the absence of objective evidence of organic disease, have been estimated to account for 50% of the cost of the Kaiser–Permanente Health Plan prepaid practice.[18] It is one of the assumptions of a systems approach to health care as practiced at Kaiser that integration of mental and physical health care reduces the enormous cost of unnecessary medical services. There is a widespread tendency in our society to define problems in living as problems of health and to seek medical consultation for them. Sociocultural factors favor presenting discontent and emotional distress in the form of somatic complaints.[19]

People who have experienced recent life changes or long-standing dissatisfaction with their life conditions (mostly family and work) use medical care facilities very often.[20] This tendency contributes to the staggering cost of medical care in the United States. Unnecessary laboratory tests and therapeutic procedures, overutilization of medical facilities, and misplaced sanctioning of the sick role by physicians are among the relevant factors.

Psychosocial screening and brief therapeutic intervention by mental health professionals acting as consultants in medical settings can help contain the cost resulting from needless tests and medical visits. As early as 1941 Billings had reported that introduction of liaison psychiatrists to a general hospital resulted in reduced diagnostic and therapeutic procedures, shortened hospitalization, and thus created savings for patients and community.[21] Short-term outpatient psychiatric therapy offered to selected patients in a prepaid group practice medical program in Washington, D.C., in 1970 resulted in the reduction of visits, laboratory tests, and X-ray procedures by about 30%.[22] Introduction of social workers and casework to a hospital-based primary care program has been shown to result in greater cost effectiveness of ambulatory care[23]; the crucial element was the early detection and management of psychosocial problems.

RATIONAL DEPLOYMENT OF CONSULTANTS

The above facts and figures document the need for mental health consultants in all health care settings. Liaison psychiatrists, social workers, nurses, and psychologists are needed to help with diagnostic assessment, patient management, rehabilitation, and teaching psychosocial aspects of medicine to medical students and physicians. By virtue of their medical training, psychiatrists ought to play a key role as consultants and integrators.[2,3]

Geographic and conceptual separation of mental health care from medical health care is a costly anachronism.[8] It ignores results of epidemiological studies and contributes to fragmented and thus inferior patient care. Availability of psychiatric consultation and liaison services to other health professionals in both hospital and community could contribute to the prevention of psychiatric morbidity, psychogenic invalidism, and unwarranted assumption of the sick role. This could result in better patient care, avoidance of needless disability, and reduction in the cost of health care. To achieve these goals we need to train future consultants and provide economic and intellectual incentives to make their work satisfying.

TRAINING OF CONSULTANTS

Preparing psychiatrists for the consultant role should be one of the main objectives of residency training programs.[24] A recent survey showed that only 10% of the total residency training time is spent in consultation–liaison work.[25] This is inadequate. The Psychiatry Education Branch of NIMH has recognized this and assigned high priority to the support of consultation–liaison services,[26] which offer not only direct service but also teaching for psychiatric residents, medical students, and other health professionals.[2,3]

PSYCHIATRIC RESIDENTS

Rotation on a consultation–liaison service has become an integral component of psychiatric residency.[25] To be effective this rotation should occur not earlier than the second year and should be full-time for a minimum of 3 months. It should encompass clinical experience on an organized liaison service and teaching in the form of clinical conferences and theoretical seminars devoted to psychosomatic medicine and the theory of consultation. Psychosomatic medicine provides an indispensable conceptual framework for liaison work.[2] Without it the liaison psychiatrist would lack the broad perspective and intellectual challenge in his work that are essential for professional satisfaction.

Clinical skills that the residents need to acquire during their rotation include eliciting and integrating information about patients along several dimensions: psychological, sociocultural, medical, and economic.[27] The resident also learns to formulate conclusions clearly and expeditiously, to communicate them in plain English, to mediate between patients and those taking care of them, and to render consultation that is therapeutic for the patient and useful to the consultee.[2,3] Medical wards provide a setting in which the resident can put to a rigorous test his knowledge of psychiatry, ability to apply it under time pressure, and ability to interact with other health professionals.

MEDICAL STUDENTS

Increasing numbers of students spend part of all of their psychiatric rotation on a liaison service.[25] The students will be the consultees of the future. The psychiatric liaison service rotation not only exposes them to the psychosocial problems and psychiatric disorders with which they will have to deal as physicians but also teaches them how to refer patients for psychiatric consultation, what to expect from it, and how to implement the consultant's advice.[24]

POSTRESIDENCY FELLOWS

The number of postresidency fellowship programs in consultation–liaison psychiatry is growing.[24] This training is designed for future practitioners and teachers in this area, and the curricula differ from program to program. Some appear to stress liaison in juxtaposition to "mere" consultation; this is a mistake. Both consultation and liaison are integral aspects of the same clinical activity.[2,3] To separate them would be divisive and misleading. A liaison service that fails to provide routine psychiatric consultations is as inadequate as one that ignores the value of extended contacts with the consultees and the mediating function of the consultants.[2,3]

A fellowship typically involves 1 year of full-time work on a liaison service and has three components: clinical experience, teaching, and research. Clinical work should involve both exposure to a wide range of referrals and liaison with a medical or surgical ward of a special unit such as a coronary care unit, oncology, or neurology. Teaching involves supervision of psychiatric residents and medical students and seminars for medical residents and nurses. A clinical research project should be undertaken by fellows to expose them to research techniques and help them acquire an investigative or scholarly bent. The program should also include seminars on psychosomatic medicine in its broad sense.[28,29]

NEED FOR EVALUATION

Evaluation of the effectiveness of consultation is of crucial importance. Only a handful of evaluative studies of psychiatric consultation in general hospitals have been published.[3] Several criteria for evaluating the outcome of consultation–liaison work may be suggested, such as patient satisfaction, consultee satisfaction, relief of symptoms, length of hospitalization, utilization of laboratory tests, social functioning after discharge, degree of compliance with consultant's advice, and, last but not least, reduction in the cost of medical care. A related task is the assessment of the impact, if any, of the teaching of psychiatry and psychosocial aspects of medicine on medical practice. The relevant criteria of effectiveness should include the quality of medical records, timeliness and appropriateness of referrals for consultation, enhanced diagnostic and psychotherapeutic skills of the consultee, utilization of the services of liaison nurses and social services, consultee compliance with consultant's advice, and greater patient satisfaction with medical care and hospitalization.

With increasing scrutiny of the cost effectiveness of all aspects of medical practice, consultation–liaison work needs to demonstrate its effectiveness as a clinical and teaching activity. Only reasonable proof of its effectiveness will secure funding of liaison services in the future. Studies must start now.

CONCLUSIONS AND PROPOSALS

I have compared and contrasted two major current models of consultation in psychiatry. I have pointed out areas of controversy and advocated a point of view that is based on the conviction that psychiatry is first and foremost a medical specialty and its place is in the health care delivery system. Psychiatrists are not social reformers or engineers, nor are they magic healers offering solutions for all dilemmas of the human condition. Consultation is one of their main professional activities. To meet current social needs, psychiatric consultations should be offered primarily in the context of health care delivery. Community mental health consultation has a place in schools, factories, or courts. Its goal should be primarily preventive.

The following propositions summarize my discussion:

1. Two distinct conceptions of consultation in our field vie for recognition and influence: psychiatric–therapeutic consultation and community mental health consultation. These differ in their goals, participants, settings, and methods.

2. To enhance the value of consultation for the consultees and to avoid misleading them, the consultant should restrict his area of operation to that for which he has been trained and can legitimately claim to be an expert.

3. Current social needs, coupled with a limited supply of consultants, call for priority of psychiatric consultation provided within comprehensive health care over that promoting mental health. The psychological–biological training of psychiatrists is their unique asset and should not be squandered in professional activities for which such training is not essential.

4. Consultation and liaison should be adequately taught in all psychiatric residency programs.

5. There is a pressing need for the clarification of concepts and formulations concerning the criteria of outcome of psychiatric consultation so that evaluation of its effectiveness can be advanced.

6. Psychiatrists should avoid posing as experts in all spheres of human behavior and functioning and as potential fixers of all psychological malfunctioning. They should explicitly define the limits of their expertise and distinguish between consultation in the service of health and consultation that could help manipulate people's attitudes to suit political, religious, or business interests.

REFERENCES

1. Arnhoff FN, Kumbar AH: *The Nation's Psychiatrists–1970 Survey.* Washington, DC, American psychiatric Association, 1973.
2. Lipowski ZJ: Consultation–liaison psychiatry: An overview. *Am J Psychiatry* 131:623–630, 1974.
3. Lipowski ZJ: Consultation–liaison psychiatry: Past, present, and future, in Pasnau RO (ed): *Consultation-Liaison Psychiatry.* New York, Grune & Stratton, 1975, pp 1–28.

4. Mannino FV, MacLennan BW, Shore MF: *The Practice of Mental Health Consultation.* Adelphi, Md, National Institute of Mental Health, 1975.
5. Caplan G: *The Theory and Practice of Mental Health Consultation.* New York, Basic Books, 1970.
6. Jahoda M: *Current Concepts of Positive Mental Health.* New York, Basic Books, 1958.
7. Favazza AR: A sociodynamic model of consultation. *Int J Soc Psychiatry* 19:129-135, 1973.
8. Coleman JV, Patrick DL: Integrating mental health services into primary medical care. *Med Care* 14:654-661, 1976.
9. Gardner EA: Emotional disorders in medical practice. *Ann Intern Med* 73:651-653, 1970.
10. Lipowski ZJ: Psychiatry of somatic diseases: Epidemiology, pathogenesis, classification. *Compr Psychiatry* 16:105-124, 1975.
11. Locke BZ, Gardner EA: Psychiatric disorders among the patients of general practitioners and internists. *Public Health Rep* 84:167-173, 1969.
12. Shepherd M: the extent of mental disorder. *Can Psychiatr Assoc J* 21:401-409, 1976.
13. Spaulding WB: The psychosomatic approach in the practice of medicine. *Int J Psychiatry Med* 6:169-181, 1975.
14. Bellin SS, Locke BZ, New M: The neighborhood health center as a mental health diagnostic service. *Public health Rep* 91:446-451, 1976.
15. Lipowski ZJ: Review of consultation psychiatry and psychosomatic medicine: II. Clinical aspects. *Psychosom Med* 29:201-224, 1967.
16. Moffic HS, Paykel ES: Depression in medical inpatients. *Br J Psychiatry* 126:346-353, 1975.
17. Shevitz SA, Silberfarb PM, Lipowski ZJ: Psychiatric consultations in a general hospital: A report on 1000 referrals. *Dis Nerv Syst* 37:295-300, 1976.
18. Harrington RL: Systems approach to mental health care in an HMO. Presented at the 102nd annual meeting of the American Public Health Association, New Orleans, La, Oct 20-24, 1974.
19. Mechanic D: Social psychologic factors affecting the presentation of bodily complaints. *N Engl J Med* 286:1132-1139, 1972.
20. Burnell GM: Determining health needs in an HMO. Presented at the 102nd annual meeting of the American Public Health Association, New Orleans, La, Oct 20-24, 1974.
21. Billings EG: Value of psychiatry to the general hospital. *Hospitals* 15:140-144, 1941.
22. Goldberg ID, Krantz G, Locke BZ: Effect of short-term outpatient psychiatric therapy benefit on the utilization of medical services in a prepaid group practice medical program. *Med Care* 8:419-428, 1970.
23. Nason F, Delbanco TL: Soft services: A major, cost-effective component of primary medical care. *Soc Work Health Care* 1:297-308, 1976.
24. Reichsman F: Teaching psychosomatic medicine to medical students, residents and postgraduate fellows. *Int J Psychiatry Med* 6:307-316, 1975.
25. Schubert DSP, McKegney FP: Psychiatric consultation education—1976. *Arch Gen Psychiatry* 33:1271-1273, 1976.
26. Goldberg RL, Haas MR, Eaton JS, et al: Psychiatry and the primary care physician. *JAMA* 236:944-945, 1976.
27. Lipowski ZJ: Physical illness, the patient and his environment: psychosocial foundations of medicine, in Reiser MF (ed): *American Handbook of Psychiatry,* ed 2, Arieti S (ed-in-chief). New York, Basic Books, 1975, vol 4, pp 3-42.
28. Lipowski ZJ: Psychosomatic medicine in the seventies; An overview. *Am J Psychiatry* 134:233-244, 1977.
29. Lipowski ZJ, Lipsitt DR, Whybrow PC (eds): *Psychosomatic Medicine: Current Trends and Clinical Applications.* New York, Oxford University Press, 1977.

Consultation–Liaison Psychiatry   *23*

Past Failures and New Opportunities

Liaison psychiatry has recently become one of the fastest growing areas of special interest within the field of general psychiatry. A major factor in this development has been a decision by the Psychiatry Education Branch of the National Institute of Mental Health to increase funding for the training of psychiatrists in liaison work. In fiscal year 1978, support for liaison programs accounted for one fifth of the total funds at the Branch's disposal. Since 1974, 272 postresidency fellowships in liaison psychiatry have been funded (J. S. Eaton, personal communication, August 10, 1978). About 80% of the psychiatric residency programs surveyed in 1976 offered some training in consultation–liaison work, although only 10% of the residents' time was reportedly devoted to such training. Liaison services have been established, or reestablished, in a growing number of teaching general hospitals.

Such expansion is remarkable in view of the fact that only 10 years ago, the very term "liaison psychiatry" was seldom heard, opportunities for postresidency training were almost nonexistent, and certainly not subsidized, and liaison work was carried out unobtrusively by a handful of interested people on the fringes of psychiatry. Whatever its sources, the present popularity of liaison psychiatry calls for a sober reappraisal of its goals, objectives, and current state. These issues may be seen more clearly when viewed from a historical perspective: The history of the rise and fall and a second rise of liaison psychiatry may help us to avoid its second fall.

Definition and Brief History of Liaison Psychiatry

The *term* "liason psychiatry" first appeared in the literature in a paper by Billings[2] published in 1939 and generally refers to that area of psychiatric practice which involves consultation to and collaboration with nonpsychiatrist physicians and other health workers in all types of medical care settings, but especially in general hospitals.[3] The collaboration encompasses patient care, teaching of psychiatry and psychosocial aspects of medicine, and research at the borderland between medicine and psychiatry. Consultation refers to the provision of expert advice on the diagno-

Reprinted from *General Hospital Psychiatry* 1:3–10, 1979. Copyright © by Elsevier North Holland, Inc., 1979. Reprinted by permission of Elsevier Science Publishing Co., Inc. Based on a paper read at the Biennial Meeting of the New York State Psychiatric Association, New York, November 5, 1978.

sis, management, and prevention of mental disorders, psychological distress, and deviant illness behavior among patients treated by nonpsychiatrist physicians. The physically ill, injured, or disabled are a special focus of this consultative activity. Liaison
in this context implies regular contact by a psychiatrist or other mental health worker
with the clinical staff, for the purpose of enhancing psychosocial aspects of patient care.
Such liaison involves participation in ward rounds and meetings, and mediation between patients and staff to prevent disruption of care by interpersonal conflicts and
inadequate communication. Furthermore, efforts are made to sensitize staff members
to those psychological and social issues that add to the burden of illness for the patients and to the stress of taking care of them for the staff.

The *concept* of liaison psychiatry is not new. On the contrary, it is half a century
old. In 1929, George W. Henry, a psychiatric consultant at Cornell Medical School
who became the founder of what later came to be called liaison psychiatry, wrote:

> On the staff of every general hospital there should be a psychiatrist who would make regu-
> lar visits to the wards, who would direct a psychiatric outpatient clinic, who would continue
> the instruction and organize the psychiatric work of interns and who would attend staff con-
> ferences so that there might be a mutual exchange of medical experience and a frank discus-
> sion of the more complicated cases.[4]

While Henry pioneered liaison work, a document of far-reaching importance was
taking shape. The Commission on Medical Education, organized by the Association
of American Medical Colleges in 1925, presented its Final Report (the Lowell Report)
in 1932,[5] in which were discussed issues that remain a matter of concern and debate
today: rapid growth of medical knowledge and technology; excessive specialization;
maldistribution and inequality of health care; overuse of laboratory tests; rising cost
of medical care; and inadequate teaching of psychosocial and preventive aspects of
medicine. The Commission concluded that "sound medical care requires that the physician understand the importance and influences of social, economic, and psychological factors as they contribute to the causation, treatment, and prevention of disease in
the individual." One could hardly express more succinctly the biopsychosocial model
of medicine. The Commission also offered thoughtful comments on psychiatry, observing that no other branch of medicine has been so riddled by "dangerous fadism."
It recommended that psychiatric teaching and research be integrated with that in general
medicine, pediatrics, and neurology, if future physicians were to deal with the ubiquitous psychological factors in disease.

Of uncommon contemporary relevance, the Lowell Report offered a penetrating
analysis of the flaws of American medicine, presented guidelines on how to remedy
them, and provided an explicit and cogent formulation of the biopsychosocial model
of medicine. Why is it that half a century later we are preoccupied with the very same
problems? Does it mean that they are insoluble, or that their solution takes centuries,
or that our attempts to solve them have been faulty? Psychiatry has, of course, changed
since 1932. In that year, there were 546 psychiatrists in this country; this year there
are about 27,000, an increase of some 5000%. By comparison, the total number of
physicians has grown by only about 250%. In 1932, only eight medical schools in

North America reported psychiatric liaison with the clinical departments of teaching general hospitals. In 1977, there were about 1000 general hospital psychiatric units in this country alone. Fifty years ago, psychiatry was hardly taught at all in medical schools; today, psychiatric teaching accounts for a sizable proportion of the curriculum. Despite these dramatic changes in the scope of psychiatry, its impact on medical practice and on the quality of medical care from the psychosocial viewpoint has been modest indeed. Perhaps some additional historical information may throw some light on this paradox.

In 1934, the Rockefeller Foundation granted funds for the development of five psychiatric departments in general hospitals. The idea was to bring psychiatry closer to medicine. One of these experimental units, that at the Colorado General Hospital, was called "psychiatric liaison department."[6] Billings[7] reported in 1941 that during the 5 years after its establishment, the average stay of the psychiatric patient at the hospital was reduced by about half, and that the number of X rays and laboratory tests was also reduced. The overall savings per patient amounted to $43.00 (daily cost per patient in 1938–39 was $4.89). Billings concluded that the introduction of psychiatry to the general hospital was of value because "the integration of the principles of psychiatry with those of the other branches of medicine reduces diagnostic and therapeutic floundering, shortens the hospital stay for the patient and thereby saves the hospital, patient and community money."

In addition to these economic advantages there were other benefits, listed by Hunter[8] in her survey of the first 12 years of psychiatric liaison at the Colorado General. During that period, 5000 patients were referred to the liaison department; liaison was extended to all services and personnel connected with the hospital; close contact was developed with the community; teaching hours increased four times by "popular demand" from the students; research into personality factors in various illnesses flourished; and the psychosocial aspects of training of general practitioners increased in response to their growing demand for it. The dean of the medical school expressed the hope that a full-time psychiatrist would be associated with every major service in the hospital to correlate the teaching of psychiatry and comprehensive medicine. Despite these truly impressive achievements, Hunter noted that the psychiatrists were still often in the position of outsiders and remarked that "this attitude will continue until psychiatry is accepted and accepts itself as an integral part of a more comprehensive whole in the program of a general hospital." This remark may hold a key to the fact that, 30 years after it was made, we are still talking about the "new" biopsychosocial model[9] and read articles on the "Obstacles to Effective Psychiatric Liaison"[10] and on "The Educational Challenge of Consultation–Liaison Psychiatry."[11] Fifty years ago, an explicit biopsychosocial model was formulated, and drastic changes in the medical school curricula and a rapidly growing role of psychiatry in medical teaching followed. Liaison services sprouted and gradually grew into full-fledged general hospital psychiatric units, the number of which has grown by leaps and bounds. Yet despite this growth, liaison between medicine and psychiatry has hardly flourished, and its early rise was followed by benign neglect on the part of the leaders of both disciplines. What went wrong?

OBSTACLES TO LIAISON

Greenhill,[12] in his comprehensive and thoughtful review of liaison psychiatry, reflects on its changing fortunes, asserting that the main obstacles to its development have been the resistance of the physicians and psychiatrists and, to a lesser extent, poor logistics and the resistance of the patients.

The resistance to liaison on the part of nonpsychiatrist physicians may be related to their personality and nature of their work. Walton[13] has documented differences between what he called physically minded and psychologically minded doctors. The personality variable that differentiated the two was thinking-introversion—that is to say, the doctors who were interested more in physical than in psychological aspects of illness were less reflective and less interested in abstract ideas. But to expect all physicians, regardless of their personality, to embrace the biopsychosocial model of illness and to deal with patient's psychological problems is both unrealistic and presumptuous. A doctor has the right to work in a manner consonant with his personality.

Another difficulty is related to the common human tendency to reduce complexity and to avoid the disorganizing and distressing effects of information overload.[14] Proponents of the biopsychosocial model, including liaison psychiatrists, urge physicians at large to make their tasks more complex than many of them seem to be able to endure. Psychiatrists, incidentally, have no monopoly on tolerence of complexity: They tend to espouse monolithic theories, to interpret behavior from a restricted viewpoint, and to embrace a single therapeutic technique. All physicians have to cope with the relentless information onslaught and growing complexity. Their attempts to contain this input and avoid distressing confusion deserve empathy.

Greenhill suggests that one of the principal aims of the liaison programs, and a premature one, has been the "conversion" of physicians. Others have written of indoctrination or proselytizing in this context. This choice of words suggests an apostolic zeal, if not fanaticism; it implies that liaison psychiatrists possess superior truths and the right to impose them on others. Such an approach is not in any sense "liaison" but rather a crusade, one that is liable to provoke justified resistance.

Finally, developments in psychiatry were until quite recently distinctly unfavorable to any meaningful collaboration with medicine. Emphasis on psychodynamics and on social aspects of behavior, to the relative neglect of biological factors, marked the field for 30 years. It is only lately that the pendulum has been shifting, with the usual danger that it might shift to the other extreme. Liaison with medicine is still ranked by mental health workers quite low on the list of priorities in psychiatric training, clinical assignments, allocation of funds, and general esteem. A recent large-scale opinion survey on priorities in mental health carried out among community mental health and state hospital workers reflects this.[15] Although responses to the survey are not, of course, representative of American psychiatry, they do reflect the views of community mental health workers whose affinity to medical issues is open to question.

All in all, a number of factors operating within the profession have impeded collaboration with medicine in the past 30 years. Issues of territoriality, focus on community mental health, the preferred modes of practice, and the specific emphases in psychiatric training have all combined to favor retreat from medicine rather than to endorse liaison with it. Perhaps the fate of liaison psychiatry is really not so surprising after all. Physicians and psychiatrists work in close proximity but are protective of their respective territories and ambivalent about collaboration. Outside pressure was needed to bring them together. In this rather chilly climate, the liaison psychiatrists made attempts to maintain an open boundary between medicine and psychiatry. It has been said, however, that a man who runs along the boundary between two countries is liable to be shot at by both sides.

It is no wonder that, as a consequence of this precarious position, relatively few people have remained in the field and that much of the literature and research produced has been mediocre. Scholarship and investigative work do not flourish under conditions of lukewarm support, brief tenure, and preoccupation with the need to justify one's professional existence. In turn, relative lack of solid scientific and intellectual achievement provides critics with cogent arguments against supporting an activity showing such a marginal yield.

Until recently, only a sense of either mission or intellectual curiosity, or, occasionally, both, could keep people in liaison psychiatry. Although a sense of mission may provide sustaining motivation, it also tends to encourage a certain intrusiveness, a desire to convert others, to indoctrinate them, or to buttonhole potential converts, and other strategies which may bring some initial success in spreading the doctrine but may also mobilize the very resistance that it aims to overcome. On the other hand, intellectual curiousity, or just a wish to do a good job and stand on one's record, is a more appropriate attitude for a respectable craftsman than for a missionary, and one that is more likely to be effective in the long run.

NEW PERSPECTIVES FOR LIAISON PSYCHIATRY

Despite the obstacles enumerated above, an emerging constellation of forces offers new prospects for liaison psychiatry and calls for a reappraisal of its role, functions, and modes of operation. It is these forces—predominantly economic, political, and social, and, to a lesser extent, intellectual, ideological, and scientific—that have likely prompted the initiative of the Psychiatry Education Branch to support liaison programs. The economic burden of health care is staggering and is estimated to exceed $180 billion this year. Any measure that could help contain the cost of health care without unacceptably lowering its quality needs to be applied. Excessive utilization of health care facilities, needless hospitalization, overuse of laboratory facilities, inadequate preventive medicine, and psychogenic invalidism are some of the targets for remedial action.

It is reasonable to postulate that psychosocial and behavioral aspects of medicine and illness influence the cost of health care. In a survey of 1000 consecutive referrals of medical and surgical inpatients for psychiatric consultation at the Dartmouth–Hitchcock Medical Center, 27% of the patients referred could not be assigned a medical diagnosis.[16] This suggests that these 270 patients may well have been needlessly hospitalized and that more effective screening could have prevented the consequent expenditures.

Study after study has documented that a high proportion of those seeking medical help and complaining of physical symptoms do not suffer from any physical illness. Rather, such symptoms reflect psychosocial stress and subjective distress, which need to be identified and managed by nonmedical means to prevent repeated medical consultations and investigations and the adoption by the patient of a fixed sick role. Furthermore, study after study has documented a positive association between physical and psychiatric morbidity in most of the populations studied.[17] Regardless of how one views these findings in terms of causal relationships, it seems clear that adequate health care should involve proper attention to both these types of morbidity, through collaboration between medical and mental health workers. Studies have documented that the two most common psychiatric problems among the physically ill are depression and organic brain syndromes.[16] It follows that recognition and adequate management of these problems need to be taught to all health workers, and this again calls for interprofessional collaboration.

The whole field of psychiatric complications of physical, including cerebral, disease has been largely neglected by psychiatrists, as reflected in the relative dearth of informative literature and therapeutic guidelines. Until recently, psychiatric aspects of physical illness, whether cancer or heart disease or head injury, have been largely ignored in both medical and psychiatric English literature.

Heart disease is the number one cause of death in this country, responsible for about 600,000 deaths annually. Of the 400,000 or so survivors of heart attack, some 60% are estimated to display significant depression and anxiety, or both, during the acute hospitalization, and 20 to 30% are found to be depressed 1 year later. Studies have shown that 15 to 20% of victims of a heart attack fail to return to work and that psychosocial factors play a major role in this. Cardiac rehabilitation is gaining ground in this country and elsewhere, and liaison psychiatrists are beginning to play a part in rehabilitation teams.[18] Rehabilitation of the victims of strokes, head and spinal cord injuries, and other disabling conditions is a matter of growing concern and a fitting area for psychiatric liaison.

Considering the major role of psychosocial factors in increasing the economic burden of illness and health care, to what extent are physicians prepared by training and willing to deal with psychiatric problems encountered in medical practice? Epidemiologists tell us that some 15% of the American population is affected by mental disorders in 1 year and about three fifths are identified and/or receive treatment in the primary care sector.[19] About one fifth is served by the specialty mental health sector and one fifth by the general hospitals and nursing homes. These figures underscore four points: (1) the key role of primary or family physicians as providers of mental health care; (2) the need for adequate training for these physicians in diagnosis, appropriate referral, and management of mental disorders; (3) the desirability of integration of medical and mental health care services; and (4) the opportunity for liaison psychiatry to integrate the relevant clinical and teaching activities.

Hyams and associates[20] surveyed a large group of primary physicians and reported that about 40% would not be willing to treat their patients' emotional problems under any circumstances, while most of the others would be willing to do so if they had more time and training. These authors conclude that psychiatry should provide new services that would take over primary responsibility for the treatment of emotional problems presented by patients of physicians not willing to treat them, and offer a backup service for those who are willing to do so.

Fisher[21] has written recently about what the family physician expects from psychiatrists, emphasizing the importance of improved referral procedures aimed at better communication, learning experience, and patient care. Fisher asserts that one of the best ways to improve learning opportunities for family physicians is to provide them with psychiatric liaison service experience. This contention is supported by one survey of general practitioners in which the respondents expressed preference for teaching of psychiatry in outpatient settings and on medical and surgical wards.[22]

Has psychiatry responded to the challenge implied in the survey findings and related postulates? Yes, to some extent, but only very recently. It has taken the initiatve of the Education Branch of NIMH and concomitant economic incentives to implement some of the postulates put forth by the students of primary practice. Eaton and associates[11] noted that only in the past few years had psychiatric educators accepted the notion that liaison psychiatry should be an integral part of psychiatric residency training. It has been reported that about one third of medical students are given some education, albeit varying greatly in extent, in liaison work[1]; it is likely that a majority of the students still learn clinical psychiatry by rotating on inpatient psychiatric wards of general hospitals, where they can hardly learn how to deal with psychiatric aspects of general medical practice.

One obvious reason for providing this form of training is the relative scarcity of liaison psychiatrists and the heavy teaching load that they are expected to carry.[23] The policy of the NIMH promises a change. Goldberg and associates[24] wrote recently that the Psychiatry Education Branch had given high priority to consultation–liaison psychiatry and to its role in medical student education for comprehensive primary care. Economic factors influence political decisions and they, in turn, influence medical training and practice. Current emphasis on primary care—a political decision—has consequences for both medicine and psychiatry. Both professions are under pressure to revamp their priorities in training. In addition, there is currently a strong tendency in psychiatry to develop an entente cordiale with medicine in the interest of self-preservation as a profession. Liaison psychiatrists have found themselves at the growing edge of this rather ambivalent courtship.

Thus, after half a century, combined economic, political, and social forces have created a favorable climate both for the biopsychosocial approach to medicine and for liaison psychiatry. Their fate will largely depend on the extent to which they are shown to be effective in improving the quality of health care and containing its rising cost.

CLINICAL OBJECTIVES OF LIAISON PSYCHIATRY

First, it is important to stress that consultation and liaison constitute integral aspects of liaison work, despite the recent tendency of some to downgrade consultation and extol liaison as the only valid approach. Psychiatric consultation is still a necessary service for liaison psychiatrists to offer to other physicians and, if properly carried out, involves liaison and teaching. How much liaison is involved depends especially on the needs of the consultee. To discourage potential consultees from referring patients just for consultation would mean that some patients would be denied this service for reasons irrelevant to their needs. Liaison in the context of consultation implies discussion of the patient with the consultee, interpretation of the patient's mental state and behavior, and mediation between patients and staff. Liaison, in the sense of regular contacts with a particular clinical service, complements consultation. Because it is highly time consuming, liaison should be confined to areas where it is especially needed or desired, such as intensive care units, oncology, and rehabilitation services. These areas contain much psychiatric morbidity and their staffs are likely to welcome liaison to help them deal with the patients and with their own work-related stresses.

Second, it is important to emphasize the team approach to liaison psychiatry. A team, including psychiatrists and other mental health workers, provides a cohesive group sharing a common purpose. Experiences, information, and frustrations can be shared and support offered. Teaching and research can be coordinated more easily if the liaison service functions as an organized unit. Roles within the team overlap but should be defined, because some functions require medical training and others do not. Work involving differential diagnosis and the use of psychotropic drugs for the physically ill are issues requiring psychiatric knowledge; liaison and brief supportive therapy as well as the initial screening of patients may be carried out by the liaison nurse; a social worker may choose to focus on family interviews, liaison with social agencies, and the follow-up of patients.

Third, the need for the follow-up of patients by the liaison team, both during and after hospitalization, should be addressed. Follow-up provides not only some continuity of care but also an opportunity to evaluate the effectiveness of the consultation.

Finally, extension of consultation–liaison work beyond inpatient services to hospital outpatient clinics and other settings for primary care is in order. Several recent papers describe this type of liaison.[25, 26] For example, Slaby and his colleagues[26] report on the pattern of psychiatric liaison evolved at the Primary Care Center of the Yale–New Haven Hospital and observe that continued psychiatric consultation and education are needed if primary physicians are to assume more responsibility for their patients' psychosocial and psychiatric problems. It is the continuity of liaison that is the crucial factor. Such continuity is most readily achieved if the liaison person becomes a member of the primary care team. In rural areas, consultations should be offered in small hospitals.

TRAINING OBJECTIVES OF LIAISON PSYCHIATRY

With regard to training, the first need is for more teachers of liaison psychiatry. As the demand for clinical service and teaching of various groups mounts, the years of neglect of this area of psychiatry begin to show. Our main hope lies in postresidency fellows in consultation–liaison psychiatry, of whom there are 58 this year. There is an urgent need to review their training to find out how much consensus there is regarding its content, and what skills a fellow should demonstrate at the end of the training. A related problem is that of existing faculty. Ideally, at least one full-time liaison psychiatry teacher should be available in every psychiatric residency program, as well as visiting, part-time colleagues to teach various aspects of liaison psychiatry.

The second proposed priority is the teaching of medical students, who should have exposure to consultation–liaison work as part or all of their psychiatric rotation. Unless departments of psychiatry make this sort of teaching a priority, an opportunity will be missed and we will once again hear that over one half of family physicians found their psychiatric training to be more or less inadequate. It is obvious that we cannot afford to spread ourselves too thin; as McKegney has stated,[27] too much effort has been expended on trying to teach medical residents and senior staff. Such teaching is as a rule unwelcome and serves little purpose. What informal teaching occurs in the conduct of consultation and liaison must suffice.

RESEARCH OBJECTIVES OF LIAISON PSYCHIATRY

Much clinical research has been carried out by liaison psychiatrists over the past 20 years. Studies of psychiatric complications of open-heart surgery, hemodialysis, and myocardial infarction are well-known examples. There is a pressing need for more high-quality clinical research on such problems as the incidence, nature, and pathogenesis of psychiatric disorders found in association with the most highly prevalent chronic diseases—cardiovascular, neoplastic, pulmonary, and so forth. Another neglected area of growing importance because of the increasing number of old people is that of organic brain syndromes. The whole problem of somatic complaints not accounted for by physical illness has barely been touched by psychiatric investigators. We are constantly asked to evaluate complaints of pain, for example, and still lack reliable methods of estimating the extent of the contribution of psychological factors to its causation.

Last but not least, evaluative research is almost nonexistent, yet without it, the future of liaison programs will hang in the balance. After all, the ultimate work is whether it makes a difference in the well-being and illness behavior of patients. The study by Payson and Davis,[28] showing that patients seen in consultation had better psychosocial adjustment 6 months later than those who had been thought to need referral but were not referred, has not been replicated. The same holds for Billings'[7] study indicating that liaison work reduced hospital stay and use of laboratory tests and X rays for certain categories of patients, a work published in 1941 and most relevant today.

To address these needs, every liaison service in the country should aim at conducting at least one clinical research or scholarly project. Every liaison fellow should be required to carry out such a project as part of his fellowship. The quality of the literature on liaison subjects must be raised. Clinical anecdotes and high-sounding verbiage will hardly attract superior young people to the field.

CONCLUSION

Liaison psychiatry has been given a chance to prove its worth as a clinical activity and an agent for teaching the psychosocial approach to medicine. Furthermore, this approach has been given legislative blessing as a way to improve the quality of heatlh care and reduce its cost. There are predictions that a major change in American medicine over the next decade will be the growing government intervention and pressure aimed at controlling cost.[29] This suggests that the value of liaison psychiatry and what it stands for will be assessed by the government in terms of dollars saved, an unpalatable but realistic forecast. Meanwhile, we have been given extended credit, as it were, and an opportunity to expand the scope of our clinical, teaching, and research activities. It is on the quality of our record in these areas over the next 5 to 10 years that our contribution to medicine and psychiatry will ultimately be judged.

REFERENCES

1. Schubert DSP, McKegney FP: Psychiatric consultation education—1976. *Arch Gen Psychiatry* 33:1271–1273, 1976.
2. Billings EG: Liaison psychiatry and intern instruction. *J Assoc Am Med Coll* 14:375–385, 1939.
3. Lipowski ZJ: Consultation-liaison psychiatry: An overview. *Am J Psychiatry* 131:623–630, 1974.
4. Henry GW: Some modern aspects of psychiatry in general hospital practice. *Am J Psychiatry* 9:481–499, 1929–30.
5. *Final Report of the Commission on Medical Education.* Office of the Director of Study, New York, 1932.
6. Billings EG: The general hospital; its psychiatric needs and the opportunities it offers for psychiatric teaching. *Am J Med Sci* 194:234–243, 1937.
7. Billings EG: Value of psychiatry to the general hospital. *Hospitals* 15:305–310, 1941.
8. Hunter H: Psychiatric liaison work: A twelve-year survey. *J Assoc Am Med Coll* 23:305–312, 1948.
9. Engel GL: The need for a new medical model: A challenge for biomedicine. *Science* 196:129–136, 1977.
10. Schubert DSP: Obstacles to effective psychiatric liaison. *Psychosomatics* 19:283–285, 1978.
11. Eaton JS, Goldberg R, Rosinski E, Allerton WS: The educational challenge of consultation-liaison psychiatry. *Am J Psychiatry* 134 (suppl):20–23, 1977.
12. Greenhill MH: The Development of Liaison Programs, in Usdin G (ed): *Psychiatric Medicine.* New York, Brunner/Mazel, Inc., 1977, pp 115–191.
13. Walton JH: Differences between physically-minded and psychologically-minded medical practitioners. *Br J Psychiatry* 112:1097–1102, 1966.
14. Lipowski ZJ: Sensory and information overload: Behavioral effects. *Compr Psychiatry* 16:199–211, 1975.
15. Norris EL, Larsen JK: Critical issues in mental health service delivery: what are the priorities? *Hosp Commun Psychiatry* 27:561–566, 1976.
16. Shevitz SA, Silberfarb PM, Lipowski ZJ: Psychiatric consultations in a general hospital. A report on 1,000 referrals. *Dis Nerv Syst* 37:295–300, 1976.
17. Lipowski, ZJ: Physical illness and psychiatric disorder: a neglected relationship. *Psychiatr Fen* (Suppl. 1979), pp. 32–57.
18. Soloff PH: The liaison psychiatrist in cardiovascular rehabilitation: An overview. *Int J Psychiatr Med* 8:393–402, 1977–78.
19. Regier DA, Goldberg ID, Taube CA: The de facto U.S. mental health services system. *Arch Gen Psychiatry* 35:685–693, 1978.
20. Hyams L, Green MR, Haar E, et al: Varied needs of primary physicians for psychiatric resources. *Psychosomatics* 12:36–45, 1971.
21. Fisher JV: What the family physician expects from the psychiatrist. *Psychosomatics* 19:523–527, 1978.
22. Hendrie HC, Grisell JL, Hudson J: The views of general practitioners and psychiatrists on psychiatric teaching in medical school. *Mich Med* 72:155–159, 1973.
23. Reichsman F: Teaching psychosomatic medicine to medical students, residents and postgraduate fellows. *Int J Psychiatr Med* 6:307–316, 1975.
24. Goldberg RL, Haas MR, Eaton JS, Grubbs JH: Psychiatry and the primary care physician. *JAMA* 236:944–945, 1976.
25. Rittelmeyer LF, Flynn WE: Psychiatric consultation in an HMO: A model for education in primary care. *Am J Psychiatry* 135:1089–1092, 1978.

26. Slaby AE, Pottash ALC, Black HR: Utilization of psychiatry in a primary care center. *J Med Educ* 53:752–758, 1978.

27. McKegney FP: Consultation-liaison teaching of psychosomatic medicine: opportunities and obstacles. *J Nerv Ment Dis* 154:198–205, 1972.

28. Payson HE, Davis JM: The psychosocial adjustment of medical inpatients after discharge: a follow-up study. *Am J Psychiatry* 123:1220–1225, 1967.

29. Ginzberg E: How much will U.S. medicine change in the decade ahead? *Ann Intern Med* 89:557–564, 1978.

Liaison Psychiatry, Liaison Nursing, and Behavioral Medicine

24

Liaison psychiatry has emerged in the past several years as a major subdivision, some would say a subspecialty, of psychiatry. Its rapid emergence from relative obscurity reflects changing trends in medicine and psychiatry, and in health care delivery. More specifically, it owes much to a 1974 decision of the Psychiatry Education Branch at NIMH to give high priority to the development of consultation–liaison services in the general hospitals.[1] That decision was apparently based on two sets of premises: (1) Medicine is shifting its focus to primary care and primary care physicians identify and treat (or fail to treat) about three fifths of psychiatric disorders. Medical students and nonpsychiatric physicians should be prepared for that task, and liaison psychiatrists are the right persons to help with the preparation. (2) Psychiatry's drift away from medicine needs to be arrested if the specialty is to be salvaged.[1,2] Since liaison psychiatry represents the main viable bridge between medicine and psychiatry, it is logical to expand it.

The above premises and decisions were no doubt inspired by the government's growing concern about the escalating cost of health care. To contain the cost, primary care had to be emphasized and more efficient management of psychosocial and psychiatric problems by primary care physicians fostered. Such combined economic, political, social, and educational considerations have propelled liaison psychiatry into prominence after 50 years of benign neglect. Herein lies an opportunity for it to grow and prove its worth, but also a risk that the new popularity and economic incentives could encourage a drive for short-term gains at the expense of long-term goals. For example, research projects could be undertaken with an eye on the current predilections of the granting agencies rather than for the sake of new knowledge. Furthermore, a bandwagon could be readily created with the usual accompaniment of promotional blarney and undeliverable promises. A familiar sequence of disavowal and decline of liaison psychiatry would likely follow its heyday. To prevent this, its development should be from now on carefully planned and monitored, its goals realistically formulated, and apostolic zeal of its advocates tempered. The author proposes several measures aimed at ensuring liaison psychiatry's continued growth. For the sake of clarity its scope will be defined first.

Reprinted from *Comprehensive Psychiatry* 22(6):554–561, 1981. Copyright © 1981 by Grune & Stratton, Inc. Reprinted by permission. This article is based on a paper presented to the Maryland Psychiatric Society, Baltimore, Maryland, October 11, 1979.

DEFINITIONS

Liaison psychiatry may be defined as that area of psychiatry which is concerned with the diagnosis, treatment, study, and prevention of psychiatric morbidity in the physically ill, of somatoform and factitious disorders, and a psychological factors affecting physical conditions. In a narrower sense, the term designates the realm of psychiatric consultation to and collaboration (or "liaison") with nonpsychiatric physicians and other health workers in all types of medical care settings, but especially in the general hospitals.[3, 4]

Much confusion surrounds the word "liaison" in this context. It cropped up first in the psychiatric literature in the 1920s when Barrett[5] wrote that psychiatry had gained "the position of liaison between medicine and social problems," while Pratt[6] predicted that psychiatry would become "the *liaison* agent" integrating and clarifying all available knowledge concerning the patient. The term reappeared in 1934, when the Psychiatric Liaison Department was established at the Colorado General Hospital.[7] Billings[7] was probably the first writer to use the term "liaison psychiatry."

More recently, "liaison" has been used in two related senses: (1) as an abbreviation for "consultation–liaison psychiatry"; and (2) as a designation of regular contacts by a psychiatrist (or other mental health worker) with a medical or surgical ward or unit for the dual purpose of assisting and teaching staff to identify and manage psychosocial and psychiatric problems, and of mediating between patients and staff to maintain communication and resolve conflicts.

Liaison, in the second sense, denotes a *strategy* of providing clinical service and teaching, one that involves standing out by being there. The liaison person may spend from a few hours a week to as much as one half of every working day on the ward to which he is assigned. This issue has recently become a bone of contention when some workers in the field began to extol liaison as the only worthwhile service and to contrast it with consultation as an allegedly obsolete and inferior activity. I will take up this controversy later on.

CLINICAL SERVICE

CONSULTATION AND LIAISON INTEGRATED

Provision of service implies organization. This writer has consistently advocated a *team concept* of liaison work.[3,4,8,9] One or more psychiatrists and liaison nurses comprise the core team, to which social workers or psychologists may be added if funds are available.

Both consultation and liaison (in its narrower sense) are integral components of clinical service rendered by liaison workers.[3] Consultation on matters of personality assessment, diagnosis, and management is the cornerstone of liaison psychiatry, which would lose its reason for existence without it. Thus, to devalue consultation, as is the current fad, amounts to undercutting the branch on which liaison workers must sit. This writer has proposed that liaison is best carried out *in the context of consultation*.[3]

This implies that the consultant makes an effort to discuss every consultation with the consultee and other members of the medical team involved in the patient's care. Such a comprehensive consultation, encompassing the patient, the consultee, and the clinical team, represents, in this writer's view, the most economical and effective way of providing service in this area of psychiatry. It integrates consultation with liaison, has educational potential, and takes into account the fact that liaison psychiatrists are scarce.

In the heady 1930s, Dunbar and associates[10] predicted that "the time should not be too long delayed when psychiatrists are required on all our medical and surgical wards, and in all general and special clinics." When one considers that there are some 6000 community general hospitals and about 25,000 psychiatrists in this country, and that the proportion of medical students choosing to specialize in psychiatry has declined by more than 300% in the past several years, the absurdity of Dunbar *et al.*'s prediction is compelling. Today's proponents of liaison, in its highly time- and labor-intensive form, as *the* working model for all settings ignore those stubborn facts. By advocating the impossible they undermine liaison psychiatry's credibility and expose it to the risk of being dismissed by the planners of health care delivery as an idealistic luxury. Such a verdict would amount to the death knell for the subspecialty.

Two organizational changes to strengthen the service aspect of liaison psychiatry are proposed: (1) expanding the role of liaison nurses; and (2) the merger of liaison services with those of behavioral medicine.

EXPANSION OF THE ROLE OF LIAISON NURSES

Our experience with liaison nursing over the past 5 years suggests that much of the day-to-day liaison function may be carried out by a properly trained liaison nurse. She is well suited to be consultant to the medical and surgical nurses and thus to help raise the standards of psychosocial patient care. A liaison nurse can help the other nurses heighten their sensitivity to the patients' psychological needs and increase their tolerance for the patients' deviant or disturbing behavior. As a result, conflicts and crises related to unorthodox behavior can be either avoided or better handled, and psychiatric complications either prevented or promptly identified and referred. Furthermore, the medical and surgical nurses can in turn influence the attitudes, practices, and psychiatric referral habits of the house staff. After all, it is often the nurses who trigger such referral by virtue of their observations or complaints.

Our recent study of referral patterns for psychiatric consultation of two patient samples of 1000 each, referred before and after the employment of a liaison nurse, bears out the above assertions.[9] Since the nurse joined our team in 1975 a statistically significant drop has occurred in the number of patients referred for disposition (usually transfer to psychiatry), in the frequency of the psychiatrists' intervention in patient–staff conflicts, and in transfers to the psychiatric unit. We believe that these findings reflect the impact of our liaison nurse's work.

It is proposed that liaison should be focused on those areas, such as oncology or critical care units, where it is most needed, and that it be largely delegated to liaison nurses, members of the liaison team. Liaison psychiatrists should concentrate instead on difficult consultations requiring integration of knowledge from several fields for diagnosis and treatment, and on teaching and research. Such a division of labor would reconcile the demand for services with the short supply of liaison psychiatrists.

MERGER WITH BEHAVIORAL MEDICINE

Behavioral medicine has been defined as "systematic application of the principles and technology of behavioral psychology to the field of medicine, health and illness."[11] Such application is a very recent but vigorously spreading development, one spearheaded mostly by clinical psychologists and already viewed by some as a "skirmish ground for turf" between them and liaison psychiatrists.[12] It would be most unfortunate if the practitioners of behavioral medicine came to view their activities as either preempting or competing with those of liaison workers. On the contrary, in the writer's opinion, those two types of activity would complement each other most effectively if they were integrated.

Formation of unified liaison psychiatry–behavioral medicine divisions would, I believe, counteract destructive competition and achieve the best utilization of psychological and psychiatric knowledge and techniques at the interface between psychiatry and medicine. Practitioners of behavioral medicine can contribute therapies for various stress-related symptoms affecting physical conditions and for somatoform disorders such as psychalgia. They also can offer proficiency in designing and conducting research which liaison psychiatrists often lack. They in turn have the advantage of broad training in medicine and psychiatry that is indispensable for diagnosis and treatment of complex clinical problems involving both somatic pathology and psychopathology. Unified divisions proposed here offer the best organizational format for clinical work, teaching, and research at the borderland between medicine and psychiatry and the behavioral sciences. At Dartmouth, a merger has been effected and the two components collaborate while retaining autonomy.

EDUCATION

Teaching has been one of the key functions of liaison psychiatrists.[3,4,8] They have been called upon with growing frequency to teach medical students and residents, primary care physicians, psychiatric residents, liaison fellows, nurses, physician's assistants, and so forth.[1] There must be a limit to what a handful of liaison psychiatrists can reasonably be expected to accomplish without spreading themselves too thin. Priorities have to be set up, taking into account educational needs and opportunities of a given clinical setting. I would propose that in general the teaching efforts should focus on medical students on the one hand, and liaison fellows on the other.

TEACHING MEDICAL STUDENTS

Liaison psychiatrists are well suited to help prepare future physicians to identify, manage, and refer appropriately the psychosocial and psychiatric problems they will encounter in their practice. For several years now some programs, including ours, have had medical students assigned to the liaison service for their psychiatric rotation.[13-15] Such practice is recommended for all training centers. Even if it were not feasible to assign all the medical students to a liaison service for the full rotation, every student should have at least some exposure to liaison work as part of his psychiatry rotation; some students may spend all of it on the service. There is evidence that students learn psychiatry as adequately on a liaison service as elsewhere.[13,15] In addition, our own experience with the liaison rotation to date suggests that the students become more effective consultees.

A student who acts as an apprentice psychiatric consultant to medicine and surgery learns at first hand those attitudes and actions of physicians which are incompatible with good psychosocial patient care and are a common source of frustration to liaison psychiatrists. The student shares, for example, the frustration of seeing a patient referred for consultation only after a serious ward crisis has developed, or of dealing with consultees who refer patients an hour before their discharge. Such direct experiences are more likely to influence the student's future professional behavior than hours of indoctrination. A student may be expected to learn during his liaison rotation how to take a psychosocial history, diagnose common psychiatric disorders, use psychotropic drugs properly, appreciate the importance of doctor–patient relationship, apply supportive psychotherapy, and refer patients appropriately for psychiatric consultation and to behavioral medicine. These are crucial skills for primary care physicians to have.[4]

LIAISON FELLOWS

The future of liaison psychiatry will largely depend on the training of sufficient numbers of liaison psychiatrists and their competence. This calls for adequate training of liaison fellows. Since 1974, NIMH has funded some 300 fellowships in liaison psychiatry, yet very little has been written about their objectives and syllabus. It is unknown what types of training the various programs offer and a need for guidelines is evident.

At Dartmouth, our fellowship comprises five interrelated aspects; (1) theoretical teaching in the form of psychosomatic seminars; (2) supervised clinical experience; (3) liaison with a selected clinical area; (4) supervision and teaching of psychiatric residents and medical students; and (5) a mandatory clinical or scholarly research project. The fellows are expected to be competent general psychiatrists skilled in dealing with psychiatric problems encountered in medical settings. They are encouraged to adopt a truly eclectic and critically common-sense approach to clinical work and psychiatric theories, and to cultivate a habit of reading the literature and contributing to it. Most of them have embarked on an academic career in liaison psychiatry, as we would have wished them to do.

Different programs are likely to offer different emphases and experiences. Our own main objective is to train future liaison psychiatrists and not psychosocially minded internists or gynecologists. We predict that the need for psychiatric consultants to nonpsychiatric physicians will continue indefinitely. The notion that liaison psychiatry's success would mean its own dissolution as all physicians would become psychosocially sophisticated strikes me as lacking any basis in reality.

Investigation

Clinical Research

Research is essential for the long-term growth of liaison psychiatry. So far the latter has struggled to justify its existence by providing service and some teaching. From now on, the liaison psychiatrists will have to, in addition, produce research of acceptable quality. They are strategically placed to expand knowledge in several neglected areas, important to both psychiatry and medicine: (1) the relationship between physical illness and psychopathology, especially between the most prevalent diseases, such as coronary heart disease, cancer, and chronic obstructive pulmonary disease, and psychiatric disorders[16]; (2) somatoform and factitious disorders; (3) organic brain syndromes, especially delirium[17]; (4) psychological factors affecting physical conditions; and (5) deviant illness behavior, that is, attitudes and actions by the sick which are incompatible with recovery or rehabilitation.

Evaluative Research

Evaluative research on liaison work, in its service, teaching, and cost-effectiveness aspects, must supplement clinical investigations on the above subjects. Efforts are already being made to address some of the most pressing questions such as these: (1) Is psychiatric consultation useful to patients and consultees? (2) Does the presence of a liaison service result in savings due to shortened hospitalization, fewer laboratory tests, and less frequent use of medical outpatient facilities? (3) Is liaison in its narrower sense effective in raising standards of psychosocial patient care? (4) Is liaison teaching of medical students effective in influencing their future behavior as physicians?[4,13,15,18-22]

Answers to the above questions are slowly accruing and will determine which particular approaches and strategies are effective in which clinical settings. There is little doubt that no single approach to clinical service and teaching can be applied indiscriminately to a large city hospital, a small rural one, and a highly specialized university center. Flexibility is needed, not rigid dogmatism. Unless liaison psychiatry documents its usefulness to the patients and consultees, no amount of propaganda will keep it in business. Studies show that physicians tend to value prompt and helpful consultative service rather than attempts to convert them to biopsychosocial ideals.[22,23] By contrast, NIMH enjoins us to be educators above all.[1,2,21] Such contrasting demands will have to be reconciled in the light of research data.

Conclusions

Liaison psychiatry is at a crossroads. Conflicting demands made on it by NIMH, consultees, hospital administrators,[24] and psychiatric educators[25,26] have created strains and controversies. What goals, priorities, and strategies should prevail? A heated panel discussion at the 1980 Annual Meeting of the American Psychosomatic Society highlighted two major contentious issues: First, should liaison psychiatry's primary function be *teaching* of psychosocial aspects of medicine and its main goal be a reform of medical practice according to the biopsychosocial model, or should it be the provision of competent clinical *service?* And second, should the basic working strategy be *consultation or liaison?*

This writer views clinical service in the form of comprehensive consultation, one that involves a measure of liaison, as the key function of liaison psychiatry. Such consultation can meet the educational goal of demonstrating to perceptive physicians the relevance of psychosocial aspects of illness and patient care, and is likely to satisfy both patient and consultee, and thus gain psychiatry a measure of much-needed respect. The current tendency to juxtapose liaison and consultation is a strategic error which could undermine liaison psychiatry's effectiveness, fiscal base, and long-term chances of survival. Its decline would in turn weaken the links between psychiatry and medicine which, precarious as they are, have taken two centuries to forge.[27]

Teaching psychosocial aspects of medicine to medical students and various health workers could not suffice as a raison d'etre for liaison psychiatry. Such teaching has to be organized around clinical service. Its impact will ultimately depend on the quality of such service and of the clinical and evaluative research liaison workers produce. Joining forces with behavioral medicine would predictably enhance the quality of both service and research, and thus the impact of teaching. The future of liaison psychiatry will be secure if its contribution to better patient care and to knowledge is found to be demonstrably valuable. Missionary zeal, unrealistic reformist strivings, and too much stress on expedience would jeopardize its long-term survival.

REFERENCES

1. Eaton JS, Goldberg R, Rosinski E, *et al:* The educational challenge of consultation–liaison psychiatry. *Am J Psychiatry* 134 (suppl): 20–23, 1977.
2. Goldberg RL, Haas MR, Eaton JS, *et al:* Psychiatry and the primary care physician. *JAMA* 236:944–945, 1976.
3. Lipowski ZJ: Consultation–liaison psychiatry: An overview. *Am J Psychiatry* 131:623–630, 1974.
4. Lipowski ZJ: Consultation–liaison psychiatry: Past failures and new opportunities. *Gen Hosp Psychiatry* 1:3–10, 1979.
5. Barrett AM: The broadened interests of psychiatry. *Am J Psychiatry* 2:1–13, 1922.
6. Pratt GK: Psychiatric departments in general hospitals. *Am J Psychiatry* 5:403–410, 1925–26.
7. Billings EG: Liaison psychiatry and intern instruction. *J Assoc Am Med Coll* 14:376–385, 1939.
8. Lipowski ZJ: Review of consultation psychiatry and psychosomatic medicine. 1. General principles. *Psychosom Med* 29:153–171, 1967.
9. Lipowski ZJ, Wolston EJ: Liaison psychiatry: Referral patterns and their stability over time. *Am J Psychiatry* 138:1608–1611, 1981.
10. Dunbar FH, Wolfe TP, Rioch JM: Psychiatric aspects of medical problems. *Am J Psychiatry* 93:649–679, 1936.
11. Blanchard EB: Behavioral medicine; A perspective, in Williams RB, Gentry WD (eds): *Behavioral Approaches to Medical Treatment.* Cambridge, Mass, Ballinger Publishing Co., 1977, pp 1–6.
12. Goldiamond I: Behavioral approaches and liaison psychiatry. *Psychiatr Clin North Am* 2:379–401, 1979.
13. McKegney FP, Weiner S: A consultation–liaison psychiatry clinical clerkship. *Psychosom Med* 38:45–54, 1976.

14. Schubert D: Teaching psychiatry to medical students on a consultation service. *Int J Soc Psychiatry* 23:282-284, 1977.
15. Weddington WW, Hine FR, Houpt JL, *et al:* Consultation-liaison versus other psychiatry clerkships: A comparison of learning outcomes and student reactions. *Am J Psychiatry* 135:1509-1512, 1978.
16. Lipowski ZJ: Physical illness and psychiatric disorder: A neglected relationship. *Psychiatr Fenn* (suppl):32-57, 1979.
17. Lipowski ZJ: *Delirium: Acute Brain Failure in Man.* Springfield, Ill, Charles C Thomas, 1980.
18. Koran LM, Van Natta J, Stephens JR, *et al:* Patients' reactions to psychiatric consultation. *JAMA* 241:1603-1605, 1979.
19. Kramer BA, Spikes J, Strain JJ: The effects of a psychiatric liaison program on the utilization of psychiatric consultations. *Gen Hosp Psychiatry* 1:122-128, 1979.
20. Payson HE, Davis JM: The psychosocial adjustment of medical inpatients after discharge: A follow-up study. *Am J Psychiatry* 123:1220-1225, 1967.
21. Reifler B, Eaton JS: The evaluation of teaching and learning by psychiatric consultation and liaison training programs. *Psychosom Med* 40:99-106, 1978.
22. Sasser M, Kinzie JD: Evaluation of medical-psychiatric consultation. *Int J Psychiatry Med* 9:123-134, 1978-79.
23. Karasu TB, Plutchik R, Conte H, *et al:* What do physicians want from a psychiatric consultation service? *Compr Psychiatry* 18: 73-81, 1977.
24. Sanders CA: Reflections on psychiatry in the general-hospital setting. *Hosp Commun Psychiatry* 30:185-189, 1979.
25. Greenhill MH: Teaching and training of the psychosomatic approach. *Biblthca Psychiatr* 159:15-22, 1979.
26. Melchiode GA: Psychoanalytic teaching in medical education. *Am J Psychiatry* 136:1071-1073, 1979.
27. Lipowski ZJ: Holistic-medical foundations of American psychiatry: A bicentennial. *Am J Psychiatry* 138:888-895, 1981.

Liaison Psychiatry

25

Referral Patterns and Their Stability over Time

WITH E.J. WOLSTON

Consultation to nonpsychiatric physicians in general hospitals and other clinical settings is the cornerstone of the clinical service rendered by liaison psychiatrists.[1] Patterns of referral for such consultations need to be recorded to help establish priorities in teaching, research, and deployment of personnel. Characteristics of the referred patients, sources of referral, and the main forms of psychiatric intervention need to be documented, and the stability of the referral patterns over time needs to be investigated.

Our purpose in this paper is to report a comparison of two samples of 1000 patients referred for consultation over two periods of 3 and 4 years, respectively.

METHOD

Sample A consisted of 1000 medical and surgical inpatients referred for psychiatric consultation between January 1975 and March 1979 for whom a properly completed statistical form was available. The only criterion for inclusion in the study was the availability of a completed form. The comparison sample (sample B) consisted of 1000 patients referred between November 1971 and October 1974; data on these patients have been reported previously.[2] Both groups of patients had been referred to the Psychiatric Consultation Service from the wards of the Dartmouth–Hitchcock Medical Center in Hanover, New Hampshire.

The Dartmouth–Hitchcock Medical Center is a 420-bed teaching general hospital that serves as both a primary and a tertiary care facility. The patient population is mostly rural and dependent on farming and small industries. The Psychiatric Consultation Service operates as a team consisting of two senior staff psychiatrists, two full-time psychiatric residents, one or two postresidency fellows, and a full-time liaison nurse (since 1975). A designated medical social worker is available for family interviews. The residents rotate on the service during their second year of training. They act as primary consultants and then present the patients to one of the staff psychiatrists or fellows, who thus see all of the patients. Referrals are made formally by the medi-

Reprinted from *American Journal of Psychiatry* 138(12):1608–1611, 1981. Copyright © 1981 by the American Psychiatric Association. Reprinted by permission.

cal and surgical resident staff. The consultation residents are required to complete a standard statistical form for every patient they have seen. Psychiatric diagnoses recorded on the forms are usually those made by the residents.

Data for sample A were obtained from the uniform statistical forms by one of us (E.J.W.) and analyzed with computer assistance. Data for sample B had been collected in the same manner.[2] The significance of the differences between the samples, when appropriate, was assessed by chi-square analyses.

Findings

Demographic Characteristics

There were no statistically significant differences between the patient groups in demographic characteristics. The profile of the referred patients in terms of age, sex, and marital status remained consistent. About 70% of the patients were between 20 and 59 years of age. Those 70 years old and older were underrepresented (i.e., they comprised slightly more than half of their percentage in the hospital population as a whole). Women were overrepresented: the ratio of women to men (1.6:1 and 1.8:1, respectively) was much higher than the ratio in the hospital population (1.2:1). The most likely patient to be referred was a young or middle-aged married woman.

Diagnostic Characteristics

Table I shows that the distribution of psychiatric diagnoses was less consistent than the demographic profile of the patients. Depressive disorders of all types were the most frequent diagnoses in both samples, but their frequency was significantly lower in sample A. Organic brain syndromes constituted the second largest diagnostic category in

TABLE 1. Diagnoses of 1000 Patients Referred for Psychiatric Consultation between January 1975 and March 1979 (Sample A) and 1000 Patients Referred between November 1971 and October 1974 (Sample B)

Diagnosis	Sample A		Sample B		Significance[a]
	N	%	N	%	
Depressive disorders	427	42.7	502	50.2	$p < 0.05$
Organic brain syndromes	139	13.9	155	15.5	n.s.
Anxiety neurosis	47	4.7	68	6.8	n.s.
Hysterical neurosis	19	1.9	52	5.2	$p < 0.001$
Schizophrenia	17	1.7	31	3.1	$p < 0.05$
Alcoholism	43	4.3	30	3.0	n.s.
Psychophysiologic disorders	7	0.7	19	1.9	$p < 0.05$
Other	204	20.4	97	9.7	$p < 0.001$
No psychiatric diagnosis	97	9.7	46	4.6	$p < 0.001$

[a]By chi-square analyses.

both samples. Depressive disorders, organic brain syndromes, and anxiety neurosis together accounted for 70% of all psychiatric diagnoses. Hysterical neurosis, schizophrenia, and psychophysiologic disorders accounted for only 4.3% of the diagnoses in sample A; all three were significantly less often diagnosed than they had been for sample B. Alcoholism (as a primary problem) and attempted suicide (8%) showed no significant change. Significantly more patients in sample A were classified as "other" and "no psychiatric diagnosis." The increased frequency of the "other" category was due to a tendency to diagnose adjustment reactions and personality disorders in sample A, neither of which were reported separately in sample B.

PATTERNS OF REFERRAL AND INTERVENTION

Table 2 shows that internal medicine consistently accounted for about 60% of all referrals, followed by surgery. Assistance with diagnosis and advice on patient management, or both, accounted for between 75% and 85% of the reasons for referral. One notes, however, a significant drop in referrals for disposition (usually transfer to psychiatry).

Psychiatric intervention patterns showed several significant differences in the more recent sample: more brief psychotherapy at the bedside, less reliance on drugs alone, less mediation by psychiatrists in staff–patient conflicts, fewer family interviews by psychiatrists (these were more often carried out by the social worker), and fewer transfers to the psychiatric unit.

TABLE 2. Patterns of Referral and Intervention for 1000 Patients Referred for Psychiatric Consultation between January 1975 and March 1979 (Sample A) and 1000 Patients Referred between November 1971 and October 1974 (Sample B)

	Sample A		Sample B		
Variable	N	%	N	%	Significance[a]
Source of referral					
Internal medicine	572	57.2	590	59.0	n.s.
Surgery	217	21.7	194	19.4	n.s.
Neurology	110	11.0	140	14.0	n.s.
Other	83	8.3	76	7.6	—
No data available	18	1.8	0		
Reason for referral					
Assistance with diagnosis	521	52.1	574	57.4	n.s.
Advice on management	508	50.8	556	55.6	n.s.
Disposition	154	15.4	277	27.7	$p < 0.001$
Intervention					
Psychotherapy	460	46.0	380	38.0	$p < 0.001$
Drugs only	220	22.0	360	36.0	$p < 0.001$
Staff mediation	50	5.0	120	12.0	$p < 0.001$
Family intervention	50	5.0	70	7.0	n.s.
Transfer to psychiary	110	11.0	163	16.3	$p < 0.005$

[a]By chi-square analyses.

DISCUSSION

COMPARISON WITH OTHER STUDIES

Caution is indicated in generalizing from the data collected in one hospital. For example, although both our study and that of the only other published sample of comparable size that we are aware of[3] found a marked preponderance of women, investigators from a New York hospital[4] reported the exact opposite. Our data suggest, however, that the demographic profile of the patients referred for psychiatric consultation for the same hospital tends to remain remarkably stable over time.

To our knowledge, only one previous study addressed the issue of consistency of psychiatric diagnoses assigned by a liaison service.[5] In 1962 it reported high consistency in two samples compared over 2 consecutive years. By contrast, our study shows that some, but not all, diagnoses were assigned consistently. Compared with the 1962 study, however, ours involved samples nearly six times larger, a much greater number of diagnosticians, and a much longer time span.

We find a fair degree of consistency with comparable reports form other hospitals in the United States and even in other countries. Depressive disorders consistently top the list of the reported diagnoses, averaging about 40% (range, 23% to 58%).[2,4,6-13] In our experience, most of these disorders would fall in the DSM-III categories of either dysthymic disorder or adjustment disorder with depressed mood. It is a practically important task for future research to establish the prevalence of the various depressive disorders among both referred and nonreferred patients.

Diagnosis of a depressive disorder in a physically ill person is difficult for two reasons. First, the somatic symptoms of depression are indistinguishable from those of chronic llness such as cancer. Second, the criteria for an adjustment disorder in DSM-III are difficult to apply in this population. DSM-III proclaims that such a disorder represents a maladaptive reaction, one manifested by impairment in the social or occupational sphere or by symptoms exceeding an expected, "normal" reaction to the stressor. Yet how is one to judge what constitutes a normal reaction to cancer or a heart attack, for example? These issues need to be addressed by researchers so that a reliable and therapeutically useful diagnosis may be assigned.

The overall prevalence of depression among medical inpatients, diagnosed by strict criteria, is reported to range from 20% to 25%.[14] It is not surprising, therefore, that depressive disorders account for close to half of psychiatric diagnoses recorded by liaison psychiatrists.

Organic brain syndromes consistently accounted for about 15% of psychiatric diagnoses in our study; this percentage is consonant with other comparable reports.[6,8-11,13,15] Only two studies gave a much lower[7] or higher[3] percentage. In our experience, delirium is by far the most common organic brain syndrome encountered on medical and surgical wards. Its prevalence in these settings is unknown but has been estimated to be about 10%.[16] Delirium and other organic brain syndromes tend to be underdiagnosed by nonpsychiatric physicians.[17] A revised classification of and explicit diagnostic criteria for the organic brain syndromes in DSM-III should result in much-needed research and improved teaching in this area. Liaison psychiatrists are well placed to contribute to both.

Schizophrenia, with few exceptions[15,18] is infrequently seen by liaison workers, even though any reference to it in the patient's record is likely to result in immediate referral.[6-11,13] Hysterical neurosis (conversion disorder) was inconsistently diagnosed in our study and in other published series, which have reported a range of 1% to 30%.[4-11,13,15,19] The new category of somatoform disorders in DSM-III may be expected to facilitate diagnosis and stimulate research in this muddled area.

CONCURRENCE OF PHYSICAL AND PSYCHIATRIC ILLNESS

Between 70% and 80% of the patients in our study were given both a psychiatric and a medical diagnosis. Such high concurrence is hardly surprising in view of the selective nature of our patient population and the well-documented positive statistical association between physical and psychiatric morbidity.[14] The reported prevalence of psychiatric disorders among medical inpatients varies widely—from 20% to 70%— but may be conservatively estimated at 30% to 50%.[14] By contrast, recently reported referral rates for psychiatric consultation average about 4% of hospital admissions.[4-6,9-3] It follows that only about 10% of patients expected to need consultation are referred. Studies show that the rates of referral do not correlate with independently assessed prevalence of psychiatric morbidity in medical populations.[20-22] The decision to refer is influenced less by the presence and severity of psychopathology than by such factors as noncompliance, unexplained somatic complaints, or disturbing behavior on the part of the patients and by the knowledge of and attitudes toward psychiatry on the part of consultees.[20-23] A liaison nurse can play a key role in helping to identify and manage emotionally disturbed medical patients.

THE ROLE OF THE LIAISON NURSE

Our study of sample A coincided in time with the addition of a liaison nurse to our team. We postulate that the observed significant reduction in requests for disposition, in psychiatrists' intervention in staff–patient conflicts, and in transfers to the psychiatric ward is causally related to this fact. The liaison nurse was not only effective in case identification but also helped ward nurses tolerate and care for emotionally disturbed and disturbing patients, thus reducing the frequency of requests for transfer to psychiatry. Furthermore, as a result of her direct work with patients and liaison with the nursing staff, psychiatric consultants were called in to help with difficult diagnostic and therapeutic problems rather than with patient–staff conflicts. A tactful liaison nurse can often help a patient who refuses to see a psychiatrist or whose physician spurns psychiatric consultation. On the basis of our experience over the past 5 years we recommend that at least one liaison nurse be included in every consultation team as an effective agent in enhancing psychosocial patient care.[24-26]

REFERENCES

1. Lipowski ZJ: Consultation-liaison psychiatry: An overview. *Am J Psychiatry* 131:623-630, 1974.

2. Shevitz SA, Silberfarb PM, Lipowski ZJ: Psychiatric consultations in a general hospital: A report on 1000 referrals. *Dis Nerv Syst* 37:295-300, 1976.

3. Kligerman MJ, McKegney FP: Patterns of psychiatric consultation in two general hospitals. *Psychiatry med* 2:126-132, 1971.

4. Karasu TB, Plutchik R, Steinmuller RI, *et al:* Patterns of psychiatric consultation in a general hospital. *Hospt Commun Psychiatry* 28:291-294, 1977.

5. Wilson MS, Meyer E: Diagnostic consistency in a psychiatric liaison service. *Am J Psychiatry* 119:207-209, 1962.

6. Anstee BH: The pattern of psychiatric referrals in a general hospital. *Br J Psychiatry* 120:631-634, 1972.

7. Fava GA, Pavan L: Consultation psychiatry in an Italian general hospital: a report on 500 referrals. *Gen Hosp Psychiatry* 2:35-40, 1980.

8. Fleminger JJ, Mallet BL: Psychiatric referrals from medical and surgical wards. *J Ment Sci* 108:183-190, 1962.

9. Ries RK, Kleinman A, Bokan JA, *et al:* Psychiatric consultation-liaison service. *Gen Hosp Psychiatry* 3:204-212, 1980.

10. Taylor G, Doody K: Psychiatric consultations in a Canadian general hospital. *Can J Psychiatry* 24:717-723, 1979.

11. Tiller JWG: Psychiatric consultations from public wards of a Melbourne metropolitan teaching hospital. *Med J Aust* 1:431-435, 1973.

12. West ND, Bastani JB: The pattern of psychiatric referrals in a teaching hospital. *Nebr Med J* 15:438-440, 1973.

13. White W, Bloch S: Psychiatric referrals in a general hsopital. *Med J Aust* 1:950-954, 1970.

14. Lipowski ZJ: Physical illness and psychiatric disorder: a neglected relationship. *Psychiatr Fenn* 1979, pp 32-57.

15. Wig NN Shah DK: Psychiatric unit in a general hospital in India: patterns of inpatient referrals. *J Indian Med Assoc* 60:83-86, 1973.

16. Lipowski ZJ: Delirium: *Acute Brain Failure in Man.* Springfield, Ill, Charles C Thomas , 1980.

17. Levine PM, Silberfarb PM, Lipowski ZJ: Mental disorders in cancer patients; A study of 100 psychiatric referrals. *Cancer* 42:1385-1391, 1978.

18. Henker FO: Psychoses in the general hospital. *South Med J* 64:1236-1237, 1971.

19. Lipowski ZJ, Kiriakos RZ: Borderlands between neurology and psychiatry: Observations in a neurological hospital. *psychiatry* Med 3:131-147, 1972.

20. Denney D, Quass RM, Rich DC, *et al:* Psychiatric patients on medical wards. *Arch Gen Psychiatry* 14:530-535, 1966.

21. Richman A, Slade HC, Gordon G: Symptom questionnaire validity in assessing the need for psychiatrists' care. *Br J Psychiatry* 112:549-555, 1966.

22. Schwab JJ, Clemmons RS, Freemon FR, *et al:* Differential characteristics of medical in-patients referred for psychiatric consultation: a controlled study. *Psychosom Med* 27:112-118, 1965.

23. Steinberg H, Torem M, Saravay SM: An analysis of physician resistance to psychiatric consultations. *Arch Gen Psychiatry* 37:1007-1012, 1980.

24. Lipowski ZJ: Liaison psychiatry, liaison nursing, and behavioral medicine. *Compr Psychiatry* 22:554-561, 1981.

25. Davis DS, Nelson JKN: Referral to psychiatric liaison nurses. *Gen Hosp Psychiatry* 2:41-45, 1980.

26. Stickney SK, Hall RCW: The role of the nurse on a consultation-liaison team. *Psychosomatics* 22:224-235, 1981.

The Need to Integrate Liaison Psychiatry and Geropsychiatry

26

Liaison psychiatry is concerned with the diagnosis, treatment, study, and prevention of psychiatric disorders among patients in nonpsychiatric health care settings, especially in general hospitals. Liaison psychiatrists provide consultations primarily for medical and surgical inpatients. Between 70% and 80% of the referred patients are physically ill, and about 30% are aged 60 years or over.[1] Those patients not found to be physically ill have usually been admitted for investigation of somatic complaints for which no organic basis could be found. The two patient groups, the physically ill and the somatizing, constitue the main target population of liaison psychiatry.

Geropsychiatry focuses on psychiatric morbidity among the elderly (those aged 65 years and older). It shares an important common ground with liaison psychiatry in that about 30% of medical and surgical inpatients are elderly. In 1980, 26.1% (or nearly 10 million) of the patients discharged from nonfederal short-term hospitals were 65 years old or over, and they accounted for 38% of the total hospital beds and had an average hospital stay about 30% longer than those under 65.[2] These figures illustrate clearly the extent of overlap between liaison psychiatry and geropsychiatry in the general hospital.

PSYCHIATRIC MORBIDITY IN THE HOSPITALIZED ELDERLY

The prevalence of mental disorders in elderly medical and surgical inpatients is estimated to be between 40% and 50%[3,4] and may actually be higher. Delirium (acute confusional states), dementia, and affective and anxiety disorders predominate. Delirium occurs in 30% to 50% of the elderly patients at some point during their hospitalization.[5-7] It is usually due to organic factors such as infection, reaction to medical drugs, and hypoxia, and may be brought on by the hospitalization itself.[6-8] Its hazards include falls and fractures, pulmonary embolism or deep-vein thrombosis due to restraints or oversedation, and removal of intravenous catheters.[7] It is associated with high mortality[8] and longer-than-average hospitalization for nonmedical reasons[9] and creates serious management problems for staff, anguish for the patient's

Reprinted from *American Journal of Psychiatry* 140:1003-1005, 1983. Copyright © 1983 by the American Psychiatric Association. Reprinted by permission. Supported in part by GP Special Training Grant MH-13172 from NIMH.

family, and the risk for the patient of being misdiagnosed as having dementia and being sent to a chronic-care facility.[10] Knowledge of delirium among medical and surgical house staff is lamentably inadequate.[11] Dementia, with or without delirium, is found in at least 10% of elderly patients.

In one study[3] affective and anxiety disorders were found in 30% of the patients over age 65 who were admitted to an acute medical ward. In the elderly these disorders are strongly associated with physical illness[3,12] and often create difficult diagnostic problems due to their clinical presentation with somatic symptoms or with cognitive impairment, i.e., pseudodementia or pseudodelirium. Furthermore, psychopharmacologic treatment of these disorders in the presence of physical illness or dementia has many pitfalls and hazards, such as precipitation of delirium or cardiovascular and other medical complications.[13] It follows that diagnosis and management of an elderly person with a functional psychiatric disorder require a thorough knowledge of psychiatric medicine, an area of expertise of liaison psychiatrists.

THE ROLE OF THE LIAISON PSYCHIATRIST

It is surprising in the face of the above facts and figures that so little has been reported about the work of liaison psychiatrists with elderly medical–surgical inpatients, even though the latter account for about 30% of referrals for consultation.[14] In the only published report known to me, Krakowski[14] stated that he had found organic brain syndromes in about 65% and depression in 25% of the referred elderly. My own experience suggests that the proportion of geriatric referrals is growing and that a liaison psychiatrist increasingly functions as a de facto part-time geropsychiatrist yet one without the benefit of appropriate training and expertise. This work involves formidable diagnostic and management problems. Diagnosis often implies the difficult task of distinguishing dementia from depression with pseudodementia, delirium from pseudodelirium, and affective illness with somatic symptoms from physical illness. Management may entail not only the choice of appropriate psychotropic drugs but also such matters as assessment of competence, contacts with the patient's family and with assorted social agencies, and liaison work with the staff. The latter often need to be persuaded that not every cognitively impaired elderly patient is hopelessly demented and in need of permanent institutionalization. To compound the problem, when transfer to a psychiatric ward is indicated one often meets with vociferous opposition on the part of its nursing staff, who argue that the patient is too ill and needs too much special medical and nursing care. The issue of where a physically ill elderly person with a treatable psychiatric disorder should be managed calls for debate and decisions on a national scale and soon, as the problem grows relentlessly.

In many cases the liaison psychiatrist must insist on additional medical workup to determine the cause of delirium, to search for a potentially reversible cause of dementia, or to look for occult malignancy in a depressed elderly patient. The liaison nurse helps with management of terminal patients and those whose disturbing behavior on the ward exasperates nursing staff. The elderly, especially those cognitively impaired, tend to be viewed by the medical and surgical staff as something of a nuisance, one difficult to manage and dispose of. The liaison psychiatrist or nurse may have to take on the roles of patient advocate, mediator between patient and staff, and educator of the latter in an area in which his knowledge is often less than expert. Furthermore, a liaison psychiatrist may help to reduce hospital stay and thus its cost, and to prevent chronic disability due to psychological factors, as has been demonstrated in the case of elderly female patients undergoing surgery for hip fracture.[15] About 40% of such patients show evidence of dementia on admission,[16] while about one half become delirious during hospitalization.[17] Delirium tends to prolong hospital stay and thus results in an increased cost and blockage of badly needed beds for orthopedic patients.[18] As the number of admissions of elderly women with hip fracture is steadily growing,[18] liaison work with this group of patients alone could result in substantial human, social, and economic benefits.

PRACTICAL IMPLICATIONS AND PROPOSALS

A recent article in *Lancet*[19] warned that the number of the oldest and most frail in Britain will increase dramatically in the next 30 years and will pose a formidable challenge to health care resources. This warning also applies to the United States. The prevalence and incidence of both physical and psychiatric morbidity are highest in the very old. This implies that the proportion of the elderly in general hospitals and the frequency of psychiatric disorders among them are likely to increase in the years to come and to call for ingenious planning now. A plan that I wish to propose involves basing psychogeriatric consultations, research, and teaching concerned with elderly medical–surgical patients on existing consultation–liaison services. This would obviate the need to create new psychogeriatric services for this patient population, would use the expertise of liaison psychiatrists, and could bolster liaison psychiatry as an integral component of health care in a modern general hospital.

Implementation of this plan would require special training for liaison psychiatrists in geropsychiatry. As a first step, at least one member of every liaison service should undergo such training. Joint postresidency liaison psychiatry–geropsychiatry fellowships should be established for young psychiatrists willing to specialize in this area. The National Institue of Mental Health, the National Institute on Aging, hospital administrations, and private foundations should be approached and persuaded to fund such training programs with the goal of meeting the needs of the hospitalized elderly for psychiatric diagnosis and treatment and of the medical and surgical staffs for geropsychiatric consultation and education.[20] An integrated liaison psychiatry–geropsychiatry service could provide an excellent vehicle not only for clinical service and teaching but also for conducting badly needed geropsychiatric research. Far too little is known about the epidemiology of psychiatric disorders among the physically ill, and especially hospitalized, elderly; the etiology and pathogenesis of transient cognitive disorders; the natural hisotry of primary dementias; and the differentiating features of pseudodementia and pseudodelirium.[8] These are but a few subjects that properly trained liaison psychiatrists would be strategically placed to investigate in collaboration with their medical colleagues or gerontologists.

CONCLUSIONS

Liaison psychiatry has grown rapidly in the past decade, thanks largely to financial support by the National Institute of Mental Health, which has funded a considerable number of liaison services and fellowships since 1974.[21] Continuation of this critical support is currently in doubt, and liaison services and education may have to be curtailed at the very time when demand for geropsychiatric consultations in general hospitals is expected to increase and to continue growing. If this dilemma is to be resolved and a crisis avoided, several measures need to be taken. First, the existing liaison services should be reformed so as to be able to function in part as psychogeriatric consultation services for medical and surgical inpatients. Second, appropriate education of liaison psychiatrists and other liaison workers in geropsychiatry needs to be undertaken and sponsored jointly by the National Institute of Mental Health and the National Institute on Aging. And third, the chief emphasis on liaison psychiatry should be shifted from education of nonpsychiatrists to clinical service and research and should include geropsychiatry. Teaching efforts should become more narrowly focused than in recent years and presented as an ancillary rather than primary function of liaison psychiatrists.[22]

Linking liaison and geropsychiatric services in general hospitals would have the double advantage of satisfying the need for psychiatric assistance for elderly medical and surgical patients on the one hand and of strengthening the role of liaison psychiatry as an indispensable component of general hospital psychiatric services on the other.

REFERENCES

1. Lipowski ZJ, Wolston EJ: Liaison psychiatry: Referral patterns and their stability over time. *Am J Psychiatry* 138:1608–1611, 1981.
2. US Department of Health and Human Services: *Utilization of Short-Stay Hospitals: Annual Summary for the United States, 1980.* Series 13, number 64. Washington, DC, National Center for Health Statistics, 1982.
3. Bergmann K, Eastham EJ: Psychiatric ascertainment and assessment for treatment in an acute medical ward setting. *Age Ageing* 3:174–188, 1974.
4. Schuckit MA, Miller PL, Hahlbohm D: Unrecognized psychiatric illness in elderly medical-surgical patients. *J Gerontol* 30:655–660, 1975.
5. Chisholm SE, Deniston OL, Igrisan RM, et al: Prevalence of confusion in elderly hospitalized patients. *Gerontol Nurs* 8:87–96, 1982.
6. Gillick MR, Serrell NA, Gillick LS: Adverse consequences of hospitalization in the elderly. *Soc Sci Med* 16:1033–1038, 1982.
7. Warshaw GA, Moore JT, Friedman SW, *et al:* Functional disability in the hospitalized elderly. *JAMA* 248:847–850, 1982.
8. Lipowski ZJ: Transient cognitive disorders (delirium, acute confusional states) in the elderly. *Am J Psychiatry* 140:1426–1436, 1983.
9. Glass RI, Mulvihill MN, Smith H, *et al:* The 4 score: An index for predicting a patient's non-medical hospital days. *Am J Public Health* 67:751–755, 1977.
10. Glassman M: Misdiagnosis of senile dementia: denial of care to the elderly. *Social Work* 25:288–292, 1980.

11. Berkowitz HL: House officer knowledgeability of organic brain syndromes: a pilot study. *Gen Hosp Psychiatry* 3:321-326, 1981.
12. Lader M: Differential diagnosis of anxiety in the elderly. *J Clin Psychiatry* 43 (9, section 2):4-7, 1982.
13. Salzman C: A primer on geriatric psychopharmacology. *Am J Psychiatry* 139:67-74, 1982.
14. Krakowski AJ: Psychiatric consultations for the geriatric population in the general hospital. *Bibl Psychiatr* 159:163-185, 1979.
15. Levitan SJ, Kornfeld DS: Clinical and cost benefits of liaison psychiatry. *Am J Psychiatry* 138:790-793, 1981.
16. Haljamae H, Stefansson T, Wickstrom I: Preanesthetic evaluation of the female geriatric patient with hip fracture. *Acta Anaesthesiol Scand* 26:393-402, 1982.
17. Williams MA, Holloway JR, Winn MC, *et al:* Nursing activities and acute confusional states. *Nurs Res* 28:25-35, 1979.
18. The old woman with a broken hip (edtl). *Lancet* 2:419-420, 1982.
19. Acheson ED: The impending crisis of old age: A challenge to ingenuity, *Lancet* 2:592-594, 1982.
20. Hall GG, Starkman MN: Incorporation of gerontology into medical education. *J Am Geriatr Soc* 27:368-373, 1979.
21. Eaton JS Jr, Goldberg R, Rosinski E, *et al:* The educational challenge of consultation-liaison psychiatry. *Am J Psychiatry* 134(March suppl):20-23, 1977.
22. Lipowski ZJ: Liaison psychiatry, liaison nursing, and behavioral medicine. *Compr Psychiatry* 22:554-561, 1981.

Current Trends in
Consultation–Liaison Psychiatry

27

HISTORICAL BACKGROUND

THE BEGINNINGS: 1930–1945

Liaison psychiatry was launched in the United States in the early 1930s as part of the drive to bring psychiatry closer to general medicine after decades of their geographic and conceptual separation.[1] In the 1920s and 1930s, psychiatric units became established in a growing number of general hospitals so as to strengthen the links between psychiatry and medicine in matters of patient care, education, and clinical investigations. As a logical outgrowth of this development, efforts were made to provide psychiatric consultations to the nonpsychiatric physicians working in the various divisions of the hospital. In 1929, George W. Henry, a pupil of Adolf Meyer, the founder of psychobiology, published a pioneering paper in which he spelled out the advantages and difficulties of establishing regular professional contacts or liaison between a psychiatric consultant and his medical and surgical colleagues.[2] In the years to follow, a number of teaching hospitals began to feature such liaison in an organized manner. In a few cases, a hospital psychiatric unit was nothing but a liaison service, operating without beds set aside for psychiatric patients, whose function was to offer psychiatric consultations and teaching throughout the general hospital.[1,3] In addition to providing clinical service and education to other physicians, liaison psychiatrists engaged in research at the interface of medicine and psychiatry. The emergence of psychosomatic medicine as an organized movement in the early 1930s stimulated interest in such research. Three persons pioneered psychosomatic medicine in America from about 1932 on: Helen Flanders Dunbar, Franz Alexander, and Harold G. Wolff.[1] Dunbar initiated a study, in a general hospital setting, on psychosocial aspects of several physical illnesses and hence became one of the first liaison researchers.[4] She advocated a holistic approach to medical practice, theory, and research, an approach which was the hallmark of both Meyer's psychobiology and psychosomatic medicine. Liaison psychiatry evolved as an organized endeavor by psychiatrists to apply and teach this approach in their work in nonpsychiatric divisions of general hospitals. The term "liaison psychiatry" was probably first used by Billings in 1939,[5] but was not widely used until recently.

PERIOD OF CONCEPTUAL DEVELOPMENT: 1945-1969

After 1945, liaison services continued to be organized in a growing number of teaching hospitals in the United States. In Canada, probably the first such service was set up by this writer at the Royal Victoria Hospital in Montreal, in 1959. The most important development of this period, however, was the growth of the literature on the conceptual aspects of liaison psychiatry.[6] Formulations of its objectives and modes of operation appeared, while the first comprehensive review of it was published in 1967,[7,8] and attracted considerable interest. The approach to and the conduct of psychiatric consultations in medical settings became increasingly more comprehensive and sophisticated. In its simplest form, such a consultation involves a diagnostic assessment of a patient referred by a nonpsychiatric physician and advice on management. Such a consultation is patient-oriented, involves little, if any, contact with the consultee, and is concerned neither with the interpersonal issues nor with teaching. In the 1950s and 1960s many liaison psychiatrists concluded that such a narrow approach to psychiatric consultations in medical settings could not do justice to the problems at hand, and proposed several major modifications[7,8]: (1) A patient-oriented consultation, one which included a psychodynamic assessment of the patient's personality, symptoms, and reaction to illness; (2) a crisis-oriented, therapeutic consultation involving a rapid assessment of the patient's predicament and bedside psychotherapy by the consultant; (c) a consultee-oriented consultation, whose main target was the consultant and his problems with a given patient; (4) a situation-oriented consultation, which focused on the interaction between the patient and the clinical team; and (5) an expanded psychiatric consultation in which the inquiry included not only the patient but also the clinical team and the patient's family.

These proposed new models of consultation were not to be viewed as mutually exclusive. Rather, it was left to the consultant's judgment which approach to follow in a given case. They highlighted, however, the importance of taking into account the social interactions of the disturbed patient, the importance of viewing a medical ward as a social milieu, and the needs and attitude of the consultee. Clearly, the new approaches to consultation went far beyond the traditional medical model of diagnostic assessment and advice on management. They reflected the dominant trends in psychiatry of those years, notably psychodynamics, emphasis on the interpersonal relationships, crisis theory, and biopsychosocial conceptions of disease elaborated by psychosomatic writers.

A major development was the formulation of two related yet distinct models of operation of liaison services, that is, the consultation and the liaison models; they will be discussed later. The emerging services were called "liaison" or "consultation" or "consultation-liaison" ones, presumably reflecting the organizers' predilection for one or the other model, or for the integration of both of them.

Despite these conceptual advances, and the increasing role of liaison psychiatrists in teaching and research, the growth of liaison psychiatry prior to 1970 was rather unobtrusive. Relatively few psychiatrists entered the field and stayed in it more than several years. Training in liaison psychiatry was almost nonexistent, as I discovered when in 1957 I began to look for an opportunity to embark on it. As in 1958 I became one of the first two fellows on the Psychiatric Consultation Service at the Massachusettts General Hospital, the service was only 2 years old and training was mostly by apprenticeship rather than formal. One had to learn liaison work by trial and error.

PERIOD OF RAPID GROWTH: 1970 TO PRESENT

In the 1970s things began to change. The National Institute of Mental Health (NIMH), concerned about the growing rift between psychiatry and medicine that followed the launching of community mental health centers and the blurring of the boundaries between the work of psychiatrists and other mental health workers, decided to intervene. In the early 1970s it began to promote the establishment or expansion of liaison services in the general hospitals throughout the country and to enable young psychiatrists to train in liaison psychiatry. Since 1974, a few hundred liaison fellows have been trained thanks to NIMH grants; the number, size, and prestige of liaison services have grown substantially and the teaching of liaison psychiatry has become an integral part of psychiatric training in many American departments. The liaison literature has flourished. Two new journals, *General Hospital Psychiatry* and *Psychiatry in Medicine* (now *International Journal of Psychiatry in Medicine*), were founded and devoted largely to subjects concerned with liaison work. Research by liaison psychiatrists has increased rapidly in volume and displayed growing methodological sophistication, thanks no doubt to the entry into the field of a sizable number of young psychiatrists, some of them well trained in research methodology and eager to investigate the many clinical problems encountered at the boundary between medicine and psychiatry. New medical therapies have spawned substantial numbers of psychosocial and psychiatric problems that needed to be investigated and managed. Hemodialysis, cardiac surgery, cancer chemotherapy, critical care medicine, organ transplantation, surgery for obesity, intravenous hyperalimentation—these are but the most prominent innovations which have resulted in psychiatric problems and casualties. Liaison psychiatrists have not only had to keep abreast of these therapeutic advances but also to offer advice on the diagnosis, management, and prevention of related psychiatric problems. The growing number of psychotropic drugs has forced the liaison psychiatrist to learn their application to and hazards for the various categories of the physically ill patients. Last but not least, the new medical technology has given rise to ethical problems related to the selection of patients for certain treatments, to a patient's right and competence to refuse a treatment, and other issues. Liaison psychiatrists have often been called upon to act as advisers on such matters.

Thus, in a matter of only a decade or so, liaison psychiatry has become transformed from a relatively marginal area of special interest into a full-fledged subspecialty of psychiatry, one of growing scope and complexity. The very term "liaison psychiatry" that was hardly a household word prior to 1970 has gained widespread currency and familiarity. It is this recent rapid growth of the field that justifies writing the present overview of current trends as an effort to chart its scope and development.

DEFINITION OF LIAISON PSYCHIATRY

Liaison psychiatry may be defined as a subspecialty of psychiatry, one concerned with (1) diagnosis, treatment, study, and prevention of psychiatric morbidity among the physically ill patients and those who somatize, that is, communicate their emotional distress in the form of somatic symptoms and seek medical help for them; and (2) the provision of psychiatric consultations, liaison, and teaching for nonpsychiatric health workers in all types of health care settings, but especially in the general hospitals.

This two-part definition may seem a bit cumbersome, yet it makes explicit the area of expertise and activities of liaison psychiatrists. It implies that liaison psychiatry is not merely an administrative concept, one referring simply to a setting in which psychiatry may be practiced, but rather a designation for a special area of knowledge, clinical work, and educational and investigative concerns within psychiatry. Furthermore, my definition implies the need for special training for liaison psychiatrists.

MEANING OF LIAISON

Confusion and controversy has surrounded the use of the word "liaison" in this context.[9] The term has been used in two main senses: (1) as a convenient abbreviation for consultation–liaison psychiatry; and (2) to refer to regular contacts by a liaison psychiatrist, or another liaison worker, such as a nurse, with members of a medical or surgical ward or specialized unit. The purpose of liaison, in this narrower sense, is to assist and teach nonpsychiatric health workers to recognize and manage psychosocial and psychiatric problems occurring among patients under their care. Liaison may also include efforts at mediation between patients and staff, with a view to maintaining adequate communication and avoiding or resolving disruptive conflicts between these two groups. The extent to which liaison should play a role in a consultant's work has lately become a matter of sharp controversy and I will return to this later.

ORGANIZATION OF LIAISON SERVICES

THE IMPORTANCE OF ORGANIZED SERVICE

It has become an accepted premise that in order to provide efficient clinical service and teaching, and to facilitate research, it is essential to have an organized liaison service, one based on the department of psychiatry in a given hospital. In the past, such services were relatively few and mostly confined to teaching hospitals, and psychiatric consultations were provided on an ad hoc basis by psychiatrists who were often neither experienced nor interested in work at the interface of medicine and psychiatry. Such consultations tended to be perfunctory and hasty and usually lacked any element of liaison to the consultees. As a result, the consultations got a bad name and did little to encourage collaboration between psychiatrists and other physicians, or to fulfill a teaching function. Clearly, only an organized liaison service, one consisting of psychiatrists, liaison nurses, and in some cases clinical psychologists or social workers, can provide an adequate link between psychiatry and medicine.

According to the American Hospital Association, in 1978 there were about 1200 general hospital psychiatric units in this country and all of them offered consultation and education services.[10] While it is not clear how many of these units featured a separate liaison service, there is no doubt that the number of such services has increased lately.

A liaison service offers distinct advantages. Consultations can be provided efficiently and promptly, teaching and liaison can be organized on a regular basis, research projects can be undertaken and statistical data gathered, and negotations with department heads and administrators can be conducted. None of these advantages is feasible where no organized service exists. Last but not least, such a service is a team of psychiatric workers who share special interests and expertise, play complementary roles, and support one another in the kind of work which is at times difficult and frustrating. The frustrations are related to attitudes of indifference, if not outright rejection and hostility, towards such workers that are still encountered in medical settings.

ORGANIZATIONAL MODELS: CONSULTATION AND LIAISON

If one accepts the premise that an organized liaison service or team is an optimal arrangement, than how could it best fulfill its function as a vital link between the psychiatric unit and the other divisions of a general hospital? The answer to this question will largely depend on what one views as being its main goals. Opinions are divided regarding this crucial point. All liaison psychiatrists would probably agree that their main goal is to raise the standards of psychosocial patient care.[7,11] They hold different views, however, about what the best strategy to achieve this goal should be. Some writers stress education of the nonpsychiatric staff and prevention of psychiatric morbidity among medical and surgical patients as the chief objectives.[11] Others emphasize the provision of clinical service in the form of consultations and bedside psychotherapy, where indicated, as the primary functions of liaison psychiatrists.[9] This approach puts less stress on teaching and on interpersonal issues involving patients and staff.

Greenhill[6] has described several operational models of liaison services which boil down to two basic ones; the consultation and the liaison model, respectively. The former implies that liaison psychiatrists largely confine themselves to providing consultations at the request of their medical and surgical colleagues, but do not attempt to educate the latter in any ongoing and systematic manner. The liaison model, by contrast, envisages the assignment of one or more liaison workers to a particular ward or special unit to consult, case find, and teach.[6] The liaison person is expected to meet regularly, sometimes even daily, with the clinical team to which he has been assigned and become its member. He is concerned not only with provision of patient-oriented consultations, but also with the interactions within the team as well as between its members and the patients under their care. The advocates of this model stress its value in teaching, conflict resolution, and early case detection and hence prevention of psychiatric morbidity.[11] This model comprises all three basic forms of consultation: patient-oriented, consultee-oriented, and situation-oriented.[7]

The liaison model has lately gained considerable popularity and also stirred up lively controversy. Lack of agreement on the precise operational meaning of the term "liaison" has helped to confuse the polemic. In the opinion of some liaison psychiatrists, the liaison model should be the preferred one because of its alleged educational and preventive potential. Critics, however, argue that implementation of this model calls for commitment of so much personnel, time, and financial resources that few services can afford it.[12] On the other hand, they assert, provision of competent psychiatric consultations is necessary in every hospital and should be the main clinical function of a liaison service.

This divisive controversy remains unresolved. The contrast between the two models has been carried by some writers so far that they even speak of consultation psychiatrists and liaison psychiatrists, respectively, as if these were two distinct and opposed professional groups.[11] This is misleading and causes needless divisions within the subspecialty. The question is not whether one should practice consultation or liaison, but rather how much liaison can be usefully employed and afforded in a given setting at a point in time. Consultation remains the cornerstone and *raison d'être* of liaison psychiatry, and to devalue its function is a grave error, one likely to undermine the subspecialty as a whole. There is as yet no published evidence to support the claim that intensive liaison is an effective means of preventing psychiatric morbidity or of helping physicians to be more sensitive to and better able to cope with psychosocial and psychiatric aspects of their practice. Two studies have shown that "active" liaison, involving extensive daily contact with medical staff, has resulted in substantial increase in referrals for psychiatric consultation.[13,14] Such an increase, however, may also follow the introduction of one weekly conference for the medical staff.[15] Clearly, the issue of how much liaison is needed to achieve what goal has never been resolved, and remains a matter of personal conviction. Physicians reportedly expect liaison psychiatrists to provide prompt and practically helpful consultations on matters of diagnosis and treatment, and show little interest in liaison and its educational objectives.[16,17] Advocates of intensive liaison as *the* working model for liaison psychiatry tend to disregard these wishes, and downplay shortage of trained liaison workers and general lack of funding for liaison activities. A satisfactory resolution of this contentious issue is necessary if liaison psychiatry is to continue to develop. This writer has proposed the following compromise.[9]

INTEGRATING LIAISON AND CONSULTATION

First, intensive liaison should be largely confined to selected areas of the hospital where it is most needed because of high incidence of serious psychosocial and psychiatric problems, and because of stress on the staff. Critical care and hemodialysis units, oncology, and rehabilitation divisions represent such priority areas par excellence.[6] Second, every consultation should be *comprehensive* and contain a measure of liaison.[7,9] Comprehensiveness implies that the consultant evaluates not only the referred patient's mental state, but also his interactions with the clinical staff, and the specific needs of the consultee. Moreover, the patient's family relationships and social supports are taken into account. Liaison in this context implies that the consultant takes care to discuss the patient with the consultee and other members of the clinical team, and provides regular follow-up as long as the patient remains in the hospital.

Done in this way, the consultation is truly comprehensive and may be expected to have some educational value for all concerned. Third, liaison nurses should be employed to carry out the day-to-day liaison with medical and surgical nurses.[8,18] In my opinion, such an approach can do more to improve the quality of psychosocial patient care, to facilitate early case detection, and even to prevent psychiatric and interpersonal crises from arising on the wards, than intensive liaison involving psychiatrists and physicians. And fourth, the question of how much liaison should be offered by a given service needs to be decided on the basis of availability of liaison workers and of proper funding, as well as by appraising the need for it on the part of the medical staff.

Linking Liaison Services and Behavioral Medicine

Liaison services should be linked with those of behavioral medicine.[9] The latter has emerged in the last decade as an organized effort, launched mostly by clinical psychologists, to apply the tenets and techniques of behavioral psychology to medical problems. Practitioners of behavioral medicine have developed a whole range of preventive and therapeutic methods in such areas as management of chronic pain, noncompliance with medical treatment, prevention of cardiovascular diseases, and amelioration of stress-related disorders.[19] The recently established Yale Behavioral Clinic provides an example of a joint effort by liaison psychiatrists and behavioral psychologists to apply this new approach in a medical setting.[20] One may hope that their collaboration will enhance the efficacy of psychosocial approaches to the prevention and management of physical illness, and will raise the volume and quality of research at the interface of medicine and the behavioral sciences, including psychiatry.

Linking Liaison Services and Geropsychiatry

Another proposed organizational change involves integration of liaison psychiatry and geropsychiatry.[21] The elderly constitute about one third of admissions to the general hospital and referrals for psychiatric consultations.[21] The incidence of mental disorders, mostly delirium, dementia, and affective disorders, in this patient population is high, estimated to be a least 40% to 50% and requires collaboration between liaison psychiatrists and other physicians in matters of diagnosis and treatment. Neither the former nor the latter are usually experts in geropsychiatry. To meet the growing need for mental health care of the elderly, especially those who are both psychically and psychiatrically ill, at least some liaison psychiatrists need to be trained in geropsychiatry and hence prepared to offer expert advice.[21] Liaison services would thus appropriately function, in part, as geropsychiatric consultation services to the elderly medical and surgical patients.

Dilemmas of Funding

Lastly, an organizational issue which has never been properly resolved concerns the funding of liaison services.[22,23] It is generally accepted that such services are not self supporting financially and have had to depend on government grants to operate.[22]

As these grants are expected to be discontinued in the near future, alternative sources of funding will have to be found. Proposed solutions have included a special tax on hospital beds, contracts with the administration of the hospital, and reimbursement by insurance companies for liaison activities.[22,23] No generally accepted and workable method of funding has emerged so far, and a search for it will no doubt preoccupy liaison psychiatrists in the next few years.

LIAISON EDUCATION

The teaching of psychiatry and the psychosocial aspects of medicine has been one of the key functions of liaison psychiatrists from the beginning. As early as 1942, a report on psychiatric education asserted that liaison teaching in the general hospitals was "one of the most valuable means of emphasizing the total aspect of the patient and of breaking down the barriers between psychiatry and other clinical subjects."[24, p. 229]

In the past decade the educational role of liaison psychiatry has come into prominence once more. Changing trends in health care delivery, marked by growing emphasis on primary care, have highlighted the need for teaching medical students and primary physicians how to recognize and deal with the psychosocial and psychiatric problems presented by patients seeking medical care. Epidemiological studies have found that about 15% of the American population are affected by mental disorders in any one year and that about 60% of the cases are seen and managed, for better or worse, by the primary care physicians.[25] Despite the remarkable increase in general hospital inpatient units in the last few decades, about two thirds of patients with primary psychiatric diagnosis reportedly occupy medical and surgical, rather than psychiatric, beds.[26] Impressed by such findings, the Education Branch of the NIMH decided to give high priority to the development of liaison services and teaching.[27] Liaison psychiatrists, on account of their experience with working at the interface of medicine and psychiatry, were deliberately selected as prospective teachers of medical students, nonpsychiatric physicians, and other health workers. As the exact number of liaison psychiatrists was unknown but presumed to be relatively small, efforts were undertaken to encourage young psychiatric trainees to enter this field. Since 1974, NIMH has provided training grants to support liaison services in their teaching activities and made available stipends for liaison fellows. The future availability of these grants is currently uncertain in view of the budgetary cuts for medical education generally. A reappraisal of liaison teaching is called for in order to preserve those aspects of it which are believed to be effective in influencing medical practice in the direction of a more holistic approach. As the documented evidence of such effectiveness is still unavailable, however, one has to rely largely on subjective impressions.

Engel, one of the most outspoken advocates of teaching the biopsychosocial model of disease and medical practice, has asserted recently that psychiatrists have taken on "by default" the task of teaching both the psychiatric *and* the psychosocial aspects of medicine; that is two distinct domains.[28] He claims that this has led to the spread of a false notion that all that is psychosocial in medicine falls within the scope of psychiatry rather than being the proper concern of all physicians. Engel accuses psychiatrists of having thus "conspired with the rest of medicine to sustain the dualism that separates the psychosocial from the rest of biology, and psychiatry from the rest of medicine."[28, p. 804] Despite this criticism, he recommends that psychiatrists should continue to educate the nonpsychiatric physicians as few other qualified teachers of the biopsychosocial approach exist yet, and ought to try to identify and cultivate those of them (he calls them "mutants") who would be willing to spread this approach among their colleagues.

Engel thus challenges psychiatrists, specifically the liaison ones, to play a demanding educational role which not all of them are eager to pursue. Some of them, including this writer, tend to agree with Greenhill,[6] that the missionary zeal and efforts to convert other physicians have been carried too far and that the primary roles of liaison psychiatrists should be to assist in direct patient care and to build a database which might provide empirical support for the biopsychosocial conceptions. This does not imply the abandoning of all teaching efforts, but rather points to the need to focus them on clearly defined objectives and groups.[9] The teaching of medical and surgical nurses is best left to properly trained liaison nurses.[9,29] Liaison psychiatrists should concentrate their teaching efforts on three groups of trainees: medical students, psychiatric residents, and liaison fellows.[9] These proposed teaching priorities do not preclude education of nonpsychiatric physicians but would limit it to manageable proportions. Liaison activities, especially those connected with patient-oriented consultations, as well as participation in various clinical conferences and in continuing education for nonpsychiatric physicians provide a forum for teaching of the latter.

Teaching Medical Students

Medical students constitute an important group on which to focus teaching efforts. They tend to be more open minded with regard to the importance of psychosocial aspects of medicine than are practicing physicians. For the past several years a number of liaison services have provided opportunity for medical students to spend part or all of their psychiatric clinical clerkship on such a service.[30,31] There is evidence that students learn psychiatry in this setting no less well than on other psychiatric services in a general hospital.[32] Acting as an apprentice on a psychiatric liaison service, a student has a chance to observe the role of psychosocial factors in disease and to appreciate the importance of the doctor–patient relationship for the patient's illness behavior, and especially for his compliance with prescribed therapy. Such direct learning experience is apt to be more influential in shaping the student's professional attitudes than are formal lectures and seminars.[33] A student on a liaison rotation can learn such crucial knowledge and skills as how to take a psychosocial history, identify and manage common psychiatric disorders, use psychotropic drugs properly, apply brief psychotherapy as a means of crisis intervention, and refer patients appropriately for psychiatric consultation.[9] All medical students should have exposure to, and ideally spend part or all of their psychiatric clerkship on, a liaison service.

TEACHING PSYCHIATRIC RESIDENTS

Nearly 30 years ago, Barnes et al.[34] drew attention to the severe shortage of experienced psychiatric consultants and recommended that psychiatric residents should spend a period of time on a liaison service so as to learn crucial consultative skills. In the past decade this postulate has been largely implemented and teaching of liaison psychiatry has become an integral part of psychiatric training in the United States, even though its extent varies considerably from program to program.[35] It is only recently, however, that clear objectives for training residents in liaison psychiatry have been formulated.[36] They include the learning of the following aspects of the field: (1) the consultation process, (2) the biopsychosocial approach to medical practice, (3) the diagnosis and treatment of psychiatric disorders most often encountered in medical settings, and (4) how to gather data and communicate them to the consultees.[36]

In most training programs residents are now required to spend a period of full or part time work on a liaison service.[35] Such a rotation is likely to become mandatory in all programs, as it provided trainees with an opportunity to learn a body of knowledge and skills that every properly trained psychiatrist should possess. They include such items as the causative role of physical illness and its various treatments in psychopathology, the influence of body functioning and experience on psychological processes and vice versa, proper use of psychotropic drugs in the physically ill patient, and the communicative skills in dealing with the whole range of health workers.

TEACHING LIAISON FELLOWS

The future of liaison psychiatry will depend on the training of sufficient numbers of liaison psychiatrists able to provide clinical service and teaching, and to engage in research. Until the early 1970s little opportunity for systematic training in psychiatric liaison work had been available, and what there was consisted mostly of a clinical apprenticeship. The situation changed radically in 1974, when NIMH began to provide grants for liaison psychiatry which offered stipends for liaison fellows. Since then a few hundred young psychiatric trainees have availed themselves of this opportunity. The follows are, as a rule, psychiatrists who have already completed most or all of their psychiatric training and wish to specialize in liaison psychiatry. The duration of the fellowship has ranged from 1 to 2 years. The main objective of these fellowships has been to train future liaison psychiatry practitioners, teachers, and clinical investigators who possess proper expertise in psychiatric medicine. This objective presupposes the existence of a body of knowledge and skills to be acquired. The definition of liaison psychiatry given earlier in this chapter provides a broad frame of reference for what needs to be learned in order to be competent in this area. The latter has grown in scope and complexity to such an extent that special training in it has become mandatory for those who wish to call themselves liaison psychiatrists.

The literature contains virtually no detailed accounts of, or guidelines for, the contents of liaison fellowships. One may assume that while the general objectives and curricula adopted by the training programs offering such a fellowship overlap considerably, they are likely to differ in the contents of teaching and clinical experience provided for the fellows. This writer has listed elsewhere the main aspects of the liaison fellowship offered at the Dartmouth Medical School.[9] They include the following features: (1) theoretical teaching in the form of psychosomatic seminars, (2) supervised consultative experience, (3) liaison with a selected clinical area, usually oncology or intensive care, (4) supervision and teaching of medical students and psychiatric residents, and (5) conduct of a clinical or scholarly research project.

It is essential that liaison fellowships continue to be provided in the future if the subspecialty is to develop, or even survive. One cannot look to the government institutions to fund such training indefinitely, as such funding is subject to the unpredictable vagaries of economic policies. One viable solution may be to offer such a fellowship to selected psychiatric residents in their last year of training and hence to fund it from the same sources as the other residency positions.

LIAISON RESEARCH

Clinical research at the interface of medicine and psychiatry has constituted one of the main activities of liaison psychiatrists from the beginning. One of its pioneers, Dunbar, embarked on psychosomatic studies of the medical and surgical patients in the early 1930s.[4] She was interested in the role of personality factors in the etiology, course, and therapeutic response of illness, as well as in the impact of the latter on the patient's personality. Thus her studies were both etiologic and somatopsychic, in the sense that she was concerned as much with the causative role of psychological factors in physical illness as with its psychological consequences. By contrast, other prominent psychosomatic researchers, such as Alexander, focused almost entirely on a search for the putative psychogenesis, that is, psychological causation, of several diseases, which they studied and theorized about employing the psychoanalytic method and theory, respectively. The overly narrow focus had characterized much of the clinical psychosomatic research until the early 1960s.[37] Failure of this approach to yield clinically useful therapeutic and preventive measures for medical practice had contributed to its demise. In the past 20 years the orientation of psychosomatic studies has become increasingly psychophysiological and somatopsychic.[37] This shift of research focus and methodology has paralleled the growth of liaison psychiatry. Psychiatric consultants in the general hospitals have been faced with a wide range of clinical problems at the interface of psychiatry and medicine, such as the psychiatric complications of new medical and surgical therapies, which clamored for investigation. Psychosomatic clinical research has largely become liaison research, in the sense of being conducted by liaison psychiatrists in the general hospitals.

Liaison research falls into two main general categories: (1) Evaluative studies of the outcome of psychiatric consultation and teaching in medical settings. To this category also belong studies of the prevalence of psychiatric morbidity in various medical patient populations as well as those of referral patterns for psychiatric consultation. And (2) research at the interface between medicine and psychiatry, that is to say studies of the interaction of biological and psychosocial factors in the etiology, course, outsome, therapeutic response, and prevention of disease. Included here are investigations of psychosocial reactions to and psychiatric complications of a whole range of physical illnesses and injuries.

It would be well beyond the scope of this article to attempt a comprehensive review of liaison research. I will try instead to outline major areas of investigation and give a few illustrative examples. For more detailed information readers are referred to other sources.[36-42]

EVALUATIVE STUDIES

This type of research has increased in volume and quality in the last decade, but much more of it is still needed. McKegney and Beckhardt[41] have recently reviewed studies in this area, while Trent et al. have published a survey of relevant methodology.[36] The former authors rightly emphasize that whatever the intrinsic merits of the biopsychosocial model might be in the eyes of its protagonists, its wider acceptance will depend on "scientific demonstration that psychological and social factors influence biologically defined medical illness."[41, p. 198]

Epidemiological studies of the prevalence of psychiatric morbidity in medical and surgical patient populations, while not strictly speaking evaluative, are crucial in that they provide data on which to base evaluation of the effectiveness of liaison services and teaching.[39,43] These studies have demonstrated positive statistical association between physical and psychiatric disorders. They have also largely documented high prevalence of psychiatric morbidity in medical populations, both in and out of hospital.[39,43] Published estimates of such morbidity among general hospital inpatients have ranged from 20% to 70%.[39,43] This wide discrepancy in the reported prevalence reflects unresolved problems in the definition of psychiatric cases and the related difficulties with reliable case-finding.

Studies of referral patterns provide information on the demographic characteristics of the medical patients referred for psychiatric consultation, on the distribution of psychiatric diagnoses among them, and on the types of intervention undertaken by the consultants.[18] Only about 4% of patients admitted to the general hospitals are referred.[18] Thus, even if one accepts the most conservative estimate of the prevalence of psychiatric morbidity in this population, only about one in five of the patients believed to be in need of psychiatric consultation is actually referred for it. Of those referred, about 30% are aged 60 years or over and 70% to 80% are physically ill.[18] About 20% to 30% of the referred patients are those hospitalized for investigation of somatic symptoms which could not be accounted for on medical grounds, or following attempted suicide. Depressive disorders, organic brain syndromes, and anxiety disorders account for about 70% to 80% of the assigned diagnoses.[18] One awaits the results of the application of the DSM-III diagnostic criteria to this patient population.

Outcome studies represent evaluative research in the strict sense. They involve assessment of various outcome indicators of clinical and teaching activities of liaison psychiatrists.[36,41] One notes a welcome increase in the number of such investigations in the last decade, but there are still too few of them to allow definitive conclusions. Several tentative ones, however, may be drawn from the published reports.[41] First, despite a common belief that medical patients are averse to being referred for psychiatric consultation, findings do not support this contention. Second, consultees prefer prompt and practically useful consultations to liaison teaching, while their compliance with a consultant's recommendations in a given case varies considerably and depends on the nature of the advance given and the effectiveness of the communication between consultants and consultees. Third, intervention by a liaison psychiatrist may result in reducing the length and cost of hospitalization as well as in a more favorable long-term outcome for the patient. And fourth, active liaison with a given ward may lead to a marked increase in timely referrals to consultants.[41]

McKegney and Beckhardt[41] have concluded on the basis of their comprehensive review that (1) Sensitive and reliable screening devices for psychiatric case finding in medical populations are badly needed. (2) Evaluative studies should in the future focus on patient outcomes and on cost effectiveness of consultation liaison work, rather than on results of liaison teaching. And (3) educational efforts by liaison psychiatrists should become more narrowly focused and aim at more modest objectives than in the recent past.

RESEARCH AT THE INTERFACE OF MEDICINE AND PSYCHIATRY

Clinical studies by liaison psychiatrists are to a large extent influenced by the nature of the patient population with which they work clinically and by the setting where their work is carried out.[44-47] The physically ill and the somatizing patients constitute the two main populations involved. The clinical work with them takes place mostly on the medical and surgical wards, and in the intensive and other special care units, of a general hospital. The majority of liaison psychiatrists operate in this setting, although some of them work in outpatient and emergency clinics, primary practice groups, rehabilitation centers, and other health facilities. Thus, consultation–liaison clinical work tends to center on medical and surgical inpatients, that is, individuals who are acutely ill, or suffer an acute exacerbation of a chronic illness, or are hospitalized for diagnostic investigations. Moreover, liaison psychiatrists are concerned primarily with the psychological attributes and reactions, social interactions, and psychiatric disorders exhibited by these patients.

Although published studies by liaison psychiatrists cover a wide range of topics, several major research themes may be distinguished:

1. Studies of psychosocial reactions to various diseases, injuries, and therapeutic procedures. A growing number of medical and surgical conditions and therapies have been studied from this angle. Reactions to myocardial infaction,[48] cancer,[49] chronic obstructive pulmonary disease,[50] rheumatoid arthritis,[51,52] diabetes,[55] and renal dialysis[56] provide ready examples of the more important research endeavors in this area. (Of course, not all of these studies have been carried out by liaison psychiatrists, but it would be difficult to base this survey on research actually done by the latter). The key psychological variables studied in this context have included the personal meaning of illness for the patient as well as the cognitive, emotional, and behavioral or coping responses to it.[8,11,37-40,42-45]

2. Studies of psychopathological reactions to physical illness or injury, and to assorted treatments. Included in this group are investigations mostly of depressive and anxiety disorders occurring in response to the personal meaning of illness and its personal, social, and economic consequences for the individual.[39,43]

3. Studies of organic mental disorders, that is, those psychiatric conditions which are due to cerebral damage or dysfuntion.[57] This is an area largely neglected by psychiatric researchers in the past and one especially important to liaison psychiatry on account of the high frequency of organic brain syndromes, especially of delirium,[58,59] in the general hospitals. A thoroughly revised classification of these disorders in DSM-III represents an input of liaison psychiatry to this area of psychiatric nosology.[60] Considering that the elderly constitute about one third of referrals for psychiatric consultation from medical and surgical wards[18] and that organic mental disorders are most common in this age group, liaison psychiatrists are strategically placed to contribute new knowledge in this important field.

4. Studies of abnormal illness behavior. The focus of this research is on two distinct groups of patients: first, those who seek medical help for somatic symptoms in the absence of organic pathology[61-63]; and second, those who are physically ill but behave in a manner incompatible with optimal recovery or with successful rehabilitation. This latter category includes noncompliance with medical treatment.[64,65]

5. Studies of the application of psychological and psychopharmacological therapies to medical problems. These are two large and fast-growing areas of clinical research at the interface. Application of behavioral concepts and methods to health problems has flourished in the past decade under the label of "behavioral medicine."[19,66] While much of the clinical and research activity in this field is carried out by clinical psychologists, their work overlaps with that of liaison psychiatrists.[9,67,68] A typical example of research in this area involves essential hypertension.[69] The most important example of research on the use of psychotropic agents in medical conditions are the studies on the effectiveness of tricyclic antidepressants in the treatment of chronic pain.[70]

The methodology of liaison research has ranged from anecdotal and descriptive clinical accounts to sophisticated design employing the latest investigative tools. Notable examples of the latter type of studies were presented at the Annual Meeting of the American Psychiatric Association in Toronto, in May 1982. Liaison psychiatrists working at the Clinical Center of the National Institutes of Health in Bethesda, Maryland, organized a Symposium on Research at the Interface of Medicine and Psychiatry.[46] They reported studies on such subjects as depression associated with Cushing's disease, neurobiology of anorexia nervosa, relationship of plasma cortisol and beta-endorphin immunoreactivity to surgical stress and requirement for analgesics after surgery, and neuropsychological status of patients with CNS systemic lupus erythematosus treated with pulse methylprednisolone therapy.[46] Most noteworthy is the fact that those studied illustrate the application of the newest investigative techniques to research at the interface. Moreover, the researchers have shown an effective strategy in setting up such high-quality research. They utilized consultations to and liaison with physicians and surgeons at the Clinical Center as a springboard for collaborative studies chosen for their good fit with the available clinical material and technical facilities. This is a strategy which liaison psychiatrists everywhere could emulate for the dual purpose of contributing to knowledge and to strengthen the links with their colleagues in clinical work.[47]

CONCLUSIONS

Liaison psychiatry has grown rapidly in the past decade. It has shown impressive gains in the numbers of personnel and services and in the scope of clinical, educational, and research activities. It is impossible, however, to assess how much impact it has had on medical practice and teaching, on the quality of psychosocial patient care, and on the relations between medicine and psychiatry. While hardly sufficient as evidence, the published comments by an anesthesiologist may be quoted as an example of a measure of acceptance of liaison psychiatry on the part of other physicians: "In psychiatry a major subspecialty has arisen.... More and more departments have organized a liaison service whose members are assigned the responsibility, on a day-to-day basis, of seeing and treating those patients who have come to the hospital because of physical problems and have acquired an additional set of psychiatric problems.... prompt attention to the psychiatric problems often can have a salutary effect on resolving the original medical problems, thus sparing the patients much anguish...."[71, p. 191] The author of these remarks proposed formation of anesthesiology liaison services modeled after the psychiatric ones!

Liaison psychiatry is likely to move in the direction of expanding clinical service beyond the confines of teaching hospitals to the community ones, to the nursing homes, and to primary care practitioners. Clinical research is likely to grow in volume and methodological sophistication. Teaching will probably concentrate on medical students and psychiatric trainees. The latter have shown growing interest in liaison psychiatry in recent years, as the subspecialty offers opportunities for stimulating clinical work and research on a wide range of subjects related to the mind–body relationship. Some of the most challenging research enterprises fall in this area today.

Liaison psychiatry has come a long way to becoming an integral part of general hospital psychiatry and of clinical services offered by a modern general hospital. Liaison psychiatrists have contributed significantly in recent years to the literature of psychosocial and psychiatric aspects of medical practice and of many physical illnesses and their treatments. Liaison psychiatry's future growth will depend on its ability to provide clinical service and research of high quality. Missionary zeal, unrealistic efforts to convert other physicians to the biopsychosocial model, and exaggerated claims of clinical effectiveness could arrest its progress and should be tempered.

REFERENCES

1. Lipowski ZJ: Holistic-medical foundations of American psychiatry: A becentennial. *Am J Psychiatry* 138:888–895, 1981.

2. Henry GW: Some modern aspects of psychiatry in a general hospital practice. *Am J Psychiatry* 86:481–499, 1929.

3. Lipowski ZJ: Consultation-liaison psychiatry: Past failures and new opportunities. *Gen Hosp Psychiatry* 1:3–10, 1979.

4. Dunbar FH, Wolfe TP, Rioch JM: Psychiatric aspects of medical problems. *Am J Psychiatry* 93:649–679, 1936.

5. Billings EG: Liaison psychiatry and intern instruction. *J Assoc Am Med Coll* 14:376–385, 1939.

6. Greenhill MH: The development of liaison programs, in Usdin G (ed): *Psychiatric Medicine.* New York: Brunner/Mazel Inc., 1977, pp 115–191.

7. Lipowski ZJ: Review of consultation psychiatry and psychosomatic medicine. I. General principles. *Psychosom Med* 29:153–171, 1967.

8. Lipowski ZJ: Review of consultation psychiatry and psychosomatic medicine. II. Clinical aspects. *Psychosom Med* 29:201–224, 1967.

9. Lipowski ZJ: Liaison psychiatry, liaison nursing, and behavioral medicine. *Compr Psychiatry* 22:554–561, 1981.

10. American Hospital Association: *Hospital Statistics, 1979.* Chicago, AHA, 1979.

11. Strain JJ, Grossman I: *Psychological Care of the Medically Ill: A Primer in Liaison Psychiatry.* New York, Appleton-Century-Crofts, 1975.

12. Hackett TP: Consultation psychiatry. Paper read at the Annual Meeting of the Academy of Psychosomatic Medicine, Dallas, December 1981.

13. Kramer BA, Spikes J, Strain JJ: The effects of a psychiatric liaison program on the utilization of psychiatric consultations. *Gen Hosp Psychiatry* 1:122–28, 1979.

14. Torem M, Saravay SM, Steinberg H: Psychiatric liaison: benefits of an "active" approach. *Psychosomatics* 20:604–611, 1979.

15. Lipowski ZJ: Psychiatric liaison with neurology and neurosurgery. *Am J Psychiatry* 129:136–140, 1972.

16. Karasu TB, Plutchik R, Conte H, et al: What do physicians want from a psychiatric consultation service? *Compr Psychiatry* 18:73–81, 1977.

17. Sasser M, Kinzie JD: Evaluation of medical-psychiatric consultation. *Int J Psychiatry Med* 9:123–134, 1978–79.

18. Lipowski ZJ, Wolston EJ: Liaison psychiatry: Referral patterns and their stability over time. *Am J Psychiatry* 138:1608–1611, 1981.

19. Williams RB, Gentry WD (eds): *Behavioral Approaches to Medical Treatment.* Cambridge, Mass, Ballinger Publishing Co, 1977.

20. Weiss SM: News and developments in behavioral medicine. *J Behav Med* 5:275–281, 1982.

21. Lipowski ZJ: The need to integrate liaison psychiatry and geropsychiatry. *Am J Psychiatry* 140:1003–1005, 1983.

22. Fenton BJ, Guggenheim FG: Consultation-liaison psychiatry and funding. *Gen Hosp Psychiatry* 3:255–260, 1981.

23. Hales RE, Fink PJ: A modest proposal for consultation-liaison psychiatry in the 1980's. *Am J Psychiatry* 139:1015–1021, 1982.

24. Ebaugh FG, Rymer CA: *Psychiatry in Medical Education.* New York, Commonwealth Fund, 1942.

25. Regier DA, Goldberg ID, Taube CA: The de facto U.S. mental health services system. *Arch Gen Psychiatry* 35:685–693, 1978.

26. Bachrach LL: General hospital psychiatry: Overview from a sociological perspective. *Am J Psychiatry* 138:879–887, 1981.

27. Eaton JS, Goldberg R, Rosinski E, Allerton WS: The educational challenge of consultation-liaison psychiatry. *Am J Psychiatry* 134 (suppl):20–23, 1977.

28. Engel GL: The biopsychosocial model and medical education. *N Engl J Med* 306:802–805, 1982.

29. Lewis A, Levy J: *Psychiatric Liaison Nursing.* Reston, Va; Reston Publishing Co, 1982.

30. McKegney FP, Weiner S: A consultation-liaison psychiatry clinical clerkship. *Psychosom Med* 38:45–54, 1976.

31. Schubert D: Teaching psychiatry to medical students on a consultation service. *Int J Soc Psychiatry* 23:282–284, 1977.

32. Weddington WW, Hine FR, Houpt JL, *et al:* Consultation-liaison versus other psychiatry clerkships: A comparison of learning outcomes and student reactions. *Am J Psychiatry* 135:1509-1512, 1978.
33. Markham B: Can a behavioral science course change medical students' attitudes? *J Psychiatr Educ* 3:44-54, 1979.
34. Barnes RH, Busse EW, Bressler B: The training of psychiatric residents in consultative skills. *J Med Educ* 32:124-128, 1957.
35. Schubert DSP, McKegney FP: psychiatric consultation education—1976. *Arch Gen Psychiatry* 33:1271-1273, 1976.
36. Trent PJ, Houpt JL, Eaton JS: *Consutation-Liaison Psychiatry: Evaluating Its Effectiveness.* Rockville, Md, National Institute of Mental Health, 1982.
37. Lipowski ZJ: Psychosomatic medicine in the seventies: An overview. *Am J Psychiatry* 134:233-244, 1977.
38. Creed F, Pfeffer JM (eds): *Medicine and Psychiatry: A Practical Approach.* London, Pitman Books, 1982.
39. Lipowski ZJ: Physical illness and psychiatric disorder: a neglected relationship. *Psychiatr Fenn* (suppl):32-57, 1979.
40. Lipowski ZJ, Lipsitt DR, Whybrow PC (eds): Psychosomatic Medicine: Current Trends and Clinical Applications. New York, Oxford University Press, 1977.
41. McKegney FP, Beckhardt RM: Evaluative research in consultation-liaison psychiatry. Review of literature, 1970-1981. *Gen Hosp Psychiatry* 4:197-218, 1982.
42. Christie MJ, Mellett PG (eds): *Foundations of Psychosomatics.* New York, John Wiley and Sons, 1981.
43. Usdin G (ed): *Psychiatric Medicine.* New York, Brunner/Mazel, 1977.
44. Lipowski ZJ: Physical illness, the patient, and his environment, in Reiser MF, Arieti S (eds): *American Handbook of Psychiatry,* ed 2. New York, Basic Books, 1975, vol 4, pp 3-42.
45. Weiner H: The prospects for psychosomatic medicine: Selected topics. *Psychosom Med* 491-517, 1982.
46. Symposium: Research at the interface of medicine and psychiatry. *Gen Hosp Psychiatry* 5:79-114, 1983.
47. Lipowski ZJ: Liaison psychiatry and the quest for new knowledge. Discussion of the Symposium Research at the Interface of Medicine and Psychiatry. *Gen Hosp Psychiatry,* 5:111-114, 1983.
48. Denolin H (ed): *Psychological Problems before and after Myocardial Infarction.* Basel, S. Karger, 1982.
49. Holland JC: Psychologic aspects of cancer, in Holland JF, Frei E (eds): *Cancer Medicine,* ed. 2. Philadelphia, Lea and Febiger, 1982.
50. Dudley DL, Glaser EM, Jorgenson BN, Logan DL: Psychosocial concomitants to rehabilitation in chronic obstructive pulmonary disease. *Chest* 77:413-420, 1980.
51. Baum J: A review of psychological aspects of rheumatic diseases. *Semi Arthritis Rheumatol* 11:352.
52. Rogers MP, Liang MH, Partridge AJ: Psychological care of adults with rheumatoid arthritis. *Ann Intern Med* 96:361, 1982. 344-348, 1982.
53. Whitlock FA: *Psychophysiological Aspects of Skin Diseases.* Philadelphia, WB Saunders, 1976.
54. Baretz RM, Stephenson GR: Emotional reponses to multiple sclerosis. *Psychosomatics* 22:117-127, 1981.
55. Hauser ST, Pollets D: Psychological aspects of diabetes mellitus: A critical review. *Diabetes Care* 2:227-232, 1979.
56. Levy NB (ed): *Psychonephrology I.* New Yok, Plenum Medical Book Co, 1981.
57. Lipowski ZJ: Organic mental disorders: introduction and review of syndromes, in Kaplan HI, Freedman AM, Sadock BJ (eds): *Comprehensive Textbook of Psychiatry,* ed 3. Baltimore, Williams and Wilkins, 1980, pp 1359-1392.
58. Lipowski ZJ: *Delirium: Acute Brain Failure in Man.* Springfield, Ill, Charles C Thomas, 1980.
59. Lipowski ZJ: Transient cognitive disorders (delirium, acute confusional states) in the elderly. *Am J Psychiatry,* 140:1003-1005, 1983.
60. Lipowski ZJ: A new look at organic brain syndromes. *Am J Psychiatry* 137:674-678, 1980.
61. Ford CV: *The Somatizing Disorders.* New York, Elsevier, 1983.
62. Mechanic D: Effects of psychological distress on perceptions of physical health and use of medical and psychiatric facilities. *J Hum Stress* 4:26-32, 1978.
63. Barsky AJ, Klerman GL: Overview: hypochondriasis, bodily complaints, and somatic styles. *Am J Psychiatry* 140:273-283, 1983.

64. Garrity TF: Medical compliance and the clinician–patient relationship: A review. *Soc Sci Med* 15:215–222, 1981.
65. Zisook S, Gammon E: Medical noncompliance. *Int J Psychiatry Med* 10:291–303, 1981.
66. McNamara JR (ed): *Behavioral Approaches to Medicine.* New York, Plenum Publishing Co, 1979.
67. Goldiamond I: Behavioral approaches and liaison psychiatry. Psychiatr Clin *North Am* 2:379–401, 1979.
68. Morgan CD, Kremer E, Gaylor M: The behavioral medicine unit: a new facility. *Compr Psychiatry* 20:79–89, 1979.
69. Luborsky L. Crits-Christoph P, Brady JP, *et al:* Behavioral versus pharmacological treatments for essential hypertension—A needed comparison. *Psychosom Med* 44:203–213, 1982.
70. Blumer D, Heibronn M, Pedraza E, Pope G: Systematic treatment of chronic pain with antidepressants. *Henry Ford Hosp Med J* 28: 15–21, 1980.
71. Schotz S: An anesthesiology liaison service. *Anesthesiology* 52:190–191, 1980.

Index